AF711680

MEASURING ATTACHMENT

Also Available

Attachment from Infancy to Adulthood: The Major Longitudinal Studies
Edited by Klaus E. Grossmann, Karin Grossmann, and Everett Waters

Metacognition, Strategy Use, and Instruction
Edited by Harriet Salatas Waters and Wolfgang Schneider

MEASURING ATTACHMENT

Developmental Assessment across the Lifespan

EDITED BY

Everett Waters
Brian E. Vaughn
Harriet Salatas Waters

Foreword by L. Alan Sroufe

THE GUILFORD PRESS
New York London

Copyright © 2021 The Guilford Press
A Division of Guilford Publications, Inc.
370 Seventh Avenue, Suite 1200, New York, NY 10001
www.guilford.com

All rights reserved

No part of this book may be reproduced, translated, stored in a retrieval system, or transmitted, in any form or by any means, electronic, mechanical, photocopying, microfilming, recording, or otherwise, without written permission from the publisher.

Printed in the United States of America

This book is printed on acid-free paper.

Last digit is print number: 9 8 7 6 5 4 3 2 1

Library of Congress Cataloging-in-Publication data is available from the publisher.

ISBN 978-1-4625-4647-3 (hardcover)

About the Editors

Everett Waters, PhD, is Emeritus Professor of Psychology at Stony Brook University, State University of New York. A graduate of the University of Minnesota's Institute of Child Development, he is a coauthor of Mary Ainsworth's classic volume *Patterns of Attachment.* He is a recipient of the 2009 Bowlby–Ainsworth Award for contributions to attachment theory and measurement and a Lifetime Achievement Award from the Society for Emotion and Attachment Studies.

Brian E. Vaughn, PhD, holds the Human Sciences Professor of Human Development Chair in the Department of Human Development and Family Science at Auburn University. A graduate of the University of Minnesota's Institute of Child Development, he has published widely on attachment and temperament and the relation of infant attachment to social competence in early childhood. He is a recipient of the 2011 Bowlby–Ainsworth Award for advancing ethological methods in attachment study.

Harriet Salatas Waters, PhD, is Emerita Professor of Psychology at Stony Brook University, State University of New York. A graduate of the University of Minnesota's Institute of Child Development, she has made significant contributions to research on attachment narratives in middle childhood, adolescence, and adulthood. She is a recipient of the 2021 Bowlby–Ainsworth Award for contributions to the theory and measurement of attachment representations.

Contributors

Joseph P. Allen, PhD, Department of Psychology, University of Virginia, Charlottesville, Virginia

Lianne Bakkum, MSc, Institute of Public Health, Cambridge University, Cambridge, United Kingdom

Kristin Bernard, PhD, Department of Psychology, Stony Brook University, Stony Brook, New York

Annie Bernier, PhD, Department of Psychology, University of Montreal, Montreal, Quebec, Canada

Elizabeth A. Carlson, PhD, Institute of Child Development, University of Minnesota, Minneapolis, Minnesota

David Corcoran, PhD, Colleges Ontario, Toronto, Ontario, Canada

Judith A. Crowell, MD, Department of Child and Adolescent Psychiatry, Stony Brook University, Stony Brook, New York

Robbie Duschinsky, PhD, Institute of Public Health, Cambridge University, Cambridge, United Kingdom

Christopher R. Facompré, MA, Department of Psychology, Stony Brook University, Stony Brook, New York

Brooke C. Feeney, PhD, Department of Psychology, Carnegie Mellon University, Pittsburgh, Pennsylvania

Carol George, PhD, Department of Psychology, Mills College, Oakland, California

Kathryn A. Kerns, PhD, Department of Psychology, Kent State University, Kent, Ohio

Markus Maier, PhD, Department of Psychology, Ludwig-Maximilians University, Munich, Germany

Greg Moran, PhD, Department of Psychology, Western University, London, Ontario, Canada

David R. Pederson, PhD, Department of Psychology, Western University, London, Ontario, Canada

German Posada, PhD, Department of Child Development and Family Studies, Purdue University, West Lafayette, Indiana

Carlo Schuengel, PhD, Clinical Child and Family Studies, Vrije Universiteit, Amsterdam, The Netherlands

Ashley Seibert, PhD, Department of Psychology, Shippensburg University, Shippensburg, Pennsylvania

Judith Solomon, PhD, Greater New Haven Counseling and Family Therapy Center, Hamden, Connecticut

Douglas M. Teti, PhD, Department of Human Development and Family Studies, The Pennsylvania State University, University Park, Pennsylvania

Brian E. Vaughn, PhD, Department of Human Development and Family Science, Auburn University, Auburn, Alabama

Everett Waters, PhD, Department of Psychology, Stony Brook University, Stony Brook, New York

Harriet Salatas Waters, PhD, Department of Psychology, Stony Brook University, Stony Brook, New York

Theodore E. A. Waters, PhD, Department of Psychology, New York University—Abu Dhabi, Abu Dhabi, United Arab Emirates

Malcolm L. West, PhD, Department of Psychiatry (retired), University of Calgary, Calgary, Alberta, Canada

Foreword

Attachment theory and research have created a revolution in developmental psychology. They have moved us from the study of infants, children, and parents governed by prevailing contingencies of reinforcement to the study of relationships and meaning. They have also moved us from theories based on drive reduction to a biologically based theory focused on goal-directed behavior, behavioral systems, and the organization of behavior. Attachment theory has proven to be an enormous success and the research yield has been massive. Not as widely appreciated, attachment study has revolutionized research methods and strategies.

Prior to Mary Ainsworth's work, convention largely limited researchers to one of two equally unsatisfactory measurement approaches. They could rely on frequency counts of discrete behaviors that, while seen to be objective, had very limited convergent and discriminative validity, or they could employ subjective, global ratings that tended to have poor reliability and uncertain validity. Mary Ainsworth's use of the ethological method to develop parent–infant interaction scales, and her system for capturing infant attachment relationships, pointed to a third, more powerful approach (see Chapters 1 and 2). Close, careful observation in naturalistic settings is at the core of the Ainsworth system. Rather than focusing solely on the presence–absence or frequency of behaviors, her scales also attend to the social, behavioral, and emotional context that make behavior meaningful to a caregiver and child. Based on transcripts of detailed ethological observations, Ainsworth's rating scales highlight behavior as it actually occurs and emphasize that constructs such as desire for proximity or contact with caregivers can be manifest in multiple ways. Mary Ainsworth taught developmental psychologists to prioritize the organization of behavior (Chapter 3).

The development and validation of the measures included in this volume led to an outpouring of research on representation and to work linking external behavior to the inner world of the mind. They also initiated a bridge between developmental and social psychology.

Important empirical contributions have come from these measures. One of the most impressive concerns intergenerational transmission. Disorganized attachment in infancy predicts disorganized attachment in the next generation (modestly, of course, but astounding nonetheless). Although this empirical finding itself has been highly influential, the real accomplishment has been filling in the links in the chain of transmission, something that has not been done before in developmental research (Chapter 4). Very careful research has demonstrated that disorganized attachment predicts a tendency to dissociate in the face of trauma or loss. This tendency then predicts unresolved status on the Adult Attachment Interview (AAI). Unresolved AAI status predicts frightening parental behavior directly observed in the home. Such frightening parental behavior is a key influence on disorganized infant attachment. The cycle is complete.

Of course, there is much work ahead to confirm, clarify, and contextualize this monumental set of findings. Still, without decades of work on measurement, none of this would have been possible. Moreover, the road ahead is not smooth; attachment measures remain difficult to use and often require hands-on training or a virtual apprenticeship (Chapter 5). Through our Minnesota Attachment Training workshops, we have worked hard for decades to make training on measures such as the Strange Situation available. Individual researchers, especially Mary Main and her group of certified AAI trainers, have done yeoman's work as well. Nonetheless, it remains a significant undertaking to make the necessary training available.

Measurement issues are always important in psychological research. Without a degree of precision and standardization in measurement, it is not possible to properly compare and communicate research findings, to resolve disagreements that arise in the field, or to be confident that theoretical propositions have been adequately tested. Measurement and standardization issues are especially important in a field such as attachment research for two reasons: (1) Attachment research has been extraordinarily popular, inevitably leading to a proliferation of "new" or "alternative" or "modified" measures; and (2) attachment measures are so familiar that we easily assume that, by now, everyone must be using and interpreting them correctly. Moreover, attachment, as a relationship construct, remains more complex than it first appears. It is not at all easy to adequately capture qualitative aspects of relationships, such as effectiveness of the relationship or degree of confidence of the infant in the attachment figure. Yet capturing the qualitative aspects of attachment in a way that they are open to quantitative analysis and summary is precisely what we wish to do.

Well-grounded criteria are necessary for validating any measure of attachment. Foremost among these is that it directly assess, or be related to, actual observations of attachment–exploration balance in the natural environment. Closely related to this are use of attachment figure as a secure base and preferential treatment of the attachment figure under stress, that is, seeking out this person in particular when frightened or distressed. (Reactions to loss would be distinctive for genuine attachment figures, but studies based on such a criterion would be impractical.)

With infants, observing the attachment–exploration balance and other secure base behavior in the home can be done adequately with several hours of observation over multiple visits. The Ainsworth Sensitivity Scales, described in this volume (Chapter 1) and elsewhere are useful for this, as are the Maternal Behavior Q-set and the Attachment Q-set (Chapters 1 and 2). With adult–adult attachment relationships, direct observation of secure base use and support is a useful criterion (e.g., Chapter 11). In the absence of such criteria, the final option for researchers (and the one most widely used) is to relate the purported attachment measure to another already established measure. This commonly used approach brings measurement issues to the fore. There are two separate kinds of problems to discuss.

Take first the case in which someone introduces a new (or modified) laboratory measure. Ideally, researchers will directly anchor the new measure to field observations. Short of that, they would check whether it related to previously validated measures, such as the Strange Situation or the Attachment Q-set (Chapters 2 and 3). The evaluation of new measures cannot depend on face or content validity. Criterion-related validity is essential. Nor is the presence of other correlates, such as later behavior problems or social acceptance alone, convincing. Such correlates are useful for extending the nomological net of the new measure, but they cannot substitute for ties to secure base behavior. Many things besides attachment predict such outcomes. And, in fact, it has been important to show that attachment measures are not simply tapping sociability, IQ, or other third variables, as well as directly validating any new attachment measure against variations in attachment–exploration balance. Many proposed measures in use today do not meet these important criteria. The chapters in this volume describe both well-validated measures and well-thought-out validation strategies.

More subtle issues arise with the widespread application of even well-validated measures. For example, what can we make of anomalous findings or null findings with measures we have come to trust? With replication currently a significant, and sensitive, issue, null findings can be important. They might indicate a need to revise or temper conclusions or even raise questions about accepted aspects of theory. However, null results can also mean that the outcome measure was not properly conceptualized or adequately assessed or, even more troublesome, that the attachment measure itself was not obtained or scored according to established criteria. Null findings always raise these questions, because they are so easy to produce.

When we encounter a research report claiming that a well-validated attachment measure fails to replicate a previously reported result, there are questions to be asked before calling the original attachment measure into question. Was the measure in the new study scored the same way? Was the attachment measure in the new report related to an established network of other relationships? If home observational data are available, was the presumed attachment measure related in particular to these? Did the measure in fact correlate with anything? If not, this singularly reported null result is meaningless. In the absence of these kinds of data, one cannot take nonreplication at face value. The particular attachment assessment itself, as measured, may have been invalid, not the original measure, the construct in general, or the aspect of theory in question. Without evidence that the current measurement was valid, a large sample, agreement within a lab, credentials of investigators, and prestige of the study do not matter. These are very important measurement issues, because a carefully constructed nomological network of findings could be cast into doubt simply because measurements were not done correctly in a new study. Such difficult issues are discussed throughout this volume, but they are not easily resolved. The editors return to these and related issues in Chapter 14.

One of the hardest problems in attachment research concerns the measurement of attachment in the years between infancy and adulthood (Chapters 6–8). In the early years, one can directly look at secure base behavior in the infant–caregiver dyad. In adult couples, one can directly assess support seeking and support giving. These can be used to validate adult narrative measures. But this is considerably more difficult to do in child and adolescent samples. It is possible to examine high-stress situations (periods of illness, hospitalizations, etc.) that would call forth clear attachment behavior, but these are rare and would require a major research effort. Short of that, the best approach is a longitudinal investigation, wherein one obtains established measures in the early years and shows them to be related to later observational measures, drawings, narratives, or projective measures of attachment. These longitudinal data can perhaps be supplemented with contemporary correlates. Still, it would take considerable time to gain confidence in middle childhood or adolescent measures, because any correlation could be due to another parenting or child variable. Chapters 6 and 7 provide the best view to date of these matters.

The measures surveyed in this volume are widely used. Several also illustrate methodological innovations. In many cases they highlight what Paul Meehl referred to as the "bootstrap" effect; that is, they were derived from theory, then examined with new data leading to refinement and further testing. Of course, validation is an ongoing process. Without doubt, improvements to existing measures and development of new valid measures lie in the future of attachment research. For now, this volume will be useful as a guide for deciding which current measures to use in a particular research project.

In conclusion, many of the most difficult issues in attachment measurement are addressed in this volume. There is no sugarcoating of the complexities in this work. Beyond pointing to problems, new directions for research are suggested throughout. New methods of assessing attachment are discussed, primarily drawing on important work in cognitive psychology (Chapters 8, 10, and 12). Chapter 13 even adapts projective methodology to provide an innovative perspective on narrative and defensive processes underlying attachment representations. The editors are as knowledgeable about the range of attachment measures as anyone in the world. Indeed, they have done important work validating standard attachment measures, as well as working to develop new ones. They have assembled an excellent array of contributors and worked closely with them to produce an exceptionally coherent volume. *Measuring Attachment* is a fine tool for primary attachment researchers, students, clinicians, and experts from other disciplines who need to understand the measures and issues underpinning attachment literature. This is not to say that *Measuring Attachment* is light reading. It brings together a great deal of detailed material that, for too long, has been unavailable outside attachment research circles. However, as Mary Ainsworth taught us, the answers are often in the details.

L. ALAN SROUFE, PhD
Professor Emeritus
University of Minnesota

Acknowledgments

Many individual researchers have contributed to the Bowlby–Ainsworth tradition by mentoring and training in attachment theory and measurement. Attachment study is especially indebted to Alan Sroufe and Elizabeth Carlson, whose Minnesota Attachment Measurement workshops have provided comprehensive Strange Situation training to hundreds of students, colleagues, and practitioners over three decades. We are similarly indebted to Mary Main and Erik Hesse, whose rigorous, yet uniquely personal, format for AAI training workshops set an equally high standard for training in attachment assessment. In addition to training hundreds of prospective attachment researchers and practitioners in the use of the AAI, they have established an international network of skilled workshop leaders to meet the demand and ensure the continuity of this valuable training. We hope both teams are making video recordings of some of their training workshops for future reference. In addition to providing invaluable training material and documenting an important era in attachment history, these would also preserve and allow us to share with new generations something of the enthusiasm and esprit that Mary Ainsworth instilled in her students and closest colleagues.

We also want to thank the Cox-Steiner family and their Center for Mental Health Promotion. For over two decades, they have helped sustain the Bowlby–Ainsworth tradition through their support for the New York Attachment Consortium, memorable receptions for the attachment community at the Society for Research in Child Development, and the Bowlby–Ainsworth Award program. Their multifaceted support has done much to make this volume possible.

Contents

CHAPTER 1

Mary Ainsworth, Ethology, and Maternal Sensitivity

German Posada, Everett Waters, Brian E. Vaughn, David R. Pederson, and Greg Moran

John Bowlby viewed attachment as the product of biases in an infant's learning abilities interacting with a complementary caregiving system. The key dynamic was not drive reduction but the behavior of one or a few individuals serving as a template around which the infant's attachment behavioral system became organized. Two of the most important issues in attachment study have been the kind of caregiving environment that is required for attachment to develop and the impact of individual differences in early care on attachment patterns during and after infancy. In early research, specific responses such as separation distress were taken as markers of the onset of attachment (e.g., Spitz, 1965; Schaffer & Emerson, 1964). Unfortunately, such behavior proved very sensitive to context (e.g., Waters, Matas, & Sroufe, 1975) and thus unsuitable as a marker of attachment onset. This led researchers to focus instead on how patterns of care influence individual differences in infant security once attachment is well established.

In her classic Uganda and Baltimore studies, Mary Ainsworth took up the challenge of exploring and sorting through the many aspects of "mothering" to identify key influences on attachment security (Ainsworth, 1967; Ainsworth, Blehar, Waters, & Wall, 1978/2015). Based on arduous ethological observations and an exceptional sense for behavioral detail, pattern, and context, Ainsworth's insights continue to influence conceptualizations of caregiving influences on infant attachment. In addition, her work on caregiving constructs has proved quite useful in age-appropriate conceptualizations of secure base support in childhood (Posada, Kaloustian, Richmond, & Moreno, 2007; Posada & Waters, 2018) and even in marriage (Crowell et al., 2002).

We review in this chapter the theoretical underpinnings, history, and methods of maternal sensitivity assessment. We begin with Bowlby's departure from traditional psychoanalytic models and methods, and his emphasis on ethological methods and prospective longitudinal studies. We then give a brief overview of Ainsworth's Uganda and Baltimore studies—both of which are impressive to read and generously repay careful study. We then present more recent approaches to assessing infant–caregiver interaction in naturalistic settings. Also, we briefly discuss measurement issues central to the cross-cultural generality in the study of child–parent attachment relationships. This is followed by a discussion of how constructs developed in infancy research have been elaborated and adapted for research on attachment in early childhood. Finally, we describe important considerations to ensure the quality of observational and Q-sort data.

CAREGIVING IN ATTACHMENT THEORY: THE IMPORTANCE OF ACTUAL EXPERIENCE

Much of our understanding of attachment development is built upon Bowlby's insight that, in addition to the well-demonstrated effects of trauma, attachment behavior and representations, depend very much on the cumulative effect of ordinary variations in actual care and family experiences.

As a practicing child psychiatrist, Bowlby saw children in real families, facing separations, suffering losses, and interacting with parents who often experienced real problems of their own. Indeed, one of the goals of attachment theory is to explain how everyday experiences that are not manifestly traumatic can create significant difficulties for children. The answer, Bowlby decided, is in their effect on the child's expectations about parent's availability, responsiveness, and efficacy as sources of support and havens of safety. Accordingly, Bowlby's view of psychopathology assigned an important etiological role to "ordinary" experiences that children (and adults) experience or feel as threatening. These include fear of the dark, fear of separation and of novelty, looming objects, and other sensitivities that, although not objectively or frequently dangerous today, reflect useful adaptations rooted in our evolutionary heritage. In particular, he emphasized the attributions and expectations about parents, safety, and security that arise from such experiences (Bowlby, 1988).

Of course, some children do encounter traumatic experiences—sometimes a single instance, sometimes repeatedly over years. Bowlby recognized the significance of such experiences. But they were not evident in every case. Finding little evidence that infants and young children could fantasize truly traumatic experiences, Bowlby concluded that a child's sense of safety and security, and mental representations of relationships in general, owe much to real and in many respects ordinary experience. This was a significant departure from psychoanalytic thinking and clinical practice and resulted in naturalistic observation replacing the clinical case study as the primary source of attachment data. But Bowlby was a theorist, not a field researcher. So it fell to Mary Ainsworth to provide the proof of concept, the demonstration that naturalistic observation could inform an emerging attachment theory independent of psychoanalysis.

THE UGANDA AND BALTIMORE STUDIES: MATERNAL SENSITIVITY

Mary Ainsworth was a keen and patient observer, genuinely fascinated by behavior. Moreover, she was gifted with an eye for both patterns and details—and a tremendous capacity for hard work. In a word—a born ethologist. She also had a keen sense of what kinds of data would be decisive for the future of attachment theory (Ainsworth & Bowlby, 1991; Ainsworth & Marvin, 1995).

Ainsworth brought her considerable talents to bear in two definitive longitudinal studies. In Uganda and then in Baltimore she asked,

1. "Does Bowlby's description of attachment relationships fit the facts of caregiver and infant behavior in infancy?"
2. "What aspects of caregiver behavior are most important to the development and quality of infant secure base behavior?"
3. "How can we quantify phenomena as complex as maternal care and infant attachment behavior for empirical analysis?"

Combining traditional ethological methods with the conceptual framework of Bowlby's attachment theory, Ainsworth sought not only to describe caregiver and infant behavior but also to make clear the importance of context (Hinde, 2005; Main, 1999). In doing so, she moved away from traditional ethological focus on specific behavioral elements to focus on more organized behavior patterns that shared functions. And as the target behaviors were increasingly familiar, well described, and well understood, she moved from frequency counts toward the use of behaviorally anchored but conceptually defined rating scales as the most satisfactory method for quantifying her observations (Main, 1999). This has been a defining model for developmental attachment study in the Bowlby–Ainsworth tradition.

Uganda: Exploring Infant–Mother Relationships

Impressed by Robertson's exemplary fieldwork with hospitalized children, Ainsworth took her 2-year stay in Uganda as an opportunity to design and conduct the kind of observational study needed to consolidate Bowlby's hypotheses about the importance of real behavior, early experience, and the caregiver's role in support of both exploration and security (Bretherton, 2003; Karen, 1994). Working from her base in Kampala, she undertook a short-term longitudinal study of 26 mothers and their 28 unweaned Ganda infants (two sets of twins) in villages about 15 miles away (Ainsworth, 1963, 1964, 1967). She had been led to expect that Ugandan mothers routinely sent their infants away to relatives in order to wean them. This seemed an interesting opportunity to observe reactions to separation and reunion. But she soon realized that her study participants no longer followed this practice. Accordingly, she focused her observations on routine care, the normative course of attachment development, and individual differences in patterns of infant–mother interactions.

Mothers were paid for 2-hour visits at 2-week intervals, conducted along with a native social worker, Ms. Chibuka. When observations began, the youngest infant was 3 days old and the oldest, 19 months, with most of the sample between 7 and 39 weeks of age. The span of observations ranged from 6 to 38 weeks. In addition to observing maternal and infant behavior in and around the home, Ainsworth took full advantage of the mothers as informants about their own and their babies' behavior.

Their reports, as well as her own detailed notes, were transcribed for later analysis. Excerpts from these transcripts illustrate the range and depth of her observations (see Table 1.1).

TABLE 1.1. Sample Observations from *Infancy in Uganda*

Sulaimani (28 weeks old) was held by his mother. Even while he sat on his mother's lap he made faces as if about to cry. Finally he quieted. I wished to photograph him sitting by himself and suggested that his mother put him down on the mat. As soon as he was put down he screamed. I suggested that his mother give him something to distract him that might induce him to crawl. His mother returned with a small tin of shoe polish and gave it to him. He fingered the tin and stopped crying. But when we took it away in order to use it as an incentive for crawling, he cried again and would not try to get it. I suggested, finally, that his mother come nearer. When she did, he crept toward her, and stopped crying as soon as she took him up. (p. 221)
Mother as informant:
Sulaimani's mother discussed her concern about Sulaimani's crying so much. Soon she shifted her attention to (discussing another child and his mother). She criticized the other mother for giving (her infant) too much attention; she should just let him cry. Because of this, I wondered whether Sulaimani's mother was, in fact giving him too little attention and asked when she held him. She replied that she held him when she was not working and that his father also played with him sometimes. She said that she used to play with him more when he was younger, before he could sit alone. She reported that she never carried him on her back—only on her hip—and that no one else carried him. She did not make a practice of taking him to the garden with her; she either left him in the house alone or with someone else. During this interview the mother answered inquiries straightforwardly, and often, when talking about Sulaimani, her face would light up in a smile. (p. 221)

Note. From Ainsworth (1967).

Key Results

The Uganda study was a career-defining research experience. During the course of the study, Ainsworth described the emergence of 21 different attachment behaviors at different points in time during the first 2 years. These included differential smiling, differential crying, crying when the mother leaves, following, burying the face in mother, clinging, greeting (lifting arms and clapping), use of the mother as a secure base, and flight to the mother as a haven of safety (Ainsworth, 1967). Her observations highlighted the limitations of theories that viewed attachment in terms of simple reinforcement of dependency behaviors or of feeding and drive reduction.

On reviewing her field notes, Ainsworth noticed that the infants "do not always stay close to the mothers but rather make little excursions away from her, exploring other objects and interacting with other people, but returning to the mother from time to time" (Ainsworth, 1967, p. 345). She particularly noted the apparently paradoxical fact that although secure infants come back to their attachment figures, keep track of them, and share with them their discoveries, their bond does not interfere with the development of competence and independence. Bowlby's view of infants supported by their mothers in a balance between exploration and proximity seeking, what became known as the *secure base phenomenon,* was a much better description than the traditional views from psychoanalysis and learning theories.

Finally, an important and often overlooked aspect of Ainsworth's observations in Uganda concerns her success at placing maternal and infant behavior in context. Both maternal care and infant behavior are sensitive to context. Whether maternal care was described as more or less optimal, and whether infants were described as secure or insecure, the dyads' immediate context provided a better understanding of the reasons that might explain behavior. The specific circumstances surrounding dyads and families that favored or impeded caregiving practices were also noted.

Lessons from the Uganda Study

The Uganda study was an important first step toward understanding the infant–mother dyad. The information collected about maternal behavior associated with security provided clues about the importance of variables such as the quality and quantity of care, excellence of the mother as an informant, and maternal warmth, among others. Those insights were to be systematically investigated in Baltimore.

WHAT MOTHERS AND BABIES ACTUALLY DO

The study's detailed ethnographic descriptions of each mother and infant illustrate Ainsworth's openness to letting the phenomenon under study define itself, rather than rigidly imposing an a priori theoretical scheme or scoring system. Her extensive home observations demonstrated the value of studying the meaning and function of behavior in its natural context. The Uganda study was a singular contribution to Bowlby's attachment theory. It provided both Bowlby and Ainsworth with tangible evidence and encouragement that they were on the right track and encouraged them to forge ahead. Aside from this, the most useful results from the study were descriptive, a virtual ethogram summarizing the behaviors underpinning the infant–mother bond. These were the foundations on which the subsequent Baltimore study was built. Toward the end of her career, Ainsworth lamented that the rigors of ethological observation seemed to be losing out to the conveniences of laboratory assessment (Ainsworth & Marvin, 1995, p. 12).

YOU HAVE TO START SOMEWHERE

Ethological studies typically involve only one or two observers and the observations focus on a wide range of target behaviors that are occurring in the same time frame. This limits the possibilities for independence among observations and variables. The Uganda study was conducted in a remote location, with limited resources. Ainsworth was the sole observer and data manager. She necessarily knew the identities of the mothers and infants she was observing. Nor could she be unaware of previous observations when she visited the same family in subsequent months. As in any ethological research, the only guarantees are in the quality of the observations, the coherence of the results, and ultimately in replication (e.g., Goodall, 1986). Indeed, most of the statistical analyses from the project are descriptive, not aimed at testing specific hypotheses. Thus, the Uganda study is best viewed as an essential first look at the infant–mother relationship, a trial run for measurement strategies, and a source of hypotheses (see Bretherton, 2003).

The Baltimore Study: A More Systematic Look at Infant Care

Joining the psychology faculty at Baltimore's Johns Hopkins University gave Mary Ainsworth the needed access to laboratory space and students to build on her insights and results from Uganda. It was to be an intensive longitudinal study combining naturalistic observation with systematic laboratory assessments. As in Uganda, she would study a relatively small sample in great detail. Again, a central focus was the role of maternal care. But now the focus was sharper. She had a much clearer sense of how maternal behavior is organized, the notion of attachment strength had been discarded in favor of attention to patterns of secure base behavior, and her observational methods were both more refined and more systematic (Ainsworth et al., 2015).

Mothers were first contacted through pediatricians in private practice, usually before the baby's birth. Infant–mother interaction and exploratory behavior were observed in the course of 4-hour visits at 3-week intervals from birth through the end of the baby's first year. To assist with the home observations, Ainsworth trained and supervised Barbara Wittig, George D. Allyn, and Robert S. Marvin. Each proved to be a notable observer. Developmental level was assessed approximately every 9 weeks using the Griffiths Scale of Infant Intelligence. The last visit, at about 12 months, took place in a laboratory in which each infant–mother pair was observed in what would become known as the Strange Situation Procedure.

The evolution of Ainsworth's observational style is evident in sample transcripts from the Baltimore study (e.g., see Table 1.2). As in Uganda, she was exceptionally sensitive to the context in which infant and maternal behavior occurred. But whereas the Uganda observations focused on providing a rich narrative, the Baltimore observations were made with an eye toward quantification.

Assessing Maternal Behavior

A key advance in the Baltimore study was the development and refinement of methods for quantifying narrative records. It was clear from the Uganda study that frequency counts of discrete behaviors, irrespective of context, could not capture the complexity of close interactions and secure base support. Accordingly, Ainsworth made sure that measures based on frequencies and percentages were always carefully contextualized—abrupt or interfering *when picking baby up*; acknowledges baby *when entering the room*, and so forth. The level of detail at which the observations were conducted is evident from the list of variables in Table 1.3.

TABLE 1.2. Mary Ainsworth as an Observer: Sample Observations from the Baltimore Study

As soon as M picked baby up, she stopped crying and put one arm over mom's shoulder as she carried her into the bedroom. B had lost her pacifier. M finds it and takes it with her into the bedroom. M talks and smiles at B, and pats her face. B laughs. M then puts baby down in the crib and removes the pacifier from her mouth. B jiggles up and down as she lies supine in her crib and she cries. M offers her the pacifier again. B takes it and stops crying. B, herself, puts the pacifier in her mouth. M starts to remove her overalls and tights, and B waves her feet and coos and reaches towards her toes. M asks her, "Where's your piggies?" and begins to play with B's toes a little bit. B likes this. M then removes waterproof pants and her diapers. B seems very happy and pats her hands together. M notices this and says "pat-a-cake." B pats a little bit more. B has had a hard bowel movement and M comments that this may have been bothering her. She wipes B off with a Kleenex. B continues to pat her hands, and M again says, "Pat-a-cake." M powders B's diaper rash, which is slight, and B claps her hands again. She continues to clap her hands as M begins to put clean diapers on. Then, for some reason or other, she turns and stares at me.

Note. From original narrative transcripts, courtesy of Robert S. Marvin.

TABLE 1.3. Maternal Care Variables Scored from Baltimore Home Observation Transcripts

A. General attitude of M toward B and her role	
MA-1	**Mother's perception of baby:** Extent to which the mother's perception of the baby is realistic versus distorted by her own needs, feelings, fantasies in a way that impacts on care.
MA-2	**Mother's delight in baby:** Extent to which the mother expresses (intensely or quietly and gently) enjoyment of her baby. Expressed in response to the baby's behavior. Delight in the baby being himself (as opposed to mere pride in having a baby).
MA-3	**Mother's acceptance of baby:** Degree to which the mother insightfully accepts the responsibilities associated with having a baby versus overtly or covertly resenting or rejecting that such responsibilities unduly encroach on other spheres of her life.
MA-4	**Mother's attitude toward baby as evidenced by her excellence as an informant:** Extent to which the mother is a good observer and reporter of the details and subtleties of baby's signals, preferences, and idiosyncrasies. Reports these readily, with interest and enthusiasm versus little information or reports are markedly discrepant with what is observed.
B. Feeding	
MB-1	**Synchronization of mother's interventions with baby's rhythms:** Extent to which baby is fed when but not before he is ready versus overly rigid, scheduled feeding or erratic irregular feeding, seemingly in response to intense demands or the mother's needs.
MB-2	**Determination of amount of food and end of feeding:** Extent to which the mother is adaptable and sensitive in meeting the baby's nutritive needs versus arbitrary determinations that result in under- or overfeeding.
MB-3	**Mother's regard for baby's preferences in kind of food:** Extent to which the mother recognizes baby's solid food preferences and manages to tactfully present less preferred foods versus intrusive disregard for the baby's preferences.
MB-4	**Mother's synchronization of rate of feeding to baby's pace:** Extent to which feeding is something the mother does with the baby rather than to the baby.
MB-DI	**Mother's attitude to non-nutritive sucking:** Indulgence and facilitation versus restrictiveness and impatience.
C. Availability and interaction	
MC-1	**Mother's availability to baby:** The extent to which the mother is available to the baby for some kind of physical, visual, or auditory contact in the course of the day.
MC-2	**Total availability of caretakers to baby:** The extent to which a caregiver (mother, father, or others) is available to the baby for physical, visual, or auditory contact in the course of the day (i.e., the extent to which maternal availability is "covered" by availability of other caregivers).

(continued)

TABLE 1.3. *(continued)*

MC-3	**Amount of interaction offered by mother:** Extent to which the mother offers or affords opportunities for interaction. In addition to offering ample opportunities for interaction, the mother enriches routine caregiving interactions with opportunities for playful interaction versus little contact or little interactive content in the contacts that do occur.
MC-4	**Appropriateness of mother's initiations or interactions:** Extent to which the timing and manner of the mother's behavior is appropriate to the baby's state and current activity. Exquisitely sensitive to infant cues versus overstimulation, intrusiveness, or ill-timed interactions that preclude extended bouts of smoothly coordinated enjoyable interaction.
D. Physical contact	
MD-1	**Amount of physical contact:** Amount of physical contact including contact over and above that required for routine care.
MD-2	**Quality of physical contact in holding baby:** The quality of physical contact when holding, carrying, and feeding the baby. The extent to which the contact is close, comfortable, and mutually accommodative versus rigid and unaccommodating (too close for comfort or loose, dangling, careless).
MD-DI	**Mother's sensuousness in care of baby:** No rating because mothers in the sample tended to be neither unusually sensuous nor notably avoidant in contact or stimulation. Note is made of specific instances of sensuous contact, mothers' attitudes toward such behavior, and reactions to baby's response.
E. Response to crying	
ME-1	**Effectiveness of mother's response to baby's crying:** Mother's effectiveness in heeding cries, correctly interpreting the cause, responding appropriately, and responding in a timely manner.
F. Social contact	
MF-1	**Amount of visual contact:** Extent to which the mother deliberately or otherwise makes it possible for the baby to sustain visual contact with her and/or other members of the household during the day.
MF-2	**Amount of auditory and vocal contact:** Extent to which the mother actively engages baby vocally during interactions and routine care, and uses vocalization to maintain contact when she is out of sight versus often leaving baby alone and out of contact, and little vocal accompaniment to routine care.
MF-3	**Frequency of play interaction (8 weeks and later):** Extent to which interactive play with baby is mixed into routine care and becomes an integral part of the day versus infrequent play and predominantly matter-of-fact manner during routine care.
MF-4	**Appropriateness of play interaction (8 weeks and later):** Extent to which playful interactions are enjoyable for the baby versus controlling, overstimulating, inappropriate to the baby's age, or more geared to the mother's than to the baby's enjoyment.

(continued)

TABLE 1.3. *(continued)*

G. Facilitation of sensorimotor development	
MG-1	**Stimulus potential of the physical environment (6 weeks and later):** Extent to which mother arranges the baby's physical environment to facilitate sensorimotor development.
MG-2	**Mother's encouragement of achievement (8 weeks and later):** Extent to which mother, through play or direct training (intentionally or unintentionally) facilitates and encourages sensorimotor development versus understimulating, letting baby remain helpless and undemanding as long as possible.
MG-3	**Appropriateness of mother's encouragement of achievement:** Extent to which the mother is flexible and sensitive in her engagement and stimulation of the baby versus providing only basic care and/or overly intense (even frightening) or age-inappropriate interaction.

Capturing such detailed information in naturalistic observations, without video recordings, demands stamina, sustained attention, and a choreographer's sense of how infant–mother interactions are organized.

Using the Strange Situation as a criterion, Ainsworth sorted through a wide range of early (first quarter) and later (fourth quarter) variables to identify at different ages and in different levels of detail the aspects of maternal behavior that were most related to attachment outcomes. Both positive (e.g., responsiveness to crying, behaving affectionately during pickups, contingent responsiveness in face-to-face interactions) and negative behaviors (e.g., holding babies ineptly, aversion to physical contact) assessed in the first quarter significantly predicted security at age 1. Similar markers of contingent responsiveness, skillful interaction, and affective sharing during the last quarter were also significantly related to security at age 1 (Ainsworth et al., 1978/2015, Chapter 8).

Importantly, Ainsworth's focus on behavioral detail allowed her to detect consistent individual differences even as the forms of maternal behavior changed with the babies' ages. Despite discontinuity in specific behaviors, her observational records revealed the continuity of behavioral organization. At the same time, she sensed that there were important aspects of behavioral organization and maternal styles that could not be captured at this level of detail. This led her to develop broader, behaviorally anchored but more conceptually defined measures as well.

Quality of Care Scales

Based on a thorough examination of maternal behavior recorded in the transcripts, Ainsworth developed a set of four scales that reflected more general qualities of maternal behavior in caregiving routines during the last quarter of the infant's first year. She labeled these scales (1) sensitivity versus insensitivity to the baby's signals and communications, (2) cooperation versus interference with the baby's ongoing behavior, (3) acceptance versus rejection of the baby's needs, and (4) physical and psychological accessibility versus ignoring and neglecting (Ainsworth et al., 1978/2015).

Each of these constructs is rated on a 9-point scale with conceptual and behavioral anchors for points 1, 3, 5, 7, and 9. Brief summaries of the scales are included in *Methods* sections of numerous empirical reports and in chapters. However, the full text, which includes a lengthy conceptual treatment of each construct, as well as the anchor points, was only circulated in mimeograph. Fortunately, the full text is now available as Appendix IV in the 2015 reissue of *Patterns of Attachment* online at *www.psychology.sunysb.edu/attachment/measures/content/ainsworth_scales.html*. The experience with mother–infant interaction, sensitivity to detail and context, and to the role of cognition, motivation, and defensive processes in maternal behavior reflected in these materials is unsurpassed in attachment study to this day. They should certainly be read (and enjoyed) by every student of attachment.

Sensitivity versus insensitivity to the baby's signals and communications refers to a mother's ability to "see things from her baby's point of view. She is alert to perceive her baby's signals, interprets them accurately, and responds appropriately and promptly, unless no response is most appropriate under the circumstances. She tends to give the baby what he seems to want, and when she does not, she is tactful in acknowledging his communication. Furthermore, she makes her responses temporally contingent on the baby's signals" (Ainsworth et al., 1978/2015, p. 140).

Sensitive mothers detect their infant's signals even when such signals are subtle and understated. They treat infant signals as if they have meaning and tend to correctly interpret such meaning by realistically (not egocentrically according to their own wishes and moods) judging the baby's behavior and signals, and they empathize with the baby's feelings and wishes. Overall, they provide their babies what their communications suggest they want; if the baby initiates social interaction, then she responds socially; if he wants to play, she responds playfully, if he wants to be picked up, she picks him up, and she puts him down if he wants to explore; if he is distressed, she knows what to do and how to calm him down.

Toward the end of the first year, when limit setting becomes more salient in infant–mother exchanges, sensitive mothers acknowledge babies' wishes, although they do not unconditionally accede to them (Ainsworth, Bell, & Stayton, 1974). Typically, sensitive mothers are able to generate well-resolved interactions with their infants. The quality of maternal behavior during exchanges with her baby is likely to be the most important index of sensitivity. Finally, sensitive mothers are prompt in responding to their infants' signals and communications.

Overall, arbitrary and very rigid timing during interactions are typically insensitive to the infant's rhythms and signals. Insensitive mothers often seem, at a certain level, to be unaware of their babies' behavior; they either ignore or fail to perceive in the infant's activity the subtle and hard to detect communications. Moreover, insensitive mothers tend to distort or misconstrue those aspects of their infants' behavior of which they are aware. Even if they have an accurate perception of the infant's moods and activities, they do not empathize with him or her. Because they appear to lack empathy and understanding of their infants' behavior, mothers of insecure infants improperly time their responses to the infant, and often the kind and quality of their responses is inappropriate.

Cooperation versus interference with the baby's ongoing behavior refers to a mother's ability to respect her baby as a separate person; thus, she plans to "avoid situations in which she might have to interfere with his activity or to exert direct control over him. When she does intervene, she is skillful at 'mood setting,' so that the baby is persuaded that he wants to do what she wants him to do" (Ainsworth et al., 1978/2015, p. 140). The core issue here is the extent to which a mother's behavior in interaction with her baby is geared in timing and quality to the baby's current interests, activities, state, and mood.

Cooperation refers to cooperation with an infant's ongoing behavior. The key is coordination and support for exploration expanding the infant's activities in time and space; it is not permissiveness. Mothers with high scores on this scale guide rather than control the infant's activity. Both members determine the dyad's interactions and change of activities. Cooperative mothers do not interrupt the baby's behavior, but wait for a natural break in the infant's activity. These mothers invite their infant to participate rather than impose what they have in mind upon the infant.

Highly *interfering* mothers overwhelm their infants physically. They often disregard the infant's activities and pick him up, move him around, restrict and restrain his movements. Interference is also evident when mothers' primary mode of interacting involves instructing, training, directing, eliciting, and controlling. Interfering mothers show little appreciation for the infant as a separate, active, and autonomous individual whose activities have a validity of their own.

Acceptance versus rejection of the baby's needs refers to "the balance between the mother's positive and negative feelings about her baby and the extent to which she has been able to integrate or to resolve her conflicting feelings" (Ainsworth et al., 1978/2015, p. 140). Note the importance of spelling out and taking into account the entire label; using just *acceptance versus rejection* may lead to misunderstandings. High scores on this scale reflect maternal behavior indicative of acceptance that overrides frustrations, irritations, and limitations brought about by the infant even when he is angry or unresponsive. Although she may occasionally feel irritated by his behavior, she does not cast him as an opponent, nor does she resent the temporary limitation her maternal role places on her other activities.

Low scores are indicative of anger, resentment, irritation in conflictive interaction, and limited positive feelings that result in more or less rejection of the baby. Rejection might be manifest in mothers' comments about the baby, as well as their behavior, or both. The rating of this scale assumes that child–mother relationships include both positive and negative elements, and it reflects the extent to which a mother has integrated such elements, and whether negative feelings permeate her interactions with the infant. Central to its assessment is an explicit consideration of the mother's own needs and goals as they intersect with infant–mother interactions, and the emotional resolution as expressed in both maternal behavior and language.

Scoring acceptance versus rejection depends on maternal comments, as well as behavior. Because social norms dictate that mothers (and caregivers in general) love and enjoy their babies, comments during initial visits are often quite positive and should not be taken at face value. Evidence of mothers being critical with their babies, commenting negatively or complaining about how difficult the baby is, being easily irritated with the baby's activities, harshly reprimanding the infant, and/or getting angry with the baby, among others, tend to emerge, if at all, over time. To further complicate matters, the context of observation (laboratory, home, playgrounds) is likely to influence maternal manifestations of acceptance versus rejection.

Accessibility versus ignoring/neglecting refers to "the mother's psychological accessibility to her infant when she is at home and in this sense physically accessible to him. . . . The accessible mother . . . seems able to attend to her baby's signals and communications, despite distraction by other demands on her attention" (Ainsworth et al., 1978/2015, p. 141). Highly accessible mothers are aware of their babies at all times and keep their infants within reach, at least through distance receptors. They are aware of their infants' signals and activity, and respond to them. Although accessible mothers typically respond to their babies most of the times, the issue here is not how accurately and appropriately a mother responds, but her awareness and accessibility. An accessible mother is able to divide her attention among matters other than those concerned with her infant, yet remain aware of him, his location, and activities.

Inaccessible mothers may ignore their babies, and because of this may neglect them psychologically and/or physically. Thus, for instance, a crying baby is tuned out and the mother does not hear him or she deliberately does not respond to his cry. From the infant's point of view, either case is experienced as the mother being inaccessible. This mother responds to her baby only when she deliberately intends to do something to or for the baby; that is, her interventions are typically at her own desire and convenience, so they are not contingent on her baby's behavior.

As in the case of the acceptance–rejection scale, gathering information about accessibility requires extended or multiple observations. Context is also important, as laboratory assessments tend to momentarily liberate mothers from other demands or, alternatively, place demands on their attention that due to the nature of the task at hand (the meaning of doing research and wanting to please the researchers) alter the mother's priorities regarding attention deployment. As with the acceptance–rejection scale, accessibility versus ignoring has not often been scored in recent research.

Clearly, these four scales are more integrative and conceptual than measures based on specific caregiving practices. The emphasis is not on content per se but on the organization of maternal behavior over time and context. Importantly, observers need to focus on the content and structure of interactions. These are not to be vague ratings of *"warmth," care, love, general positivity, or other nonspecific socially desirable traits*. Indeed, it is better to think of them as summaries of naturalistic observations than as mere "ratings." It is also useful to consider how a baby might experience the behavior over time. A particularly insensitive or intrusive behavior may sometimes suggest looking for a similar pattern of behavior. Scorers should look for convergent evidence for their ratings. Babies' expectations about availability and responsiveness are generally built on more than an isolated miscue or an awkward moment.

Key Results

Not surprisingly, scores on the four maternal behavior constructs tend to be highly intercorrelated, often .80 or higher (e.g., Bretherton, 2013). To some extent, this reflects the fact that maternal behavior is organized by schemas and superordinate goals (e.g., to be a secure base) that reflect the mother's own attachment-related experiences and internal working models. In addition, stressful circumstances tend to undermine each of the facets covered by the Ainsworth scales. Thus, substantial correlations are to be expected across a wide range of maternal behaviors. Still, convergence at such high levels suggests also an element of the "halo" effect due to the fact that all four scales are scored from the same observations.

In light of these high intercorrelations, and the fact that the criteria for scoring the sensitivity to the baby's signals and communications, and cooperation versus Interference with the baby's ongoing behavior are somewhat easier to observe and are more often supported by multiple indicators, most often just these two scales are employed. Indeed, the label *maternal sensitivity* is now widely used in referring to the full range of maternal contributions to attachment development. This is a useful term, as long as we keep in mind that it is shorthand for quite a wide range of behaviors patterned in a particular manner. However, insights from the acceptance versus rejection of the infant's needs and psychological/physical accessibility scales are important in thinking about prevention and intervention and in evaluating change in applied research.

Information about links between maternal behavior and infant security are among the key results from the Baltimore study. Table 1.4 summarizes the links of first quarter maternal behaviors and fourth quarter maternal sensitivity ratings and infant security in the Strange Situation at age 1. These results support Bowlby's contention that the roots of infant security are in real (as opposed to fantasized) experience. They also help sort out which aspects

TABLE 1.4. First- and Fourth-Quarter Correlates of Maternal Behaviors and Infant Security at Age 1

	Secure ($N = 13$)	Insecure ($N = 10$)	p
First-quarter behavior			
Ignoring infant crying	1.60	2.48	n.s.
Unresponsiveness to crying (minutes/hours)	3.64	7.80	<.01
Mean duration of pickup episodes (minutes)	8.70	6.24	<.10
% of pickups in which mother behaves affectionately	16.90	7.40	<.05
% of holding time in which mother is tender, careful	55.00	14.10	<.001
% of holding time in which mother is inept	5.00	33.20	<.001
Aversion to physical contact	2.28	5.07	<.01
Provides baby with an unpleasant experience	1.45	4.57	<.005
Contingent pacing (in face-to-face interaction)	52.90	16.78	<.01
Silent, unsmiling initiation (face-to-face interaction)	12.20	21.74	n.s.
Routine manner	11.00	28.02	<.01
Timing of initiating feeding	6.40	2.60	<.001
Timing of terminating feeding	6.54	3.03	<.001
Dealing with baby's food preferences	6.70	3.85	<.01
Pacing according to baby's rate of intake in feeding	6.85	3.38	<.01
Lack of emotional expression	2.69	5.10	<.02
Rigidity	2.15	3.70	<.02
Fourth-quarter Maternal Behavior Scales			
Sensitivity–Insensitivity	6.48	2.40	<.01
Cooperation–Interference	7.62	4.40	<.01
Acceptance–Rejection	7.30	3.85	<.01
Accessibility–Ignoring	6.62	3.70	<.01

Note. From Ainsworth et al. (1978/2015).

of maternal behavior are most important in attachment development—highlighting motivation, emotional engagement, and contingent responsiveness rather than stimulation per se or specific methods of feeding or routine care.

In addition to clarifying the salient features of maternal care, these results have had a significant impact on how we understand attachment security. If sensitivity to signals and cooperation with ongoing behavior are the antecedents, then expectations of availability and responsiveness, and thus confidence to explore and open communication, are the necessarily salient outcomes. Bowlby, of course, placed great emphasis on the role of appraisal processes as a key factor in emotionality. And such expectations can be associated with a rich range of emotional accompaniments when they are confirmed or violated. Thus, while affording emotion a central role in attachment relationships, these results are an important step toward a more cognitive view of infant security.

Inevitably, this important work has been the focus of replication studies and its generality explored in different contexts and with different methodologies. de Wolff and van IJzendoorn (1997) conducted a meta-analysis of 66 studies that follow-up on Ainsworth's original findings. Twenty-six of these employed Ainsworth's scales. The remainder used conceptually similar measures. Results consistently supported her conclusions regarding links between early maternal care and infant security. However, even among the studies using the Ainsworth scales, the combined effect size was r (835) = .24, $p < .0001$. Although moderate by conventional standards (Cohen, 1988), this level of association is considerably lower than that found in the Baltimore study.

Several factors likely contribute to this difference. Most obviously, not all the researchers had formal training in the use of Ainsworth's scales. And many of the observations were conducted during single visits, over much briefer intervals (often as little as 15 minutes), and/or in a restricted range of contexts. As de Wolff and van IJzendoorn (1997, p. 577) point out, "study quality" is very difficult to assess in assembling data for meta-analytic research. And while excluding potentially weaker studies might increase the validity of the analysis, it can equally well open the door to overrepresenting studies with more positive results. Thus, it is hard to fault their inclusion of all 66 studies in their report. Nonetheless, it is instructive to note that a number of more recent studies employing Pederson and Moran's Maternal Behavior Q-set and Posada and colleagues' Maternal Behavior with Preschoolers Q-set, very experienced scorers, and lengthy observation intervals have reported results more similar to those of Ainsworth (see below).

Even in this research, quite a bit of infant security variance remains unexplained. Of course, moderate, even small, correlations can result in substantially different cumulative experiences for high- and low-scoring individuals when extrapolated through countless interactions (e.g., Abelson, 1985). Nonetheless, the study of early influences on infant security remains a high priority in attachment research.

Lessons from the Baltimore Study

THE ETHOLOGICAL NARRATIVE

Ainsworth's use of a narrative rather than time sampling methodology allowed her to capture a wide range of behaviors and contexts. With the narrative transcripts in hand, she could then develop rating scales that were much more relevant to mothers' and infants' actual behavior than scales made up a priori (i.e., by the "armchair" method). These could then be used to summarize and quantify information from the narrative records and to bring psychological/psychodynamic insights into play at a later stage in the analyses.

Of course, there are limits to the behavioral detail that can be captured in narrative records. Clearly, they cannot support the kind of microanalyses that have proved so useful in the work, for example, of Beatrice Beebe and her colleagues (2010) on infant–mother face-to-face communication. Unfortunately, our own experience is that in indoor naturalistic settings, the video camera is not as quick or as steady (or as unobtrusive) as the human eye.

MULTIPLE LEVELS OF ANALYSIS

The Baltimore study benefited greatly from Ainsworth's willingness to look at behavior at different levels of analysis. At the most detailed level, she was an ethologist recording behavior as she observed it. Alert to the importance of context, she systematically included information about it in her observations. Recognizing that behaviors can serve a variety of functions, she recognized the limitations of discrete behaviors as operational definitions of theoretically defined constructs and grouped behaviors (in context) into functionally defined categories. And sensitive to the fact that maternal behavior affects infant expectations over time and context, she developed rating scales that summarized behavior in terms of constructs such as sensitivity to signals and cooperation with ongoing behavior.

There is no easy way to do all this. It is physically demanding and conceptually challenging. It is only tolerable if one finds behavior interesting (see Waters, Vaughn, & Bernard, Chapter 3, this volume). The modest effect sizes found between maternal behavior and infant security in some studies remind us that there are no shortcuts. They also caution us about the difficulties inherent in transferring such methodologies across laboratories and in scaling up work from small studies for use in larger scale projects.

OBSERVING ORDINARY AND EMERGENCY BEHAVIOR

Ainsworth also found it useful to combine naturalistic observation with structured laboratory assessments. Had she focused solely on structured interaction settings (in which infants often become impatient or distressed) and the often stressful Strange Situation, calming and comforting would likely have been the most salient feature in the mothers' behavior. In such contexts, it is easy to imagine that the function of attachment is to extinguish negative emotions. However, the rich narrative descriptions of infant–mother in "ordinary," nonemergency interactions made clear that the mother's role entails *both* comforting/calming and support for exploration (see Marvin, Cooper, Hoffman, & Powell, 2002; Posada et al., 1999; Waters, 2008; Waters & Cummings, 2000). A simpler, less demanding methodology might have obscured the organization of attachment behavior and undermined one of Bowlby's key insights into the nature of the child's tie to its mother.

MOTHERS AS INFORMANTS

Ainsworth's use of mothers as informants raises interesting issues. They are certainly selective and subjective; therefore, it is better not to use them as the only source of information when possible. At the same time, she found mothers quite informative regarding the typicalness of the baby's behavior on a given day, as a source of behaviors and situations to put on an intuitive "look out for" list, and as clues to mothers' goals and attributions, and so forth. Interestingly, Ainsworth found that the mother's excellence as an informant was closely related to the quality of infant–mother interactions and to infant security (see Ainsworth, 1967, p. 45; Bretherton, 2013, pp. 467, 469). Thus, Ainsworth's openness to such data proved to be a significant advantage.

FURTHER DEVELOPMENTS

The Uganda and Baltimore studies speak eloquently of Mary Ainsworth's skills and the skills of mothers. They also illustrate the advantages and difficulties of naturalistic observation. As Ainsworth noted, in a research environment that values productivity and favors high-tech methods, the low-tech rigors of the ethological method place it at a significant disadvantage (Ainsworth & Marvin, 1995, p. 12). Not surprisingly, a great deal of effort has gone into making naturalistic observation more learnable, more economical, and more quantifiable.

The Maternal Behavior Q-set

David Pederson and Greg Moran at the University of Western Ontario were greatly influenced by the Uganda and Baltimore studies. However, they recognized that Ainsworth's narrative methods were too costly and too difficult to be widely adopted. They had worked for several years with traditional ethological methods, checklists, handheld digital recorders, and rating scales without finding a satisfactory alternative. The simpler methods did not adequately take the organization and context of behavior into account. Handheld devices freed observers from the distraction of taking detailed notes but simply introduced different kinds of distractions. And without underlying narrative records, the limitations and biases of human memory undermined the effectiveness of global rating scales. Following Waters and Deane's (1985) work on secure base behavior, Pederson and Moran turned to the Q-sort method as an economical alternative to Ainsworth's methodology.

The Q-sort method was originally developed for use in personality and psychiatry research (see Block, 1978, 2008). A Q-set is a set of descriptive items printed on small cards. Instead of rating each item individually, scorers sort the cards into piles according to a fixed distribution on the basis of how characteristic the item is of the target individual (e.g., 9 piles of 10 items each). The pile into which an item is placed determines its score. Thus, items placed high in the sort (Pile 9) are assigned a score of 9. Items placed low in the sort (Pile 1) are assigned a score of 1. The use of a fixed distribution forces the scorer to attend to the content of each card and make thoughtful comparative judgments. It also restricts the possibilities for socially desirable responding, because not all "good" items can be placed high in the sort.

The primary advantages of the Q-sort method for attachment research include the following: (1) Familiarity with the Q-set items gives a sense of what to focus on during observations; (2) this, and the fact that the items serve as powerful retrieval cues during sorting, allows observers to spend more time observing and less time taking detailed notes; (3) Q-sort data lend themselves to a wide range of strategies for assessing agreement, reliability, items, scales, and broadly defined constructs; and (4) "criterion sorts" used as templates for scoring constructs such as security or sensitivity to infant signals make scoring criteria explicit, as well as open to revision and criticism. (See Vaughn, Waters, & Teti, Chapter 2, this volume, for additional details on the rationale, scoring, and analysis of Q-sort data.)

Working from Ainsworth's maternal sensitivity scales and their own extensive observations of mother–infant interaction, Pederson and Moran (e.g., Pederson et al., 1990; Pederson & Moran 1995; Smith & Pederson, 1988) developed the Maternal Behavior Q-set (MBQ) for use in research on mother–infant interaction. They began with an initial pool of 150 items. They reduced this to 90 items by eliminating items that were redundant, ambiguous, unlikely to be observed, or that could not be sorted reliably.

The MBQ items address the general domains and many of the more specific behavioral categories that Ainsworth suggested in her Uganda and Baltimore studies, often employing several items to address the same behavior in different contexts. Thus, they tap a mother's tendency to (1) detect and recognize signals or situations that might require her response, and to respond promptly and appropriately to these situations, (2) participate in and cooperate with her infant's activities, (3) accept her infant's needs, and (4) be accessible and skillful in detecting her baby's signals and communications despite other demands on her attention and behavior. Items also refer to a mother's affect when interacting with her infant, as well as when talking about her infant.

TABLE 1.5. MBQ Items Judged by Experts to Be Most and Least Characteristic of the Prototypical Sensitive Mother

Item no.	Item content
Most characteristic	
6	Interactions appropriately vigorous and exciting as judged from baby's responses
9	Responds consistently to baby's signals
12	Interprets cues correctly, as evidenced by baby's response
29	Slows pace down; waits for baby's response in face-to-face interactions
53	Well-resolved interactions with baby—interaction ends when baby is satisfied
54	Interactions revolve around baby's tempo and current state
60	When baby is distressed, is able to quickly and accurately identify the source
63	Monitors and responds to baby even when engaged in some other activity
Least characteristic	
2	Unaware of or insensitive to baby's signals of distress
4	Delays response; baby cannot connect mother's response with the action that initiated it
7	Responds only to frequent, prolonged, or intense signals
52	Fails to interrupt activity by her baby that is likely to be dangerous
57	Overwhelms baby with constant, unphased barrage of stimulation
68	Often appears to "tune out" and not notice distress or bids for attention
73	Interaction pace/content set by mother rather than according to baby's response
74	Often misses "slow down" or "back off" signals from baby during face-to-face play

Faculty and graduate students familiar with home observations, and with attachment theory and research, sorted these 90 items to describe a prototypical sensitive mother. The items that anchor the high and low ends of this criterion sort are presented in Table 1.5. This "criterion sort" is used as a template against which to score individual mothers on maternal sensitivity.

Key Results

In an initial study (Pederson et al., 1990), interobserver agreement on MBQ sensitivity scores was quite satisfactory (r (38) = .75, p < .001). As indicated in Table 1.6, subsequent studies from more than one laboratory, culture, and

TABLE 1.6. Maternal Behavior and Infant Security in More Recent Studies

			Behavior		
Study	***N***	**Sample**	**Mother**	**Child**	***r****
Pederson et al. (1990)	40	Canadian middle class	MBQ[a]	AQS[b]	.52
Moran et al. (1992)	19	Canadian, dev. delay	MBQ	AQS	.49
Pederson & Moran (1995a)	89	Canadian pre- and full-term	MBQ	AQS	.61
Pederson et al. (1998)	60	Canadian middle class	MBQ	SS[c]	.51
Posada et al. (1999)					
Study 1	41	Colombian middle class	MBQ	AQS	.48
Study 2	43	Colombian low SES	MBQ	AQS	.55
Posada et al. (2002)					
Study 1	61	Colombian middle class	MBQ	AQS	.46
Study 2	60	U.S. middle class	MBQ	SS	.33
Posada et al. (2004)	30	Colombian middle class	MBQ	AQS	.42
			Ethnography	AQS	.61
Posada et al. (2007)					
Study 1	50	U.S. middle class	MBPQ[d]	AQS	.31
Study 2	40	U.S. middle class	MBPQ	AQS	.49
Posada et al. (2016)	237	Overall sample (4 cultures)	MBPQ	AQS	.36
Posada et al. (2018)					
Time 1 (3.5 years)	74	U.S. middle class	MBPQ	AQS	.42
Time 2 (5.5 years)	74	U.S. middle class	MBPQ	AQS	.34

*All correlation indices are statistically significant, $p < .05$.
[a]Maternal Behavior Q-set.
[b]Attachment Q-set.
[c]Strange Situation.
[d]Maternal Behavior with Preschoolers Q-set.

social class have reported substantial correlations between MBQ sensitivity scores and infant attachment security assessed with the Waters (1995) Attachment Q-set (AQS) and in the Strange Situation (e.g., Moran, Pederson, Pettit, & Krupka, 1992: Pederson & Moran, 1995, 1996; Pederson, Gleason, Moran, & Bento, 1998; Pederson et al., 1990; Posada et al., 1999, 2002; Posada, Carbonell, Alzate, & Plata, 2004) (see Table 1.6). Notably, the results are quite consistent from Canadian samples of healthy middle-class and developmentally delayed infants to a Colombian sample of mothers from very low socioeconomic status (SES) whose infants were hospitalized for nutritional problems and gastrointestinal illnesses (Posada et al., 1999). Thus, from the beginning, the MBQ seemed suitable for research in a wide range of contexts. It offers an empirically sound alternative to assess maternal sensitivity. It is worth noting that these studies, which use a methodology closer to that of Ainsworth (e.g., long observation periods in naturalistic contexts and experienced observers) report levels of associations more similar to those found by Ainsworth than suggested in meta-analytic studies.

Pederson and Moran have undertaken several revisions to the original MBQ to address some conceptual and empirical issues that emerged in the course of the initial studies with the measure. For example, they have ensured that all the items focus on interactive behavior or on how the infant experiences it. Items that drew attention to trait-like characteristics of the mother rather than to interactive behavior were eliminated or revised. In addition, they have added items that might help clarify the antecedents of avoidant and resistant attachment. These include items such as "Interactions are object oriented; e.g., with toys, food"; "Physically aloof when interacting with baby"; "Terminates physical contact before B is satisfied"; and "Interactions with B are characterized by conflict." The current MBQ item set is Version 3.1. Information including the MBQ items, criterion sorts, a manual, and suggestions about observing and video recording, is available online at *www.psychology.sunysb.edu/attachment/measures/content/pederson_qset.html.*

The Sensitivity Construct and Culture

Bowlby placed great emphasis on the notion that both maternal care and infant attachment are shaped in part by our primate evolutionary endowment. Indeed, he described the mother and infant as coadapted, in the sense that attachment development depends on an interaction between biases in learning abilities that guide how behavior becomes organized and species-general patterns of maternal care. At the same time, openness to learning and cultural influence is one of the hallmarks of human behavior. This raises the question, can constructs like "maternal sensitivity" and measures like the MBQ be used across cultures without major revisions?

Posada et al. (2004) addressed this question in a sample of 30 lower-middle and middle-class Colombian families. They recruited Colombian ethnographers, unfamiliar with the MBQ and the AQS, to observe infant–mother interactions and prepare narrative transcripts of their observations. Then, experts, who were not familiar with Ainsworth's measures, used ethnographic methods described by Spradley (1980) and Strauss (1987), to develop 11 content-based scales that captured, in their view, the most salient aspects of infant–mother interaction. These were then compared with sensitivity and security scores based on independent home visits by observers who were familiar with attachment theory and experienced with the MBQ and AQS.

The Colombian ethnographers highlighted the promptness, consistency, and effectiveness of maternal responses, and the level, diversity, quality, and enjoyment of physical contact and interaction, and the mothers' ability to balance competing demands. Conceptually these are very similar to the variables Ainsworth noted in the Uganda and Baltimore studies, and to the items in the MBQ. Moreover, as indicated in Table 1.7, most of their scales were substantially correlated with independent MBQ sensitivity scores and AQS security scores.

TABLE 1.7. Associations between Ethnographic Scales and Sensitivity and Security Scores

Ethnographic scale	Sensitivity (MBQ)	Security (AQS)
Overall quality of care	.47**	.61**
Specific domains of early care		
1. Promptness of response	.61**	.51**
2. Response effectiveness	.55**	.63**
3. Behavioral consistency	.45**	.51**
4. Balance between responding to the baby and other demands	.51**	.33*
5. Balance between physical care and social interaction with baby	.30*	.57**
6. Enjoyment of interaction	.43**	.76**
7. Interactive smoothness	.49**	.55**
8. Frequency of physical contact	.40*	.55**
9. Quality of physical contact	.42**	.65**
10. Frequency of verbalizations	.30†	.53**
11. Diversity of functions in maternal verbalizations	.30†	.53**

Note. MBQ, Maternal Behavior Q-set; AQS, Attachment Q-set. Reprinted with permission from Posada, Carbonell, Alzate, and Plata (2004, p. 515). † = $p = .0$; * = $p < .05$; ** = $p < .01$.

This is a very useful approach to assessing the generality of attachment theory concepts and measures across culture and social class. It deserves to be used more widely in support of claims about attachment and culture, and in research on attachment at older ages.

Sensitivity and Secure Base Support in the Preschool Years

Sensitivity to early signals is not an inoculation that ensures good outcomes throughout development. It is the first step in an ongoing process of support that plays an important role in building a human nervous system, a self theory, and skills in some (though not all) important aspects of social relationships. As locomotor and cognitive abilities expand, so do the infant's world and the kinds of help an attachment figure provides. Thus, the support termed *maternal sensitivity* when provided for an infant is perhaps better termed *secure base support* thereafter.

German Posada and colleagues have adapted and elaborated Ainsworth's conceptualization of sensitivity to signals, cooperation with ongoing behavior, accessibility, and acceptance for research on parent–child interactions after infancy. Drawing on the work described earlier, Posada and colleagues developed the Maternal Behavior with Preschoolers Q-set (MBPQ; Posada & Waters, 2018, Appendix A), with the aim of investigating secure base support during toddlerhood and the transition to early childhood (Posada, Kaloustian, Richmond, & Moreno, 2007; Posada & Waters, 2018; Richmond, Posada, & Jacobs, 2001). The MBPQS was based on theoretical and empirical work on attachment relationships in infancy and early childhood, interviews, and observations of mothers of preschoolers in naturalistic settings (Ainsworth, Bell, & Stayton, 1971, 1974; Ainsworth et al., 1978/2015; Bowlby, 1969/1982; George & Solomon, 2008; Greenberg, Cicchetti, & Cummings, 1990; Pederson & Moran, 1995; Pederson et al., 1990; Posada et al., 1999, 2002; Waters & Gao, 1998; Waters, Kondo-Ikemura, Posada, & Richters, 1991). An initial pool of 142 items was reduced to 90 items that refer to specific domains of maternal behavior (e.g., contributions to harmonious interactions, secure base support, supervision, and limit setting). As in development of the AQS and the MBQ, pilot data were used to identify redundant, ambiguous, and difficult-to-observe items for elimination.

Four Ph.D. developmental psychologists and graduate students familiar with attachment theory and experienced in naturalistic observation of preschool-age children used the MBPQS items to describe the prototypical parent who is most sensitive (in the broad sense) and most skilled at providing secure base support. Interobserver reliability among the experts was satisfactory; all pairwise correlations were >.86. The sorts were averaged to obtain a criterion sort against which to score parents on the sensitivity/secure base support construct (Posada et al., 2007).

In addition, Posada et al. (2007) identified subsets of MBPQS items that could be summed to provide scores on four content-based scales:

1. *Contributions to harmonious interaction* focuses on maternal behavior that facilitates smooth exchanges with the child and cooperates with child behavior. The scale comprises 20 items that refer both to maternal behavioral and affective involvement in the transactions with the child. Some example items include "Participates in play with child, e.g., plays in the sand, runs with child"; "Mother behaves as part of a team, exchanges with child are harmonious"; "Is overcontrolling, intrusive, in interactions with child, e.g., provides excessive instructions, or physically reorients child" (reverse-scored); and "When child expresses positive affect, mother joins in."

2. *Secure base support* comprises 22 items that summarize the mother's support for exploration and her effectiveness in serving as a haven of safety and a source of comfort when needed. Example items include "When child goes back to mother, she is unresponsive or business-like in acknowledging child's returns" (reverse-scored); "When child cries or signals, mother delays in responding or checking what's going on" (reverse-scored); "Makes sure that child explores available toys or activities (including peers)"; "Smoothly facilitates explorations away from and returns to her"; and "When child shows her something he is playing with, mom asks about it, comments positively on it, encourages child to do something with it."

3. *Supervision/monitoring* combines eight items that refer to the caregiver's skill at keeping track of the child, anticipating problem situations, and maintaining supervision while participating in the child's activities. Examples of items in this scale are "Follows or moves to a better location to supervise/monitor as child moves from place to place"; "Is two steps ahead of child, anticipates conflictive situations and does something to prevent escalation"; and "Balanced in her role as supervisor of and participant in child's activities."

4. *Limit setting* includes five items that refer to how a mother sets rules and boundaries for her child's activities, whether she considers the child's wants and desires, and how she handles violations of those rules and expectations. Examples of items in this scale include "In limit setting, mother negotiates with child until a mutually satisfying solution is achieved"; "When setting rules and prohibiting an activity to child, explains reasons"; and "Enforces rules she sets."

The full set of MBPQS items and the criterion sort values for scoring maternal sensitivity are available in Posada and Waters (2018, Appendix A) Scoring for the four content-based scales is available from the first author.

Key Results

Posada et al. (2007) report that in two initial studies of mothers and their 3- to 5-year-old children (*n*'s = 50 and 40), all four scales had high internal consistency (alpha = .74–.89). Correlations among the first three scales ranged from .55 to .82, $p < .01$). As indicated in Table 1.6, several studies in different cultural contexts have reported that MBPQS scores, based on the sensitivity/secure base support criterion sort, are significantly correlated with preschool AQS security scores. In each case, the effect size was comparable to that of studies with the MBQ. Further empirical evidence in different social and cultural contexts is provided by Posada et al. (2016).

These initial results with the MBPQS point to the relevance of maternal sensitivity and secure base support beyond infancy. This is an important research direction. Just as maternal Adult Attachment Interview (AAI) classifications leave a great deal of infant security unexplained (van IJzendoorn, 1995; Verhage et al., 2016), early maternal sensitivity leaves a great deal of infant and preschool attachment security, and their developmental correlates, unexplained. Conceptualizing the issue in terms of "the effects of early experience." most of this research has focused on a single assessment of maternal sensitivity. Although suitable for research on the early phases of attachment onset, such designs entirely miss the importance of continuity in the caregiving environment for attachment and social development beyond infancy. Insofar as maternal sensitivity presents us with a "transmission gap," the first and most obvious candidate to explain the missing variance is maternal sensitivity (and secure base support) at later ages (Posada, Trumbell, Lu, & Anaya, 2018).

Results to date suggest that MBPQS is a productive approach to study caregiver sensitivity in the preschool years. Both the AQS and the MBQ improved over time as their authors accumulated the experience and results needed to fine-tune and supplement the item sets. We expect that the same will be true for the MBPQS.

ENSURING THE QUALITY OF OBSERVATIONAL AND Q-SORT DATA

Measures such as the AQS, the MBQ, and the MBPQS have helped keep naturalistic observation a viable methodology in attachment study. Of course, scores derived using the Q-sort method are only as good as the observations they summarize. Therefore, it is useful to employ "best practices" that contribute to good observation and good Q-sort data. These include aspects of training, planning visits, observational procedures, and Q-sorting.

Working with Q-Sorts in Naturalistic Settings

Becoming Familiar with the Q-Set

A good Q-set incorporates considerable expertise regarding a particular behavior domain. Indeed, trainees often describe the process of becoming familiar with the MBQ and MBPQS items as a mini-seminar on maternal behavior. In addition, the Q-sort method greatly facilitates naturalistic observation by putting bounds on what is to be observed and cueing the observer's attention to relevant events and contexts. Accordingly, one of the first tasks in training to use the MBQ or MBPQS is to become familiar with the items and the sorting procedure. This is easily accomplished by having trainees read and discuss each item with an experienced observer, and perform practice sorts (e.g., describing the observer's idea of a typical mother, a most sensitive mother, the ideal mother when providing secure base support). As trainees become familiar with the Q-set items, it is also useful to watch videotapes (if available) and to accompany an experienced observer who can comment on what they are noticing during an actual observation. It is also useful to have an expert observer explain his or her thinking while sorting the items after a visit.

Setting, Number, and Duration of Visits

The MBQ and MBPQS were developed for observation of relatively unconstrained behavior over significant periods of time and fluid contexts. The MBQ has been used successfully in home settings (Pederson & Moran, 1995, 1996; Pederson et al., 1998; Posada et al., 2002, 2007) and in hospitals (Posada et al., 1999). The MBPQS has been used primarily during free play on public playgrounds and at home (Lu, Posada, Trumbell, & Anaya, 2018; Posada et al., 2002, 2007, 2016, 2018). In most instances, it is advantageous to have two researchers observing and sorting independently.

The appropriate number of visits depends on the research design. In correlational studies, it is important to have a good estimate of the typical behavior of each individual subject (e.g., studies on the associations between maternal secure base support and child secure base behavior). Poor estimates reduce the size of correlations and suggest lower correlations than would be obtained with more reliable data. The *alpha* reliability of overall Q-sort descriptions, based on the mean correlation between Q-sort descriptions that are averaged into a composite, is a useful indication of whether a given set of observations has converged on a representative picture of a subject's typical behavior.

One of the advantages of the Q-sort method is that the multi-item descriptions make it possible to estimate this within individual subjects rather than across a full sample. Thus, the criterion for "enough data" can be evaluated case by case. If two visits have not yielded a reliable estimate of a subject's typical behavior, then an additional visit can be scheduled. In studies that focus on group differences, the primary goal is to obtain a good estimate of the mean behavior of each group (e.g., studies comparing maternal sensitivity across contexts such as cultures of socioeconomic groups). Single observations that provide rather noisy estimates of individuals' behavior can in combination provide quite adequate descriptions of group members' typical behavior. The noise simply reduces statistical power, which can be recovered by using a larger sample. Thus, single visits to a larger number of homes can be a good strategy for some designs; for others, it is important to study each subject repeatedly.

Observations generally last from 1 to 2 hours. Although the duration of observations is usually fixed (i.e., 1–2 hours), the information density of observation intervals is not constant. The rate at which scorable behavior occurs and the amount of time needed to obtain what seems a representative picture of an individual's behavior varies from one visit to the next. One mother and child may interact frequently and across a variety of contexts, and provide a rich behavior sample in as little as 45 minutes. Another dyad, or the same dyad on a different day or context, may fill the time with fewer and less informative interactions. Sometimes the mother will occupy herself away from the infant for significant intervals, with the infant amusing him- or herself in a highchair or infant seat while mother talks on the telephone, does housework, or engages the interviewer. In such contexts scorable events can be rather infrequent and the range of scorable content observed rather limited.

Although such interactions should be sampled, it is sometimes useful to suggest a change of activities or some sort of interaction, such as reading a story or playing with a favorite toy or going outdoors, to increase the information flow during at least a portion of the visit. After all, the naturalistic home environment most often involves tasks for the mother (e.g., siblings, preparing meals, dealing with visitors) that compete with her caregiving of her child (see Pederson & Moran, 1995). Thus, the inclusion of structured elements to the visit (e.g., completing questionnaires, engaging in a brief interview regarding demographic information) may usefully complement periods in which observers attempt to play the proverbial "fly on the wall."

It is important to ask the mother early in the visit whether the baby has felt well, slept well, and whether the observer is seeing reasonably typical "day in the life." If mother or child has been ill or is overly tired, if there are unusual demands or unusually hectic traffic in the house, or if the visit seems to be an inconvenience, the visit should be rescheduled. In doing so, visitors should make it clear that the mother has not disappointed or inconvenienced them, that they appreciate the family members' time and are quite happy to be accommodating.

Even under seemingly ordinary conditions, visits sometimes seem uninformative or observers take away rather different perspectives on what happened. This usually results in low (<.6) agreement across items. Under these circumstances, it is useful to try to schedule an additional observation. Averaging this into the Q-sort descriptions of the initial visits provides a more representative description of the target behaviors.

Observer Number and Behavior

It is generally useful to have two researchers observe in tandem but without discussing their observations. Behavior is complicated, and the duration of typical home visits is long. Thus, two sets of eyes, two perspectives on a particular event, someone to interact with or assist the mother can all be helpful.

People behave differently when there are strangers about, sometimes restricting their behavior, other times becoming more active, more sociable than usual. Adults' behavior often tends toward politeness, socially desirable norms and "visitor rituals" (feeling that it is necessary to converse, offering food, etc.). Although much of this passes with time and familiarity, there remain significant individual differences in how easy it is to access "typical" behavior. Accepting courtesies, explaining one's interest in typical behavior, and maintaining an informal manner while appearing busy are helpful. Being overly formal, task-oriented, or busy, failing to show ordinary social interest, often makes mothers feel they are being evaluated. The best way to minimize observer impact on participants is to behave unremarkably.

A comfortable informal manner is important during home visits. It puts mother and child at ease and increases the chances of observing typical behavior. However, inexperienced observers, unfamiliar with what exactly is to be observed or uncomfortable in the observer role, sometimes become absorbed in conversation with the mother, who may enjoy the company or find conversation a pleasant distraction. Observers need to be alert to this temptation, as it simply cuts into observation time. Similarly, observers are often tempted to engage infants well beyond what is necessary to get them past initial wariness. This, too, cuts into observation time and affects the infant's or child's behavior by making the observer more attractive as a playmate; it also affects maternal behavior. Some of the motivation here comes from the observer. Socializing defers the hard work involved in making extended naturalistic observations. A useful maxim for observers is that if one is not experiencing the visit as hard work, one is not working hard enough.

Taking Notes

Trainees and novice observers are well advised to make written notes of the time, content, and context of particularly informative interactions. These are then a useful guide in discussing the observations with a more experienced observer. They can also be reviewed before sorting. The tendency is to take too many notes, at the expense of watching closely. Thus, it is useful for an experienced observer to provide some pointers about the level of note taking that is manageable.

Experienced observers differ in their approach to note taking. Some find it unnecessary and feel that mothers never become entirely comfortable with such overt signs that they are being watched. Others find it useful to make light notes that point to specific Q-set items. With care, notes can be informative enough to serve as reminders of key events, yet be innocuous enough to show mothers ("Just some reminders to myself, some things I have to remember, some things I might forget"). Openness is disarming; officiousness is annoying. Importantly, empirical results from studies that used (e.g., Pederson & Moran, 1995) and did not use (e.g., Posada et al., 2004) notes do not seem to differ. Associations between sensitivity and security, both significance and size of correlation indices reported, are very similar.

Video Recording

The availability of high-resolution, low-light, battery-powered video recorders opens the door to video recording in homes and on playgrounds. Our experience using video in homes, however, suggests that real-time observations are markedly preferable. Rooms typically are much smaller than one imagines. Brightness is dramatically different from one angle to the next. Small cameras are difficult to hold steady, and tripods are awkward and conspicuous. It never looks like it does in the movies. In addition, the audio track on most consumer recorders does not provide a good representation of the mother's or the child's auditory experience. A poor audio record makes it difficult to tell whether the mother or child could have heard all the sounds captured in the recording, much less judge the child's and parent's sense of distance and accessibility.

Video recording inevitably makes the experience of being observed more salient to the mother and sometimes to the child as well. Especially in homes, mothers' self-consciousness is evident in their fleeting glances at the cameras, references to being photographed, and general unease. Filming at playgrounds and parks (e.g., Posada et al., 2007) is generally more manageable, because open spaces allow the camera operator to move into the background and avoid, to an extent, being detected at every move members of a dyad make. Though still a challenge, recording outdoors has been more satisfactory. Over the years, we have made limited use of video records in the home for pilot work, training, and teaching. Aside from this, we feel we get better data working from direct observations. Nevertheless, with recent advances in digital video technology, careful planning, and experience, video recording remains a useful strategy for training and for keeping coders blind to information that would be evident if they had visited the home themselves (e.g., Tarabulsy et al., 2009).

From Observations to Data

Q-set items' value as retrieval cues during scoring diminishes quickly over time. Thus, Q-sorting is always performed promptly after each visit. If the same individuals are to be observed on multiple occasions, a sort is performed after each visit, and the data from the several visits are averaged.

Pederson and Moran (1995) have developed a "debriefing procedure" to help observers reflect on their observations before sorting the Q-set items. Their observers always take notes during the visit. During the debriefing, they discuss the notes with an expert blind to the identity of the individuals who were observed. Together they reconstruct the course of the visit, highlighting and discussing specifics of the mother's behavior in key contexts (e.g., infant distressed, secure base behavior, signals to mother, occasions for proximity seeking, monitoring the infant over time and from one location to another, detecting and responding to infant signals, and indications of her physical and psychological availability).

These debriefing interviews serve several important functions. For novice observers, it is an important aspect of developing their observational and note-taking skills. The debriefer directs attention to key events, asks probing questions about the context and details of the mother's and the infant's behavior, and comments on the level of detail and completeness of the observer's notes. In this way, observers learn to be attentive to behavior from the moment they arrive at a home, to pay special attention to transitions from one activity to another, and to make distinctions based on the context in which behavior occurs. They also learn that in sorting the Q-set items, it is important to avoid placing too much weight on isolated events and to look for convergent evidence in support of item placements.

After a summary of the visit, the interviewer feeds back impressions of the mother's behavioral strategies, and these impressions are either validated or corrected by the observer. Similarly, the interviewer describes the mother's availability, monitoring, cooperation, and acceptance, as well as her caregiving strategies. After the debriefing (and perhaps adding some comments or clarifications to the observation notes), the observer sorts the Q-set items to describe the behavior he or she observed during the visit.

Posada and colleagues (1999, 2002, 2007, 2016, 2018) use a more traditional procedure. Immediately after a visit, the two observers describing maternal behavior independently sort the Q-set items. They then evaluate agreement by computing the correlation between their two sorts and also identifying and discussing items on which they disagreed by more than 2 points.

Discussing item disagreements serves several roles. It provides an opportunity for observers to reconsider and modify (or not) individual item placements. It also helps minimize observer drift into idiosyncratic use of particular items. And, perhaps most importantly, the discussions serve an ongoing training and over time sharpen both observers' skills.

Overall agreement (prior to discussing any large discrepancies) in the range of .70 or more is considered acceptable. This is the level of agreement reported in publications. After discussion, the observers' sorts are averaged, and this composite is the description used for scoring item-based scales and criterion sorts. Most trainees achieve this level of agreement in the course of as few as three to five visits. The few who do not are usually assigned to other roles in the research.

Whichever approach is used, it is very important for observers to keep in mind that their task is to describe what they observed. They should not be making broad good–bad, sensitive–insensitive evaluations, then using the Q-set items to draw a picture consistent with their evaluation. Q-sort descriptions are multifaceted descriptions, not focused evaluations of a single construct. They are an image of maternal behavior observed during the visit, not of a theory. Although the immediate goal might be to derive a score on maternal sensitivity using a particular criterion sort, the same Q-sort data description might later be used to score additional constructs or used in an entirely different research project. See Waters (2013) and Vaughn, Waters, and Teti (Chapter 2, this volume) for additional discussion of observing infant–mother interaction and the Q-sort method generally.

CONCLUSION

In proposing his developmental model of attachment, Bowlby placed caregiving at the heart of his analysis and suggested that the construction and elaboration of a child's bond to primary caregivers, usually but not exclusively the mother, are rooted in the vicissitudes of countless ordinary interactions. Although traumatic experiences were expected to have an impact on attachment relationships, Bowlby considered that everyday, real-life experiences in interactions would be central in the formation and maintenance of child–caregiver attachment relationships.

Ainsworth articulated the caregiving construct in attachment theory through careful empirical research of infant–mother interactions during the first year of life (Ainsworth, 1967; Ainsworth et al., 1978/2015). She described a model of care that focuses on the quality rather than quantity of care. This is the significance of the maternal sensitivity construct. Her studies were a turning point for research about the influences of maternal caregiving on children's development of attachment relationships. In addition, her methodological strategy and assessments remain unparalleled in the field and an example of developmental research. Her studies stand out for the thoroughness and extent to which she probed child–mother interactions. The Q-sort method has helped make her insights more explicit and her observational approach more accessible. It has also helped extend research on maternal sensitivity and the secure base phenomenon well beyond infancy. In doing so, it is helping us appreciate the scope and coherence of the developmental perspective underlying Bowlby's and Ainsworth's attachment theory.

REFERENCES

Abelson, R. P. (1985). A variance explanation paradox: When little is a lot. *Psychological Bulletin, 97,* 129–133.

Ainsworth, M. D. S. (1963). The development of infant–mother interactions among the Ganda. In B. M. Foss (Ed.), *Determinants of infant behavior* (Vol. 2, pp. 67–104). London: Methuen.

Ainsworth, M. D. S. (1964). Patterns of attachment behavior shown by the infant in interaction with his mother. *Merrill–Palmer Quarterly, 10,* 51–58.

Ainsworth, M. D. S. (1967). *Infancy in Uganda: Infant care and the growth of love.* Baltimore: Johns Hopkins University Press.

Ainsworth, M. D. S., Bell, S. M., & Stayton D. F. (1971). Individual differences in Strange Situation behavior of one-year-olds. In H. R. Shaffer (Ed.), *The origins of human social relations* (pp. 17–57). London: Academic Press.

Ainsworth, M. D. S., Bell, S. M., & Stayton D. F. (1974). Infant–mother attachment and social development: Socialization as a product of reciprocal responsiveness to signals. In M. P. M. Richards (Ed.), *The integration of a child into a social world* (pp. 99–135). New York: Cambridge University Press.

Ainsworth, M. D. S., Blehar, M. C., Waters, E., & Wall, S. (2015). *Patterns of attachment: A psychological study of the Strange Situation.* New York: Taylor & Francis (Psychology Press). (Original work published 1978)

Ainsworth, M. D. S., & Bowlby, J. (1991). An ethological approach to personality development. *American Psychologist, 46,* 331–341.

Ainsworth, M. D. S., & Marvin, R. S. (1995). On the shaping of attachment theory and research: An interview with Mary D. S. Ainsworth. In E. Waters, B. E. Vaughn, G. Posada, & K. Kondo-Ikemura (Eds.), Care giving, cultural, and cognitive perspectives on secure base behavior and working models: New growing points of attachment theory and research. *Monographs of the Society for Research in Child Development, 60*(2–3, Serial No. 244), 3–21.

Beebe, B., Jaffe, J., Markese, S., Buck, K., Chen, H., Cohen, P., . . . Feldstein, S. (2010). The origins of 12-month attachment: A microanalysis of 4-month mother–infant interaction. *Attachment and Human Development, 12,* 1–135.

Block, J. (1978). *The Q-sort method.* Palo Alto, CA: Consulting Psychology Press.

Block, J. (2008). *The Q-sort in character appraisal: Encoding subjective impressions of persons quantitatively.* Washington, DC: American Psychological Association.

Bowlby, J. (1969). *Attachment and loss: Vol. 1. Attachment.* New York: Basic Books.

Bowlby, J. (1988). *A secure base.* New York: Basic Books.

Bretherton, I. (2003). Mary Ainsworth: Insightful observer and courageous theoretician. In G. A. Kimble & M. Wertheimer (Eds.), *Portraits of pioneers in psychology* (pp. 317–331). Hillsdale, NJ: Erlbaum.

Bretherton, I. (2013). Revisiting Mary Ainsworth's conceptualization and assessments of maternal sensitivity–insensitivity. *Attachment and Human Development, 15*(5–6), 460–484.

Cohen, J. (1988). *Statistical power analysis for the behavioral sciences* (rev. ed.). New York: Academic Press.

Crowell, J. A., Treboux, D., Gao, Y., Fyffe, C., Pan, H., & Waters, E. (2002). Secure base behavior in adulthood: Measurement, links to adult attachment representations, and relations to couples' communication and self-reports. *Developmental Psychology, 38,* 679–693.

de Wolff, M. S., & van IJzendoorn, M. H. (1997). Sensitivity and attachment: A meta-analysis on parental antecedents of infant attachment. *Child Development, 68,* 571–591.

George, C., & Solomon, J. (2008). Attachment and caregiving. In J. Cassidy & P. R. Shaver (Eds.), *Handbook of attachment: Theory, research, and clinical applications* (2nd ed., pp. 649–670). New York: Guilford Press.

Goodall, J. (1986). *The chimpanzees of Gombe.* Cambridge, MA: Harvard University Press.

Greenberg, M. T., Cicchetti, D., & Cummings, E. M. (1990). *Attachment in the preschool years.* Chicago: University of Chicago Press.

Hinde, R. (2005). Ethology and attachment theory. In K. E. Grossmann, K. Grossmann, & E. Waters (Eds.), *Attachment from infancy to adulthood: The major longitudinal studies* (pp. 1–12). New York: Guilford Press.

Karen, R. (1994). *Becoming attached: First relationships and how they shape our capacity to love.* New York: Oxford University Press.

Lu, T., Posada, G., Trumbell, J. M., & Anaya, L. (2018). Maternal sensitivity and co-construction skills: Concurrent and longitudinal associations with preschoolers' secure base behavior. In G. Posada & H. S. Waters (Eds.), The mother–child attachment partnership in early childhood: Secure base behavioral and representational processes. *Monographs of the Society for Research in Child Development, 83*(4, Serial No. 331), 74–90.

Main, M. (1999). Mary D. Salter Ainsworth: Tribute and portrait. *Psychoanalytic Inquiry, 19,* 682–730.

Marvin, R., Cooper, G., Hoffman, K., & Powell, B. (2002). The Circle of Security project: Attachment-based intervention with caregiver–preschool child dyads. *Attachment and Human Development, 1*(4), 107–124.

Moran, G., Pederson, D. R., Pettit, P., & Krupka, A. (1992). Maternal sensitivity and infant–mother attachment in a developmentally delayed sample. *Infant Behavior and Development, 15,* 427–442.

Pederson, D. R., Gleason, K. E., Moran, G., & Bento, S. (1998). Maternal attachment representations, maternal sensitivity, and the infant–mother attachment relationship. *Developmental Psychology, 34,* 925–933.

Pederson, D. R., & Moran, G. (1995). A categorical description of infant–mother relationships in the home and its relation to Q-sort measures of infant–mother interaction. In E. Waters, B. E. Vaughn, G. Posada, & K. Kondo-Ikemura (Eds.), Care giving, cultural, and cognitive perspectives on secure base behavior and working models: New growing points of attachment theory and research. *Monographs of the Society for Research in Child Development, 60* (2–3, Serial No. 244), 111–132.

Pederson, D. R., & Moran, G. (1996). Expressions of the attachment relationship outside of the Strange Situation. *Child Development, 67,* 915–927.

Pederson, D. R., Moran, G., Sitko, C., Campbell, K., Ghesquire, K., & Acton, H. (1990). Maternal sensitivity and the security of infant–mother attachment: A Q-sort study. *Child Development, 61,* 1974–1983.

Posada, G., Carbonell, O. A., Alzate, G., & Plata, S. J. (2004). Through Colombian lenses: Ethnographic and conventional analyses of maternal care and their associations with secure base behavior. *Developmental Psychology, 40*(4), 508–518.

Posada, G., Jacobs, A., Carbonell, O. A, Alzate, G., Bustamante, M. R., & Arenas, A. (1999). Maternal care and attachment security in ordinary and emergency contexts. *Developmental Psychology, 35,* 1379–1388.

Posada, G., Jacobs, A., Richmond, M., Carbonell, O. A., Alzate, G., Bustamante, M. R., & Quiceno, J. (2002). Maternal care giving and infant security in two cultures. *Developmental Psychology, 38*(1), 67–78.

Posada, G., Kaloustian, G., Richmond, M. K., & Moreno, A. (2007). Maternal secure base support and preschoolers' secure base behavior in natural environments. *Attachment and Human Development, 9,* 391–411.

Posada, G., Trumbell, J. M., Lu, T., & Kaloustian, G. (2018). The organization of attachment behavior in early childhood: Links with maternal sensitivity and child attachment representations. In G. Posada & H. S. Waters (Eds.), The mother–child attachment partnership in early childhood: Secure base behavioral and representational processes. *Monographs of the Society for Research in Child Development, 83*(4, Serial No. 331), 35–59.

Posada, G., Trumbell, J., Noblega, J., Plata, S., Peña, P., Carbonell, O. A., & Lu, T. (2016). Maternal sensitivity and child secure base use in early childhood: Studies in different cultural contexts. *Child Development, 87,* 297–311.

Posada, G., & Waters, H. S. (2018). The Maternal Behavior with Preschoolers Q-set. In G. Posada & H. S. Waters (Eds.), The mother–child attachment partnership in early childhood: Secure base behavioral and representational processes. *Monographs of the Society for Research in Child Development, 83*(4, Serial No. 331), 135–140.

Richmond, M., Posada, G., & Jacobs, A. (2001, April). *Maternal behavior and attachment security in 3-year-olds: A naturalistic study.* Poster presented at the meeting of the Society for Research in Child Development, Minneapolis, MN.

Schaffer, H. R., & Emerson, P. E. (1964). The development of social attachments in infancy. *Monographs of the Society for Research in Child Development, 29*(3, Serial No. 94), 1–77.

Smith, P. B., & Pederson, D. R. (1988). Maternal sensitivity and patterns of infant–mother attachment. *Child Development, 59*(4), 1097–1101.

Spitz, R. A. (1965). *The first year of life: A psychoanalytic study of normal and deviant development of object relations.* New York: International Universities Press.

Spradley, J. P. (1980). *Participant observation.* New York: Holt, Rinehart & Winston.

Strauss, A. L. (1987). *Qualitative analysis for social scientists.* New York: Cambridge University Press.

Tarabulsy, G. M., Provost, M. A., Bordeleau, S., Trudel-Fitzgerald, C., Moran, G., Pederson, D. R., . . . Lemelin, J. P. (2009). Validation of a short version of the Maternal Behavior Q-Set applied to a brief video record of mother–infant interaction. *Infant Behavior and Development, 32,* 132–136.

van IJzendoorn, M. H. (1995). Adult attachment representations, parental responsiveness, and infant attachment: A meta-analysis on the predictive validity of the Adult Attachment Interview. *Psychological Bulletin, 117*(3), 387–403.

Verhage, M. L., Schuengel, C., Madigan, S., Fearon, R. M., Oosterman, M., . . . van IJzendoorn (2016). Narrowing the transmission gap: a synthesis of three decades of research on intergenerational transmission of attachment. *Psychological Bulletin, 142*(4), 337–366.

Waters, E. (1995). The Attachment Q-Set (version 3). In E. Waters, B. Vaughn, G. Posada, & K. Kondo-Ikemura (Eds.), Care giving, cultural, and cognitive perspectives on secure base behavior and working models: New growing points of attachment theory and research. *Monographs of the Society for Research in Child Development, 60* (2–3, Serial No. 244), 234–246.

Waters, E. (2008). Live long and prosper: A note on attachment and evolution. (Original work published 2002). Retrieved January 28, 2020, from *www.psychology.sunysb.edu/attachment/gallery/live_long/live_long.html.*

Waters, E. (2013). Assessing secure base behavior and attachment security using the Q-sort method. Retrieved from *www.psychology.sunysb.edu/attachment/measures/content/aqs_method.html.*

Waters, E., & Cummings, M. (2000). A secure base from which to explore relationships. *Child Development, 71,* 164–172.

Waters, E., & Deane, K. (1985). Defining and assessing individual differences in attachment relationships: Q-methodology and the organization of behavior in infancy and early childhood. In I. Bretherton & E. Waters (Eds.), Growing points of attachment theory and research. *Monographs of the Society for Research in Child Development, 50* (1–2, Serial No. 209), 41–65.

Waters, E., Gao, Y., & Elliot, M. (2003). *Parental Secure Base Support and Supervision Q-Set.* Unpublished manuscript, Department of Psychology, State University of New York at Stony Brook, Stony Brook, NY. Retrieved from *www.psychology.sunysb.edu/attachment/measures/content/parent_support_qset.html.*

Waters, E., Kondo-Ikemura, K., Posada, G., & Richters, J. E. (1991). Learning to love: Mechanisms and milestones. In M. R. Gunnar & L. A. Sroufe (Eds.), *Minnesota Symposia on Child Psychology: Vol. 23. Self processes and development* (pp. 217–255). Hillsdale, NJ: Erlbaum.

Waters, E., Matas, L., & Sroufe, L. A. (1975). Infants' reactions to an approaching stranger: Description, validation, and functional significance of wariness. *Child Development, 46,* 348–356.

CHAPTER 2

Assessing Secure Base Behavior in Naturalistic Environments

The Attachment Q-set

Brian E. Vaughn, Everett Waters, and Douglas M. Teti

Ainsworth defined *attachment security* in terms of an infant's confidence in its caregiver's availability and responsiveness. This was manifest in the infant's secure base behavior across time and context in naturalistic settings (Ainsworth, Blehar, Waters, & Wall, 1978/2015). Accordingly, the Strange Situation's validity rests on its links to secure base behavior at home (Ainsworth, Bell, & Stayton, 1971). As use of the Strange Situation expanded beyond Ainsworth's laboratory and yielded interesting results in scores of studies, its validity was increasingly taken for granted. It was accepted as "the attachment situation," valid on its face, the "gold standard" of attachment measurement, and many attachment researchers turned away from naturalistic observation.

By the early 1980s, research articles reporting Strange Situation data completely eclipsed those reporting on naturalistic observations. For a time, the very success of the Strange Situation obscured the fact that behavior in the Strange Situation is not a "snapshot" of behavior at home, but rather a sign of rather different kinds of behavior than the more "natural" context of the home (e.g., Sroufe & Waters, 1977; Sroufe, Fox, & Pancake, 1983). The field also seemed to have forgotten (or to have chosen to ignore) that the critical link to secure base behavior at home had been demonstrated only once and in a small sample. The Attachment Q-set (AQS; Waters & Deane, 1985; Waters, 1987) was developed with two specific goals in mind. First, its developers hoped to facilitate research on links between attachment behavior at home and behavior in the Strange Situation. Second, they wanted to reawaken interest in naturalistic observation as a method of assessment and discovery.

The AQS has succeeded in focusing attention on the link between laboratory and home behavior. Within a decade of its publication, links between home behavior and the Strange Situation had been examined in dozens of studies (e.g., Vaughn & Waters, 1990; van IJzendoorn, Vereijken, Bakermans-Kranenburg, & Riksen-Walraven, 2004). Today, researchers are increasingly alert to the importance of checking links to home behavior when using the Strange Situation outside Western, home-reared, middle-class samples, where the validity of the Strange Situation cannot be taken for granted. Adaptations of the AQS are even helping to rebuild bridges to primatology research, where naturalistic observation has always been a mainstream methodology, often closely coordinated with laboratory and biological methods (e.g., McCormack et al., 2007; Warfield, Kondo-Ikemura, & Waters, 2011).

THE ETHOLOGICAL OBSERVATIONAL FOUNDATIONS OF ATTACHMENT THEORY

Like Freud, and unlike many of Freud's followers, John Bowlby was trained as a scientist. At Cambridge he studied biology with Edgar Adrian, the 1932 Nobel laureate in Physiology and Medicine, and memory and cognition with the eminent psychologist, Fredrick Bartlett. Both Adrian and Bartlett were excellent experimentalists and eclectic theorists, and both taught the value of careful observation (van Dijken, van der Veer, van IJzendoorn, & Kuijpers, 1998). Bartlett's (1932) work on schemas and reconstructive processes in memory, and in the early 1940s his student Kenneth Craik's (1943) work on mental models and control systems, were important starting points for modern cognitive psychology and are clearly reflected in Bowlby's ideas about attachment representations.

Notwithstanding Bowlby's training in rigorous scientific methods, he also valued psychoanalysts' insights about the importance of early experience. However, he was uncomfortable with their emphasis on intrapsychic events and their method of studying early experience through retrospective reconstruction from therapeutic sessions. At Cambridge, he had learned that a theory should be empirically accessible. He also learned that Konrad Lorenz, Nikolaas Tinbergen, and other ethologists (behavioral biologists) had gained insights into the motivation and relationships of nonverbal animals through painstaking observations of their behavior in natural settings.

Ethology became prominent with the work of Lorenz and Tinbergen in the 1930s and flowered during the decades of the 1950s to the 1970s, the period during which attachment theory emerged. A central tenet of ethology is that discovering the biological meaning of behavior requires the study of behavior in natural contexts. Despite its low-tech methodology, the value of ethological studies was acknowledged by the 1973 Nobel Prize awarded to Karl von Frisch, Konrad Lorenz, and Nikolaas Tinbergen "for their discoveries concerning organization and elicitation of individual and social behavior patterns."

Ethology's orienting principles include the following:

1. *Behavior has more meaning and is more interesting than generally appreciated.* Not simple, obvious, or mundane. It is as distinctive a characteristic of a species as its anatomy. Studied in detail, it reveals a story about how an animal lives in the world. Thus, the first step toward understanding behavior is to describe it in detail, to identify its elements and organization.
2. *Behavior is organized.* The form and organization of behavior is determined by both the environment in which it evolved and the environment in which it occurs.
3. *Behavior serves adaptive functions.* Species-specific patterns of behavior are organized so as to facilitate survival and (ultimately) reproductive goals in historical and current environments experienced by the individual.
4. *Behavior develops.* Development is an important mechanism through which behavior becomes adapted to the environment.
5. *Behavior evolves.* Thus, it is best understood in the evolutionary context provided by cross-species comparisons.

Ethology provided Bowlby an alternative to psychoanalytic ideas about motivation and development. Of special importance was the notion that behavior is organized into distinct systems, with distinct structure, motivational underpinnings, function, and developmental course. Viewing attachment as a distinct behavioral system with evolutionary underpinnings was a major departure from the psychoanalytic view that all motivation is rooted in satisfaction of libidinal drives. Ethology also provided a rationale and methodology for direct observation and longitudinal prospective study of development.

Like his mentors Adrian and Bartlett, and his hero Charles Darwin, Bowlby was a keen observer. He found behavior interesting and knew how to make the most of the decidedly low-tech method of simply watching what was happening around him (see Table 2.1). Moreover, in conceptualizing attachment as a distinct behavioral system, he drew heavily on research and examples from classical ethology (e.g., Baerends, 1959, 1972; Beer, 1961; Hinde, 1966; Tinbergen, 1951) and comparative psychology (e.g., Harlow, 1958; Harlow & Suomi, 1971; Harlow & Zimmerman, 1959). Indeed, in their last paper together, Ainsworth and Bowlby (1991, p. 333) described their commitment to an ethological perspective as the distinguishing feature of their theory.

Significantly, naturalistic observation was compatible with Bowlby's emphasis on the importance of ordinary, as opposed to traumatic, experiences in shaping personality development. Psychoanalysis focused on the pathogenic effects of intense but relatively low-frequency and in many cases unique experiences. Of course, Bowlby recognized the power of such intense experiences, especially loss and abuse. But he also saw that children built expectations from and attached meaning to countless "ordinary" interactions in which parents

TABLE 2.1. John Bowlby as an Observer

My father was a keen observer and a skilled photographer. I have a picture of him completely absorbed in the moment as he watched some primates at the London Zoo. He was very visually oriented, very alert, not just to the physical aspects but also to the context in which things occurred. As a young man, he became keen on ornithology, and we have drawers and drawers of index cards on which he recorded his observations of each bird: the setting, where he found it, what time of year it was, the plumage, the behaviour, and any other significant facts. I remember when we used to go out for a walk he always had a pair of binoculars around his neck. He was always the last one along—constantly keeping an eye out for any birds or animals he might see.

As you know, he didn't conduct many empirical studies, but I think he must have been a very good observer in his clinical work. He didn't have the patience to conduct observational studies of the type Jane Goodall or Mary Ainsworth did, but he greatly appreciated and valued all their contributions. I think he knew how accurate and relevant their observations were, and he often said how much he depended on their findings for his own work.

Note. From Richard Bowlby, conversation with Everett Waters (August 20, 2010).

were thoughtful, nurturing, selfish, insensitive, or misleading. Moreover, there was no need to study such experiences retrospectively. They are quite observable in garden-variety child–caregiver interactions. Indeed, because of their ordinariness and low intensity, children (and adults) find them very difficult to recall in clinical sessions. Thus, they are often more accessible to the ethological observer than to the diagnostician or therapist. This was a salient issue for Bowlby, because he had been forbidden to interview parents or visit families at home during his psychoanalytic training (Bowlby, quoted in Grosskurth, 1977, p. 402).

Mary Ainsworth: Gathering Information on How Infants Actually Behave

As a researcher at the Tavistock Clinic, Mary Ainsworth's first assignment was to help James Robertson organize and analyze observational notes from his study of children separated from their parents by brief stays in hospital or substitute care. Like Bowlby, Robertson was a skilled photographer and keen observer (Robertson & Robertson, 1990). Impressed by Robertson's skills and the richness of the data that could be had by simply observing, Ainsworth decided that she would someday employ similar methods in her own studies (Bretherton, 2003). The opportunity to do so presented itself when she accompanied her husband on a 2-year assignment in Kampala, Uganda.

Infancy in Uganda (Ainsworth, 1967) is a classic in developmental psychology, developmental ethnography, and human ethology. The sample comprised 26 mothers and their 2- to 9-month-old infants recruited from several villages near Kampala. They were visited for 2 hours every 2 weeks. Rather than making up a priori checklists or rating scales, Ainsworth followed ethologists in opting for detailed narrative notes, which she transcribed and annotated after each visit. She felt this allowed her to include behavior that might not have been anticipated in a checklist or time sampling protocol and allowed her to include detailed information about the context in which behaviors occurred. The excerpts in Table 2.2 illustrate the level of detail and the sensitivity to context Ainsworth captured in her observations.

Describing behavior in such detail, in real time, is a skill, an art, and very hard work. Thus, it is not surprising that John Bowlby found these observations so evocative and so valuable as support for his ideas about the child's tie to its mother, as descriptions of attachment development, and as portraits of individual differences. For Ainsworth, they were the foundation for empirically grounded measures that served well in her future research.

The primary goal of the Uganda study was to describe normative patterns and individual differences in attachment development. Understandably, Ainsworth initially looked for specific behavioral markers of attachment onset and intensity. Such markers would be very helpful in trying to identify aspects of early experience that accelerate or delay attachment onset. But she soon recognized that attachment onset is not marked by the emergence of a particular behavior.

> When one attempts to identify the use of the mother as a haven of safety one realizes how interlocked all these attachment patterns are and how the same general behavior may mean different things in different contexts. Thus, for example, the child, when put down on the floor, may crawl to his mother in a purposive but non-anxious way. If she arrives after an absence, he may greet her enthusiastically

TABLE 2.2. Sample Observations from *Infancy in Uganda*

Paolo (forty-two weeks) sat on his mother's lap for the first half of our visit. When his two sisters got up and left the house he scrambled down from his mother's lap and followed them as far as the doorway. He stood up holding onto the doorjamb. Then he became more active, creeping about, playing with a little string of celluloid balls happily and noisily. Occasionally he smiled across the room at his mother who did not like to let him out of her sight. And yet Paolo often made a big fuss if mother left the room and he was prevented from following her. (p. 346)
Muhamidi (thirty-two weeks) wanted to be with mother all the time. Whenever he was parted from her for even a moment, he cried and tried to follow. He was said to have been doing this ever since he could crawl (twenty weeks). At thirty-four weeks, I tried to photograph him by himself, but whenever his mother moved away, he cried and tried to follow her. (p. 337)
William (eighteen weeks) was given to me to hold. He smiled at his mother across the room. He became increasingly restless, giving me the impression of wanting to get to his mother, with every muscle oriented toward her, although he did not cry. Once back in his mother's lap he gave me a brilliant smile. (p. 339)

Note. From Ainsworth (1967, Chapter 20).

> and creep toward her. If he has been exploring, he may occasionally return to her and make contact. But all of these approaches can be distinguished from the flight to her as a haven of safety, perhaps more because of context than because of actual behavior although there is both speed and absence of delight in the flight. Similarly, a baby may scramble over his mother and occasionally bury his face in her person, and the impression that is given is affectionate attachment. He may venture around the room, return to her, and bury his face. The impression is the same. But he may also bury his face and give the distinct impression that he is using his mother as a haven of safety. (Ainsworth, 1967, p. 347)

Of course, this does not diminish the value of Ainsworth's descriptions of the emerging behavioral integration and coordination with maternal behavior. It simply marks a shift in her thinking—from focusing on the form of attachment behavior to focusing on its organization and function—as her insights were carried over into the Baltimore study and her work on the Strange Situation. This is typical of the way that ethological studies progress.

In Baltimore, Ainsworth recruited 15 infant–mother pairs through pediatricians in private practice, usually before the baby's birth. She and assistant Barbara Wittig visited the families every 3 weeks from 3 to 54 weeks after the baby's birth. She then recruited two additional assistants, Robert Marvin and George Allen, and added 11 more dyads to the sample. Each visit lasted for approximately 4 hours, resulting in about 72 hours of observation for each dyad. As in Uganda, she used narrative notes rather than checklists or time sampling. She also supplemented her observations with information from the mother. Transcripts from the home observations often exceeded 15–20 single-spaced, typed pages, that is, nearly 250 pages per infant over the course of the year, transcribed using a manual typewriter and multiple sheets of paper interspersed with carbon paper to make multiple copies. Finally, when the infants were a year old, they were seen with their mothers in the Strange Situation.

By the fourth quarter of the first year, all the infants were making exploratory excursions away from their mothers and returning to her when they were bored or distressed. This was the same secure base phenomenon Ainsworth had observed in Uganda. Translating observations of such behavior into a format that could be analyzed empirically proved difficult.

> The task of assessing the infants' attachment/exploration balance in the home environment was extremely complex. Classification—rather than quantification—of separate behavioral dimensions again seemed best to represent the configural quality of the behavioral phenomena. The basic concept is that a child can who use his mother as a secure base for exploration can move away from her freely, and yet tends to return to her on his own initiative from time to time, to play at her feet or to make brief contact before moving off again. (Ainsworth, Bell, & Stayton, 1971, p. 34)

Ultimately, Ainsworth settled on a classification scheme that assigned infants to one of five groups on the basis of an overall assessment of how effectively they negotiated cycles of exploration away from and back to the mother. The categories were as follows:

- *Group I.* A consistently smooth balance between exploratory and attachment behavior.
- *Group II.* Some use of mother as a secure base, mixed with occasional mismatches between mother's and infant's goals and consequent disruptions of secure base behavior.
- *Group III.* Little evidence of consistent secure base use. Baby explores actively, with little concern for mother's whereabouts.
- *Group IV.* Little evidence of consistent secure base use. Baby sometimes explores actively away from mother, if only briefly. More frequently, he seeks contact with his mother. He may become quite distressed if prevented from following her. Proximity and contact often lead to difficult interactions with fussing and ambivalence rather than the comfortable interactions and returns to play characteristic of Group I.
- *Group V.* Little evidence of consistent secure base use. The infant seems passive both in contact seeking and exploration. He often seems concerned with the mother's whereabouts, and often engages in self-comforting behaviors.

These complex and ultimately subjective classifications would not have found favor for very long in increasingly rigorous and empirically oriented journals. Moreover, Ainsworth herself was "not altogether satisfied with this classificatory system" (Ainsworth et al., 1978/2015, p. 241), believing that it could be improved in light of ongoing data analyses. Ultimately though, refining the classification of secure base behavior in naturalistic settings would have required extended observation in much larger samples. This was not a project to initiate in the midst of an already ambitious longitudinal study, and perhaps not a manageable project using traditional paper-and-pencil ethological methods. It is not surprising, then, that once behavior in the Strange Situation had been validated by links to home behavior, most of the measurement research in the Baltimore project (and in much subsequent attachment study) focused on the more circumscribed setting provided by the Strange Situation. Nonetheless, Ainsworth retained her sense that the core phenomenon is ultimately in naturalistic behavior. Focusing exclusively on laboratory behavior marked "a turning away from 'fieldwork,' and I don't think it's wise" (Ainsworth & Marvin, 1995, p. 12; Waters, Bretherton, & Vaughn, 2015).

This is the context in which the AQS was developed. The Q-sort method, to which we now turn, does not eliminate the need for sharp eyes and considerable stamina. However, it does help new observers learn how attachment and exploratory behaviors are organized. It eliminates the daunting task of transcribing lengthy narratives, and perhaps most importantly, it provides an economical and rigorous method for translating observations into quantitative data.

THE Q-SORT METHOD

The Q-sort method has a long and colorful history in the social sciences. The conceptual foundation for the method was conceived and first elaborated by William Stephenson (1953), who intended it to provide a means for assessing the individual's subjective view of various aspects of the world. Block (e.g., 1961/1978, 2008) realized that the convergence of views/perceptions made using Q-sort methods should result in an objective view of that same world, and he made extensive use of Q-sort data in studies of adult personality and personality development (Block & Block, 1980). In addition to assessing adult personality traits, the Blocks developed sets of Q-sort items (Q-sets) to assess parental practices, goals, attitudes, and values regarding childrearing, and as descriptions of specified social environments (e.g., the household as a support for children's development). Many of these Q-sets are still used by developmental and personality/social psychologists (e.g., Block, Block, & Keyes, 1988; Lanning, 1994; McCrae, Terracciano, Costa, & Ozer, 2006; McNally, Eisenberg, & Harris, 1991; Santos et al., 2020; Vaughn et al., 2016; Waters, Garber, Gornal, & Vaughn, 1983; Waters, Noyes, Vaughn, & Ricks, 1985). The principles involved in developing Block's Q-sorts were also used when developing items and protocols for the AQS.

Nuts and Bolts of Developing and Using Q-Sorts

In most applications to observational research, the Q-sort method proceeds in five key steps: (1) constructing an appropriate Q-set, (2) naturalistic observation by researchers familiar with the Q-set items, (3) applying a sorting procedure to assign a score to each Q-set item to reflect how characteristic the item is of the subject's typical behavior, (4) combining data from multiple observers and/or multiple occasions to increase and evaluate the psychometric reliability, and (5) using Q-set items to provide theoretical definitions of broadly defined constructs such as "secure attachment," and using these (or scales that comprise subsets of items) to assign scores to individuals.

Constructing a Q-Set

When developing a new Q-set, initial observations typically yield quite a few ideas for items. Subsequent observations yield somewhat fewer new items, eventually reaching a point of diminishing returns at which additional observations, distributed over different families and settings, no longer yield new content or details or information about context. This preliminary item set is likely to provide good coverage of the target domain. The items are then edited, tested in additional observations, and revised before the Q-set is finalized. Pilot observations often suggest a few additional items or reveal items that are so strongly related that they are redundant. Moreover, because most behaviors (in both human and nonhuman species) serve multiple functions (e.g., Hay, 1980; Baerends & Drent, 1982), and because context plays such a significant role in the meaning of behavior, it is often necessary to write multiple items to represent a given behavior in importantly different contexts.

The number of items in a Q-set depends primarily on the scope of the target behavioral domain, the need to take the context in which behaviors occur into account, and the range of content required to define higher-level constructs. Experience suggests that the most useful and manageable Q-sets comprise at least 40, and not more than 100 items. The current version of the AQS includes 90 items.

As explained below, observations are quantified by sorting the Q-set items into piles (categories/bins) ranging from *Most characteristic* to *Most uncharacteristic* of the individual being described. For clarity, the main text of an item is often supplemented with an item note (or footnote) indicating what would be implied by scoring an item as very uncharacteristic (i.e., placing the item low in the Q-sort). This is useful, because many behaviors do not have an obvious or logical opposite. Matters are clear enough when the item "Smiles when greeted" is *characteristic* of an infant at home. But what if an observer reports that the item is quite *uncharacteristic*. Is this to say that the infant is impassive when greeted? Or is it that the infant is positively rejecting or avoidant? Either interpretation makes sense. It is necessary that observers, sorters, and those who would use such data understand which meaning is intended. Item notes are used, not to force a theoretical issue but to ensure consistent use. Like the items themselves, item notes are developed through a process of pilot observations.

A well-constructed Q-set encodes considerable expertise and sophistication about the target behavioral domain, including key behaviors, what distinctions are worth making, and how the behaviors function in combination and in relation to context. Novice observers often report that simply becoming familiar with the Q-set items is like completing a mini-seminar on the behavioral domain they will be observing. In addition, using a Q-set to describe even a small number of individuals communicates a great deal about what to observe and how.

By focusing observers' attention on key behaviors, eliminating transcription costs, and facilitating quantitative analyses (see below), the Q-sort method makes it easier to employ naturalistic observations as primary data. The price of these economies is the effort entailed in developing a suitable Q-set. And, of course, a limitation of the Q-sort method is that once data have been translated into the language of Q-set items, the underlying observations cannot be reconstructed. Initial observations of unfamiliar behavior domains or contexts, or research in which sequential information or frequency counts are required, call for narrative or video records.

Observing

Ethologists have long recognized that narrative records best capture the details and the temporal structure of behavior in naturalistic settings. Unlike checklists and time sampling, narratives are open to unanticipated behaviors and sequences, and preserve (if often coarsely) the frequency and duration of events. Before the advent of compact, economical video recording, narrative records were the preferred format for extended observations, especially when observing novel behaviors or contexts. Observations were either captured as notes, which were later transcribed and elaborated, or transcribed from audio recordings.

Rather than attempting to maintain every behavioral detail in short-term memory and alternating between observing and writing, Q-sort observers can watch continuously for behaviors or contexts that are mentioned in the Q-set items. Employing a well-designed Q-set, an observer can focus on the flow of behavior without having to alternate between observing and note-taking. In addition, familiarity with the Q-set items creates something of an attentional filter, which makes observation more manageable. Although some observers prefer to take light notes, most find this unnecessary or even distracting. Finally, when sorting Q-set items after a period of observations, each Q-set item, having played a role in noticing scorable behaviors, supports accurate item placements by acting as a useful retrieval cue (see "Sorting the Q-set items" below). As a result, reliability is typically quite high even after as much as 1–3 hours of observation.

Mary Ainsworth's observations in Uganda and in her Baltimore project attest to the potential richness of narrative records. At the same time, her work also illustrated how demanding the task can be, especially if observations are conducted over long intervals. Narrative records are also very expensive to transcribe and edit. Perhaps most significantly, they are very difficult to quantify. The Q-sort method preserves some of the key advantages of the observation/narrative methodology, while making the task easier for observers and formalizing the transition from observation to quantitative data.

VIDEO RECORDING

In principle, Q-sorts can be based on real-time observations or video recordings. Where access and effective concealment are possible, video records can be very useful. Interactions in both human and nonhuman primate infant–mother dyads are often rapid and subtle; videotaping allows the observer to slow down or take a second look at interactions about which the observer is initially uncertain. In addition, if a behavior pattern occurs that was not initially included or well-integrated into scoring systems, researchers can return to the original video record as an aid to revising scoring materials and/or rescoring the observations.

Although video recordings provide an accurate and enduring record of what was recorded, they are not necessarily preferable to simple observation. In addition to paying close attention to the competing demands for context (field of view) and behavioral detail, skilled videographers have to be alert to action taking place outside the video frame. They also need to maintain enough situation awareness to realize when it would be useful to pan away from the target individual in order to provide context that will be useful during scoring. Unfortunately, the seemingly simple task of keeping an individual in frame makes significant demands on an observer's attention. Indeed, it is a tedious, exhausting vigilance task that, along with monitoring whether equipment is operating properly, capturing sound, and maintaining power, largely precludes accomplishing anything useful in the way of supplementary observation.

Videographers are often surprised or lack specific recall of content they recorded only hours ago. Although we have occasionally used video to supplement ordinary observations when developing Q-set items or rating scales, and for collecting materials to illustrate our research, we generally prefer observation to recording for primary data. Exceptions include constrained settings such as the Strange Situation or secure base interactions between adults in couple problem-solving interactions. In these constrained contexts, good recordings can be obtained with a fixed camera or with minimal camera control guided by monitoring an external display. Video recordings are useful in such research, because they allow multiple observers to view the behavior at their convenience.

Unfortunately, unconstrained behaviors of infants and children (or child–parent dyads) rarely meet these conditions. We are reminded of advice we received as graduate students from the eminent primatologist, Stuart Altmann, when we asked his opinion of some ideas for automated data recording. He said, rather sternly, "If you want to do observational research get yourself a pencil and paper, sit behind a tree, and get to it." In adapting the Q-sort method for behavioral data, we feel we have brought some economics to naturalistic observation without too many attendant costs. At the same time, Altmann's point remains—naturalistic observation is hard work. But just as there is no getting around the economics of it, there is no getting around the rationale Bowlby and Ainsworth asserted for studying behavior on its own terms.

HOW MANY OBSERVATIONS AND HOW LONG SHOULD OBSERVATIONS LAST?

Observations should be long enough to get a good estimate of individual differences in key behaviors. In addition, a sufficient number of participants should be observed to get a good idea of the range of individual differences. Both criteria depend on the frequency and context sensitivity of the target behaviors. Statistical power alone is not a sufficient criterion. The reliability/representativeness of the data collected is equally important.

One of the important insights of the psychometric paradigm is that accuracy per se does *not* guarantee reliable assessment (e.g., Viswanathan & Berkman, 2011). When observation intervals are too brief, observations can be accurate but not representative of an individual's typical behavior (Waters, 1978; Heyman et al., 2001). Traditional designs evaluate reliability across an entire set of test items. One of the advantages of the Q-sort method is that it allows researchers to assess the reliability/representativeness of observation intervals on a *per* individual basis rather than only across individuals (see below). We strongly recommend this procedure.

One of the most troublesome problems in observational research is that different behaviors occur at different rates. As a consequence, an individual's scores on frequently occurring behaviors may be estimated quite reliably, while individual differences on relatively rare behaviors are not reliable/reproducible at all. An advantage of the Q-sort method is that it allows sorters to assign significance to behaviors that seem important in context, even if their absolute frequency is too low to reliably estimate mean rates for individuals. For example, it is rather rare for an infant to hit at its mother. Even in the course of 2–3 hours of observation, the frequency is likely to be less than one occurrence per infant. If we observed one infant hitting at its mother twice and another only once, we could not reliably infer that the first typically hits twice as often as the other, or even that either infant hits at least once every 3 hours. There is simply too little information in 3 hours of observation to reliably estimate individual rates of such rare behaviors. Because less frequent behaviors are less reliably assessed than more frequent behavior in a given observation interval, correlations and group comparisons are subject to greater attenuation due to measurement error in statistical analyses. This can dramatically distort the pattern of results when multiple behaviors are evaluated as correlates or indicators, or effects in observational studies.

As explained below, the Q-sort method focuses not on the frequency of behaviors but on their role in the organization of an individual's behavior. Thus, an observer might note that the infant who hit at mother twice was responding to particularly intrusive behavior and discount the behavior altogether, while attaching great significance to the single hit if it seemed out of context or was accompanied by angry expressions or additional angry behaviors. Thus, the Q-sort method is less susceptible than traditional frequency counts to the problem of low frequency behaviors. The subjectivity introduced by having observers focus on the importance of behavior in context rather than solely on frequency can be kept under control by employing multiple observers and averaging their Q-sort descriptions to create a more reliable consensus sort with significant observer idiosyncrasies averaged out.

Finally, in deciding on the number and duration of observations, it is important to keep in mind that (low) reliability affects correlational results and group comparisons differently. Low reliability reduces the size of the correlation statistic (r). Increasing the sample size lowers the threshold for calling the (attenuated) correlation significant, but it does not bring the size of the correlation closer to the correct value. In contrast, low reliability does not reduce the apparent mean difference between two groups. Instead, the effect is seen in an increase in the error term for the comparison. As with correlational data, then, low reliability reduces the likelihood of calling comparisons of group means statistically significant but without attenuating the mean difference. Thus, increasing sample size retains the correct mean difference and counteracts the effect of low reliability on statistical power. Reliability calculations are discussed below.

The important implication here is that in correlational designs, resources are better spent on additional observation time and multiple observers than on increasing sample size. In group comparisons, resources might be better spent on larger samples. Taking the availability of time, additional observers, additional observation opportunities, and additional participants into account, it is often wise to consider whether a given question is better approached using a correlational or group comparison strategy.

SORTING THE Q-SET ITEMS

After observing a target individual for the specified interval(s), the individual's behavior is summarized by assigning a score to each Q-set item. One could hardly assign individual ratings to a large number of Q-set items without massive halo effects distorting the result. Instead, the items are sorted into a predefined (fixed) distribution (e.g., for the AQS, a distribution of nine piles of 10 items each is used) on the basis of how characteristic the item is of the child's behavior. *Characteristic* refers not to the frequency of a behavior but to whether it is central to describing the organization of the individual's behavior, whether it would distinguish this individual from others, whether the individual would work for the opportunity to perform the behavior or, if *Uncharacteristic*, to avoid it. Behaviors can occur at very high frequency (e.g., turning to look at unexpected noises) but not tell much about an individual's overall behavior or distinguish him or her from others. Similarly, slapping at mother when she tries to be helpful is a very low-frequency behavior but could be considered quite telling with regard to the organization of a child's behavior. Most observers quickly become comfortable making and reaching agreement on such judgments.

Q-sorting should be performed promptly after observing the target individual and, whenever possible, before any other individual is observed. Most observers require some time to become familiar and comfortable with the sorting procedure (i.e., make certain that the observer understands what "high" and "low" in the sort means, the meaning of "middle placements"). This should be worked out in pilot/training observations in which an experienced observer/sorter accompanies one or two trainees. Trainees should be familiar with the Q-set items in advance of the pilot observations. Initially, the more experienced observer may point out or briefly comment on behavior that corresponds to particular Q-set items, then explain the rationale for his or her item placements while sorting. Subsequent observations are carried out with minimal commentary. Then the trainee sorts the Q-set items with comment and advice from the more experienced sorter.

Q-Sorts Should Be Descriptions, Not Evaluations. A Q-set serves as a vocabulary for summarizing observations on a target individual. Although any Q-set is designed to survey a defined behavior domain, Q-sets are not as narrowly focused on specific constructs as traditional intelligence and personality tests. Instead, the Q-sort serves as a description from which a wide range of different constructs might be scored. Observer/sorters are explicitly instructed that their job is to *describe* what they have observed. They must not make their observations through the lens of a particular construct or sort the items with an eye toward portraying the target individual in such narrow terms. Moreover, the advantages of the Q-sort method include opportunities to (1) collect and quantify observations from observers who can be blind of the constructs that will be scored, (2) revise construct definitions even after the descriptive data have been collected, and (3) score a set of descriptions on constructs that were not anticipated in the original design (e.g., for discriminant validity or to test alternative interpretations after planned analyses are completed). These advantages depend on the observers observing and describing rather than judging and diagnosing.

Most good observers become proficient sorters after a few practice trials. Nonetheless, for observations in naturalistic settings, we generally obtain Q-sorts from two concurrent, independent observers. Working in pairs and comparing results motivates both observers and helps cover oversights that may occur in the course of an extended observation. Averaging the independent sorts (see below) provides a more reliable composite sort. In addition, identifying and discussing major discrepancies in item placements helps sharpen and maintain observation and sorting skills. Figure 2.1 summarizes the three-step procedure for sorting a 90-item Q-set such as the AQS into a rectangular distribution.

Sorting in Three Steps. Conceptually, the Q-sort method scores an item on the basis of how many items it would surpass in pairwise comparisons. However, with typical Q-sets, this would entail far more comparisons than are practical (1,225, 4,005, and 4,950 for item sets of 50, 90, and 100 items, respectively). The procedure described below and summarized in Figure 2.1 divides the Q-set items roughly into three piles: those that are most obviously *Characteristic* and those most obviously *Uncharacteristic,* with the remainder being Neither/Not salient/Not observed. Subsequent steps focus on comparisons within these three piles. Each pile is subdivided into three (for a total of nine). These are arranged from *Most uncharacteristic* (Pile 1) on the left, through items that are Neither Characteristic nor Uncharacteristic/Not

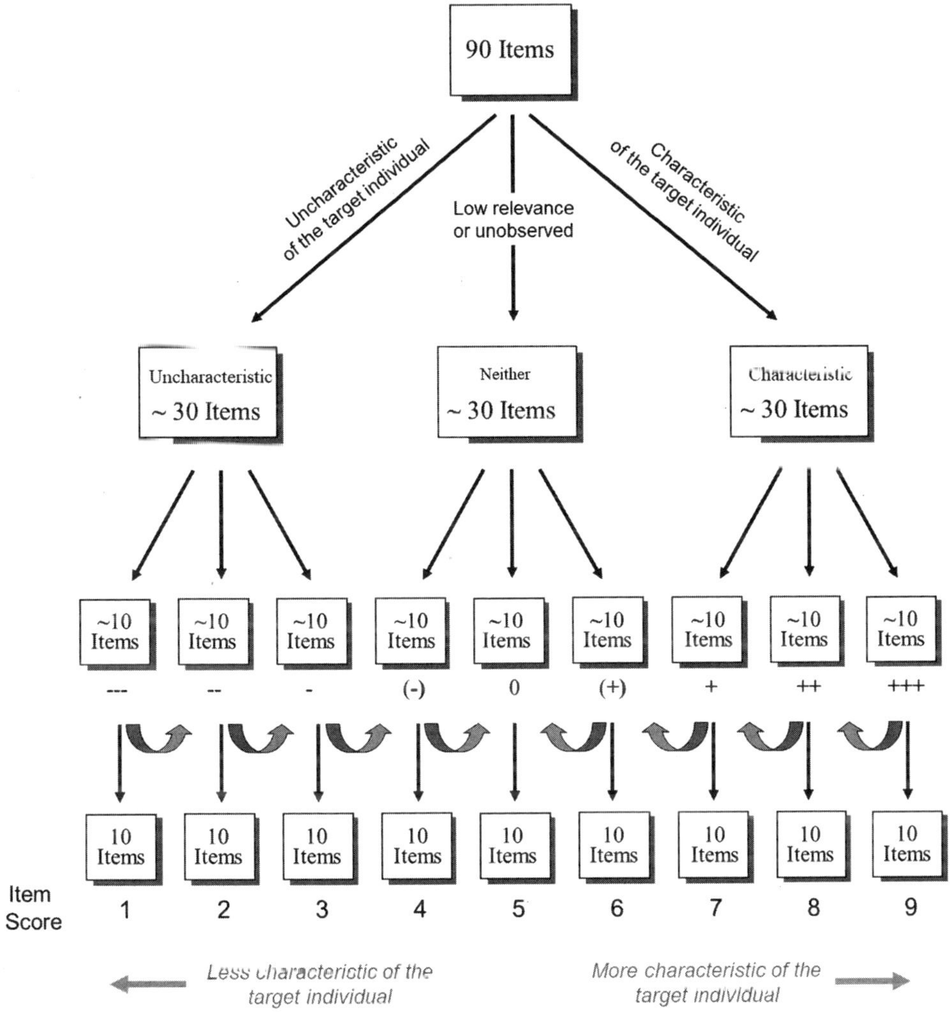

FIGURE 2.1. Sorting diagram.

salient/Not observed *(Piles 4, 5, and 6)*, to *Most characteristic (Pile 9)* on the right. Finally, comparisons within each of the piles (and occasionally with items in adjacent piles) fine-tune the sort and match the number of items in each pile to a predefined rectangular or quasi-normal distribution.

Sorting the items into nine piles along a dimension from *Most uncharacteristic* to *Most characteristic*) is much more economical than performing every possible pairwise comparison and keeping track of wins and losses for specific items. Moving from preliminary to increasingly finer item discriminations at each step increases the reliability of the sort and allows item placements to be revised. The sorting procedure is described in greater detail below and in Figure 2.1.

▶ *Step 1: Sort into three initial piles.* Sort the Q-set items into three categories. On the left, place items that are *Uncharacteristic* of the target individual (or that the individual seemingly avoids, perhaps by avoiding contexts in which the behavior might arise). On the right, place items that are *Characteristic* of the target individual. The remaining items (i.e., those that would not distinguish the target individual among others or behaviors that are not observed during the observation interval) fall, by default, into the middle pile. Although it is not necessary to place equal numbers of items in each pile at this stage, subsequent steps are somewhat easier if approximately equal numbers of items are placed in each of the three initial piles.

This step roughly organizes the items in terms of descriptiveness and relevance to the target individual. Decisions at this stage are only preliminary. As the items compete for higher or lower placement in the subsequent steps, a misplaced item can migrate to a more appropriate final placement. Experienced sorters can anticipate where an item is likely to end up in the final sort and make these initial placements accordingly. This facilitates the more refined sorting in Steps 2 and 3.

▶ *Step 2: Expand the sort into nine piles.* Sort the items in the leftmost (*Uncharacteristic*) pile into three, with the very most uncharacteristic items *on the far left* and the more moderately uncharacteristic items in the piles closer to the center of the overall sort. Then the items initially placed in the right (*Characteristic*) pile are divided into three, with the very most characteristic items *on the far right.* Finally, the middle pile (*Neither Characteristic nor Uncharacteristic*) is divided into three, with mildly uncharacteristic items on the left, mildly characteristic items on the right, and the remainder (neither characteristic nor uncharacteristic, or unobserved) in the middle. (Note that observers are sometime justified in judging that an unobserved behavior is consistent (or inconsistent) with the target individual's overall behavior, despite not having observed it during a given interval. In such cases, it is appropriate to place the item somewhat outside of the center pile. Although this is unlikely to make much difference at all in scoring, this allows observer/sorters to feel more comfortable with the Q-sort summaries of their observations.)

As we mentioned earlier, it is not necessary to assign equal numbers of items to each pile at this stage. But the final step is easier if the numbers in each pile are somewhat similar (within five or six items).

▶ *Step 3: Fine-tune the sort and finalize the number of items in each pile.* In Step 3, the final item comparisons are made, pile placements are finalized, and the number of items is set to match the predefined distribution (e.g., 10 items in each of nine piles for the AQS). Beginning with the items in the *rightmost pile,* compare the items and select the number required by the predefined distribution. These become Pile 9 in the final sort, the items that are *Most characteristic* of the target individual. Remainders are mixed with the items in next pile closer to the center of the sort (i.e., Pile 8) for sorting. As illustrated in Figure 2.1, this procedure is repeated for items in Piles 8, 7, and 6—selecting the items necessary to fill a pile and moving any remainder toward the center of the sort.

At each step, if a pile initially contains fewer items than required for the predefined distribution, combine them with the items from the adjacent pile closer to the center, compare the combined items to identify the required number, and place the remainder in the pile closer to the center. When combining adjacent piles in this way, items should be shuffled before selecting among them; that is, ignore that some of the items were previously judged less characteristic or uncharacteristic. Allow them to compete on an equal basis for placement in the current pile. When the required number of items has been identified, the remainder, having lost in competition to fill the current pile, are placed in the pile closer to the center and participate in competition to fill that pile.

Finally, beginning with the pile on the far left (Pile 1), finalize the sorting of *Uncharacteristic* items into Piles 1, 2, 3, and 4. Having worked from both ends of the sort toward the middle, Pile 5 will necessarily contain the correct number of items without sorting. The process of working from the outside piles toward the center takes advantage of the fact that items in the outer piles are the most or least characteristic of the target individual and thus lend themselves to the easiest sorting decisions. Allowing the middle pile to be determined by default relieves the sorter from having to make fine distinctions among items that are less relevant and thus more difficult to sort reliably.

SORTING INTO A RECTANGULAR VERSUS A QUASI-NORMAL DISTRIBUTION

Q-items can be sorted into a rectangular (equal number of items in each pile) or a quasi-normal (more items in the center of the sort) distribution (Block, 1961, 2008). Sorting into a quasi-normal distribution spares sorters the task of making numerous comparisons among the less descriptive items that find their way toward the center of the sort. It has nothing to do with distribution theory or significance testing. Consider that in order to sort 90 items into 90 piles requires comparing each item to each other item. Sorting 90 items into nine piles of 10 requires far fewer discriminations, because it foregoes making comparisons among the ten items within each pile. This is a compelling rationale for sorting N items into far fewer than N piles. Sorting into larger piles toward the center of the distribution further simplifies the task by additionally foregoing comparisons among items that, as mentioned above, are less salient, less obvious, less reliably sorted descriptors of the target individual.

Perhaps because many of Block's (1961/1978) California Q-set and California Child Q-set items were more psychological than behavioral and thus somewhat more subjective, he generally preferred sorting items into a peaked (quasi-normal) distribution (e.g., 5, 9, 11, 16, 18, 16, 11, 9, 5 for his 100-item Q-sets), thus reducing the number of difficult comparisons in the center of the sort. We initially followed suit in our own work with the Q-sort method (e.g., Waters et al., 1985). However, in our subsequent work (e.g., Posada, Waters, Crowell, & Lay, 1995; Vaughn et al., 2007), we have come to prefer a rectangular sort. This allows sorters to focus on item comparisons without having to match different pile sizes across the sort. The rectangular sort also seems to have been preferred in studies reviewed by (van IJzendoorn et al., 2004). In the end, both approaches preserve the many advantages of the Q-sort method and yield entirely comparable data.

ASSIGNING SCORES TO INDIVIDUAL Q-SET ITEMS

After completing the Q-sort, each item in Pile 1 is assigned a score of 1, each item in *Pile 2* is assigned a score of 2, and so forth, through Pile 9. Thus, in a typical 90-item Q-set, 10 items receive a score of 1, 10 items receive a score of 2, and so forth. As illustrated in Table 2.3, the scores assigned to Q-set items are typically entered into a spreadsheet or database in item order (i.e., score for Item 1, score for Item 2, . . . score for Item 90). This array is one observer's Q-sort description of the target individual. The data can be entered in either horizontal (row) or vertical (column) formats, although data entered in horizontal formats will be transposed for purposes of calculating rater agreement

TABLE 2.3. Data Format for Displaying and Averaging Q-Sort Descriptions of an Individual

	Observer			Item average (composite)
	Obs_1	Obs_2 . . .	Obs_n	
Item 1	4	1 . . .	2	3.1
Item 2	8	6 . . .	7	6.8
Item 3	7	5 . . .	6	5.5
Item 4	1	1 . . .	3	1.7
	⋮	⋮	⋮	⋮
Item *n*	2	4 . . .	4	3.8

Note. Columns represent independent observers' Q-sort descriptions of a single individual or Q-sort descriptions of an individual observed on different occasions. Average item scores across each row to obtain a composite description of the target individual over observers or occasions. Subsequent analyses (e.g., assessing stability or scoring constructs from criterion sorts) can be performed on the array of *n* averaged item scores.

and criterion scoring (see below). Multiple observers can be entered as additional rows or columns, and these can be averaged to obtain a more reliable composite sort. Similarly, Q-sort descriptions (or averaged descriptions) of multiple individuals can be entered as adjacent rows or columns of *N* item scores. Although behavioral researchers traditionally think of individuals in terms of single scores (e.g., a trait rating or a behavior count), the advantages of working with arrays of Q-sort scores soon become apparent and appealing.

Observer Agreement versus Reliability of Q-Sort Descriptions

Two kinds of "reliability" questions arise in research with the Q-sort method. First, do two or more observers report the same things after watching a target individual over a fixed observation period? This is the question of *observer agreement*. Second, how representative of the individual's typical behavior are these observations? This is the issue of *reliability/reproducibility* of the description.

OBSERVER AGREEMENT

Observer agreement can be assessed on the entire array of Q-set scores that describe an individual, or on individual Q-set items. For research that focuses on construct scores derived from entire Q-sorts (see the section following that describes scoring using criterion sorts), a separate observer agreement score is computed on a given construct for each target individual. The Pearson correlation between the two arrays of item scores (i.e., between columns in Table 2.3) is suitable for this purpose. Intraclass correlation is not necessary, because Q-sort descriptions should not differ in means or variances. Correlations ≥ .6 are considered acceptable levels of agreement when, as in most cases, the primary data analyses will be conducted using the averaged sorts of two or more observers. It is also useful to examine item placement discrepancies greater than 2 points. Very large discrepancies may reflect errors that can be corrected. For example, sorters occasionally reverse scores or misread items. If such errors can be identified, simply assign the correct score to the single misscored item. It is not necessary to re-sort the entire Q-set, as revising a single item has little impact on scoring. Unexplained errors and smaller discrepancies are best resolved by the averaging process. Nonetheless, trying to understand them can sharpen and maintain observational and sorting skills.

If primary analyses are to be conducted on individual Q-set items, observer agreement should also be assessed at the item level. This is accomplished by computing, for each item, the correlation between pairs of observers across individuals. Intraclass correlation is the appropriate index for item-level analysis because, unlike entire Q-sorts, individual items can have different means and variances from one observer to the next. As discussed earlier, it is also useful to examine item placement discrepancies greater than 2 points to clarify the nature of disagreements and maintain observing and sorting skills.

Before trainees are assigned to work without supervision, they should consistently produce sorts that correlate > .6 with experienced observer/sorters' Q-sorts, with no item disagreements greater than 3 points. With appropriate mentoring and feedback, most trainees achieve this level of agreement after fewer than 10 trials of supervised pilot observation and sorting. Not every researcher has the profile of cognitive, attentional, pattern matching, and analytic skills to become a skilled observer/sorter. The occasional individual who does not make progress toward a high level of agreement should be assigned some other role in the project.

RELIABILITY

Although agreement and reliability are often confused, they address quite distinct questions. Two observers can agree completely (suggesting that their observations were accurate and according to protocol), yet their results might not be entirely representative of the target individual's typical behavior. This is particularly the case for behaviors with low base rates or when an observation interval includes an unusual circumstance. In that case, the data, though accurate, would not be reproducible in subsequent observations.

Reliability assessment has a long history in intelligence and personality research. One approach readily applied to Q-sort data focuses on internal consistency across multiple Q-sort descriptions. If an *n*-item Q-sort description is representative of an individual's typical behavior, then it will necessarily be correlated with a similarly representative description from a comparable observer or occasion. If, on the other hand, the description is not representative of the individual's typical behavior, it will not be highly correlated with another, similarly unrepresentative description. Cronbach's alpha is a reliability/representativeness index based on the average correlation (i.e., internal consistency) among a set of measurements (Ghiselli, Campbell, & Zedeck, 1981). It can be usefully applied to naturalistic observations (e.g., Waters, 1978; Heyman et al., 2001) and to Q-sort data (e.g., Block 1961/1978, 2008). It is easy to compute and can be used to evaluate the reliability of both Q-sort descriptions and composites (Ghiselli et al., 1981, p. 232, Equation 9-1).

Because traditional intelligence and personality assessment focus on one measurement (trait) at a time, the reliability of such data is necessarily computed across an entire sample. Different individuals make different (unknown) contributions to the overall reliability. In Q-sort research, individuals are measured in terms of multiple items. Consequently, as with observer agreement, a separate reliability statistic for each individual allows researchers to identify individuals on whom additional observations are required. The data format and basic calculations are summarized in Table 2.4.

Traditional reliability methods can also be used to estimate how many additional observations or occasions would be required to reach any desired level of reliability–representativeness–reproducibility (Ghiselli et al., 1981, p. 236, Equation 9–3). Reliability assessment can help researchers determine how much observation is enough, and the point at which additional effort would yield little incremental advantage.

TABLE 2.4. Data Format for Computing Internal Consistency Reliability of Q-Sort Data: One Individual Described by Multiple Observers or on Multiple Occasions

	Observer or occasion			
	0_1	0_2	0_3 . . .	0_n
Item 1	2	2	2 . . .	2
Item 2	7	6	7 . . .	5
Item 3	6	7	6 . . .	6
Item 4	4	5	5 . . .	3
	. . .	. . .	. . .	. . .
Item *n*	3	2	2 . . .	4

Note. Internal consistency reliability (Cronbach's alpha) is based on the number of Q-sort descriptions (columns) and the mean of the pairwise Pearson correlations among them. Alpha = the number of observers or occasions (*n* columns) times the mean correlation (*r*) among the observers or occasions, divided by 1 + [(*n* – 1) (*r*)]. Thus, if the mean correlation among the four Q-sorts (columns) above were .50, then the reliability of a composite of the four would be alpha = 4(.5)/1 + [(4 – 1).5] = 2/2.5 =.80. (Conveniently, for two observers or occasions, this reduces to 2*r*/1 + *r*.) This can be interpreted as the correlation between the available data and a completely reliable/reproducible description of the same individual (Ghiselli et al., 1981, p. 233).

Defining and Scoring Constructs Using Criterion Sorts

Before a construct can be scored from a Q-sort description of a target individual, the meaning of the construct must be made explicit in terms of the Q-set items. Multiple experts are asked to formalize their understanding of the construct (e.g., attachment security, dependency, ego control) by sorting the Q-set items to describe a hypothetical individual who would score highest on the target construct. These construct definitions can be averaged to obtain a consensus construct definition in terms of the *n* Q-set items (see Block, 1961/1978, 2008; Block & Block, 1980). Such construct definitions are termed *criterion sorts* and serve as scoring templates to which Q-sort descriptions of individuals can be compared; that is, the (averaged) description of a hypothetical highest scoring individual is the *criterion* against which each individual is measured.

The data format for defining criterion sorts from experts' Q-sort descriptions is illustrated in Table 2.5. The format is the same as for multiple observers describing an individual, except that observer descriptions are replaced by experts' descriptions of a hypothetical highest scoring individual. Cronbach's *alpha,* based on the number of experts and the average pairwise correlation

TABLE 2.5. Data Format for Combining Experts' Q-Sort Construct Definitions to Create a Criterion Sort

	Experts			Criterion sort (item means)
	Ex_1	Ex_2 . . .	Ex_n	
Item 1	4	4 . . .	3	3.7
Item 2	8	6 . . .	7	7.0
Item 3	7	7 . . .	6	6.7
Item 4	4	5 . . .	5	4.7
	. . .	. . .	. . .	. . .
Item *n*	5	3 . . .	4	4.0

Note. Consensus Q-sort definition of the target construct (criterion sort) is constructed by computing item means across experts' descriptions of the hypothetical highest scoring individual for the target construct. Alpha reliability of the criterion sort can be computed from the average Pearson correlation among the individual experts' criterion sorts.

among their sorts, reflects the reliability/representativeness of the averaged (consensus) sort. Agreement among experts' criterion sorts for familiar constructs is usually quite high. Pairwise correlations are typically in the range of .8–.9. Thus, criterion sort reliabilities of .80 or greater are easily obtained by averaging the sorts provided by as few as five to seven experts.

SCORING CONSTRUCTS FROM CRITERION SORTS

Scores on a construct are based on the similarity between the Q-sort description of an individual and the criterion sort definition of the theoretically defined "highest scoring individual." Any of a number of profile similarity indices (Cronbach & Glaser, 1953) could be used to assess similarity between the *n*-item array describing an individual and a criterion sort. However, because the fixed distribution eliminates mean-level differences between Q-sorts, most researchers simply compute the Pearson correlation between the (composite) description of an individual and the criterion sort (Block, 1961/1978, 2008). The data format and procedure for computing individual's scores on constructs are summarized in Table 2.6. Using the Pearson correlation coefficient as an index of an individual's similarity to the criterion sort yields scores ranging between –1.0 and +1.0. Because the Pearson correlation is a nonlinear association index, some researchers adjust the scores using Fisher's *r*-to-*z* transformation. This usually has little effect, because the adjustment is

TABLE 2.6. Data Format for Computing Several Individuals' Scores on a Criterion Sort (Construct)

	Averaged Q-sort descriptions			Criterion sort (item means)
	Ind 1	Ind 2 . . .	Ind *n*	
Item 1	2.3	4.1 . . .	2	2
Item 2	7.6	6.3 . . .	7.0	5.3
Item 3	6.6	7.8 . . .	3.2	6.6
Item 4	4.2	5.1 . . .	7.3	3.2
	. . .	. . .	. . .	. . .
Item *n*	3.1	2.9 . . .	2.4	4.8

Note. Columns 1–3 are averaged Q-sort descriptions of individuals. The Pearson correlation of each composite Q-sort description (Columns 1–*n*) with the criterion sort (far-right column) serves as the individual's score on the criterion sort construct.

very small within the range of criterion sort scores typically observed for most constructs (–.10 to +.70 for Attachment Security).

Subsets of Items (Content-Based Scales)

Q-sort data also lend themselves to analysis of scales based on selected subsets of items and even to item-level analyses. Combining subsets of Q-set items into scales can be a useful way of reducing the complexity of an *n*-item Q-sort and extracting descriptive information without (or before) committing to broad constructs defined by criterion sorts. Cluster and components analysis are obvious strategies for identifying coherent subsets of items. However, Q-sets are not especially good candidates for such analyses, because highly correlated items are typically revised or eliminated when the Q-set is constructed (Block, 1961/1978, 2008). As a result, the number of clusters or factors tends to be quite large; thus, many represent only a small number of items—too many primary clusters or variates to work with and too few items per cluster/variate to yield reliable scores. A more useful alternative is to use a combination of rational and item-analytic methods to construct content-based scales. For example, an attachment Q-set inevitably includes content from domains such as exploration, proximity seeking, and response to separation, and so forth. Selecting items on the basis of these domains, then conducting item analyses to ensure internal consistency and reliability frequently yields a manageable number of content-based scales that can be used for descriptive and exploratory studies.

Note that Q-set items are not all phrased such that high scores imply more of a behavior. For example, in a subset of exploration-focused items, a high score on the item "Sits quietly when finished exploring a new toy" implies a *low* level of exploratory investment or activity. Thus, it is necessary to recode (reflect) it before summing "Sits quietly . . . " with items such as "Quickly identifies new toys and hurries to explore them." Recoding involves subtracting the assigned item score from one plus the maximum item score. Thus, for a nine-category Q-sort, a score of 9 is recoded to 1, a score of 6 is recoded to 4, and a score of 9 is recoded to 1, and so forth. (*Note:* Do not simply reverse the *sign* of an item.) After reflecting relevant item scores, as necessary, to ensure that every item "points in the same direction," scale scores are computed by summing an individual's scores on the items associated with a particular scale. The *alpha* reliability of scale scores is easily calculated, as described earlier, from the number of items and the mean Pearson correlation among them.

Item-Level Analysis

Individual Q-set items can provide useful descriptive information when correlated with or used for group comparisons involving theoretically interesting variables. Such analyses can help clarify the underpinnings of significant results obtained with criterion sorts or scales based on subsets of items. They can also be a useful source of new hypotheses. In addition, as mentioned earlier, item-level analyses can also play a useful role in training observers and maintaining the quality of observations.

SIGNIFICANT ITEM CORRELATES EXPECTED BY CHANCE

If the Q-set items were uncorrelated with one another, the expected number of significant correlations would be the number of correlations with the dependent variable (i.e., the number of Q-set items) times the designated significance level (e.g., .05). However, the correlations among Q-set items are never uniformly zero. Therefore, if one item is significantly correlated with a dependent variable, there is a greater than chance likelihood that others will be correlated with that dependent variable as well. Corrections that adjust for multiple *independent* significance tests are no solution here (Block, 1960).

A Monte Carlo-type analysis can be used to determine the probability of obtaining a specific number of significant correlations by chance (see Block, 1960). In a typical 90-item Q-set, as many as 5–15 items might be significantly correlated with random numbers on a single trial. Examining the number of such results over 10,000 trials provides a good estimate of the number of significant results that would be expected to occur by chance in Q-sort data with the observed pattern of item intercorrelations. The data format and procedure for this type of analysis is summarized in Table 2.7.

If the number of significant correlations in a study is greater than expected by chance, it is then useful to look at the individual items to see what

TABLE 2.7. Data Format for Computing the Number of Item-Level Correlates Expected by Change in a Set of Q-Sort Data

	Q-set items			Random numbers (1–9)
	Item_1	Item_2 . . .	Item_n	
Indiv. 1	4	4 . . .	3	3
Indiv. 2	8	6 . . .	7	7
Indiv. 3	7	7 . . .	6	6
Indiv. 4	4	5 . . .	5	4
	. . .	. . .	. . .	. . .
Indiv. *n*	5	3 . . .	4	4

Note. Compute the Pearson correlation of each item (column) with the column of random numbers and count the number of correlations ≥ magnitude that would be considered significant at a given significance level (e.g., .05) with sample size of *n* individuals. This is the number of significant correlations by chance on this trial. Repeat this through 10,000 trials with a new set of random numbers on each trial. Tabulate the number of trials on which 1, 2, 3, 4, . . . *n* items were large enough to meet the target significance criterion. The number of items per trial at the cutoff for the top 5 (or 1) percentile is the number of item-level correlations expected by chance at the .05 (.01) level in a set of Q-sort items with the observed item intercorrelations. This is ordinarily more than expected if the number of items is simply multiplied by the nominal significance level.

kinds of content is associated with the dependent variable. Although the item-level correlates identified in a particular analysis would not likely replicate in detail, it is reasonable to expect that a pattern of results in multiple items with related content (if not necessarily all the same items) deserve attention. If there are enough significant correlates, separate cluster or factor analyses can be a useful way of organizing the significant correlates and noncorrelates of a particular dependent variable into coherent subsets. Internal consistency reliabilities can be computed for cluster or factor scores, and their correlations with a dependent variable are more replicable than individual correlations. For item-level analyses, the rule then is to focus on results that are supported by a convergence of indications, not on individual item correlations.

Advantages of the Q-Sort Method

We noted earlier that Q-sort data afford multiple scoring options, and each of these is amenable to agreement, reliability assessment, and validation using conventional psychometric methods. The Q-sort method is also advantageous when key constructs are defined in terms of profiles or suites of behavior rather than discrete behaviors. At the same time, the Q-sort method allows low-frequency behaviors to play an important role in assessment.

As outlined in Table 2.8, the Q-sort method also has important advantages in relation to desirability biases and halo effects, which are notorious for undermining the validity of rating scales and creating false-positive results. The sorting procedure itself plays an important role in this. As mentioned earlier, sorters are forced to make decisions about each Q-set item, often at several points before finalizing the sort. The attention required to make these decisions, and the fact that they are at a level of detail far removed from

TABLE 2.8. Advantages and Limitations

Behavior and clinical judgment

- Q-set defines an important domain of behavior in detail.
- Takes context of behavior into account.
- Sorting ensures that full range of content is considered in assigning each subject's score.
- Sorting formalizes observer clinical judgment for empirical analysis.

Measurement

- Yields continuous variables.
- Doesn't try to operationalize constructs in terms of single behaviors. Generally better to measure constructs as convergence of indicators. In addition, multiple indicators give more reliable fix on individuals' score.
- Does not equate frequency with importance. Allows low-frequency behaviors to play a significant role.
- Forced-choice procedure reduces desirability bias.
- Keeps observers at arm's length from constructs to be scored.
- Does not require observers to have detailed normative information.

Research strategy

- Allows construct definitions to be made public and to be revised on the basis of data.
- A wide range of data analytic procedures are applicable.
- The ability to score several different constructs from the same Q-sort description encourages attention to discriminant validity, alternate interpretations, and refined construct definitions.

Limitations

- The sorting procedures and data formats initially strike researchers as novel and complex.
- Doesn't preserve behavioral detail or temporal structure of observations. Like ratings, checklists, and time sampling (and unlike Ainsworth's narratives) cannot reconstruct what happened from the data. Not good for primary data collection. This requires detail that can be captured only in narratives or video recordings.
- Cannot capture new behaviors or descriptive insights.

judgments about security or dependency, appears to attenuate broadly defined response sets such as desirability.

Finally, using criterion sorts has several advantages. It makes the definition of a construct explicit and public. Constructs are made explicit in terms of the scores assigned each item in the criterion sort. This allows us to study and debate experts' construct definitions that usually remain implicit in work with traditional rating scales, often with surprising results. Making constructs explicit and mapping them into specific behaviors and contexts can help us get past the labels we associate with constructs and focus instead on what observed targets actually do and on what develops. By separating data collection from construct scoring, criterion sorts also make it possible to score variables that represent alternative interpretations or to score mediating and moderating variables that were not initially anticipated. We simply develop criterion sorts for the confounding or alternative constructs (assuming that the original set of Q-items is relevant to those constructs), use them to derive scores from the original Q-sort descriptions, and use regression or covariance analysis to test the alternative hypotheses. Thereby we gain new information from the same observations and *p*-values instead of polemics. This is a particular advantage in longitudinal research, in which theory and hypotheses continue to advance and often outrun measures and designs that are established years, even decades, earlier.

Some Obstacles and Limitations of the Q-Sort Method

It is said that controversy is good for theories and bad for methods. Thanks to Jack and Jeanne Block's Berkeley longitudinal studies, the Q-sort method has moved past early controversies regarding subjectivity and *Q versus R*-type data. As used today, it is simply a method for scaling personality and behavioral items. The obstacles and limitations we have encountered are primarily practical.

Researchers considering the Q-sort method are often deterred by the unfamiliarity of the sorting and scoring procedures, and the need to construct a Q set for a particular range of behavior. As explained earlier, the sorting and scoring procedures are more unfamiliar than complex. This is easily overcome. Developing a Q-set encourages intimate familiarity with a personality and/or behavioral domain, and a unique perspective that is rarely, if ever, gained from reading theory and research reports or from working with rating scales. Over time, the dividends from knowing a behavior domain in detail and in context far outweigh the costs of observation time, item development, and collecting criterion sorts. Nonetheless, there is no denying that constructing a new Q-set takes time, a great deal of observation and thought, and, inevitably, several iterations between observation and writing/revising items.

It is important to keep in mind where the Q-sort method fits into a research program. Q-sort descriptions do not preserve the frequency, sequence, or context of individual behaviors or behavior interactions. Nor can an existing

Q-set take into account novel behaviors. Thus, first observations of unfamiliar populations or contexts are best preserved as video or narrative recordings. The Q-sort method comes into play once the full range of behavior is identified. Only then is it possible to construct a satisfactory Q-set or employ (or perhaps adapt) and existing one.

THE AQS

Our primary goal in developing the AQS was to replicate Ainsworth's findings that linked home behavior to the Strange Situation (e.g., Ainsworth et al., 1971, 1978/2015), and stimulated interest in observing attachment behavior in naturalistic settings. We also hoped that a well formulated Q-set would provide an accessible summary of the full range of behaviors Ainsworth had in mind when she spoke of the secure base phenomenon, thus helping observers see infant behavior through her eyes as it plays out across time and contexts. Finally, the AQS was designed to bring into attachment assessment characteristics that are important to the "goodness" of any developmental measure. Waters and Deane (1985) discussed these in terms of (1) fitting the measure to the construct (what Jane Loevinger [1957] called "structural fidelity"); (2) reference to behavior; (3) taking context into account; (4) integrating affect, cognition, and behavior; (5) the ability to describe qualitative change; (6) coherence of adaptive functioning in the face of behavioral change; and (7) attention to discriminant validity.

Traditionally, the Q-sort method had been employed to obtain trait ratings in personality and psychiatric research (Block, 1961/1978, 2008). To employ it for attachment study, we explicitly turned away from trait- and symptom-based language to focus on behavior, including emotional expression and regulation, as well as indicators of social-cognitive maturation. In addition, whereas trait and diagnostic ratings are used to summarize behavior across contexts, the AQS items were designed to explicitly take into account the context in which behavior occurs.

Developing and Refining the AQS Item Pool

Block (1961/1978) described a *Q-set* as the vocabulary for describing individuals and the *sorting procedure* as the grammar that defines how the individual words (items) are used. We have described the AQS items as being akin to an ethogram, in that it is rooted in direct observation and attempts to catalogue the full suite of behaviors associated with the secure base behavioral system for infants and young children. Items were designed to register both ordinary and emergency behaviors as they play out in naturalistic (as opposed to laboratory) situations. Ordinary secure base behaviors involve (1) exploring away from the caregiver, (2) evaluating and maintaining caregiver access and availability, (3) seeking information or assistance while exploring or manipulating objects or locations, and (4) returning to her when exploration is no longer productive. Emergency secure base behaviors are those employed to (1) signal distress, (2) retreat to the caregiver when distressed, and (3) establish and maintain contact until comfortable enough to resume exploration.

AQS Version 1.0 (100 Items)

In the course of developing the initial AQS item set, we consulted John Bowlby's and Mary Ainsworth's books and articles. The most useful of these, by far, was Ainsworth's (1967) *Infancy in Uganda*. Her instructions for scoring maternal and infant behavior at home, transcripts from her fourth-quarter Baltimore home observations, and transcripts of Strange Situation reported in *Patterns of Attachment* (Ainsworth et al., 1978/2015) also proved very useful. We also generated a list of constructs that might help us achieve good coverage and perhaps make the preliminary Q-set more useful. These included security, dependency, self-efficacy, several aspects of object orientation, communication skills, predominant mood, response to physical comforting, fearfulness, anger, and trust.

We then spent several months visiting infant–mother and toddler–mother dyads in their homes to evaluate and revise the preliminary items. In the process, we edited the items to better match observed behavior, to achieve greater clarity and specificity, and to improve observer agreement. We also added items to remedy omissions and deleted reference to behaviors that rarely occurred. We asked mothers to try using the items to describe their own infant or toddler and also asked about the kinds of behavior they had in mind when placing particular items high or low, or when an item proved difficult to use. This, too, resulted in some clarifications and useful distinctions.

Finally, we added items to broaden the range of constructs that could be scored from the Q-set. We were particularly interested in being able to assess the discriminant validity of security scores in relation to dependency, mood states, general sociability, and social desirability. Finally, we also added some non-attachment-related "filler" items. If a Q-set focuses too narrowly on one or a few constructs or domains, it becomes difficult to sort, because too many related items end up competing for the positions at the *Characteristic* or *Uncharacteristic* extremes of the sort. For example, if all the items in the AQS were indicative of good secure base use, sorters would have too few items to place in the middle and low ranges of the sort. Including 15–20 "filler" items minimizes this problem. It also helps avoid the problem of observers/sorters becoming too narrowly focused on the security construct and beginning to make trait-like security evaluations rather than observing and reporting behavior.

In the end, the 100-item AQS (Version 1.0) owed more to our own naturalistic observations, *Infancy in Uganda,* and Ainsworth's observational measures and transcripts than to any other source. Waters and Deane (1985) published the initial AQS, along with some preliminary research demonstrating its usefulness. They also enlisted an impressive group of experts who provided criterion sorts for security, dependency, and sociability at 12 and 36 months, and also social desirability (Waters & Deane, 1985, p. 60, note 2). Each of these constructs was construed as a continuous dimension rather than as discrete categories. For example, security was conceptualized in the criterion sorts as a dimension ranging from consistently skillful to less consistently skillful at using mother as a secure base for exploration and haven of safety. Experts reported no difficulty sorting the items to describe a hypothetically most secure, dependent, or sociable child at either age.

AQS Version 2.0 (100 Items): Refinements and Revisions

Our own experience, and that of early adopters, led to some revisions of the Version 1.0 Q-set. We clarified items that, in wider use, proved ambiguous or were a source of sorting disagreements. This involved adding reference to specific contexts, refining some difficult vocabulary, and eliminating double negatives. Using these items, we collected data to evaluate item intercorrelations and information about item variances, and evaluated item wording with novice observers. These changes, informally designated Version 2.0, facilitated observation and made the AQS easier to sort, without requiring new criterion sorts.

Current Version: AQS 3.0 (90 Items)

With further use, it became clear that some of the Version 1 edits had worked quite well and should be applied to the full item set. One such change was adding information about the context in which behaviors occur. We also found that sorters were having difficulty agreeing on when to place an item low in a sort. In particular, sorters found it difficult to agree on the meaning of placing some items very low in a sort; that is, what was the opposite of the behavior described on the card? For many items, this is obvious enough. The opposite of "Pays attention to toys" is "Ignores toys." It is less obvious whether the opposite of "Approaches mother" should be "Does not approach mother" or "Actively avoids mother." Similarly, is "Does not cry when mother leaves the room" or "Laughs when the mother leaves the room" the opposite of "Cries when mother leaves the room?" The issue here is not so much determining an item's true opposite as agreeing on one alternative or another, so that sorters can use the items in a meaningful and consistent way.

It also seemed useful to vary the valence of item phrasing within domains, for example, rephrasing/reflecting an item such as "Often asks mother for help" to "Rarely asks mother for help." This made themes such as positive interaction less obvious and thus further reduced social desirability response set in sorting. It also helped anchor both the high and low ends of constructs such as security and dependency.

Finally, we had by this time collected enough information to identify items that were highly intercorrelated and thus tended to move together in sorts. Such items are, in effect, synonyms in the Q-set vocabulary and do not add information to a sort. Indeed, they crowd out items that are competing for similar placement. Accordingly, we either eliminated such items or revised them to capture somewhat different content (e.g., similar behavior in a meaningfully different context). This reduced the AQS to 90 items. These revisions (Version 3.0) required us to develop new criterion sorts for security and dependency. Sociability and social desirability were not included, because the item set does not include enough items specific to these constructs to ensure good discriminant validity. The AQS 3.0 items are available, along with the security and dependency criterion sorts, online in the Measurement Library section of *www.johnbowlby.com*. In order to maintain comparability of scores across existing and new studies, we have ruled out further revisions.

AQS 3.0 items have a consistent format that identifies an act plus a contextual (situational, behavioral, affective) qualifier and (for most items) a statement regarding the kind of behavior that would lead to the item being placed low in a sort (i.e., the *opposite* of the behavior that defines the item). Figure 2.2 illustrates the structure of typical AQS 3.0 items. We ordinarily format the items, eight to a page, into a four-row by two-column template (2.5 × 4 inches), with a rectangular outline around each item. This template can be printed on letter-size 20- to 24-pound paper and cut along the card outlines whenever an additional Q-set is needed.

90. If mother moves very far, child follows along and continues his play in the area to which she has moved.

> (Child doesn't have to be called or be carried along; doesn't stop play or get upset.)
>
> Middle: Place in the center of the sort if the child isn't allowed or doesn't have room to move very far away.
>
> Low: Child may or may not continue play but does not change location when mother moves.

Rationale: This behavior is one aspect of the child's active role in the secure base relationship. The child manages to coordinate play with active efforts to monitor and maintain access to the mom. There is no negative connotation (e.g., clinginess or dependency) attached to this behavior. The child moves along without getting upset. This is competent secure base behavior in a child who (for trait or situational reasons) prefers to play in proximity to mother.

This behavior is most often seen in unfamiliar settings or if the child is wary of the visitor. Do not give much weight to the absence of following or moving play if the observations are limited to locations in and around the home and the child seems comfortable with the visitor.

FIGURE 2.2. AQS item format.

Item Rationales

To facilitate learning and consistent use, we have written a rationale for each AQS item (Waters, 1987). The item rationales address the relation of the target behavior to attachment theory and the secure base concept. In a few instances, this includes comparing or contrasting it to similar behavior in the Strange Situation. Where relevant, we also point out that one does not necessarily expect phenotypically similar behavior in the Strange Situation and at home. For example, Sroufe et al. (1983) reported that avoidance in the Strange Situation is associated with dependency (as rated by teachers) rather than avoidant-seeming behavior in preschool settings. Indeed, behavior seen in the Strange Situation seems quite specific to the challenges of separation and reunion in an unfamiliar setting. Although the item rationales are too lengthy to be included on the cards used for sorting the AQS, they should be consulted during learning (below) and, as needed, during sorting. Even experienced researchers find that they help maintain consistent use over time and across observers.

Here, we should add an important caveat. New adopters too readily assume that each AQS item implies or requires some sort of attachment-related attribution. Observers/sorters should not think of each item as somehow pointing to an overall security evaluation. Their task is to observe and describe, not to make trait ratings or construct-based evaluations. As illustrated below, the items cover a wide range of social and exploratory behaviors that are not specifically or exclusively related to attachment security. Indeed, these and the "filler" items included to facilitate sorting comprise almost half of the Q-set. Observers/sorters should remain agnostic with respect to the kinds of criterion sort scores that might someday be derived from their descriptions.

In combination, the AQS items and the rationale statements provide a detailed look at infants in naturalistic settings through the lens of attachment theory. Simply becoming familiar with the items is a significant step toward becoming a sophisticated observer. This is as close as we can get to seeing infant secure base behavior through Mary Ainsworth's eyes.

Training

Experience has shown that the AQS can be used properly and consistently without workshop-based training. However, acquiring expertise requires a clear understanding of the intent/rationale behind each item, as well as experience and mentoring. At first blush, any set of 90 Q-set items is likely to give the impression of overwhelming complexity. Familiarity with the AQS items is best accomplished through initial discussions of item content with an experienced user. Familiarity with the item set provides powerful cues for anticipating and observing behavior in real time. Thus, the goal of initial study is not to memorize but to understand the referents and rationales for each item. This is then consolidated through pilot home observations in the company of an experienced observer.

It is also useful for new users to see the AQS items presented in terms of content domains and contexts in which reportable behaviors often occur. Table 2.9 summarizes AQS 3.0 item content and points to representative items.

Although AQS behaviors can occur at any point in an observation, many of the items refer to specific contexts. In addition, experienced observers become alert to the contexts in which specific behaviors might be expected or most telling. For example, reactions to strangers are most often (though not exclusively) observed when observers first arrive or when an observer is offering a toy. Similarly, keeping track of the mother's location is most evident

TABLE 2.9. Content and Contexts Sampled in the 90-Item Attachment Q-set (Version 3.0)

1. Exploration from a Secure Base (13 items)
   Child keeps track of mother when playing around the house.
   Child uses mother's facial expressions as a source of information when uncertain or afraid.
2. Indications of Availability and Responsiveness-Related Expectations (11 items)
   Child laughs when mother teases him.
   Child acts like he expects mother to interfere with his activities when she is only trying to help. (negative)
3. Smooth Interaction with Caregiver (8 items)
   Child quickly greets mother when she enters the room.
   When child returns to mother after play, he is sometimes fussy for no clear reason. (negative)
4. Physical Contact (5 items)
   Child puts his arm around mother or puts hand on her shoulder when picked up.
   Child enjoys relaxing in mother's lap.
5. Distress and Comforting (5 items)
   If help in mother's arms, child quickly recovers after being frightened.
   When something upsets the child, he sits where he is and cries. (negative)
6. Behavior toward Home Visitors (7 items)
   Runs to mother with a shy smile when new people visit the home.
   Child easily grows fond of adults who visit the home and are friendly to him.
7. Other Domains and Filler Items (41 items)
   Child acts like an affectionate parent to dolls, pets, or infants.
   Child is more interested in people than things.
   Child ignores most bumps, falls, and startles.
   Child is lighthearted and playful most of the time.

when she moves from room to room (rather than within a room). New observers often find it helpful to see the AQS items clustered by the contexts in which they are most likely to be scored. Teti, Sakin, Kucera, Corns, and Eiden (1996) presented the items in an annotated spreadsheet that organized AQS items according to context. The contexts (items) are the following: Upon arrival (49, 50, 80); Child with home visitor/stranger (7, 12, 15, 17, 48, 51, 58, 66, 67,72, 78); Child is upset, fussing, or crying (2, 3, 6, 8, 10, 13, 20, 33, 38, 65, 74, 81, 88); Playing with the mother (1, 14, 27, 35, 36, 47, 54, 56, 60, 61, 63, 64, 77, 79, 86, 87, 90); Close interaction with the mother (11, 23, 28, 31, 43, 44, 53, 71); Compliance with the mother (18, 19, 24, 32, 41); Mother as the primary focus of child's attention (25, 42, 55, 59, 69, 70, 83); Mother or child leaves the room (21, 26, 34, 75); Play and exploration (4, 16, 22, 30, 39, 40, 52, 73, 76, 82, 85, 89); and Trait-like characteristics (5, 9, 29, 37, 45, 46, 57, 62, 68, 84).

New observers find this that this kind of structure helps focus their efforts during training and pilot observations. Once they are familiar with the AQS item set and how behavior unfolds in the course of a home visit, experience, context, and content guide attention, and reliance on such training devices fades away. Experienced observers find that they can anticipate behavior in a variety of contexts and notice when their expectations are not met. At the same time, they manage to notice scorable behaviors whenever and wherever they occur.

Observing and Describing Behavior with the AQS

It is not necessary to be an expert in attachment theory to be a good observer. It is more important that observers have a clear and shared understanding of what each AQS item means and how it manifests itself in behavior. It is worth reemphasizing that the observer's goal is to describe, not to formulate trait ratings or clinical evaluations. Expert observers do sometimes have a clear sense of whether a child is skilled (or not) at using the mother as a secure base. However, they just as often find themselves curious to see that their observations reproduce as a score on a particular construct, or find the result surprising. Such is the observer's immersion in the task at hand. At the same time, it is important to maintain a degree of situational awareness. For example, it is important to recognize signs that an observation might not be sampling a typical day. It is often wise to ask whether a child is feeling ill or whether his or her reaction to the visitor is typical. If a child has been (or is becoming) ill or is not well rested, we typically offer or suggest rescheduling the observation. We occasionally ask whether we can schedule an additional observation "just to make sure we're getting a look at his or her typical behavior." It is also important to hear parents' comments on the child's behavior—taking them not so much as valid explanations (though they often are) but as context that can be taken into account in describing what has been observed.

Observation Settings

The AQS was designed to assess the secure base behavior of infants and young children in naturalistic settings. *Naturalistic,* here, has to do with ecological validity. The key is to observe in the kinds of environments in which infants and children (in whatever culture or community) live their lives, without laboratory constraints that limit expressing the full repertoire of attachment-related and exploratory behaviors. In general, this means an environment that offers opportunities for behavioral choice and exploration, and for communication and proximity seeking. Most often, this means at home. However, the AQS has been used successfully in a variety of settings, including outdoor areas near the home, neighborhood parks, and indoor recreation centers. Researchers have also obtained useful data by combining home observations with observations from medical waiting rooms and shopping areas visited during a scheduled visit. As Block (1961/1978) pointed out, the ability to integrate multiple sources of information is one of the strengths of the Q-sort method. Experienced observers find it easy to tell whether information gathered outside the home contributes to their understanding of the child's behavior. They also recognize when contexts such as preschool classrooms or hallways in which brief reunions take place after preschool are too busy or to brief to inform a reliable AQS sort. The suitability of AQS observations in such settings should be evaluated in pilot data, and perhaps be related to data from home observations or laboratory assessments, before pinning an entire study on such data.

Age Range

Like the Strange Situation, the AQS assumes that a child has the locomotor skills necessary to explore, moving away from their primary caregivers and returning to them on their own. Although many 9- to 10-month-olds have the necessary locomotor skills, it is important not to confound motor maturity with secure base skills. Thus, we have generally considered a child's first birthday as the lower limit for AQS studies. As for an upper limit, the AQS items are relevant to much of the attachment and exploratory behavior of 3- to 4-year-olds (e.g., Teti et al., 1996; Posada, 2006; Posada, Jacobs, Richmond, & Kaloustian, 2007). The AQS is less useful for children over 4 years of age, because they tend to transact more of their secure base interactions verbally and over a distance, and because bouts of exploration tend to last longer and to take them away from the immediate setting. Again, experienced observers readily recognize whether the AQS items provide a satisfactory summary of what they have observed in older children.

Relating to Caregivers

When scheduling an observation, researchers should explain to the caregiver the goals of the observation and how long the visit is expected to last. It is also useful to plan a "convenience call" for the morning of the visit. Parents often hesitate to call and reschedule a visit—they promised to help and they want to follow through. It is better to reschedule than to arrive unexpectedly or inconveniently. Just explain that rescheduling is no problem at all. It is actually better for your study, and you certainly want to make the visit when it is convenient. It will not be misleading to add, "This happens all the time."

AQS observers are in the business of watching and describing. Nonetheless, it is understandable that mothers might feel self-conscious about having an observer in the house. Thus, it is useful to describe the goals of the visit in terms of observing the child (not the caregiver) and that the goal is to learn what children actually do, not to measure some sort of psychological quality. Mentioning attachment security or suggesting that you want to compare the child's standing relative to other children is likely to make the caregiver self-conscious and potentially defensive (or intrusive in interactions with the child).

Researchers sometimes feel that they need to keep the details of their measure "confidential." This makes sense for an IQ test. However, there is nothing confidential about the AQS items per se. In fact, it puts caregivers at ease to show them, early in the observation, some sample AQS items and point out that the focus is on behavior, not something "psychological" or adjustment related.

Unfamiliar visitors behaving in unfamiliar ways can put both caregivers and children off their typical behavior. Thus, it is important for both the caregiver and the child to feel comfortable. This is best accomplished by behaving informally. Always be a good guest. Even if you are shy, greet the caregiver at the door. Introduce yourself and your co-observer. Thank them for allowing you to visit. Ask some polite questions. Show an interest in the child. Ask whether the person who arranged the visit explained what the study is about. Keep in mind that this is a residence, not a museum or a market. You are not there to look at or handle objects they have displayed. If you need to use the bathroom, ask; do not go looking for it on your own. If you want to turn the TV off, ask first. If you want to find some toys for the child to play with, the caregiver will help you or show you where they can be found. If the child wants to show you his or her room or the basement, ask the caregiver first. Avoid spending long periods with the child out of the caregiver's sight. Common sense says act in the moment if the child is about to fall or pull something over. Otherwise, bring potentially problematic behavior to the caregiver's attention; ask if such behavior is safe or allowed.

When a visit is finished, be appreciative and positive. Indicate that you enjoyed the visit and that it was very interesting and very useful. Note that parents often want to ask general child development questions before the observer leaves. Be receptive—they have just done you a favor by letting you visit. At the same time, avoid commenting or offering advice on topics that are outside your experience or that are not well handled in a brief conversation without the opportunity for meaningful follow through. At the same time, do not minimize things that are beyond your expertise. Suggesting that the parents raise such issues with the child's pediatrician, and expressing confidence that they will know what to do is always a sound approach.

Monitoring Observers

In order to maintain the quality of data, it is useful for the investigator or lab manager to accompany observers on some of their visits. In our labs, we make many of our home visits ourselves, accompanied by a student or research associate as the second observer. If you are not able to participate as an observer, you can at least debrief your observers soon after each visit. Expressing interest in their results and conveying a sense that behavior in general, and attachment behavior is particular, is interesting helps observers stay motivated. Debriefing is also an opportunity to evaluate observers' engagement in the task and to find out whether any unusual circumstances arose on the visit. Also make sure observers are completing the scheduled observations in full and performing their sorts promptly. Careless observers undermine good data collection. In addition, carelessness and lack of interest are contagious. It is important to find out whether an observer can be refocused or needs to be replaced. Assigning observers to work with different partners from visit to visit often helps elevate the quality of observations and keeps observers on their toes.

When the observing team does not include a senior researcher, it is useful to contact the mother by telephone soon after the visit to thank her for participating. This is also an opportunity to make sure the visitors arrived on time and left a good impression.

Taking Notes and Discussing Observations

Most experienced observers prefer to use the AQS without making notes during the observation. Nonetheless, some prefer to take light notes indicating times and critical interactions. In our own research we leave this to observers' preferences.

Using multiple observers allows researchers to compare independent Q-sorts after the visit. Q sorts from concurrent observers should correlate at least .50. If agreement is less than this, we recommend discarding the data and looking into the source of the disagreements. Minor differences in item placements are inevitable and have little effect on scores after the sorts are averaged. Item differences greater than 3 points are worth discussing to see whether they reflect one observer noticing a behavior that the other did not see or, more significantly, one observer making too much of a single event or significant differences in how he or she is using the items. The latter need to be discussed with a more experienced observer and resolved in advance of further data collection.

Occasionally, an observer will misread an item as its opposite and wildly misplace it in the sort. Errors like this can be corrected without re-sorting the entire deck. Simply place the incorrectly scored item in the pile to which it properly belongs. Having an item or two too many or too few in one or a few piles has negligible effect on composites or criterion sort scores.

Discussions between observers play an important role in developing and maintaining familiarity with the AQS items, observation skills, and motivation. Naturalistic observation is difficult work. When working with less experienced observers, it can be useful to point out critical behaviors as they occur. This kind of coaching brings most new observers up to speed after just a few home visits. Obviously, such coached observations are not independent and should not be included in reliability assessments. Attachment behavior is complex and difficult to observe. Context and details are important. Even "expert" observers can misconstrue a particular behavior or interaction. Thus, we have come to appreciate the value of averaging Q-sort descriptions across observers and to prefer them even to our own individual sorts. It is less a matter of one observer being "right" than that four eyes are usually better than two. It is also the case that children's behaviors can be variable across days (related, but also distinct). Frequently, item placements differ for cause, and not as a mistake. This increases the value of such Q-sort descriptions as representations of actual behavior.

Additional information about observing with the AQS is available online in the Measurement Library section of *www.johnbowlby.com*.

Additional Concerns: Threats to Validity and Observations of Caregivers Other Than the Mother

Reliability

Observer agreement is primarily an indication that observers are following the observation protocol. Although this is essential, it does not indicate whether observations reliably estimate an individual's typical behavior over time and context. Low-frequency behaviors, child characteristics, changes in the observation setting, and inconsistencies in caregiver behavior contribute to day-to-day variation in child behavior. Assuming such effects are not the focus of study, they can be reduced by averaging Q-sort descriptions from multiple occasions. Traditional assessment methods assess reliability across all the participants in a study. The ability to assess reliability for each participant is an important advantage of the Q-sort method.

The number of occasions required to obtain a reliable Q-sort description of a single participant depends on how consistent their behavior is from one day to the next. The lower the correlation across occasions, the more occasions necessary to obtain a reliable composite description. In practice, we typically obtain reliable AQS descriptions (*alpha* ≥ .70) of 1- to 3-year-olds' attachment behavior by combining 60- to 120-minute observations from two occasions. In light of the time involved in recruiting participants, arranging visits, and travel, visiting for less than an hour is not economical. In about 10% of cases, we schedule additional observations to obtain good reliability.

The need for more than two visits might prove higher in studies of nonmaternal care or at-risk and clinical populations.

Observing without Others in the Home

Whenever possible, AQS observations should be scheduled when the caregiver and child can be observed alone. It is usually easy to arrange visits for times when other family members can arrange to be away. When there are older siblings, visits can often be scheduled when they are at school or playing away from home. On weekends, it is often possible for the other parent or a relative or neighbor to care for siblings for an hour or two away from the home. When other family members must be in the home, they can often find ways to occupy themselves away from the rooms in which the observations are occurring. A few comings and goings will not be a great problem. The focal caregiver will be more comfortable if he or she understands that everything does not have to be perfect.

Observing Fathers

Most infants and children direct secure base behavior toward their fathers as well as their mothers. However, if both mother and father are present, they tend to direct playful and exploratory interactions toward father and focus on mother if they need something or become upset. Moreover, mothers also step in with routine interactions (e.g., offering food or giving instructions) that would fall to the father if she were away. Observers should ask the father questions about a child's typical behavior or behavior that is not likely to arise during a single visit (e.g., Item 3—Accepts comforting from adults other than mother), just as they would the mother. If he seems uncertain (perhaps because he is not the primary caregiver), he will often suggest asking the mother. Unless an opportunity arises to check with her, and lacking direct evidence from the visit, the item should be placed in the center of the sort (i.e., Pile 5) to minimize its influence on criterion sort scores.

The Parent as a Source of Information

The AQS includes several items that are unlikely to be directly observed during the home visit, because they refer to contexts or activities that either occur at low rates or are most likely to occur in specific contexts (e.g., how the child responds when the parent leaves the house). It is appropriate to ask a parent for information about such behavior. It is also useful to ask whether an unusual behavior observed during the visit is unusual or typical. Sorters should ordinarily give more weight to a parent's response if they are confident and supported by relevant examples. Sorters should always weigh parent input, whether volunteered or elicited, against relevant behavior observed during the visit. Items that are primarily informed by parent input are necessarily uncertain, and sorters should avoid assigning them to the two highest or lowest positions in a sort.

FREQUENTLY ASKED QUESTIONS

Many of the questions about the AQS have to do with the Q-sort method itself. How do I do this? How do I do that? In the preceding sections we have addressed many of these in general and as they apply to the AQS. Many of these "How?" questions are best answered using illustrations and data templates. Here we address "When?" and "Why?" questions that have more to do with research strategy and implementation.

1 **Can the number of items be reduced?** Finding the sorting procedure unfamiliar and complex, several early adopters sought to simplify matters by (1) working with a random subset of 30–40 items and (2) dropping filler items and dependency, sociability, and desirability related items, or using only items that were placed highest or lowest in the security criterion sort. We initially encouraged such explorations. Unfortunately, they did not result in significant economies, and negative results raised doubts about whether they were attenuating the data. In practical terms, most of the investment in AQS research is in recruiting participants, travel, and observation time. Observation time is primarily a function of the frequency with which scorable behavior occurs, not the number of items to be sorted. Moreover, once observers are thoroughly familiar with the item set and sorting procedure, sorting fewer items does not save much time or effort. Subsets of items, such as the 10 highest and lowest items from the security criterion sort, can be useful for explaining constructs. However, we recommend using the full AQS item set for observational studies.

2 **Are the AQS items available in translation?** The AQS has been translated into a number of languages, including Spanish, French, Italian, Portuguese, Dutch, German, Hebrew, Turkish, Japanese, and Chinese. A Spanish translation is available on the Measurement Library section of *www.johnbowlby.com*. Other translations can be obtained from the researchers who published research with them. Translation is best accomplished using a back-translation method. Each item is translated into the new language; the translated items are blindly translated back into English and compared with the original wording, and the translation is revised to resolve differences in sense or meaning between the original and the translation. It is not necessary to validate the translated AQS, because the items are simply descriptive. Researchers have generally used the existing security and dependency sorts in order to maintain comparability in the definitions of these constructs across studies. Nonetheless, asking experts and parents from different cultures to sort AQS items to describe their sense of the typical or the ideal child's behavior

can yield interesting insights into cross-cultural differences in parenting goals, perceptions, and expectations.

3 **Can the items be rated instead of using the sorting procedure?** As explained earlier, the Q-sorting method has a number of advantages. It ensures thoughtful attention to each item. Sorting in stages also adds depth to decisions about item scores and reduces social desirability responding. And sorting into a fixed distribution facilitates the use of criterion sort scoring. Given these advantages, and compared to the time invested in recruiting participants, arranging visits, traveling, and observing, there is no real economy to rating items.

4 **Is it necessary to use two observers?** We recommend using pairs of observers whenever possible. It is an important strategy for quality control. It is also prudent for the project and, often, is more comfortable for the family. Observers are more attentive when they work in pairs. In addition to this social facilitation, it is motivating to know that assessing observer agreement is part of every observation. Even when an experienced investigator working alone might be seem to suffice (e.g., for pilot data), this is a good opportunity to begin training new observers.

5 **Can strange situation classifications be recovered from AQS assessments?** The overall quality of secure base behavior assessed at home is indeed related to one-year-old's security versus insecurity in the laboratory Strange Situation Procedure (SSP; e.g., Vaughn & Waters, 1990; van IJzendoorn et al., 2004). This is a critically important aspect of SSP validity. It also serves as an important reminder regarding the notion that attachment is primarily an emergency system. The AQS depends primarily on observing the attachment–exploration balance in nonemergency contexts (see Waters, 2008). However, we have not found distinct patterns of attachment and exploratory behavior at home that map directly into the Avoidant, Secure, and Resistant/Ambivalent (ABC) classifications; that is, infants who display confidence in their mother's availability and responsiveness at home and are skilled at using her as a secure base for exploration and comfort tend to be classified "secure" (Group B) in the SSP. Those who seem to lack confidence in their mothers' availability and responsiveness tend to be classified "insecure" (avoidant [A] or resistant [C], or D) in the SSP. Yet their difficulties using mother as a secure base do not seem to fall into a simple typology. In light of the small number of insecure infants seen in the Baltimore study (A = 6, C = 4, D = not used), perhaps this should not be surprising.

In the SSP, avoidance and resistance only occur in reunion episodes. The scoring depends on this context. The same behaviors in other episodes would not be scored and do not have the same correlates. Moreover, avoidant and resistant are rarely issues in home observations. In fact, infants who are avoidant in the SSP reunion episodes tend instead to be highly dependent in other contexts (e.g., Sroufe et al., 1983). Homotypic continuity is rarely the rule, especially across age and tasks. And there are many reasons (other than attachment-related conflict) to find something aversive but only so many ways to deal with this in behavior. Bowlby–Ainsworth attachment theory is about trust and conflict, skills and difficulty in secure base use, not about reifying or generalizing coping patterns from the SSP (Waters et al., 2015).

6 Dichotomizing criterion sort scores? Nothing in attachment theory explicitly requires discrete secure–insecure or avoidant–resistant classifications (Waters & Beauchaine, 2003; Armsden & Greenberg, 1987; Cummings, 1990). In Ainsworth's Baltimore data, even the most avoidant and resistant SSP classifications were associated with a degree of exploration at a distance, contact seeking, distance interaction, and so forth at home; that is, infants who were classified insecure in the SSP were not unattached or indifferent to their mothers at home; they were simply less skillful and consistent at using them as support for exploration and as a haven of safety (Ainsworth et al., 1978/2015). Statistical studies of structure underlying individual differences in attachment security have often suggested dimensional assessment (e.g., Fraley & Spieker, 2003; Fraley, Hudson, Heffernan, & Segal, 2015; T. Waters et al., 2015).

Dichotomizing an inherently continuous variable simply discards useful information (Fraley & Spieker, 2003; MacCallum, Zhang, Preacher, & Rucker, 2002). Nonetheless, many researchers want to formulate their studies in terms of group (secure vs. insecure) comparisons. In our experience, a security criterion sort cutoff of .30 tends to divide healthy, home-reared, 1-year-olds into the same 70:30 secure–insecure split often found in SSP data. This said, for our own research, we favor treating security criterion sort scores as a continuous variable. At the very least, consider comparing the two approaches.

7 Can the AQS be used to validate the disorganized attachment classification? Soon after the disorganized/disoriented (D) classification was identified, it was shown to have a wide range of negative correlations with early experience and subsequent adaptation. However, as Sroufe and Waters (1977) and others have repeatedly emphasized, behavior is not attachment related just because it occurs in the SSP. The same behaviors might instead reflect some sort of temperamental trait or neurointegrative disorder, and so forth. One could doubtless develop scoring systems to identify temperamental, neurodevelopmental, state-related, and perhaps even social-class-related information from the same observations. The best evidence that a behavior scored from the SSP is attachment-related is a link (positive or negative) to confidence in the mother's availability and responsiveness reflected in secure base behavior across time and context in naturalistic settings. Fortunately, several independent researchers (Seifer, Schiller, Sameroff, Resnick, & Riordan, 1996; Vittorini, 2001; van Bakel & Riksen-Walraven, 2004) independently recognized the significance of such a link for the "D" classification and undertook the necessary studies. The results are summarized in Table 2.10.

TABLE 2.10. Mean AQS Security Scores and Disorganized Classification

van Bakel & Ricksen-Walraven (2004)		Vittorini (2001)		Seifer et al. (1996)	
B (*n* = 82)	.32	B (*n* = 20)	.44	B (*n* = 29)	.43
A (*n* = 17)	.21	A (*n* = 4)	.23	A (*n* = 11)	.24
C (*n* = 18)	.10	C (*n* = 3)	.16	C (*n* = 8)	.37
D (*n* = 18)	.04	D (*n* = 6)	–.21	D (*n* = 3)	–.20

These results clearly point to an association between the "D" classification and attachment insecurity. They deserve to be cited more often in research on or that employs the classification. At the same time, they cannot be the last word on the "D" classification. Nonetheless, it would still be useful to have information on stress and coping responses of SSP "D" infants from nonattachment contexts to determine whether the classification reflects attachment-specific conflict/disorganization or a generally disorganized response to moderate stressors.

8 Is there a distinct AQS profile associated with the "D" classification? There is currently no evidence that the "D" classification is associated with a distinct pattern of secure base behavior at home. However, the data in Table 2.10 suggest that very low AQS security scores per se (which could arise from diverse patterns of item scores) could potentially be used to identify infants likely to be classified "D" in the SSP. We would need large samples of both community and risk and clinical samples to determine whether a particular AQS security cutoff score can be validated as a reliable predictor of "D" classifications in the SSP.

9 Does the AQS converge with classifications from the preschool SSP? While versions of the Strange Situation have been proposed for children ages 36–72 months (e.g., Cassidy & Marvin, 1992; Crittenden, 1994; Main & Cassidy, 1988), these tend to involve a different number of episodes, longer separations, and/or considerable modification to the criteria for scoring the interaction scales (i.e., proximity seeking, contact maintenance, avoidance, resistance, crying). Interestingly, in at least one instance (Posada, 2006), classifications from one coding system for 36-month-olds were not strongly associated with child secure base behavior at home, scored from the AQS. This suggests the possibility that "emergency" attachment measures designed for preschool-age and older children may reproduce certain features of the Strange Situation (e.g., classification categories may be similar and overlap with classifications from infancy) but not be related to secure base use at home. This should be tested in new research.

10 Can the AQS be used to assess secure base use with nonparental caregivers? The AQS has been used extensively to assess the organization of secure base behavior with caregivers other than a biological parent (e.g., day care providers/teachers, foster parents, adoptive parents). Oosterman and Schuengel (2008) reported research on foster settings and Veríssimo and Salvaterra (2006) reported research in adoptive families. Studies in group-care settings (e.g., family or center-based day care) pose special challenges to observers, because the caregiver is often tasked to meet the ordinary and emergency care demands of two to 10 or more children concurrently. Despite these formidable challenges, Howes and Hamilton (1992a, 1992b), Howes and Shivers (2006), and De Schipper, Tavecchio, and van IJzendoorn (2008) have obtained useful AQS data from observations during nonparental care.

Ideally, one would arrange to observe the child and the nonparental caregiver together, without other children present. However, this is often difficult to arrange. Observations may also be complicated by the presence of more than one caregiver, as required in many state-regulated day care settings. Researchers interested in using the AQS to study attachment and exploratory behavior in complex settings should see the Methods sections of existing reports (e.g., cited earlier and in the meta-analysis by Ahnert, Pinquart, & Lamb, 2006). It would also be useful to contact researchers who have experience arranging such observations.

11 Can the AQS be used in cross-cultural research? The AQS items are simply descriptions of observable behavior. As such, they do not present any particular obstacles to use in cross-cultural studies. If non-English-speaking observers are employed, a back-translation method should be used to prepare the required translations. A bilingual translator prepares the initial translation. Ideally, this would be a balanced bilingual speaker rather than someone who is merely conversationally fluent. This is then translated back into English by an independent, preferably balanced, bilingual translator working without knowledge of or access to the English versions of the AQS items. The back-translated English wording is then compared to the original English wording and revised to address differences in meaning or connotation. Using this method, Posada, Gao, et al. (1995) examined perspectives on infant behavior in six different language/cultural groups from Europe, Asia, Latin America, and Israel. They found that native speakers in each language group provided similar descriptions of the "ideal" child when asked to describe this child using the AQS and the forced-choice distribution format for assigning items to categories. In all language groups, the "ideal" child profile showed a significant positive association with the criterion sort for attachment security derived from sorts of North American experts.

The AQS has also been used in a range of behavioral studies of attachment in non-English-speaking groups. For example, Vereijken, Riksen-Walraven, and van Leishout (1997) and Posada et al. (2002) reported that attachment security scored from the AQS was significantly and positively associated with maternal behavior in samples from Japan and Colombia, respectively. These findings replicate results reported by Pedersen et al. (1990) and demonstrate the cross-cultural relevance of the secure base concept as suggested by Bowlby and Ainsworth.

12 **Validating new attachment measures or familiar measures in new contexts?** Observations of secure base behavior at home would seem to offer relevant convergent validation and descriptive information (item correlates) for any new security-related assessment. For example, Bretherton, Ridgeway, and Cassidy (1990) and Waters, Rodrigues, and Ridgeway, (1998) use the AQS to evaluate the secure base relevance of McArthur story stem assessments. Similarly, Monteiro, Veríssimo, Vaughn, Santos, and Bost (2008), Vaughn et al. (2007), and Veríssimo and Salvaterra (2006) used the AQS to study links between attachment security in toddlerhood and the use of a secure base "script" in storytelling by both mothers and fathers.

The AQS can also be useful as a tool for validating new applications of the SSP (e.g., beyond the age range, social class, care arrangements, cultural contexts, and clinic/risk status in which it was developed). For example, Posada (2006) used the AQS to determine whether the links between secure base behavior at home and the infant SSP established by Ainsworth et al. (1978/2015) and Vaughn and Waters (1990) apply as well to the toddler adaptation of the SSP (Cassidy & Marvin, 1992). Although rarely cited, the negative results here raise interesting questions about attachment assessment and development. See also the earlier discussion of the AQS and the "D" classification.

Surprisingly, the AQS has not been used to validate the SSP in cross-cultural studies. This would seem highly desirable in light of well-established differences in rearing conditions and priorities. Validity reflects a complex interaction between task demands, context, expectations, and the population under study and their individual histories. Thus, it would seem prudent to confirm links between SSP security and insecurity before employing it in any cross-cultural context. If the link to home behavior is established in pilot data or an initial subset of participants, this can be mentioned in support of the SSP's validity for the target population. If it is not, then researchers might consider employing the AQS as an alternative (or supplementary) measure for attachment security assessments.

REFERENCES

Ahnert, L., Pinquart, M., & Lamb, M. (2006). Security of children's relationships with nonparental care providers: A meta-analysis. *Child Development, 77,* 664–679.

Ainsworth, M. D. S. (1967). *Infancy in Uganda: Infant care and the growth of love.* Baltimore: Johns Hopkins University Press.

Ainsworth, M. D. S., Bell, S. M., & Stayton, D. J. (1971). Individual differences in strange-situation behavior of one-year-olds. In H. R. Schaffer (Ed.), *The origins of human social relations* (pp. 17–58). New York: Academic Press.

Ainsworth, M. D. S., Blehar, M. C., Waters, E., & Wall, S. (2015). *Patterns of attachment: A psychological study of the Strange Situation*. New York: Taylor & Francis (Psychology Press). (Original work published 1978)

Ainsworth, M. D. S., & Bowlby, J. (1991). An ethological approach to personality development. *American Psychologist, 46*, 333–341.

Ainsworth, M. D. S., & Marvin, R. (1995). On the shaping of attachment theory and research: An interview with Mary D. S. Ainsworth (Fall 1994). *Monographs of the Society for Research in Child Development, 60*(2–3), 3–21.

Armsden, G. C., & Greenberg, M. T. (1987). The Inventory of Parent and Peer Attachment: Relationships to well-being in adolescence. *Journal of Youth and Adolescence, 16*(5), 427–454.

Baerends, G. P. (1959). The ethological analysis of incubation behaviour. *Ibis, 101*, 357–368.

Baerends, G. P. (1972). A model of the functional organization of incubation behaviour. In G. P. Baerends & R. H. Drent (Eds.), The herring gull and its egg. *Behaviour Supplement, 17*, 261–310.

Baerends, G. P., & Drent, R. H. (1982). The herring gull and its egg: Part II. The responsiveness to egg-features. *Behaviour, 82*(1/4), i–xiii, 1–416.

Bartlett, F. C. (1932). *Remembering: A study in experimental and social psychology*. Cambridge, UK: Cambridge University Press.

Beer, C. G. (1961). Incubation and nest building behaviour of black-headed gulls: I. Incubation behavior in the incubation period. *Behaviour, 18*, 62–105.

Block, J. (1960). The number of significant findings to be expected by chance. *Psychometrika, 4*, 369–380.

Block, J. (1978). *The Q-sort method in personality assessment and psychiatric research*. Springfield, IL: Charles C Thomas. (Original work published 1961)

Block, J. (2008). *The Q-sort in character appraisal: Encoding subjective impressions of persons quantitatively*. Washington, DC: American Psychological Association.

Block, J. H., & Block, J. (1980). The role of ego control and ego-resiliency in the organization of behavior. In W. A. Collins (Ed.), *The Minnesota Symposia on Child Psychology* (Vol. 13, pp. 39–101). Hillsdale, NJ: Erlbaum.

Block, J., Block, J. H., & Keyes, S. (1988). Longitudinally fore-telling drug usage in adolescence: Early childhood personality and environmental precursors. *Child Development, 59*, 336–355.

Bretherton, I. (2003). Mary Ainsworth: Insightful observer and courageous theoretician. In G. Kimble & M. Wertheimer (Eds.), *Portraits of pioneers in psychology* (Vol. 5, pp. 317–331). Washington, DC: American Psychological Association.

Bretherton, I., Ridgeway, D., & Cassidy, J. (1990). Assessing internal working models of the attachment relationship: An attachment story completion task for 3-year-olds. In M. Greenberg, D. Cicchetti, & M. Cummings (Eds.), *Attachment in the preschool years: Theory, research and intervention* (pp. 273–308). Chicago: University of Chicago Press.

Cassidy, J., & Marvin, R. S. (1992). *Attachment organization in preschool children: Coding guidelines* (4th ed.). Unpublished manuscript, MacArthur Working Group on Attachment, Seattle, WA.

Craik, K. (1943). *The nature of explanation*. Cambridge, UK: Cambridge University Press.

Crittenden, P. M. (1994). *Preschool assessment of attachment* (2nd ed.). Unpublished manuscript, Family Relations Institute, Miami, FL.

Cronbach, L., & Gleser, G. (1953). Assessing similarity between profiles. *Psychological Bulletin, 50,* 456–473.

Cummings, E. M. (1990). Classification of attachment on a continuum of felt-security: Illustrations from the study of children of depressed parents. In M. Greenberg, D. Cicchetti, & E. M. Cummings (Eds.), *Attachment in the preschool years: Theory, research, and intervention* (pp. 311–338). Chicago: University of Chicago Press.

De Schipper, J. C., Tavecchio, L. W. C., & van IJzendoorn, M. H. (2008). Children's attachment relationships with day care caregivers: Associations with positive caregiving and child's temperament. *Social Development, 17,* 454–470.

Fraley, R. C., Hudson, N. W., Heffernan, M. E., & Segal, N. (2015). Are adult attachment styles categorical or dimensional?: A taxometric analysis of general and relationship-specific attachment orientations. *Journal of Personality and Social Psychology, 109,* 354–368.

Fraley, R. C., & Spieker, S. J. (2003). Are infant attachment patterns continuously or categorically distributed?: A taxometric analysis of strange situation behavior. *Developmental Psychology, 39,* 387–404.

Ghiselli, E., Campbell, J., & Zedeck, S. (1981). *Measurement theory for the behavioral sciences.* New York: Freeman.

Grosskurth, P. (1977). *Melanie Klein: Her world and her work.* New York: Jason Aronson.

Harlow, H. F. (1958). The nature of love. *American Psychologist, 13,* 673–685.

Harlow, H. F., & Suomi, S. J. (1971). Social recovery by isolation-reared monkeys. *Proceedings of the National Academy of Sciences of the USA, 68,* 1534–1538.

Harlow, H. F., & Zimmerman, R. R. (1959). Affectional responses in the infant monkey. *Science, 130,* 421–432.

Hay, D. F. (1980). Multiple functions of proximity-seeking in infancy. *Child Development, 51,* 636–645.

Heyman, R. E., Chaudhry, B. R., Treboux, D., Crowell, J., Lord, C., Vivian, D., & Waters, E. (2001). How much observational data is enough?: An empirical test using marital interaction coding. *Behavior Therapy, 32,* 107–122.

Hinde, R. A. (1966). *Animal behavior: A synthesis of ethology and comparative psychology.* New York: McGraw-Hill.

Howes, C., & Hamilton, C. E. (1992a). Children's relationships with teachers, mothers, and child care teachers. *Child Development, 63,* 859–878.

Howes, C., & Hamilton, C. E. (1992b). Children's relationships with child care teachers: Stability and concordance with parental attachments. *Child Development, 63,* 867–878.

Howes, C., & Shivers, E. M. (2006). New child–caregiver attachment relationships: Entering childcare when the caregiver is and is not an ethnic match. *Social Development, 15,* 574–590.

Lanning, K. (1994). Dimensionality of observer ratings on the California Adult Q-set. *Journal of Personality and Social Psychology, 67,* 151–160.

Loevinger, J. (1957). Objective tests as instruments of psychological theory. *Psychological Reports, 3*(Monograph No. 9), 635–694.

MacCallum, R. C., Zhang, S., Preacher, K. J., & Rucker, D. D. (2002). On the practice of dichotomization of quantitative variables. *Psychological Methods, 7,* 19–40.

Main, M., & Cassidy, J. (1988). Categories of response to reunion with the parent at age 6: Predictable from infant attachment classifications and stable over a 1-month period. *Developmental Psychology, 24,* 415–426.

McCormack, K., Warfield, J., Dozier, M., Gunnar, M., Maestripieri, D., Waters, E., & Sanchez, M. M. (2007). *Maternal maltreatment is associated with lower attachment security in infant rhesus monkeys* (*Macaca mulatta*). Presented at the proceedings of the 30th annual meeting of the American Society of Primatologists.

McCrae, R. R., Terracciano, A., Costa, P. T., & Ozer, D. J. (2006). Person-factors in the California Adult Q-Set: Closing the door on personality trait types? *European Journal of Personality, 20,* 29–44.

McNally, S., Eisenberg, N., & Harris, J. D. (1991). Child-rearing practices and values: A longitudinal study. *Child Development, 62,* 190–198.

Monteiro, L., Veríssimo, M., Vaughn, B. E., Santos, A. J., & Bost, K. K. (2008). Secure base representations for both fathers and mothers predict children's secure base behavior in a sample of Portuguese families. *Attachment and Human Development, 10,* 189–206.

Oosterman, M., & Schuengel, C. (2008). Attachment in foster children associated with caregivers' sensitivity and behavioral problems. *Infant Mental Health Journal, 29,* 609–623.

Pederson, D. R., Moran, G., Sitko, C., Campbell, K., Ghesquire, K., & Acton, H. (1990). Maternal sensitivity and the security of infant–mother attachment: A Q-sort study. *Child Development, 61,* 1974–1983.

Posada, G. (2006). Assessing attachment security at age three: Q-sort observations and the MacArthur Strange Situation adaptation. *Social Development, 15,* 644–658.

Posada, G., Gao, Y., Fang, W., Posada, R., Tascon, M., Schoelmerich, A., . . . Synnevaag, B. (1995). The secure base phenomenon across cultures: Children's behavior, mothers' preferences, and experts' concepts. In E. Waters, B. Vaughn, G. Posada, & K. Kondo-Ikemura (Eds.), Caregiving, cultural and cognitive perspectives on secure base behavior and attachment working models. *Monographs of the Society for Research in Child Development, 60*(Serial No. 255, 2–3), 27–48.

Posada, G., Jacobs, A., Richmond, M., Carbonell, O. A., Alzate, G., Bustamante, M. R., & Quiceno, J. (2002). Maternal caregiving and infant security in two cultures. *Developmental Psychology, 38,* 67–78.

Posada, G., Jacobs, A., Richmond, M., & Kaloustian, G. (2007). Maternal secure base support and preschoolers' secure base behavior in natural environments. *Attachment and Human Development, 9,* 393–411.

Posada, G., Waters, E., Crowell, J., & Lay, K. L. (1995). Is it easier to use a secure mother as a secure base: Attachment Q-sort correlates of the Berkeley Adult Attachment Interview. In E. Waters, B. Vaughn, G. Posada, & K. Kondo-Ikemura (Eds.), Caregiving, cultural and cognitive perspectives on secure base behavior and attachment working models. *Monographs of the Society for Research in Child Development, 60*(Serial No. 244, 2–3), 133–145.

Robertson, J., & Robertson, J. (1990). *Separation and the very young.* London: Free Association Books.

Santos, A. J., Daniel, J. R., Antunes, M., Coppola G., Trudel, M., & Vaughn, B. E. (2020). Changes in preschool children's social engagement positively predict changes in social competence: A three-year longitudinal study of Portuguese children. *Social Development, 29,* 544–563.

Seifer, R., Schiller, M., Sameroff, A. J., Resnick, S., & Riordan, K. (1996). Attachment, maternal sensitivity, and infant temperament during the first year of life. *Developmental Psychology, 32,* 12–25.

Sroufe, L. A., Fox, N., & Pancake, V. (1983). Attachment and dependency in developmental perspective. *Child Development, 54*(6), 1615–1627.

Sroufe, L. A., & Waters, E. (1977). Attachment as an organizational construct. *Child Development, 48,* 1184–1199.

Stephenson, W. (1953). *The study of behavior.* Chicago: University of Chicago Press.

Teti, D. M., Sakin, J., Kucera, E., Corns, K. M., & Eiden, R. D. (1996). And baby makes four: Predictors of attachment security among preschool-aged firstborns during the transition to siblinghood. *Child Development, 67,* 579–596.

Tinbergen, N. (1951). *The study of instinct.* Oxford, UK: Clarendon Press.

van Bakel, H., & Riksen-Walraven, J. M. (2004). AQS security scores: What do they measure? *Infant Mental Health Journal, 25*(3), 175–193.

van Dijken, S, van der Veer, R., van IJzendoorn, M. H., & Kuijpers, H. J. (1998). Bowlby before Bowlby: The sources of an intellectual departure in psychoanalysis and psychology. *Journal of the History of the Behavioral Sciences, 34,* 247–270.

van IJzendoorn, M. H., Vereijken, C. M. J. L., Bakermans-Kranenburg, M. J., & Riksen-Walraven, J. M. (2004). Assessing attachment security with the Attachment Q-sort: Meta-analytic evidence for the validity of the observer AQS. *Child Development, 75,* 1188–1213.

Vaughn, B. E., Coppola, G., Veríssimo, M., Monteiro, L., Santos, A. J., Posada, G., . . . Korth, B. (2007). The quality of maternal secure base scripts predicts children's secure base behavior at home in three socio-cultural groups. *International Journal of Behavioral Development, 31,* 65–76.

Vaughn, B. E., Santos, A. J., Monteiro, L., Shin, N., Daniel, J. R., Krzysik, L., & Pinto, A. (2016). Social engagement and adaptive functioning during early childhood: Identifying and distinguishing among subgroups differing with regard to social engagement. *Developmental Psychology, 52,* 1422–1434.

Vaughn, B. E., & Waters, E. (1990). Attachment behavior at home and in the laboratory: Q-sort observations and Strange Situation classifications of one-year-olds. *Child Development, 61,* 1965–1973.

Vereijken, C., Riksen-Walraven, C., & van Leishout, F. M. (1997). Mother–infant relationships in Japan: Attachment, dependency, and *amae. Journal of Cross-Cultural Psychology, 28,* 442–462.

Verríssimo, M., & Salvaterra, F. (2006). Maternal secure base scripts and children's attachment security in an adopted sample. *Attachment and Human Development, 8,* 261–273.

Viswanathan, M., & Berkman, N. D. (2011). Development of the RTI Item Bank on risk of bias and precision of observational studies (Methods Research Report, AHRQ Publication No. 11-EHC028-EF). Rockville, MD: Agency for Healthcare Research and Quality. Retrieved from *www.effectivehealthcare.ahrq.gov/reports/final.cfm.*

Vittorini, L. (2001). *The development of the self in toddlers: Agency in social interactions and its relations with attachment security.* Poster presented at the biennial meeting of the Society of Research in Child Development, Minneapolis, MN.

Warfield, J., Kondo-Ikemura, K., & Waters, E. (2011). Measuring infant attachment security in rhesus macaques *(Macaca mulatta)*: Adaptation of the Attachment Q-set. *American Journal of Primatology, 73,* 109–118.

Waters, E. (1978). The reliability and stability of individual differences in infant–mother attachment. *Child Development, 49,* 483–494.

Waters, E. (1987). Attachment Q-set (3.0) with item rationales. Retrieved June 1, 2017, from *www.psychology.sunysb.edu/attachment/measures/content/aqs_items.pdf.*

Waters, E. (2008). Live long and prosper: A note on attachment and evolution. Retrieved September 15, 2017, from *www.psychology.sunysb.edu/attachment/gallery/live_long/live_long.html.*

Waters, E., & Beauchaine, T. (2003). Are there really patterns of attachment?: Theoretical and empirical perspectives. *Developmental Psychology, 39,* 417–432.

Waters, E., Bretherton, I., & Vaughn, B. E. (2015). Preface. In M. D. S. Ainsworth, M. Blehar, E. Waters, & S. N. Wall (Eds.), *Patterns of attachment: A psychological study of the Strange Situation* (pp. x–xxxvi). New York: Routledge/Psychology Press.

Waters, E., & Deane, K. E. (1985). Defining and assessing individual differences in attachment relationships: Q-methodology and the organization of behavior in infancy and early childhood. In I. Bretherton & E. Waters (Eds.), Growing points of attachment theory and research. *Monographs of the Society for Research in Child Development, 50*(Serial No. 209, 1–2), 41–65.

Waters, E., Garber, J., Gornal, M., & Vaughn, B. E. (1983). Q-sort correlates of social competence. *Developmental Psychology, 19,* 550–560.

Waters, E., Noyes, D., Vaughn, B. E., & Ricks, M. (1985). Social competence and self-esteem: A Q-sort analysis of conceptual and empirical similarities between related constructs. *Developmental Psychology, 21,* 508–522.

Waters, H. S., Rodrigues, L., & Ridgeway, D. (1998). Cognitive underpinnings of narrative attachment assessment. *Journal of Experimental Child Psychology, 71,* 211–234.

Waters, T. E. A., Fraley, C. R., Groh, A. M., Steele, R. D., Vaughn, B. E., Bost, K. K., . . . Roisman, G. I. (2015). The latent structure of secure base script knowledge. *Developmental Psychology, 51,* 823–830.

CHAPTER 3

The Strange Situation

Paradigm, Practique, and FAQs

Everett Waters, Brian E. Vaughn, and Kristin Bernard

John Bowlby often referred to attachment theory as a new *paradigm*, a new way of understanding the infant's tie to primary caregivers. The term can also refer to a community of theorists and researchers bound together by shared principles and methods (Kuhn, 1962/2012; Masterman, 1970). Thus, the *attachment paradigm* refers to both Bowlby–Ainsworth attachment theory and the community that shares and contributes to this perspective.

Paradigm can also refer to one or more prototypical problems or key techniques associated with a theoretical or methodological approach (Kuhn, 1962/2012; Masterman, 1970). As students become skilled in solving such problems or using a particular tool, they come to understand the practical meaning of key theoretical concepts. They also learn to recognize the contexts in which a theory or methodology is relevant. Eventually, with much experience across many trials, they acquire the expectations and fluency characteristic of experts. The Strange Situation Procedure (SSP) has served generations of students as the paradigm through which they learned about the secure base phenomenon and the ethological approach underpinning infant attachment theory. As much as any theoretical insight or empirical result, this is why the SSP endures.

The SSP's history is detailed in van Rosmalen, van der Veer, and van der Horst's (2015) insightful review in the *Journal of the History of the Behavioral Sciences* and also in Waters, Bretherton, and Vaughn's (2015) new preface to *Patterns of Attachment: A Psychological Study of the Strange Situation*. The laboratory setup and procedures for conducting SSP assessments are detailed in *Patterns of Attachment* (Ainsworth, Blehar, Waters, & Wall, 1978/2015) and outlined in the methods sections of countless research articles. Thus, there is little to add on either score. Instead, we focus in this chapter on practical matters, implicit knowledge of the SSP paradigm that rarely finds a place in scientific writing but has everything to do with learning and using the SSP in research and applied settings. We address this chapter primarily to novices and to research consumers who need to understand not only the procedures but also the goals and practical touches that underpin good quality SSP assessments. Implicit knowledge does not lend itself to consensus. It reflects individual experience. Some in the SSP community may not agree with us on every detail. We hope they will agree that our presentation reflects the kind of information necessary to turn novices into experts.

Like many skilled measurement tasks, conducting and scoring the SSP involves more than simply following a set of rules. Written procedures and scoring instructions take us only so far. They help standardize and stabilize a method over time. As well, they are valuable aids to memory for numerous and subtle instructions. However, it matters that the SSP is rooted in behavior rather than responses to test items. The rationale for both the procedure and the scoring assume a certain understanding of how behavior works. That is, how behavior in general and infant–mother interaction in particular are organized and unfold in naturalistic settings. Unfortunately, this is not part of contemporary psychology training.

Learning to use and score the SSP entails working with an experienced coder who can illustrate Mary Ainsworth's written coding instructions with multiple examples from archival SSP recordings. There is no substitute for a mentor who can point out, "This is what the instructions are referring to when they mention behavior *X*," or "Without this context, we can't say that this behavior means *Y*."[1] Fortunately, Alan Sroufe, Elizabeth Carlson, and their colleagues at Minnesota's Institute for Child Development have conducted highly successful SSP training workshops every summer for over 20 years. Their dedication to maintaining the quality of SSP assessments is widely and deeply appreciated. Although active attachment research groups occasionally provide training, the Minnesota group's training materials are exceptional. Moreover, they can host a dozen or more trainees at once. This is the only way to keep up with the constant demand for training.

Infant attachment research in the Bowlby–Ainsworth tradition is a departure from the behaviorist paradigm of the 1950s through the 1970s, which viewed physics as the model science and focused on arbitrary sequences of discrete acts and operational definitions, with little attention to the importance of context and organization. The Bowlby–Ainsworth tradition is rooted in a new paradigm, a biological approach to behavior that focuses on organization and adaptation. Understandably, psychologists steeped in the earlier paradigm find that adopting a new perspective takes some getting used to. Communication across paradigms is always difficult and requires a willingness to see with new eyes. Today, the behaviorist and psychoanalytic paradigms that so

[1]This parallels G. Frege's (1984) conclusions regarding the relation of context to meaning in mathematics, logic, and language.

complicated (and resisted) the Bowlby–Ainsworth perspective in the 1960s and 1970s are little emphasized in the psychology curriculum. This allows training to proceed with relatively less attention to unlearning old allegiances and old ways of viewing behavior. In this respect, teaching and learning to use the SSP are probably easier today than in the past.

Nonetheless, it remains difficult to conduct consistently good SSP assessments without appreciating the goals and practical considerations underlying the procedure. These range from the layout of the room to the relation between camera work and scoring, and the flow of the procedure, not just from the first episode to the last but from telephone contacts and greetings on campus to debriefing and departure. Fortunately, we have the flexibility in this chapter to address what we might call the "pragmatics" of running SSP assessments. We undertake this in three sections.

We begin with a few words about behavior. It is not an overstatement to say that much of the human and animal behavior around us goes unnoticed. Our goal is to highlight behavior *per se* as an interesting phenomenon and help novices begin to see attachment behavior through the same lens that informed Mary Ainsworth's home observations and Strange Situation assessments.

We then turn to a detailed narrative presentation of SSP procedures, designed to complement the description of procedures in *Patterns of Attachment*. The narrative format supplements the procedures detailed in *Patterns of Attachment* and in countless empirical research reports, allowing us to provide explanations and elaborations in context, and to convey something of *what it feels like* to conduct the procedure. We hope this perspective will be valuable to potential trainees in advance of SSP training workshops, and for researchers who plan to conduct the SSP themselves, then make other arrangements for scoring. It may also be useful to research consumers who need to understand, beyond what mere instructions convey, what the assessment entails.

We conclude this chapter with a discussion of more than two dozen frequently asked questions (FAQs). These are primarily issues of theory or measurement that we encounter working with students or assisting experienced researchers who are not expert in attachment but want to teach about or supervise students interested in using the SSP. They overlap quite a bit with issues we discuss among ourselves and with our close colleagues. As in the chapter's earlier sections, our goal in discussing FAQs is to convey some of the implicit knowledge that distinguishes experts and is important for a good start in attachment study. A good part of this is information about what kinds of questions to ask and what constitutes a useful answer.

"SEEING" BEHAVIOR

Ethology is the biological study of behavior in naturalistic settings. One of its key insights is that behavior is more than mere movement; it is an essential part of a species' evolutionary endowment and thus merits careful study.

Ethologists can readily describe in great detail the behavior of species they study, describing its adaptive significance and development, and contrasting it with the behavior of closely related species. Every detail is hard-won information gleaned through exhaustive and exhausting observations. In contrast, developmental psychologists depend too often on an informal understanding of behavior, underpinned by little more than having been children themselves, rearing a child or two, or noticing children in the course of other activities. We risk much when we trade in this kind of casually acquired, incidental evidence—if it is evidence at all.

Trained in the traditions of Cambridge psychology and medicine, John Bowlby found psychoanalysts' emphasis on introspection and retrospective reconstruction unsatisfying at best. Even during his psychoanalytic training, he wondered whether his supervisors' emphasis on children's fantasies and subjective experiences would have found support in parents' reports or observations in the home. However, his supervisors denied him this kind of convergent validation—an issue that significantly delayed the completion of his training. According to his son, Richard, it was only the pressure of a new family that motivated him to finally complete his certification (R. Bowlby, 2006). In later years, he would encourage the Tavistock Clinic to include observational methodology in its curriculum and recruit James Robertson to film naturalistic observations of parent–child separations in hospital and residential care (van der Horst, 2011).

Inspired, perhaps, by Darwin's (1877) *A Biographical Sketch of an Infant*, his own enthusiasm for birdwatching, and his early hospital and residential care observations, one of John Bowlby's first insights regarding infant attachment was that the clingy, crying behavior portrayed in psychoanalytic (and learning) theories hardly captured the subtlety, complexity, and planfulness of infant's actual behavior over time in naturalistic settings. For anyone who takes the time to observe (e.g., Piaget, 1936/1952), patience reveals an active, curious, mastery-oriented infant whose mother encourages and enriches exploration and serves as a haven of comfort or safety as needed.

Bowlby felt that neither drive accumulation–reduction nor patterns of reinforcement could plausibly explain the seemingly purposeful balance infants maintain between proximity seeking and exploration over time. Nor could they explain the intricate dance of face-to-face interaction. Such behavior is too rapid and context-sensitive to be explained in terms of waxing and waning drive states. Similarly, the coordination of information about aspects of the physical environment, the caregiver's recent and current behavior, proximity and other influences on accessibility, internal states, and so forth, is too complex for simple learning explanations. Not that Bowlby dismissed the importance of learning in development. He wanted a theory that could be integrated with learning theory, without being confined by learning theory (Bowlby, 1958, p. 362).

Following Niko Tinbergen's (1951, 1963) landmark descriptions of the aims and methods of ethology, John Bowlby (1957, 1958) proposed building a new theory of infant–mother bonds rooted in (1) observation and description (especially in naturalistic settings), (2) analysis of immediate causation, (3) a view to behavior's survival/adaptive value, (4) detailed developmental analysis, and (5) an evolutionary/comparative framework. From this beginning grew his and Mary Ainsworth's commitment (e.g., Bowlby, 1969; Ainsworth & Bowlby, 1991) to an attachment theory rooted in an ethological perspective and to focusing on actual behavior observed in detail over time and in meaningful (to the infant) settings (e.g., Hinde, 1966; Tinbergen, 1951; DeVore, 1963, 1965).

An "Eye" for Behavior

Attachment researchers in the 1960s and 1970s often operationalized the child's tie to its primary caregiver in terms of frequency counts on discrete behaviors such as looking, vocalizing, and touching the mother during brief laboratory observations (see Maccoby & Masters, 1970; Sroufe & Waters, 1977). This approach promised systematic, "objective" data on what otherwise seemed a very elusive phenomenon. It was also more convenient and economical than naturalistic observation. Too convenient and economical, perhaps. In the end, they counted many behaviors but learned little about behavior.

Long before Bowlby suggested approaching attachment from an ethological perspective, he had been an avid birdwatcher, filling the drawers of library-style card catalog cabinets with detailed information on the species he encountered, when, where, and the details of their behavior. He found behavior interesting and understood its complexity and sensitivity to context, and that there was meaning to be extracted at different levels of analysis. Yet he claimed to lack Mary Ainsworth's patience and stamina as an observer, and the "eye" for behavior evident in *Infancy in Uganda* (Ainsworth, 1967) and in her scales for scoring maternal behavior at home and infant behavior in the SSP (Ainsworth et al., 1978/2015).

Some of the hallmarks of an ethological perspective on behavior are outlined below and discussed in relation to attachment assessment. These include the salience, context, meaning, and organization of behavior. These are central to attachment study in the Bowlby–Ainsworth tradition. Yet, there is little space for them in research journals.

Behavior: Seeing versus Observing

It is easy to overlook behavior unless someone points it out and provides concepts and language with which to understand it. One of us (E. W.) recalls having spent years in South Florida, scuba diving on reefs and wrecks off the coast and in the Keys, and seeing an astounding array of sea life—all without noticing a single instance of territoriality, courtship, foraging, or parental behavior as it unfolded—unseen by an untrained eye. This is reminiscent of a passage from the Sherlock Holmes story "A Scandal in Bohemia" (Doyle & Klinger (2007, p. 4):

> WATSON: . . . at each successive instance of your reasoning I am baffled until you explain your process. And yet I believe that my eyes are as good as yours.
>
> HOLMES: Quite so. . . . You see, but you do not observe. The distinction is clear. For example, you have frequently seen the steps which lead up from the hall to this room.
>
> WATSON: Frequently.
>
> HOLMES: How often?
>
> WATSON: Well, some hundreds of times.
>
> HOLMES: Then how many are there?
>
> WATSON: How many? I don't know.
>
> HOLMES: Quite so! You see but you do not observe. That is just my point. Now, I know that there are seventeen steps, because I have both seen and observed.[2]

One of the key insights underpinning ethology and behavioral biology is the recognition that behavior is every bit as characteristic of a species as its anatomy. First expressed in Julian Huxley's (1914) classic study "The Courtship Habits of the Great Crested Grebe," the idea that behavior is an object, a structure, an element on which evolution can operate, a taxonomic feature, brings it to the foreground, visible and inviting inquiry. John Bowlby (1958) was initially interested in an ethological perspective because it promised an alternative to psychoanalytic drive theory. His first references to specific behaviors that bind the infant to its mother were quite preliminary, hardly the fruit of detailed ethological observations. "Those which I believe we can identify at present are sucking, clinging and following, in all of which the infant is the principal active partner, and crying and smiling in which his behaviour serves to activate maternal behavior" (Bowlby, 1958, p. 351). In contrast, Mary Ainsworth's observations in Uganda extended the list to least 16 behaviors, each described in detail, illustrated in context, and its impact on the mother noted (Ainsworth, 1967, pp. 321–350). After reading her Uganda observations, it is difficult to see infant–mother interactions in quite the same light again. Whereas, previously, adjectives such as cute, happy, clever, and warm seemed to suffice, now you see *behavior*—complex, sensitive to context, and seemingly purposeful.

The Context of Behavior

Behavior does not occur in isolation. There is always a context. Indeed, neurobiologists have demonstrated that a primary function of structures in the basal ganglia is to incorporate context into the process of selecting, initiating,

[2]See also Isaiah 42:20.

and terminating behaviors. Indeed, the smallest biologically/adaptively meaningful unit of behavior may not be "a behavior" but "a behavior + a context."

Mary Ainsworth did a great deal to highlight the influence of context on the activation/termination and meaning of infant behaviors. In particular, she illustrated that both the content and meaning of infant behavior depends on its place in the stream of the infant's ongoing behavior, the infant's mood, and its expectations regarding the content and qualities (*e.g.*, timeliness, relevance, coordination with ongoing behavior and goals) of the caregiver's behavior. This perspective is evident throughout her Uganda and Baltimore observations and in her scales for scoring maternal behavior at home and infant behavior in the SSP (Ainsworth et al., 1978/2015, Appendices II, III, and IV). Context is so important in her work that it is well worth the effort for new researchers to read through these scales, highlighting each time the description or interpretation of a behavior is conditioned on the context in which it occurs.

The Meaning of Behavior

Behavior is not merely anatomy in motion. It carries information about an individual's view and understanding of its environment and about its goals. Melville's Captain Ahab says as much when he tells his crew to look through the masks that hide reality to the "lower layer," the meaning behind mere appearances. These, he says, are revealed in behavior. "In each event, in the living act, the undoubted deed—there, some unknown but still reasoning thing puts forth the [shape] of its true features" (Melville, 1851, Chapter 36). Infants, and often adults, cannot verbalize for us which features in the environment shape their behavior, the traces left by past experiences, or their expectations. Yet their behavior often offers glimpses and hints at where to look for further clues. Mary Ainsworth showed that an infant's behavior can tell us much more than merely what it has just done.

The idea that behavior has meaning is central to the ethological perspective. This view stems from Konrad Lorenz's (1935) classic paper "The Companion in the Bird's World," in which, among other things, he first drew attention to the phenomenon we call imprinting and discussed the impact of an individual's behavior on others. One of the goals Bowlby and Ainsworth adopted from ethology was to understand infants and mothers as mutually situated in a dyadic relationship and to understand the meaning of their behavior to each other (Sroufe & Waters, 1977). Once we begin to see behavior *qua* behavior, behavior in its own right, it is hard to imagine it not containing information, some sort of meaning. Although the ethologists had made a compelling case for viewing animals in this way, regarding human infants, Ainsworth, in particular, viewed this a hypothesis to be tested. Thus, she recorded not just the occurrence of a behavior but also the physical, behavioral, and emotional context in which it occurred. She then searched in concurrent and longitudinal data for the meaning of each partner's behavior to the other. In doing so, she discovered much about the vocabulary and meaning-structure of infant–mother interactions and the time frame and levels of behavioral detail and organization at which implicit meaning is communicated within the dyad. She also learned that the meanings they take from their interactions shape subsequent behavior, and, as Bowlby predicted, developmental outcomes. Thus, for several generations now, her insights into the meaning of infant and maternal behavior have served as the predicate for attachment measurement and research. They have also served as guides for designing prevention and intervention programs. All possible only because behavior has meaning and we have the key.

Levels of Detail and Organization

Mary Ainsworth found it useful to describe behavior at different levels of detail and organization. Following the lead of Robert Hinde (1959) and other ethologists, she described infant–mother behaviors during close bodily contact and face-to-face interaction in terms of the smallest movements that might convey meaning to its partner, or help her understand the infant's or the mother's requirements or goals. The importance of behavioral organization to her view of attachment and the secure base phenomenon is evident throughout her work, especially in the measures she developed. See, for example, her preamble to the ABC classification system (Ainsworth et al., 1978/2015, pp. 55–58.) *Organization* was not just a "buzzword" in her work; it became fashionable because of her work.

Among her most surprising findings was how much meaning is communicated in fine-grained analyses of behavioral content and organization that might easily be dismissed as trivial. Examples abound in the scales she developed for scoring early maternal behavior in her Uganda and Baltimore home observations and in her scales for scoring infant behavior during SSP reunion episodes (Ainsworth, 1967; Ainsworth et al., 1978/2015, Appendices II and III). She also found it useful to describe and quantify behavior at higher levels of organization (e.g., referring to *maternal sensitivity* or *cooperation with ongoing behavior*) in order to capture the aggregate impact of even small behaviors over countless interactions. That is, once information has been extracted from behavioral details, there can be additional information in the way these details are organized over time.

Just as behavior can be described at different levels of detail, its organization too resides at different levels, from the organization of *individual motor components* that give behavior its topography and fluidity to the *coordination of several behaviors into a skilled action,* to *coordination with something in the environment or over time,* especially in relation to a goal. Behavioral organization is also evident in the *coordination of several different behaviors* during exploration of toys during the SSP. For example, smooth, systematic coordination of locomotion, posture, gaze, and manipulation, combined with positive affect, and often affective sharing, are clear signs that an infant has recovered its composure in reunion episodes. Less well-organized behavior, including manipulating toys while looking distractedly elsewhere or anger interspersed with weak exploratory behavior, or simply sitting among toys without constructively exploring them, are all indications that the infant remains distressed despite the mother's return and efforts to provide comfort. Such distress in the absence of proximity seeking or signaling is a hallmark of moderate avoidance and weighs in favor of an insecure classification. Importantly, the key is not in any one of the behaviors but in the way they are (or are not) organized into effective exploration.

Behavioral organization is also evident in the *coherence of behavioral sequences*. For example, a typical response to the mother's departure and return in the SSP is protest, seeking, approach, clambering, clinging until comforted, and return to interest in the environment (either from the mother's lap or back on the floor with toys). It is not necessary to see each of these, or that any of them take a particular form. What is important is whether the flow of behavior keeps moving forward, toward the expectable endpoint—that is, toward being picked up and effectively comforted. The behavior sequence has lost its expected organization if approach to the mother is interrupted (e.g., partial approach and then turning to toys), if the infant (after showing distress upon separation) moves away from rather than toward her, or if the infant approaches or reaches to be picked up but then wiggles to be put down (before being comforted), only to cry again.

Behavioral organization is also reflected in the *smooth intercoordination of behaviors serving different goals*, as in cycles of exploration and proximity seeking seen in the course of extended home observations and across episodes in the SSP. On a certain reading of attachment theory, we might expect that distress (over time away from the mother) is the primary trigger that initiates transition from exploration to proximity seeking. In fact, most returns are triggered when the infant detects a change in its mother's behavior and approaches to update information on her location and availability, or by exhausting possibilities for further exploration and returning to her for interaction or direction to new opportunities to explore. Thus, information about the infant's expectations lies not simply in the quality of play or the presence or absence of distress, but in the smoothness with which the infant transitions between exploration and proximity seeking. One of the hallmarks of secure attachment, then, is the ability to maintain the organization between the two behavior systems as the infant transitions from exploration to proximity seeking and back.

Maintaining a secure base relationship entails organizing *a wide range of behavior to serve several goals, over significant periods of time* (hours or days) *and across a wide range of situational, behavioral, and affective contexts*. Observers must look for (1) specific secure base behaviors, (2) indications that the infant is making its needs clear and is exploiting opportunities to learn about the environment and its own competencies and limitations, and (3) behaviors that help knit the relationship together over time (e.g., the mother remaining interested, available, and effectively scaffolding the infant's explorations). Over such long intervals and such a wide range of activities, it is inevitable that there will be rough patches. But few are frequent or disruptive enough to compromise the sense that the mother and infant are an effective, coordinated dyad, working toward the same goals. Ainsworth found this kind of organization easier to recognize than to quantify (See Ainsworth et al., 1978/2015, Appendix V). Attachment study would benefit from additional work on this level of organization.

A Word about "Disorganization"

Mary Ainsworth always considered the ABC (avoidant, secure, ambivalent or resistant) classification system open to revision. She did not expect to have identified all the significant ways in which infants organize their SSP behavior in her initial Baltimore sample of 23 dyads, or even in the extended sample of 106. Main and Solomon (1986, 1990) introduced the disorganized/disoriented (D) classification to capture behavior that seemed paradoxical or inexplicable in relation to the established ABC classifications. Ainsworth and her students had long recognized that a few infants were simply very difficult to classify using the ABC system, but they were too few to identify as a distinct group. Main and Solomon brought many of these cases together with examples of "odd" or paradoxical behavior that would never have been identified without videotape, and cases that emerged when the SSP was used in much larger and more diverse samples.

Work on the "D" classification provides excellent illustrations of the concepts we have just reviewed (see Solomon, Duschinsky, Bakkum, & Schuengel, Chapter 4, this volume). Moreover, the "D" classification has many important correlates and has proven particularly useful in at-risk and clinical samples. At the same time, the term *disorganized* has gained wide currency, to the point of being used quite outside the scope of Main and Solomon's meaning. This is particularly true when *disorganized* is used as a trait descriptor to suggest that an individual's behavior is disorganized across multiple domains and in a wide variety of contexts.

In Main and Solomon's work, the term refers to *specific lapses* in *the organization of behavior*. These include disorganization in (1) individual behaviors; (2) behavior sequences; (3) incomplete, undirected, or misdirected behaviors; (4) stereotypies, mistimed movements, or anomalous postures; (5) freezing or stilling; (6) apprehension of the caregiver; and (7) overt signs of disorientation. Though often fleeting and very subtle, the observed behavior seems at odds with the flow of behavior or expected goals. Importantly, they are only scored with respect to the caregiver and only in reunion episodes. Infants classified disorganized do not display such behaviors frequently or across a wide range of contexts. And although the "D" classification can be significantly stable over time, the evidence on this varies considerably across samples (see Carlson, Chapter 4, this volume). Moreover, some who are not classified "D" in infancy begin to display controlling behavior associated with the "D" classification in toddlerhood. Research has not yet established whether infants/toddlers display the same disorganized behavior on repeated assessments. Nor is it yet clear whether different disorganized behaviors or clusters of disorganized behaviors have similar correlates.

Behavior is complex and subject to multiple influences. Disfluencies and limited failures of organization are inevitable. It takes a long time to explore the ins and outs of any behavior pattern, not to mention when base rates are low and differ markedly in different populations. Yet there is already substantial evidence that the lapses in behavioral organization in SSP reunions point reliably to important developmental antecedents and outcomes. This should not be an invitation to lapse carelessly into trait language—using *disorganized* as an unqualified descriptor. In fact, it would be quite extraordinary for any individual, or relationship, or for that matter, any biological phenomenon, to be wholly disorganized.

STRANGE SITUATION PRACTIQUE: A NARRATIVE[3]

Ideally, learning to conduct and score the SSP begins with some exposure to the ethological perspective on behavior. Martin and Bateson (2007), Drummond (1981/2012), Tinbergen (1951, 1963), and Hinde (1959) are excellent sources. This perspective is part and parcel of understanding and scoring the SSP. It is equally important to be familiar with the secure base concept (e.g., Ainsworth et al., 1978/2015, Chapter 1; Waters & Deane, 1985; Waters & Cummings, 2000). It is also useful to have reviewed the Attachment Q-set items that are most (and least) characteristic of skillful secure base use in infancy. Finally, it always pays dividends to make several 2- to 3-hour home visits, before and after SSP training, to observe infant–mother dyads in more contexts and over longer intervals than one sees in the SSP. As the criteria against which the SSP was initially validated, these are essential to understanding and evaluating the SSP.

The instructions for conducting the Strange Situation are detailed in *Patterns of Attachment* (1978/2015, Chapter 2 and Appendix 1) and summarized in countless research articles. Although these instructions are quite complete, they do not convey much of *what it feels like* to conduct the assessment. In many respects, conducting the SSP is more like directing a play than following a set of rules. There is not only a logic but also a goal behind each step, and there are alternative paths to follow when an infant becomes inconsolable or a mother misses her cues. It is easier to respond to the complexities of working with infant–mother dyads if you have a feel for the flow of the procedure and

[3]Throughout our descriptions of infant–mother interaction in SSP, infants are referred to as "he" and mothers as "she." Attachment researchers have long adopted this convention to avoid ambiguous pronouns when referring to infants and mothers in the SSP. In other contexts we employ current usage.

understand what you are trying to accomplish in each episode. Sometimes, you have to be patient and see what is unfolding; sometimes it is important to be decisive, perhaps abbreviating or even foregoing an episode in order to preserve the possibility of scorable behavior in later episodes. The more confident and professional you can appear in the face of such surprises, the more comfortable the mother will feel. Comfortable mothers behave more naturally and are better at following instructions given in the course of the procedure. They are also more likely to enjoy participating, and less likely to feel apart from the proceedings or exploited.

SSP procedure has changed very little over time, except that we now (1) must obtain informed consent, which requires a written description of the SSP and any attendant risks; (2) abbreviate separation episodes after 30 rather than 60 seconds of hard crying; and (3) do not have the mother leave her handbag during separations. The most significant change is that Mary Ainsworth depended on expert observers to provide a play-by-play description of each episode; today, excellent equipment that combines digital video and audio recording is available from any consumer electronics store. (See FAQ 7, below, for a discussion of SSP videography.)

The presentation here follows Mary Ainsworth's instructions quite closely, except that it unfolds more like a story than a set of instructions. The narrative format allows us to provide explanations and elaborations in context, and to address difficulties (e.g., an inconsolable infant) more or less at the time and in the context in which they are likely to arise. This makes it easier to anticipate and cope when mother or baby do not behave exactly as you might have expected. At every step, we have included examples of our own style of conversing with and instructing the mother. These illustrate a style and tone that most mothers find comfortable and easy to follow. The point is to be confident and cordial, and to help the mother feel comfortable as well. *Do not try to memorize the text.* You would only end up speaking too quickly and sounding mechanical. Instead, get a sense for the tone and level of detail and bring these into your own conversational voice.

Preliminaries

Phone Call Check-In

It is useful to call the mother the day before the visit to confirm the appointment and discuss logistics (e.g., parking, the name of the person who will meet her, whether she will be bringing additional children). Let the mother know that you hope to see what her baby is like on a typical day. Explain that, now and then, a baby arrives too tired or out of sorts, in which case, we delay starting or even reschedule.

This is also a chance to briefly assess whether there are any unusual circumstances that might lead you to reschedule the visit. These include anything that might lead the baby to experience added distress and not show typical behavior, such as having a cold or ear infection, not sleeping well, experiencing a recent prolonged separation (e.g., mother having been out of town), or having a recent change in caregiving routines (e.g., child just starting to attend day care). Let her know that she can call you if anything comes up later in the day or the next morning (e.g., baby does not sleep that night).

Lead researcher:

"We are excited to see you and [Baby's name] for your visit tomorrow. [Remind the mother about details about the visit and answer any questions.] You are scheduled to come in tomorrow at [time]. Is this usually a time when [Baby's name] is awake and alert? We want to see how [Baby's name] plays in different situations. So, I want to make sure it will be a typical day for you. Has he been sick at all recently—colds, ear infections? Have there been any changes in your routine? If anything comes up before your visit tomorrow, like [Baby's name] having a difficult night sleeping, please give me a call. We can easily reschedule for another day."

Ask whether the mother would like you to call the morning of the visit to ensure that the baby slept well and that the mother is prepared for the visit.

You will already have discussed any payment for research participation. In addition to payment for participation, we always offer to reimburse public transportation or a ride-hailing service. We also offer to provide child care for siblings in rooms near our laboratory or to reimburse babysitting. This information should be shared when recruiting parents for the study and included on your informed consent form.

Meeting on Campus

Not every campus has parking or transportation adjacent to the research site. It may be useful to provide written instructions or a simplified map. In any event, on the day of the visit, someone (other than the "Stranger") should meet the mother and baby at their car or other transportation. Every minute they spend looking for parking or your building is tiring and brings you closer to the baby's nap time. It is also stressful for the mother to have to find her way through crowds of students. Meeting the mother and baby where they arrive also affords an opportunity for the mother to become familiar with you. You may have described what to expect during a previous visit or during a phone call. You can refer to those previous conversations, as appropriate.

Lead researcher or assistant:

"Thanks for coming in today for our study. I'm going to walk with you to the building where we will be today. As we discussed before, we'll be seeing how [Baby's name] plays in different situations—with you in the room, without you, and with a new person. We'll talk about the details once we get settled. Many parents find this pretty interesting, because they get to see how their baby responds to a new environment and to new people, with and without them being there.

"So, how has the day been so far? How is everybody feeling today? Did [Baby's name] sleep on the drive over? Has he had a cold or been sick at all recently?"

If the child is fussy or very tired, you should offer the mother time to walk around or a place to relax while the baby settles. Sometimes the baby needs a diaper change. If that does not address the problem, a change of scenery or a walk outside can be very calming. Calling prior to the visit usually takes care of the possibility that a baby will be unable to participate as scheduled. Rarely, you may need to reschedule the SSP.

If you feel you need to reschedule, the mother may seem ambivalent. She may not want to disappoint you, or she may be hoping to avoid a second trip. Either way, assure her that this happens when you study babies. You may be able to reschedule the SSP. Or you may be able to complete your project without it. In either case, we always make whatever payment was agreed upon for the visit (and pay again, if the visit is rescheduled).

Explaining the Procedure to the Mother

Participating in research can be anxiety-provoking. Engaging in friendly conversation while escorting the mother to the laboratory will help her feel comfortable. General conversation about the study (general topic, how many participants, how far along the project is, etc.) is appropriate. However, avoid the specifics of the study or naming the variables you will be measuring lest this affect the mother's comfort level or behavior. And wait until everyone is settled in the laboratory before beginning to explain instructions you want the mother to remember.

Ordinarily, the SSP should be the first procedure you administer during a visit. The baby will probably remain sensitized for some time to the room in which the SSP was conducted and to the assistant who served as the "Stranger." So, you should plan to use different personnel and a different room for subsequent assessments.

Before beginning the procedure, you should explain again that the purpose of the SSP is to observe the baby's exploration, play, and social behavior in different contexts. This phrasing is easier for you, and for the mother, than offering up a summary of attachment theory. It also avoids giving the mother the (incorrect) impression that you are looking at or evaluating her.

Keep your explanation brief. Lengthy descriptions end up communicating less.

Lead researcher:

"We're interested in observing how your baby plays and responds in different situations. We'll have [Baby's name] play with some toys in a new room when you are present and when you are not in the room. We'll also see how [Baby's name] plays when a new person is in the room with him. Our procedure is supposed to mimic situations babies encounter all the time. Babies behave differently in situations like this. There really isn't anything your baby can do today that we haven't seen before. There is no right or wrong, just different styles. Anything your baby does is OK."

After providing this general introduction, provide the mother with instructions for her part in the procedure. Again, it is best to avoid lengthy instructions. A lot of detail can be overwhelming. The mother might feel uncomfortable or uncertain, afraid that she will spoil your work. You will get better data if instructions to the mother are simple and clear, and she understands that things do not have to go exactly as planned.

WRITTEN INSTRUCTIONS

Mary Ainsworth provided brief written instructions for the mothers to use during the SSP (Ainsworth et al., 1978/2015, Appendix I). Over the years we have settled on a much more informal approach that works well with the wide range of participants seen in contemporary research. There is not that much that the mother needs to do, and it can be signaled with a few knocks on the observation window.

Lead researcher:

"Let me walk you through the procedure step-by-step, so you will know how things unfold. Then I'll explain your part. To start, we're going to have you and the baby go in the room and get comfortable, and then play for a couple of minutes.

"Then we're going to have my helper [Stranger's name] come in, sit for a minute, chat with you for a minute, and then start some play with the baby for a minute. That is just to get everybody comfortable. I'll be signaling to her by knocking once on the observation window—those single knocks are just for her, so you can ignore them. Then I'll signal you to leave the room and let the baby and the visitor play. I'll signal you by knocking twice on the observation window—so just remember that the double-knock is your cue to leave. You can say 'Bye-bye' or just leave in whatever way is normal for you. Once you come out of the room, you'll be able to watch your baby with me [through the observation window, or on the video]. After a few minutes, you will return to the room. I'll explain before you return. Do you have any questions?"

As with all of our examples, do not try to memorize this. You will just sound mechanical and make the mother nervous. Just get the general tone—communicate to the mother that this is simple, and if she forgets or is unsure, there will always be someone at hand to remind her. Finally, do not try to explain all this while mother stands holding the baby or when the baby is wiggling around. Have a chair available for each of you. Sit down. Make sure the baby is under control. Then the mother can understand you. Do not hurry. Before you start explaining things, ask whether the baby needs a diaper change. You get more typical behavior from clean, comfortable babies.

Episode 1: Introducing Mother and Baby to the SSP Room and Toys

Take care of jackets, purses, anything that needs to be secured, before you introduce mother and baby into the SSP room. Do not let the baby bring a pacifier, favorite toy, and so forth, into the SSP room. There are plenty of interesting toys inside.

Episode 1 begins when you bring the mother and baby into the room and lasts only until they are settled, you give a few basic instructions, and leave the room; this usually takes less than 1 minute. Point out that the mother's chair and the stranger's chair are labeled with permanent marker (so the mother and stranger return to the correct places in later episodes).

Mary Ainsworth used to have the mother bring her purse and leave it during the first separation as a sign that she will be returning. Over time, we have dropped this. Most of the babies did not pay any attention to the purse or took mother's absence as a chance to open it up and spread everything around (which can spoil the reunion).

Invite the mother to interest the baby in the toys.

Lead researcher:

"So, for the next couple of minutes, you can let [Baby's name] play with these toys. You can respond to him, but let him play on his own if he is interested in the toys. I'll send my helper, [Stranger's name], in after a few minutes. She'll sit here quietly at first, talk to you for a bit, then play with your baby. I'll be signaling her with single knocks on the observation window. You can ignore all the single knocks. When you hear a double-knock, that will be your cue to leave the room. Just leave as you ordinarily would. Say "I'll be right back." Close the door as you leave and step around to watch through the window with me."

It does not matter whether the mother sits in her chair immediately or takes a minute on the floor to interest the baby in the toys. If she is still on the floor when the stranger enters, the stranger can casually invite her to "Have a seat."

Episode 2: Mother and Baby Acclimate to the SSP Room

Episode 2 begins when you leave the mother and baby in the SSP room and lasts 3 minutes. Make sure the door latches when you leave. This episode is an important baseline against which to compare the baby's behavior after reunions.

Episode 3: Stranger Enters, Gradually Engages Mother and Baby

Episode 3 begins when the stranger enters the room. Researchers often misunderstand the purpose of this episode and the function of the stranger. The stranger is not there to stress the baby. Quite the opposite—she is there so you can see additional facets of the baby's behavior and to soften the impact of the first separation. Most babies are less distressed when left with someone (even a stranger) than when they are left alone.

When the stranger first enters the room, she should go directly to her chair and sit quietly until she hears a single knock on the observation window. Some mothers will forget your instructions and try to initiate conversation. If this happens, the stranger can just say, pleasantly, "I'm supposed to wait for a knock."

After 1 minute, a *single (distinct) knock* on the observation window cues the stranger to start talking to the mother. The stranger should chat with the mother for the full minute. She can talk about the drive to the lab, how cute the baby is, and so forth. At some point during this brief conversation, it is also helpful for the stranger to remind the mother about what is coming next.

> **Stranger:**
>
> "In a little bit, we'll hear another knock and that will be my cue to play with [Baby's name]. Then, in about another minute, you'll hear a double-knock. The double-knock is your cue to go ahead and leave the room. Leave as you ordinarily would. You can say 'Bye-bye' if you like. You'll be able to watch through the observation window."

After the second minute, another *single knock* cues the stranger to start engaging the baby. The stranger should remain alert for these knocks while chatting with the mother or playing with the baby. If the mother begins to leave the room on a single knock, the stranger should just say, "That one is for me."

On the second single knock, the stranger will approach the baby (usually moving to the floor) and attempt to engage him/her in play. Most babies are eager to engage. A few will retreat to mother timidly. The stranger should be patient. Perhaps showing the baby a toy from a distance while naming it and showing gently how the toy works. It is useful for the stranger to be mindful of which toys interest the baby. This might prove useful later in the procedure.

Note: The point of sitting quietly and then talking to the mother is to avoid upsetting the baby by being too forward. Aside from this, it is not critical that the stranger wait a full minute to talk with the mother, or a full minute to interact with the baby. If the infant approaches and wants to interact, the stranger should be responsive; it could be off-putting to the baby if she did not respond. In any event, the episode will run for 3 minutes.

Episode 4: First Separation (Stranger Remains with Baby)

Episode 4 begins with a *double-knock* on the observation window, signaling the mother to leave. You or an assistant should be standing close to the door to make sure the baby does not leave the room and to make sure the door latches when the mother leaves. Show the mother where she can stand to watch her baby through the one-way window or on a monitor. If the mother does not hear her cue or is confused, the stranger can remind her that it is time for her to leave. (If the mother does not respond, repeat the double knock. If necessary, you can open the door a bit and say, "Mom can come out now.")

Mothers occasionally have difficulty leaving. The baby may cling to her or she may hesitate if the baby gets upset. If this happens, the stranger should try to facilitate the separation by offering toys or, if necessary, picking the baby up, carrying him around for a moment, then trying to interest him in a toy. Most of the time, the stranger can facilitate a successful separation by stepping in and saying:

> **Stranger (baby trying to prevent mother's departure):**
>
> "[Baby's name] seems upset. It is all right. Let me help you. [Reach for the baby. Then reassure the mother.] If he doesn't calm down shortly, we'll have you come right back."

Even a brief separation (when the mom steps out briefly, then back in) is better than no separation. In the very rare case that the mother finds she is not comfortable leaving her baby, it makes sense to end the procedure. Let her know that this is OK; that you don't want to get a baby too upset. Also let her know that these things happen; no harm done. Give the mother as much time as needed to calm the baby. Babies often calm down quickly once they have left the SSP room. (Rescheduling is not usually an option because the baby is likely to recognize the room on a second visit and become upset again.)

Note: The stranger's behavior during separation episodes is important. It is not her job to prevent/distract the baby from getting upset. Her normal mode is simply to be responsive if the baby engages. If the baby seems upset as, or after, the mother leaves the room, the stranger should allow his response to unfold. Scorers will want to know if the baby sat and cried, searched for mother, went to the door, or looked to the stranger for comfort. Once it is clear how the baby has responded to the separation, the stranger can remain in her chair, respond to the baby's bids to interact, or if he is clearly upset, try to comfort him and reinterest him in the toys. She should maintain her composure at all times. Sometimes an upset stranger will try to rush the comforting. She should be mindful that pressing toys on a crying baby may increase its distress. This complicates scoring. She should also remain alert for a prearranged "heads up" signal indicating (see below) that the mother is about to return.

When the mother has left the SSP room, invite her to watch the baby through the observation window (or on the video screen). Mothers differ in how they feel about their baby's response to the separation. Some mothers become anxious if their baby cries; others are disappointed if their baby does not cry. Some mothers seem agreeable to continuing the separation for the full 3 minutes, despite their baby's distress; others may want to return early. By being calm and normalizing the baby's response, you can keep the procedure running smoothly and ease the mother's discomfort. Commenting on good qualities of the baby's play or interaction, or asking whether the baby's behavior seems pretty typical, can make the mother feel more comfortable watching her baby for the first time through an observation window or on a computer monitor.

Lead researcher (with mother at observation window):

"So it looks like [Baby's name] is OK with [Stranger's name] for a few minutes. We'll see. If he starts crying, we might send you in a little sooner."

Two minutes into this first separation, walk the mother to the SSP door, remind her of her instructions, then, at 3 minutes, send her in for the first reunion. Make sure the door latches after mother reenters.

Lead researcher (after 3 minutes):

"OK, you will go in in just a moment. Knock on the door and call [Baby's name]. Then, step inside the door and close it behind you. Pause inside the door and hold your hands out like you are offering to pick him up. Greet him as you would normally. If he tries to get out of the room, you can pick him up, so he does not leave the room. If he wants to be picked up or seems a bit upset, you can pick him up, if that would help. Then try to get him interested in the toys again. In 3 minutes you will hear another double-knock, that will be your cue to leave again. You can step around and watch through the observation window [or on the computer monitor]."

ABBREVIATING THE FIRST SEPARATION

If, at any point during the first separation, the baby breaks into a sustained, hard cry, you need to evaluate the situation. Explain to the mother that you will watch briefly and perhaps send her back early.

Lead researcher (baby crying hard):

"So it looks like [Baby's name] is pretty upset. Do you think there is a chance he will calm down? If he continues crying, we will send you back in. We don't want him to get too upset."

Mothers often dismiss even hard crying as routine and say you should just carry on. Nonetheless, if the baby cries hard for 30 seconds, or the mother says he is not likely to calm down, or says she wants to return early, then abbreviate the episode. There is nothing to be learned from continued crying.

Moreover, if the baby gets too upset or exhausted from hard crying, it could interfere with the second separation–reunion sequence.

Note: The baby may fuss or stop and start crying over a period of time. The criterion here is 30 seconds of sustained hard crying. If the baby is upset enough that you decide to abbreviate the episode, you will need to alert the stranger that the mother is returning early, so she can make any necessary adjustments. Settle in advance on a prearranged "Mother is returning momentarily" signal (e.g., three knocks) that will not be mistaken for an instruction to leave. This will give the stranger time to release the baby, to get from between the baby and the door, or to clear the camera's view of the reunion. If the stranger were holding the baby on her lap (between crossed legs) when the mother returned, the baby would not be able to approach her. Obviously, lifting the baby to his feet just as the mother returns might cue an approach. Either interferes with scoring. An experienced stranger will avoid these problems.

Once you have given the stranger her "heads-up" signal, walk the mother to the SSP door, remind her of her instructions, then send her in. Make sure the door latches after mother reenters.

Lead researcher (if it looks like the baby will persist in hard crying):

"OK, let's have you return a little early. We don't want to get [Baby's name] too upset. Just knock on the door and call his name. Then, step inside the door and close it behind you. Pause inside the door and hold your hands out like you are offering to pick him up. [At 3 minutes (or straight away, if the episode is being abbreviated), tell the mother she can go in. If the baby is at the door, tell mother she can pick the baby up if necessary, to prevent him from leaving the room.]

"Greet him as you normally would and help him settle down. You can pick him up if that would help. See if he can eventually become interested in the toys again. After 3 minutes, we'll give you a double-knock. That will be your signal to leave again, just as you did before."

Episode 5: First Reunion and Stranger's Departure

Episode 5 begins when the mother returns from the first separation. The episode is scheduled for 3 minutes. You can extend it a minute or two, if necessary, so the baby can regain his composure.

Stranger's Behavior during Reunion

As mentioned earlier, the stranger must be mindful of her location when the mother enters the room. If the baby has not been upset during the separation, the stranger will already be in her chair. She should remain seated and not talk or make eye contact with the baby or do anything distracting with the toys until the reunion has occurred. It is important that the stranger not distract the baby while he is approaching the mother or when the mother is first holding and greeting or comforting the baby. This would interfere with scoring (particularly avoidance, which occurs primarily during the first 30 seconds of a reunion).

If the baby was upset during separation and the stranger is still holding him as the episode ends, you should, as mentioned earlier, give the stranger a "heads up" by knocking on the window. It is important that the baby be free to look at, interact with, or to go to his mother (or not). If necessary, the stranger can move the baby away from the door in advance of the reunion (though he might go right back). The stranger should not be at or near the door, or in the way of the camera, when the mother returns.

It is important that the baby not to be distracted from his mother by the stranger's leaving. If you are going to see scorable avoidance, it will occur in the first 30 seconds or so of the reunion. This is why it is important for the stranger to sit still; any movement can cause the baby to look away from the mother and make it difficult to accurately score avoidance. It is fine if it takes 30 seconds, or even a minute, for the stranger to effect her departure. It is better for her to leave a bit late than too early.

Ideally, the baby will be settled and back to exploration before it is time for the next separation. At the end of the 3 minutes, signal the mother to leave with a *double-knock* on the observation window.

Episode 6: Second Separation (Baby Alone)

Episode 6 begins when the mother departs for the second time, leaving the baby alone in the room. The episode is scheduled to last for 3 minutes. As before, if the baby cries hard for 30 seconds, ask the mother if she thinks he might calm down. Again, mothers are likely to minimize such crying. However, there is nothing to be learned from having a baby cry hard for longer than 30 seconds. You do not want the baby to become so distressed that he cannot greet or approach when the mother returns.

Send the stranger in after 3 minutes (or sooner if the baby has cried hard for a full 30 seconds).

Lead researcher:

"So it looks like [Baby's name] is OK right now. In a couple of minutes, I will send [Stranger's name] back in. Then, we'll watch for another 3 minutes. Then I'll send you back in."

If the baby is (or begins) crying hard, and it seems like it might continue for more than 30 seconds, ask the mother if the baby might calm down on his own.

Lead researcher:

"So it looks like [Baby's name] is pretty upset. If he continues crying, we'll send [Stranger's name] back in. Do you think he might calm down and return to the toys? If not, we will send [Stranger's name] back in a little early."

After 30 seconds of hard crying, or earlier if the mother says the baby is not likely to stop crying, you should abbreviate this episode by sending the stranger back in.

Lead researcher:

"So, [Baby's name] still seems pretty upset. Let's send [Stranger's name] back in a little early. We'll see if she can help [Baby's name] calm down. If not, then we'll send you back in."

Episode 7: Stranger Returns (Baby and Stranger)

Episode 7 begins when the stranger reenters the room. This episode will last 3 minutes, unless the child continues crying hard.

Lead researcher (to mother):

"Well it looks like [Baby's name] is doing OK with [Stranger's name]. We can watch from here for a few minutes and then we will send you back in. If necessary, we can send you back in a little early."

Stranger's Behavior

The stranger's behavior during Episode 7 is similar to her behavior during Episode 4. She should adjust her behavior to the baby's needs. If he is happy playing with the toys, she can stay on her chair. If the baby initiates interaction, she should be responsive. She should not intervene simply because the baby has followed the mother to the door and is fussing or calling for her. If he is mildly fussy, she might speak to him reassuringly or offer a toy. If the baby begins to cry, she can pick him up and try to comfort him.

After 2 minutes (or less, if the episode is to be abbreviated), give the stranger her "heads up" signal. Then walk the mother to the SSP door. Remind her of her instructions. Then send her in. Make sure the door latches after mother enters the SSP room.

Lead researcher (second reunion; no persistent, hard crying):

"OK, let's have you return in just a moment here. As before—knock on the door and call [Baby's name]. Then, enter the room and close the door behind you. Reach your arms out offering to pick him up. Then go ahead and pick him up for a moment, even if he doesn't come to you on his own. Then, you can help him get back into play. If he wants to interact with you or invites you to play, that's fine, too. When [Stranger's name] gets a chance, she will leave you and [Baby's name] in the room together. She and I will watch for 3 minutes and then we're all finished."

Or, if you abbreviate the episode, tell the mother that you are going to send her back in. Reassure her that the procedure has been a good one and there is no reason she and her baby should be separated any longer.

Lead researcher (second reunion; abbreviated due to persistent hard crying):

"OK, it doesn't look like [Baby's name] is going to calm down with [Stranger's name]. We can have you return now. This has already been a good session, and there is no reason for anyone to stay upset any longer."

Give the stranger her "heads-up" signal. Then, walk the mother to the SSP door. Remind her of her instructions, then send her in. Make sure the door latches after she enters the SSP room.

Lead researcher:

"As before, knock on the door and call [Baby's name]. Then, enter the room and close the door behind you. Reach your arms out, offering to pick him up. Then go ahead and pick him up. Then, you can help him get back into play. If he wants to talk or share toys with you, that's fine, too. [If the baby is at the door, do as indicated earlier, adding that the mother can pick the baby up if he tries to leave the room.]

"When [Stranger's name] gets a chance, she will leave you and [Baby's name] in the room together. She and I will watch for 3 minutes and then we're all finished."

Stranger's Behavior during Reunion

As noted earlier, the stranger's behavior during reunions is very important. She should be alert for the mother's return. On your warning signal (a single knock), she should put the baby down if she is carrying him. If she is sitting on the floor holding the baby, she should release him as soon as she hears the "heads up" signal, so the baby is not trapped in her lap or cued to approach when mother enters. As before, she should make sure she is not between the baby and the door or the camera when mother enters. It is important that the stranger not distract the baby during the first 30 seconds or so of the reunion. She should not try to leave while the mother and baby are still at the door.

Episode 8: Second Reunion (Mother and Baby; Stranger Exits)

Episode 8 begins when the mother enters the room for the second reunion. Follow the same procedure as for Episode 5 with regard to signals to the stranger. As in Episode 5, the stranger should not leave until she can do so without interrupting the reunion (even if it takes half a minute or more).

This final episode ordinarily lasts 3 minutes (from the mother's entry into the room). At that point, the lead researcher and the stranger can enter the SSP room, very informally, and let the mother know that the procedure is finished.

Lead researcher:

"[addressing baby] OK, we're all finished! [And to the mother] Thank you so much for coming this morning/afternoon. He was so good! [and] We really appreciate your interest in our study. [Perhaps address the baby again.] We're sorry we put you through all this. [or] You have really had enough of this room haven't you? Come on, we'll all go outside."

This informal interaction affords the mother a transition from being observed. At this point, you might ask the mother if this seemed like pretty typical behavior, whether anything surprised her, and so forth. And ask whether she has any questions.

Very rarely, a baby will persist (beyond 30 seconds) in hard crying despite the mother's return. In this event, give the mother additional time (up to the full 3 minutes) to calm him. Unlike separation episodes with hard crying, you would not ordinarily abbreviate this episode, unless the mother indicates she wants to take the infant out of the SSP room. Most babies calm down promptly, once they are out of the SSP room and see that mother is retrieving coats and other baby gear.

Lead researcher (continues):

"[To the mother] Thank you so much for coming this morning/afternoon! [and] This was great. We really appreciate your interest in our study, [etc.] [Perhaps address the baby again.] What did you think when mommy left, huh?" [or] You were a brave little one today! [or] Feel better now? [or] You've really had enough of this room, haven't you? Come on, we'll all go outside."

Concluding the SSP

Although only the first 3 minutes of this reunion are scored, it can be useful to continue filming a bit longer, even as the researchers enter the SSP room, to give the baby time to settle and perhaps show renewed interest in the toys. After this, we have our videographer join us in the SSP room. This signals to the mother that the procedure is indeed over. Although the procedure per se is over, your professionalism, and that of your assistants and any student observers, is on display until the mother and baby leave campus.

At this point, you may have some paperwork to complete with the mother. Ask if she would like some coffee or if she needs to change or feed the baby. You may need to take time to discuss other aspects of her participation in your research. Finally, we always accompany research participants back to their car or wait with them until their transportation arrives.

FREQUENTLY ASKED QUESTIONS

In this final section we address some of the most frequently asked questions (FAQs) raised by students and colleagues intending to use the SSP. Most often, questions are framed in terms of "Am I allowed to do *x, y, z*?" Or, perhaps a little more often, "This is what I've done; was it OK?" Rather than yes or no answers, we try to provide information about how to think about attachment and the SSP, and let the answers follow from there. As is customary, let us concede at the outset that these are our answers. There are no official answers (who would decide?). We have sought input from colleagues, but we alone are responsible for what the reader finds here. Over the years, we have more or less settled into the advice and opinions below. Nonetheless, we reserve the right to improve on them in light of new ideas and information.

1 What is the relationship between "attachment" and attachment behavior? For this we can hardly do better than quote Mary Ainsworth (1967) from *Infancy in Uganda:*

> Attachment is manifested through these patterns of behavior [referring to her list of 16 attachment-related behavior patterns on p. 332], but the patterns do not themselves constitute the attachment. Attachment is internal. . . . We can conceive of attachment as somehow being built into the nervous system, in the course of and as a result of the infant's experience of his transactions with his mother and with other people. This internalized something that we call attachment has aspects of feelings, memories, wishes, expectations, and intentions, all of which constitute an inner program acquired through experience and somehow built into a flexible yet retentive inner mechanism which serves as a filter for the reception and interpretation of inner experience and as a kind of template shaping the nature of the outward response. (pp. 429–430)

2 What does *attachment security* mean? Answers to FAQs about the SSP are often rooted in or depend on a coherent answer to this question. The term *secure attachment* (or securely attached) is occasionally taken to mean "tightly attached," as in "the rope was securely attached to the dock." This is a misunderstanding. Both John Bowlby and Mary Ainsworth referred to security as the emotional accompaniment to an infant's appraisal of risk or danger. Indeed, Ainsworth often pointed to the etymology of the term (Latin, *sine cura*—without care) for the sense of the concept. They meant especially appraisals in light of expectations about a primary caregiver's availability, responsiveness, and efficacy. Today, the term is often used (often implicitly) to mean little more than "generally well adjusted." Moreover, it has taken on different meanings/connotations in theory, empirical research, psychotherapy, media, and child welfare (Duschinsky, 2020). Unfortunately, this does not provide the guidance needed for measurement design or validation.

The key insights underlying modern attachment theory arose from John Bowlby's observation that human infants do not behave like the clingy dependent creature imagined in psychoanalysis and learning theory. Instead, they combine a wide range of behaviors with continuous monitoring of their external and internal environment and state, and information about their mothers' past and current behavior, in order to explore their environment while maintaining a degree of access to her as a source of information and, as required, a haven of comfort/safety (Waters et al., 2015).

Within this framework, "attachment security" can be understood as referring to confidence or certainty, or positive expectation regarding an attachment figure's availability and responsiveness in the context of exploration or seeking comfort/safety. Indeed, German-speaking attachment researchers employ the term *sicherheit,* which has etymological links to *certainty* as well as to *trust* (e.g., Grossmann & Grossmann, 2017). H. Waters and Waters (2006) and H. Waters, Waters, and Waters (2021) have suggested that mental representations of secure base experience play a significant role in generating and generalizing such expectations and the emotions they engender when they are confirmed or violated.

In designing measures of attachment development and individual differences, it is useful to think of attachment behavior as a skill rather than a trait. In addition to reflecting its inherent complexity, this perspective connects attachment theory with the extensive psychological research on skills and skill acquisition (e.g., Attri, 2018; Fridland & Pavese, 2020). In turn, this suggests fruitful empirical approaches to causation, information processing, development, validation, and intervention.

3 To what does the term *secure base phenomenon* refer? Again, we can turn to Mary Ainsworth. In *Infancy in Uganda* (1967, pp. 345–347), she described "use of the mother as a secure base for exploration" and "flight to the mother as a haven of safety." She described secure base use as follows:

> Once an infant is able to crawl, it does not always stay close to the mother but rather make little excursions away from her, exploring other objects and interacting with other people, but returning to the mother from time to time. The mother seems to provide a secure base from which these excursions may be made without anxiety. The child who is attached to his mother, if he is secure in this attachment, does not need to maintain constant proximity or contact with her. He is content to move away, as long as he knows that she is there. He can even leave the room on his own initiative, and his aplomb in so doing is sometimes in sharp contrast to his consternation when his secure base gets up and moves off. Indeed, one could scarcely identify this as a pattern of attachment were it not for the fact that the child still is concerned about his mother's whereabouts. (p. 345)

Subsequently, she emphasized the close relation between these two behavior patterns, noting that aside from speed and absence of delight, it is primarily context rather than specific behaviors that distinguish exploratory approaches from retreat to a safe haven. She captured their intercoordination in her concept of the attachment–exploration balance. Attachment researchers have occasionally understood this in terms of the two behavioral systems alternately switching on and off at transitional points in attachment–exploration cycles. Of course, this raises the question, how does the attachment system know when to initiate approach unless it is actively monitoring the mother's availability even during excursions away from her? Thus, it is more useful to view both proximity seeking and exploration as behavioral systems that can serve the goals of a superordinate attachment system. (See FAQ 4, below)

Finally, when asked about the secure base phenomenon, we routinely highlight work by Crowell et al. (2002) illustrating the relevance of the secure base concept as a framework for understanding problem-solving interactions in adult relationships. There is no better illustration of attachment as an integrative lifespan perspective.

4 Are attachment and exploration one system or two? Most attachment literature associates proximity seeking when distressed with an attachment system and proximity in the absence of threat (e.g., seeking information, help, new opportunities to explore or play) with a different, exploratory system. Although this is a fair reading of the attachment literature, it seems to us out of date. Waters (2002/2008) has argued that Bowlby overestimated attachment as a predator-avoidance system and underestimated the evolutionary significance of the exploratory system. Simply put, most of our predator problems would not be materially changed by running to our mommy. In general, the dangers we handle best are those we avoid in the first place. Given our size, lack of speed, and delicate structure, we were better off depending on foresight, learning the habits of predators, and group living than retreating to an attachment figure to avoid predators.

One of the key components of any species evolutionary endowment is its "life history strategy"—how it solves the problem of when to be born, when to mature, how much to invest in offspring, and when to die. An extraordinarily long period of immaturity is one of the most distinctive features of the human evolutionary endowment. Generally considered a precondition and an accommodation to our complex brain and highly flexible behavior patterns, growing up slowly is very much at the center of growing up human. It is how we build a nervous system and behavioral repertoire adapted to our experience. Our capacity to form and maintain long-term relationships that support learning, as well as survival, helps us turn prolonged immaturity into a prolonged apprenticeship. Here, as much or more than in protection from predators, we see the evolutionary significance of secure base relationships for human development. The ability to prosper in a human society requires years, decades, of learning, experience, and supervision.

If both seeking the mother as a haven of safety and exploration from her as a secure base depend on the mother's presence, and both offer evolutionary advantages, what can be said in favor of conceptualizing them as distinct systems? Clearly, there are species in which the young engage in haven-of-safety behavior but not exploration from a secure base, and vice versa. This makes the point that in some species, at some point(s) in evolutionary history, they were separate systems. Yet a behavior's evolutionary significance can change over time. In addition, it seems likely that each has arisen independently, through convergent evolution, in more than one species at different times. However, this does not seal the argument for treating them as distinct systems in humans. After all, few, if any, of the species that show only safe haven behavior or exploration from a secure base form enduring monogamous bonds in adulthood. This rather limits the strength of arguments from such examples to the human case.

Sroufe and Waters (1977) have argued against prejudging the attachment relevance of a particular behavior without taking into account the physical, behavioral, and affective context in which it occurs. We have proximity seeking and exploratory behavior—both complex behavior patterns, both available to a variety of superordinate motivational systems or goals. In addition, evolution has provided humans with the ability to coordinate proximity and exploratory systems that exist independently in other species. From an attachment perspective, this intercoordination would seem to be the key evolutionary innovation. Why not then conceptualize "attachment" as a superordinate system that can coordinate both proximity seeking and exploratory behavior over time and contexts?

The notion that attachment refers to a system that intercoordinates proximity seeking and exploration, rather than to either system alone, has important implications for attachment theory and measurement. It is generally consistent with the systems framework presented in Bowlby's *Attachment* trilogy and suggests an interesting architecture for computational modelling (see Petters, 2019). It also avoids a bit of a paradox in convergent validity data on attachment assessments from different contexts. Simply put, if seeking a haven of safety is prototypical attachment behavior and exploration is a distinct system, the antithesis of attachment, then we would hardly expect clear convergence among measures from *emergency*, distress-laden contexts (e.g., SSP reunions; later portions of the Adult Attachment Interview [AAI]) and *ordinary* contexts (e.g., naturalistic home observations; early portions of the AAI; the Secure Base Script Assessment). Yet this is exactly what we find. Indeed, why would Mary Ainsworth have devoted so much of her observation time in Uganda and Baltimore to ordinary, largely nonstressful settings if attachment plays out primarily in emergency, threat-laden contexts? The fact that we can glean useful information from both ordinary and emergency contexts suggests we should not privilege either system/context over the other in terms of attachment relevance or measurement.

5 **What does the SSP measure, and how do we know?** Early attachment theorists conceptualized individual differences in terms of the onset

and "strength" of attachment bonds. However, by the time Mary Ainsworth was conducting her Baltimore longitudinal study, she was discarding both concepts as theoretically unsatisfactory and empirically inaccessible. Instead, she focused on an infant's ability to use its mother as a secure base at home. Increasingly, we prefer to describe the SSP as a measure of *the extent to which an infant skillfully and consistently uses a particular figure as a secure base for exploration and retreat for comfort or safety in naturalistic settings (usually at home or on excursions with the attachment figure)*. This is closer to the empirical validation criteria. It also reflects attachment theory's roots in descriptive ethology and has clear implications for further validation studies, extensions of the SSP to new age groups and populations, and to testable research hypotheses. Ainsworth validated SSP classifications against observations of secure base behavior at home (Ainsworth et al., 1978/2015, Table 20). The table reporting these results deserves careful study. Vaughn and Waters (1990) replicated this link using the Attachment Q-set.

To be sure, correlations with theoretically relevant variables (e.g., other facets of social development, mental representations, and adjustment in infancy and across age) also point to the validity of the SSP. However, taken alone, any pattern of correlates is open to alternative explanations. Even with such correlates, the SSP could hardly claim strong ties to Bowlby's and Ainsworth's work without links to secure base use in naturalistic settings. Correlations with external variables can also provide valuable information about discriminant validity. That is, demonstrating independence from variables that offer alternative interpretations. For example, the SSP has repeatedly demonstrated good discriminant validity vis-à-vis cognitive ability in concurrent and predictive data (Ainsworth et al., 1978/2015, p. 159). See also FAQ 9, below regarding temperament.

Occasionally, authors, especially experts from other disciplines, have understood the SSP as *the* attachment situation, as if specific behaviors are attachment-related or valid indicators of attachment security simply because they were observed in the SSP. In fact, Ainsworth was unambiguous on this point: The criterion is the life the infant lives, not what it does in 20 minutes in the laboratory. If an infant uses its mother skillfully and consistently across time and context in naturalistic settings, it can only be described as "secure," regardless of its classification in the SSP. Similarly, secure base difficulties at home denote attachment insecurity, regardless of behavior in the SSP.

6 How closely do I have to replicate the physical setup described in *Patterns of Attachment*? It should be clear from the preceding section, SSP Pratique, that there is more to an SSP assessment than simply replicating the physical setup. That said, the physical setup is an important factor in how infants experience the procedure and the scorability of the observations. In general, let your understanding of the secure base phenomenon and the attachment exploration balance be your guide. Avoid gratuitous departures form Ainsworth's setup. At the same time, learn from innovations (especially in recording technology) that have worked well for others.

- *Test room.* Mary Ainsworth conducted the SSP in a 9′ × 9′ test room with an adjacent observation room. Of course, she was using a pair of observers to make simultaneous audio recordings of the behavior in the test room. Today a 9′ × 9′ room would be a bit small, because it places the participants quite close to the camera and requires more panning to follow the action. At the other extreme, the room should not be so large that infants find a great deal of space to explore behind the mother's and the stranger's chairs. Aside from chairs blocking the camera's line of sight, and the temptation to zoom in and out as the action moves to different parts of the room, the primary risk is that a very large room could introduce great variety in the distance between the infant and mother during reunions. As mentioned in the previous section, less camera movement is better. Ideally, you want the door to open inward, so the infant is less likely to go out of camera view when its mother or the stranger enters. Ideally, the door should open toward the camera. This helps keep the infant in view when reunions occur right at the door. These are very practical matters. They have little to do with attachment theory.

  Aside from such practical considerations, the exact size of the room is not critical. It just needs to be large enough for the mother's and the stranger's chairs to be 6–8 feet apart (so that being with the stranger entails being away from the mother), and far enough from the door to allow infants to greet and approach the mother across a distance during reunion episodes. The room should also be large enough that participants can be kept entirely within the video frame without repeated panning and zooming.

- *Camera port.* Recording video through a window has several disadvantages. First, it requires using a tripod, which necessarily puts the camera several feet farther away from the participants and reduces the angle of view. This makes it difficult to record behavior below the window frame. In addition, some older cameras may have trouble focusing through a window pane. Finally, the camera is likely to capture reflections off the window glass. It is far preferable to have a port through a wall adjacent to the door. Ideally, this would be in a wall between the SSP test room and an adjacent observation room. The bottom of the port should be approximately 3 feet above the floor. Framing the inside of the opening with wood provides a base on which to mount a tripod head; this will allow the camera to pan left and right, as well as up and down. You can avoid the infant seeing observers through the port with a cloth baffle. Simply cut four isosceles triangles from a length of black felt fabric and sew the edges together to make a tapering sack (baffle). Attach the wide (open) end to the wall around the viewing port and tripod head. Cut the narrow (closed) end of the sack to create an opening to accommodate the camera lens. Secure it around the end of your camera (or lens) with rubber bands. The baffle should be deep enough to allow the camera to pan the full width of the room. It may be necessary to make some sort of adjustment to keep the baffle from rubbing on the camera microphone when panning.

Keep in mind that felt fabric will not do much to muffle noise from the observation room. We have generally found that the microphones on today's consumer cameras are quite good. So it is rarely necessary to mount a microphone within the test room. However, most camera microphones pick up noise from any direction. So it is important to keep sounds from the observation area to a minimum. To this end, it is useful to move away from the camera when talking with the mother or giving instructions to the stranger.

- *Lighting.* Most consumer video cameras today work quite well in low light. Overhead fluorescent lighting is usually fine. Most cameras have a white-balance adjustment to compensate for any tint introduced by fluorescent lighting. It is also useful to avoid sharp contrast between the brightness of flooring/carpet and the walls opposite the camera. This minimizes the overall image constantly going from bright to dark as the camera captures more of the floor or more of the wall.

- *Chairs and toys.* The room should be equipped with two chairs, one for the mother and one for the stranger. It can be useful to identify the mother's chair with a letter "M" in tape or permanent marker to ensure that she returns to the same location after each separation. There should also be a set of 10–12 simple, age-appropriate toys. Examples of appropriate toys include a shape sorter, stacking rings/cups, push toys (e.g., cars), plastic animals or dolls, and so forth. Toys to avoid include those that invite very vigorous play (e.g., kick balls, anything with a long handle), electronic toys that play music or make loud noise, and toys that have small or detachable parts that pose a choking risk. It is also useful to ask the mother if her child owns any of the toys you have supplied and, if so, to replace them before the SSP. The infants should be encountering novel items, not favorite playthings. We often purchase duplicate toys so they can be replaced before they show much wear or are broken. Finally, it is important to clean the toys with disinfectant wipes and to keep the floor/carpet free of visible dirt or small items. Many mothers will appreciate knowing that you have taken these steps.

In the end, the key is not reproducing Mary Ainsworth's SSP setup exactly; it is to present infants with the kind of *experience* Mary Ainsworth created. Infants should be able to explore away from mother in several directions, retreat from the stranger to the mother, make clear approaches across the room to the mother during reunion episodes, and generally show willingness or unwillingness to explore away from mother on their own initiative, while remaining close enough to her to signal or interact with her across a distance, or achieve contact promptly, if needed. This does not require a 9′ × 9′ room, or preclude a larger room. Just keep open the option of making changes if you can see that your setup is not working.

7 Are there guidelines for good SSP videography? When Mary Ainsworth was recruiting her Baltimore sample, most 8 mm film equipment recorded less than 15 minutes of behavior (without sound). In addition, it usually required supplementary lighting, which generated a lot of heat and cast sharp shadows. Film was expensive to develop and duplicate, and editing was very time consuming. Accordingly, she relied primarily on pairs of observers to narrate rapid, independent play-by-play descriptions that were recorded on office dictating equipment and transcribed. Thus, there is no mention of videography in *Patterns of Attachment* or in Ainsworth's research reports.

Today, consumer video equipment is quite capable. It easily captures hours of behavior (with sound). Digital recordings are inexpensive and easily copied, edited, and even annotated. Moreover, consumer video cameras are compact and quite easy to operate. Thus, it is surprising how often poor videography creates difficulties for scoring SSP data and makes it difficult to compile good materials for illustrating and teaching SSP technique and scoring. A good rule of thumb or goal for SSP video is that *the recording process should be invisible to the viewer.* Scorers (or trainees/audiences) should be able to see what they need and expect to see, without the distraction of inelegant camera work.

Most video problems arise because the videographer is (1) unfamiliar with the perspective on behavior outlined in the previous section, (2) unaware of the information coders need in order to make key scoring decisions, (3) prone to unnecessary zooming and panning, and/or (4) attracted to information such as close-up facial expressions that have little significance for scoring. Once recognized, these problems are easily remedied.

The best videographers are interested in behavior and invested in doing a good job. Videographers should understand how much depends on their work. They are *key* personnel. Videography is a bit of a vigilance task. For long stretches it can seem like nothing is happening. A naive videographer may be inattentive or try to make the task more interesting by focusing on the mother or the stranger while the infant is exploring, or zooming in to capture the details of facial expressions. The more a videographer understands about what he or she is looking at and how it will be used, the easier it is to stay engaged.

The first part of this chapter (on seeing behavior) should help videographers understand their task. As should basic familiarity with the scoring appendices in *Patterns of Attachment.* It is useful to show a new videographer examples and provide commentary on well-done recordings from previous or pilot SSPs. It is also helpful to have videographers sit in on a few scoring sessions in order to gain a sense for what the scorers need and where they have difficulties. This is also an opportunity for scorers to point out where a videographer's technique has been especially helpful or could be more so.

The following dos and don'ts may seem obvious but we have encountered problems related to each of them.

DOs

✓ Arrive early. Behave professionally. Have equipment tested and ready to go before the mother and infant arrive. If you do not understand something, it is important to get it clarified as soon as possible. Ask whether your recordings are proving scorable and whether there are any problems. Remember this maxim: Data quality depends more on the videographer than on the equipment.

✓ Learn how to use your camera's controls and indicators. You do not have to become an expert, but you should be familiar with basic functions and settings. It is rarely true that "all you have to do is point and shoot." Familiarize yourself with power, zoom, focus, audio, and so forth through practice before you start recording real data. Some functions, such as autofocus, can be quite useful, but they may depend on good lighting. They may have to be turned off if you are shooting through a glass window, to prevent the camera from focusing on the glass rather than targets in the room. Similarly, auto-volume control and auto-brightness sometimes produce relatively useless, but distracting, adjustments while you are recording. It is sometimes better to turn them off and set levels manually. Some settings, such as "white-balance," may be unfamiliar but can be quite useful.

✓ If possible, use line (plug-in) power rather than battery. It is just too easy to overlook a low battery and lose power at a critical moment. When using line power, tape the entire length of the power cord to the floor with duct tape. This avoids someone tripping over the cord in the dark and (1) injuring themselves, (2) distracting participants in the test area, and/or (3) pulling the power cable out of its socket.

✓ Make sure you can tell what the infant is doing if he or she is playing close to the wall on which the camera is mounted. If objects to the left or right, or below the camera, are out of sight, a wide-angle lens adaptor might be helpful.

✓ Monitor sound through an earphone throughout the SSP to make sure you are recording sound as well as video. This also lets you know whether the felt baffle hiding the camera lens is rubbing across the microphone and needs to be pushed away.

✓ Train someone as a backup videographer in case you are unavailable.

✓ During recording, think of yourself as communicating with the researchers who will be scoring your recording. Ask yourself what the scorers need.

✓ Permanently identify each video record by writing the participant's ID number, the date, and the child's first name and birthdate on a sheet of paper or a whiteboard before the participants arrive, and have an assistant inside the test area display this to the camera for 15–20 seconds at the beginning of the video record. This prevents losing track of the participant's identity in the event paper labels become faded or lost.

✓ When recording, try to keep the whole infant in the frame most of the time. Focusing too closely on the upper body or facial expressions will miss small but significant movements (e.g., tension movements or kicks while being held). The infant does not have to be centered in the frame. Maintain enough margin ahead of the infant to make context clear and to anticipate quick moves that would put it out of frame. This also reduces the need to move the camera in response to inconsequential moves. SSP scoring rarely depends on closely zoomed shots.

✓ You can pan quickly from the infant to the mother and back to show scorers where the mother is and whether she is making inviting gestures or offering a toy over a distance. Think of these as footnotes to the scorer. Pan, hold for a count, "1-2," and back to the infant. The scorer should not lose track of the infant's behavior. Much of the information about what he or she is doing over a distance can be picked up from the audio or from a pan to her after the infant has responded.

✓ Move the camera as little as possible. If you have the infant in the frame (whether in the middle of the room playing, at the mother's chair, or at the door) with some buffer area ahead of him or her, that is fine. Keep pans to a minimum; zooms near zero.

✓ Make a "footnote pan" to show key transitions in the procedure. For example, you do not need to track the mother walking across the room to leave, or keep the camera on the door, waiting for her to return. But make sure that the scorers can tell when she has left and when she returns. If the stranger delays leaving the room for some reason and is not in camera view, a quick pan and return to the infant will let the scorers know; otherwise, a look toward the stranger might be interpreted as looking away from the mother.

✓ Be sure to capture the infant's reaction to reunions. The details of an infant's response to the mother's departure are not a major factor in scoring. In contrast, some scoring (particularly avoidance of physical contact and interaction) depends critically on the infant's behavior as the mother enters and during the next 15–30 seconds. Scorers must have this in full. Other important behaviors during reunion episodes play out over the full 3 minutes; these often involve behavior when the infant is being held or squirming to be put down. Much of the key behavior, too, can be fleeting. Tight close-ups during reunion risk losing important information about posture, efforts to be put down, kicks, and so forth. Again, it can be useful for videographers to sit in on some SSP scoring in order to understand what scorers are looking for.

✓ If the infant attempts to touch the camera lens, keep it motionless; there is a chance he or she will lose interest. If the infant grasps the baffle or the camera lens, turn it all the way to one side and hold it firmly until the infant can be interested in something else. If the stranger is present, she should try to direct the infant's attention to the toys. If necessary, the videographer should speak to the mother through the camera port: "Please try to interest him (or her) in the toys." The less you move the camera, the less likely you are to attract the infant's attention in the first place. Locating the camera port approximately 3 feet above the floor and mounting the camera lens 5–6 inches above this, along with a dark cloth baffle around the lens, affords a good video angle and rarely attracts the attention of 1-year-olds. If you are working with older children, locate the camera port (or have a second port) somewhat higher.

✓ Back up your recordings and keep the backups separate from the originals! If you record to a computer hard drive or to a solid-state memory card inserted into your camera, it is a trivial matter to make copies—immediately or on a schedule. Extra media are inexpensive and there is no loss of quality in copying digital recordings.

DON'Ts

✗ Don't get bored. Stay in the game. Equipment or procedures can go off the rails at any time. Lapses risk compromising scoring. Often, there is no way to know if something is important until after the SSP is complete and scoring begins.

✗ Don't let backlighting create overly dark images. Most video cameras automatically reduce sensitivity in response to bright light. As a consequence, anyone located near or passing in front of the light source will be rendered as a dark silhouette with few details. Unless they are very high on the wall, windows to the outside should be covered with foam-core or aluminum foil, or opaque paint.

✗ Don't make noise. The infant can hear movements and conversations through the camera port. These may upset or attract him or her to the camera.

✗ Don't zoom so close that you cannot see the context in which behavior occurs.

8 Does the SSP entail any special problems related to informed consent? During her Baltimore study, Mary Ainsworth avoided media coverage of her work in order to avoid biasing recruitment or prompting participants to raise questions for which, at this early stage in her work, she did not have answers. Interestingly, she was thinking in terms of local media. National media were the farthest thing from her mind and, of course, there was no Internet or video recording. (See below for discussion of privacy issues.)

It has been quite some time since we heard of anyone's institutional review board having significant reservations about the SSP per se. Informed consent is another matter. There are clearly issues here regarding the use of video records in the months and years after the procedure. The narrowest informed consent documents simply outline the procedure and risks, and ask the parents to indicate that they agree to participate. In our experience, it suffices to explain that the mother (or other caregiver) and infant will be videotaped during a series of 3-minute episodes that allow you to observe (1) mother and infant together in a room with age-appropriate toys, (2) play with a female research assistant (in the mother's presence), (3) play with the female research assistant alone, and (4) two episodes in which mother leaves the infant alone or with the female research assistant while she watches with the experimenter through a one-way observation window or on a computer monitor. Explain that each of the episodes is designed to mimic situations a 1-year-old encounters regularly in everyday life. Explain also that approximately 50% of infants cry during one or both separation episodes and that the separations will be concluded if the infant cries continuously for 30 seconds, or upon the mother's request. It is also relevant that the SSP has been in use in Western cultures for over four decades without a single published report of an adverse effect. In other cultures it is wise to have pilot data on the suitability of SSP (see Meehan & Hawkes, 2013).

We find it helpful to mail or e-mail mothers a copy of our approved informed consent letter in advance of the SSP. We explain that we will gladly answer any questions they have about the procedure. We also explain that mothers need not memorize the details in the consent form, that we will review it with them and remind them of the procedures when they visit campus.

More difficult issues have to do with the scope of informed consent. As explained earlier, we favor a very descriptive account of the SSP when soliciting participants' informed consent. In our view, a somewhat broader formulation is required if the recordings from the SSP are to be used for educational purposes (i.e., training and/or teaching). In fact, training and teaching raise rather different issues, especially regarding confidentiality. Training is often limited to a small number of students within one laboratory, who must be instructed in their professional responsibilities regarding confidentiality. Confidentiality is even more complicated in light of the ease with which video materials can be posted (even without the researchers' permission) on the Internet.

The issue of privacy/confidentiality is complicated by the fact that students and research samples are often drawn from the same community. Thus, one or more students might be able to identify participants from SSP recordings. We cannot hold a student who identifies a research participant in class to the level of professional responsibility we assume for faculty and research trainees. The privacy issue here is best addressed by editing the recordings to obscure the mother's identity. Short of this, one can obtain SSP examples from a different community or from SSP material recorded years or decades earlier.

A final issue has to do with what, exactly, parents have agreed to even if the informed consent includes training and instruction, and even broadcast applications. The problem is that although they are aware of their own behavior, and thus have a sense of what might have been recorded, they have no idea what might be said in commentary attached to the video after their participation has ended. Researchers should be alert to the difficult issues this raises and keep in mind that Mary Ainsworth's scoring for the SSP assesses *normal individual differences*. Inferences to clinical issues require a broader assessment.

9 **Do SSP classifications measure temperament?** The idea that SSP classifications reflect infant temperament rather than confidence in a specific caregiver is rooted in the mistaken (and inexplicably persistent) belief that the SSP's secure versus insecure distinction maps closely onto crying versus not crying during the separation episodes (e.g., Chess & Thomas, 1982; Kagan, 1982). The case against this hypothesis is decisive (e.g., Sroufe, 1985). This is not to say that an eye attuned to temperament might not see some useful clues in the course of the SSP. It is, after all, a relatively rich behavior sample across a variety of contexts. Our point is merely that temperament variance is pretty much invisible when the SSP is viewed through the lens of Mary Ainsworth's interactive behavior scales and the ABC classification system.

Consider the evidence. First of all, about half of secure infants (mostly B_3 and B_4) and a similar proportion of insecure infants (mostly C's but also some A_2) cry during the separation episodes. (Interestingly, secure (B) infants cry significantly *less* than either group A or group C at home, with less crying associated with more sensitive and responsive care. This is not what temperament theorists imagine in the SSP and is the opposite of what we would expect if secure infants were temperamentally inclined to negative affect.) Second, temperament theory posits stable individual differences in behavioral/emotional style across contexts. Yet infants' SSP classifications with the mother and with the father are not significantly related (e.g., Main & Weston, 1981; Grossmann, Grossmann, Huber, & Wartner, 1981). Surely, an infant's temperament is not different when interacting with different partners. Yet different experiences with different partners can well lead to different expectations about availability and responsiveness. Third, SSP security moderates a wide range of links between temperament and socialization outcomes (Vaughn & Shin, 2011). Obviously, a variable cannot moderate itself. Finally, aside from modest correlations between SSP security and positive affect, SSP classifications are not significantly correlated with widely used temperament assessments (Vaughn, Bost, & van IJzendoorn, 2008). The modest correlation with positive affect simply reflects that infants who experience more sensitive and responsive care engage in fewer contentious interactions. In brief, though there may be some temperament correlates of specific behavior in the SSP, the ABC classifications do not measure temperament.

10 **Are SSP classifications stable across time?** Beginning in the late 1960s, the stability of individual differences in general was a major point of contention between traditional personality/developmental psychologists and learning theorists influenced by Walter Mischel's landmark critique, *Personality and Assessment* (1968). Particularly relevant for attachment theorists, Masters and Wellman (1974) published a detailed analysis and critique of attachment stability data in *Psychological Bulletin.* Their conclusion, that attachment behavior is not stable over months, days, or even minutes, was consistent with Mischel's broad critique of the individual-differences paradigm and could have been a decisive blow to attachment research. Sroufe and Waters (1977) detailed the limitations of counting discrete behaviors and the advantages of taking an organizational perspective instead. Shortly thereafter, Waters (1978) replicated Masters and Wellman's (1974) results in data from 50 infants seen in the SSP at 12 months and again at 18 months. He then scored the same data using Mary Ainsworth's interactive behavior scales and ABC classifications, and found significant stability in the full range of variables. The results in the data Masters and Wellman (1978) reviewed were artifacts of observing discrete behavior, ignoring context, and sampling too briefly to obtain reliable estimates of infants' typical behavior. Subsequently, attachment stability has been examined in nearly 30 studies. A meta-analysis indicates that "attachment security is moderately stable across the first 19 years of life" (Fraley, 2002, p. 123). In addition, multivariate modeling suggested that the data are best explained in terms of an early prototype that is activated in the context of new experiences and contributes to the quality of those interactions (Fraley, 2002, p. 135). This model corresponds closely to Bowlby's view that early experience tends to be stable over time, yet remains open to change in light of experience.

From the point of view of attachment theory and development in general, the issue has never been stability per se but the coherence of individual differences over time and context (see Sroufe & Waters, 1977). With the challenge of learning theories behind us, stability per se is of much less interest than research on how secure base use and support evolve across time, how they are represented in memory, and how mental representations influence current behavior, expectations, and emotions. On a practical note, it would be very useful know whether SSP classifications are sensitive enough to change in response to seemingly effective individual or family therapy with caregivers or even the Circle of Security (Hoffman et al., 2006) or ABC interventions (Dozier & Bernard, 2019). Or might home observations detect improvements in secure base behavior without corresponding change in ABCD classifications. Obviously, the SSP is more economical, and often more practical, than extended home observations and would be preferable, as long as the risk of false-negative results is low.

11 **Can I use the SSP to determine whether an infant is attached to a particular individual?** In brief, the SSP was designed to assess the quality of an established attachment relationship, not whether such a relationship exists. On the basis of her observations in Uganda and Baltimore, Mary Ainsworth concluded that attachment emerges over time, not at a discrete moment in time. Proposed indicators for the presence of an attachment relationship, such as recognizing the mother, stranger fear, and separation protest, proved too susceptible to the infant's state and to situational influences to serve as useful criteria. Accordingly, Ainsworth spoke in terms of attachment becoming increasingly consolidated rather than present or absent, and scheduled SSP assessments for an age (12 months) at which her healthy, home-reared infants were actively using their mothers as a secure base (and yes, as a haven of safety; see FAQ 4). Where cognitive and/or motor benchmarks are delayed, researchers have often scheduled SSP assessments somewhat later to insure developmentally appropriate assessments (e.g., Cicchetti & Serafica, 1981; Waters & Valenzuela, 2000).

If one wanted to determine whether an infant is "attached" to a particular figure, it would probably be useful to focus the question on whether home observations indicate the presence of a well-consolidated pattern of using the adult as a secure base. That is, look for exploration away from the adult, with signs that the infant continues monitoring his or her location and activities. Look for infant signaling or retreat to the adult when uncomfortable or distressed. And look for what Ainsworth called an attachment–exploration balance over time and contexts. Do not be fooled by an infant's mere momentary preference for a new person once acclimated to him or her. Infants are often quite interested in new figures, especially if they are patient and playful, and the setting is benign.

SSP behavior is not very useful for deciding whether an attachment bond exists because (1) discrete behaviors are too susceptible to state and context, (2) the episodes are too brief to reliably estimate typical behavior, and (3) mere familiarity with the adult can be enough to initiate interaction and even comfort seeking. Some researchers have assumed that the mere ability to assign an ABCD classification implies the existence of a bond, even to nonprimary caregivers. This assumes that blind coders assigned SSPs conducted with nonattachment figures, that is, adults known to the infant only through multiple, brief, noncaregiving contacts, would reliably designate them "not classifiable." (Note: It is the % classifiable, not the distribution of classifications that matters here.) Given our boundless ability to see patterns and draw analogies in all kinds of material, this might not be a good bet. Thus, secure base use in naturalistic settings seems the most compelling evidence.[4]

[4]In order to effectively keep the scorers blind of the hypothesis and conditions, the SSPs should be conducted with the same personnel and in the same settings. Unfortunately, this largely precludes using existing SSP data as the "attached" group. In addition, scorers encountering "not classifiable" cases at a rate anywhere close to 50% would almost certainly raise questions about the population under study or develop hypotheses about the nature of the manipulation. Thus, the base rate of cases seen with nonattachment figures should be kept plausibly low (e.g., 10%).

12 Can I use the SSP to assess attachment security in cross-cultural samples, samples that have experienced extensive out-of-home care, and others that are different from the participants in Mary Ainsworth's Baltimore study? If you accept Mary Ainsworth's view that home behavior is the primary criterion against which the SSP's validity is measured, then it seems logical to require that SSP data from other populations be similarly related to secure base behavior at home before interpreting it in terms of attachment security. The logic here is pretty hard to escape. And considering the effort and expense, not to mention the potential theoretical or clinical significance, of work with the SSP, it seems reasonable to collect this kind of validity data. Moreover, we can learn quite a bit from engaging infant–caregiver dyads on their own turf, that is, by not limiting ourselves to the SSP. The Attachment Q-set (AQS, Waters & Deane, 1985; Vaughn, Waters, & Teti, Chapter 2, this volume) was developed specifically to make this task easier than in Ainsworth's day and more rewarding. Nonetheless, quite a few researchers have used the SSP in new populations without validation against blind home observations in pilot work or a portion of their sample. It is hard to place much confidence in such work.

These concerns apply as well when adapting the scoring system to take age or rearing practices into account. The problem is not that this cannot work, only that one does not know whether it has worked without comparing the adapted SSP scoring to secure base behavior at home. Posada (2006) provides a useful illustration. He conducted extended home observations of healthy, middle-class, 3-year-olds with their mothers and used the AQS to assign security scores. He then conducted the SSP and arranged the authors of the MacArthur Preschool Scoring system to blindly classify each case. In the end, the adapted SSP scoring was not related to secure base behavior at home. Nonetheless, research with the MacArthur adapted SSP has identified a wide range of competence-related, if not attachment-related, correlates. While these results put on hold the notion that the adapted SSP is strictly parallel to the Ainsworth procedure, they raise interesting questions that deserve high priority in new research. The fact that a respected journal was willing to publish this validation study, even when it reported "negative" results, is an encouragement to this kind of work.

13 Can the SSP be abbreviated? We have two comments. First, why expend the resources and effort to set up appropriate laboratory space, train assistants and coders, recruit participants, and conduct the procedures, and perhaps collect extensive data using other measures, only to put the entire enterprise at risk to save a few minutes on the SSP procedure and scoring? Second, as explained in the earlier "Strange Situation Practique" section, there is a clear logic to the order of SSP episodes. In light of this, it is hard to see how dropping or abbreviating some of the episodes would be an improvement. In any event, the changes would forfeit the validation in relation to home observations, which would need to be rechecked. This hardly seems economical.

14 Are there really discrete patterns of attachment? And what are the implications of the discrete versus continuous issue for scoring and data analysis? Mary Ainsworth (1978/2015, p. xli) expressed the view that the ABC patterns observed in the SSP reflect the different ways in which infants have organized their attachment relationships. Her preference for classifications reflected her view that (1) description is a primary function of measurement, (2) some phenomena are not easily captured on a continuum, and (3) measurement of complex phenomena should reflect their many facets. She was well aware that measurement on multiple facets or dimensions could be summarized using weighted linear composites. However, she felt that, in the context of discovery, it was best to work with patterns (profiles) than with composites. There is considerable wisdom in this view and, to researchers who are expert in the ABC classification system, the classifications are more labels for behavioral profiles than entities in themselves.

The decision to represent attachment individual differences as discrete categories versus continuous variables has practical implications for research design and data analysis. If attachment security is, in fact, a continuous variable, then assuming that all infants below some cutoff score (on a single variable or a composite of several variables) are equally insecure, and all infants above the cutoff are equally secure, discards useful variance and reduces statistical power. If, however, attachment individual differences are inherently taxonomic, then much of the diversity within secure and insecure groups is irrelevant (or unreliable) and incorporating all of this diversity into a continuous variable can only reduce statistical power. Richters, Waters, and Vaughn (1988) have provided discriminant function weights for scoring secure versus insecure and avoidant versus resistant SSP classifications as continuous variables. These weights could be used to compare results based on ABC classifications with parallel analyses of the same data scored as continuous variables.

Waters and Beauchaine (2003) have argued that attachment theory neither predicts nor requires that individual differences fall into discrete categories. Like most phenomena psychologists study, attachment individual differences arise from multiple influences acting in concert. In such cases, the central limit theorem is in play. Thus, most of the constructs we study are normally distributed, continuous variables. Not knowing the "true" situation regarding discrete categories or continuous variable, the latter is usually the best bet. If this is the right choice, new analyses using continuous variables should have greater statistical power.

With the emergence of taxonomic search methods pioneered by Paul Meehl (1965; Waller & Meehl, 1997; Ruscio, Haslam, & Ruscio, 2013), several attachment researchers have examined large datasets from different age groups to learn more about the structure of attachment individual differences. Their results paint an interestingly complex picture. Fraley and Spieker (2003a, 2003b) conducted taxonomic analyses on a large sample of SSP data and concluded that attachment individual differences are best viewed as a continuous variable at this early age. This makes sense in that, at this age, most infants in Western societies have a single primary caregiver whose behavior plays a significant role in organizing and helping consolidate their secure base behavior and the attachment–exploration balance.

By middle childhood, attachment has advanced from primarily sensorimotor representations to be less dependent on context and caregiver support to use a secure base effectively. During this time, the caregiver's secure base support expands to include co-constructing script-like attachment representations (Posada & Waters, 2018; H. Waters, Steiner, Zaman, Apetroaia, & Crowell, 2018). In light of this close parent–child collaboration, and the fact that script-like representations tend to be acquired as a package rather than element by element, it is interesting that taxonomic analyses by T. Waters et al. (2019) indicated that middle childhood attachment representations fall into discrete categories (expectation of instrumental help vs. elaborated secure base script). By adolescence, greater experience with the complexities of parent–child relationship, experience in other relationships, and the opportunity to observe other children's relationships elaborates the basic secure base script to incorporate a wider range of interactions in a diverse context. Accordingly, taxonomic studies of the AAI suggest that adolescent and adult attachment representations once again fit a continuous distribution model (Fraley & Roisman, 2014; T. Waters et al., 2015).

So, what to do? In general, it makes sense to employ measures and analyses that are familiar to your target audience. Discrete categories can be useful tools (useful fictions) if you (1) value the descriptive power they offer as shorthand for behavioral profiles, (2) are seeking, or are open to discovering, new facets of attachment relationships, or (3) work in an applied context in which categories are likely to communicate more effectively. Just keep in mind that category labels are shorthand for profiles across several behaviors. If you fall into viewing them as real entities, then you had just as well combine the behaviors into a single weighted composite. Meanwhile, we look forward to theoretical and empirical research to clarify the mechanisms that consolidate attachment representations after infancy and elaborate middle childhood representations in adolescence and adulthood. It is also important to reanalyze some existing analyses of ABC classifications as continuous variables to see whether the promised increase in statistical power is great enough to be of practical significance. Finally, we look forward to new work that takes a skills and modeling approach to secure base-related phenomena (e.g., Petters & Beaudoin, 2017). Much of this work is likely to assess attachment individual differences as continuous variables.

15 **Are SSP classifications traits?** Certainly not in the classic sense, though there is probably some yet to be detailed generalization of early attachment-related expectations to some relationship contexts beyond the infant–mother relationship. The SSP classifications reflect an infant's expectations in the relationship with a particular partner. As mentioned earlier, infants' SSP classifications with the mother and with the father are not significantly related (e.g., Main & Weston, 1981; Grossman et al., 1981). In addition, the SSP is too brief to provide reliable estimates of an infant's typical behaviors. Instead, the SSP is a test situation, and the observed behaviors are best thought of as predictive signs, to be used as when as a physician, recognizing a red spot on the retina, considers the possibility of diabetes (a metabolic disorder, not a disorder of the retina). Similarly, avoidance in the SSP predicts poorly organized secure base behavior, not more avoidance, at home. Even if we limit ourselves to the relationship domain, there is little evidence that SSP behavior or classifications reflect or predict similar behavior outside the SSP or across age. Where there are similarities across context and across age, they are in skilled or less skilled secure base use, not in trait-like persistence of behavioral styles.

Generally speaking, traits are more coherent and pervasive in our thinking than in actual behavior. We see prototypes, selectively recall confirming instances, and use trait language more often than we should. Consider the verbal associates of a term such as *avoidant*—disengaged, indifferent, risk averse, and so forth. There are almost certainly studies attempting to (and marginally managing to) relate infant or adult attachment to each of these, even though the links reflect only semantic associations, not the logic of attachment theory. It is not clear how such work could advance attachment theory or guide useful applications.

16 **How do the attachment relationships of infants classified A versus C in the SSP differ?** This is a hard one. As mentioned earlier (FAQ 14) Mary Ainsworth viewed SSP classifications as reflecting different ways in which infants organize their secure base relationships with specific partners. At the same time, she was quite clear about the distinction (see FAQ 1) between the inner, representational/relational attachment phenomenon and the behaviors in which it was manifest. She knew that in many respects A and C infants' behaviors at home were more similar to each other than to infants classified B (Ainsworth et al., 1978/2015, p. 124). Moreover, we have not found distinctive AQS patterns of attachment behavior to distinguish infants classified A versus C in the SSP (e.g., Vaughn & Waters, 1990). At best, they seem similarly inconsistent and ineffective at using the mother as a secure base.

Although the published attachment literature is a treasure trove of significant statistical tests on A versus C infants, it is difficult to formulate a clear explanation of how these two patterns arise. In part, this is due to the fact that the number of infants classified A or C in a particular study is usually small compared to the B group. This might be addressed through meta-analysis, but there has to be a coherent literature to analyze. Unfortunately, foundational attachment theory (as opposed to post hoc explanation of significant A–C differences) does not provide much guidance. Indeed, as we read attachment theory, it is agnostic regarding how insecure attachment is manifest one pattern, two, or more, in home behavior or the SSP. The lack of theoretical guidance may account for the lack of programmatic research on A versus C classifications, their origins, and their external correlates.

One possibility is that the A versus C classifications are not, so to speak, patterns of attachment but something else. For example, assume infants' attachment relationships differ primarily in terms of their ability to consistently and effectively use their primary caregiver as a secure base. In addition, suppose that every infant could also be located on a separate individual-differences dimension somewhat along the lines of the internalizing–externalizing dimension familiar from personality psychology and clinical diagnosis; call it "coping style."

First, consider infants classified B (secure). Faced with threat or distress, these infants would have ready access to a well-consolidated secure base response repertoire that lets them (1) do something (being unable to act, itself, is stressful), and (2) exit the bad situation. Having escaped the situation, the secure infant's internalizing–externalizing coping style does not come into play. Thus, the difference between secure (B) and insecure (A or C) infants reflects access to secure base responses. Now, consider infants classified A (insecure–avoidant) versus C (insecure–resistant). In the face of threat or distress, none these infants has ready access to a secure base response that would facilitate escaping or coping with the situation. With no ready escape via secure base behavior, individual coping styles come into play. Some would tend more toward internalizing responses, others toward externalizing responses. Thus, the difference between B and non-B infants might be different in kind than that between A and C infants—the former related to attachment security, the latter reflecting different coping styles among similarly insecure infants.[5]

Of course, an infant's location on the hypothesized coping style dimension would not be much in evidence during home observations unless some sort of significant threat or distress arose. This happens, but not often enough to parallel the challenges built into the architecture of the SSP. Thus, the salience of the A versus C distinction in the SSP and the difficulty in finding correlates of the A versus C distinction in home observations. We are agnostic on the nature of variables that might underpin the A versus C classifications in the SSP. Our point is simply that Bowlby–Ainsworth attachment theory does not predict specific patterns of individual differences among insecure infants, and we would do well to keep an open mind about the constructs that might explain them.

17 **What to think about subgroups?** There is nothing in attachment theory, and not much empirical data regarding antecedents and correlates, to support the idea that the subgroups within the A, B, and C classifications

[5]In principle, though wholly outside the realm of ethical research design, B (secure) infants' standing on the coping style variable might become evident if they were confronted with an utterly inescapable stress (e.g., several additional separation episodes) in a modified SSP. With their secure base response option blocked, perhaps, their individual coping styles would come into play, some tending toward internalizing responses, others toward externalizing responses. That is, secure infants might tend toward A or C classifications in later reunions.

reflect substantively different ways of organizing attachment relationships. When Mary Ainsworth was developing the ABC classification system, she recognized that there would be diversity around any prototype she defined. Rather than forcing every case into one of too few categories, she assigned subgroup (subscripted) classifications to infants who did not squarely fit the ABC prototypes. With the accumulation of cases, it became clear which of these variants occurred often enough to include in the ABC classification system. One group, B_4, was only identified in cases recruited after the main longitudinal study and were thus not observed at home.

Even after *Patterns of Attachment* was published, Ainsworth was reluctant to dispense with the subgroup designations. She considered it almost inevitable that new patterns would be discovered when the SSP became more widely used, and when research expanded to include different populations. Today, over 40 years later, it seems less likely that research will discover new groups or subgroup (except perhaps in cultures very different from our own). Nonetheless, the subgroups remain a useful part of the classificatory system, if only as an aid to consistent assignment to the major ABC groups. Even infants destined for the same ABC classification are not identical. Insofar as the variations around the ABC prototype recur, it is useful for coders to know that there is more than one way to earn any of the ABC classifications. For example, some B infants who do not cry in response to separation, who show little proximity seeking and perhaps even some avoidance in the first reunion episode, seem good candidates for the A (avoidant) classification. However, infants classified A maintain or increase their avoidant behavior in the second reunion, whereas infants whose avoidance declines or disappears, and who may even show a bit of approach or even fussing, are assigned to group B_1 or B_2 if avoidance gives way to proximity seeking.

Similarly, it is useful for coders to know that an infant can show some A-like behaviors in the initial episodes, yet belong in the B group if these indications decline and more B-like behavior appears in the second, separation–reunion sequence. Of course, if subsequent research on caregiving antecedents or external correlates suggested that the early, low-keyed avoidance was a better fit to Group A, then there was option of reassigning the B_1 classification to the A group (presumably A_3). This strategy reflects Ainsworth's commitment to an ethological/observational approach. As she often told student observers, "We'll let the data fall where they may; the world is always more interesting the way it really is than in [a scorer's] theory" (personal communication between Everett Waters and Mary Ainsworth, 1972).

18 **Does *Patterns of Attachment* provide enough information for me to score SSP scales and assign classifications without other training?** No. You need to work with an expert to become a skilled coder. Not that *Patterns of Attachment* does not provide enough detail. It is one of the most detailed descriptions of infant behavior ever published. It is just that to be a good scorer, you have to (1) learn how to look at behavior (as discussed earlier in this chapter in the section entitled "Behavior: Seeing versus Observing"), (2) learn what the verbal descriptions in the coding instructions refer to in actual behavior, (3) see enough examples of relevant behaviors to make important discriminations, and (4) establish blind agreement with expert coders. These require access to a rich set of training materials and an opportunity to work with a trained coder. Fortunately, the attachment training group at Minnesota's Institute of Child Development has offered summer SSP scoring seminars every summer for over 20 years. Information about enrolling is available online at *www.attachment-training.com*. If there were an easier way, we would recommend it. Although it might be possible to develop self-training materials from video recordings of conventional training sessions, this would require quite a bit of editing and we might not have the permissions required to put the recorded examples online.

19 Is it a good idea to pay experienced coders to score my SSP videos? We don't recommend hiring SSP coders in lieu of learning something about coding yourself. You are in a better position to maintain quality control, formulate hypotheses, analyze, and report data if you know the ins and outs of both the interactive behavior scales (proximity seeking, contact maintaining, avoidance, and resistance) and the classification criteria. If you engage someone to do the scoring for you, he or she will bring back exactly what you contracted for—no insights, no surprising observations, nothing about behavior unrelated to the scoring, not even details that went into their scoring decisions. That said, the Minnesota attachment training team is a good place to turn for help locating professional scorers. This chapter and release of the first paperback edition of *Patterns of Attachment* provide useful background for those wishing to use the SSP in their research. However, as mentioned in the previous FAQ, they are not enough.

20 Can I assign SSP classifications after viewing only the two reunion episodes? The infant's level of exploration and interaction in the preseparation episodes is a benchmark against which a scorer gauges exploration in the separation episodes and recovery in the reunion episodes. Certainly, some cases can be correctly classified from reunion behavior alone. However, there would inevitably be more than a few errors. We recommend that you do not base publications or clinical assessments on reunion episodes alone.

21 Can I assign SSP classifications without first scoring interactive behavior scales? The interactive behavior scales (proximity seeking, contact maintaining, avoidance, and resistance) provide the reference points and criteria for assigning ABC classifications and subgroups. They are very interesting to work with and remind you over and over what a great eye Mary Ainsworth had for behavior. They also illustrate the advantages of building scales by organizing actual behavior descriptions rather than creating them from memory and purely rational/semantic distinctions. Working with typed vignettes that describe actual behavior allowed Mary Ainsworth to assign rather different behaviors to the same level on a scale. Consider the options for Clear-cut but not persistent avoidance: (5a) "Baby looks when mother return but gives no greeting"; (5b) Baby does not look when mother returns; she eventually gains his attention but he remains unresponsive"; and (5c) "Baby greets mother when she returns but then either markedly turns away or tries to go out the door." When the full range of reunion behavior is examined, it becomes clear that each of these deserves a lower score than marked, persistent avoidance (Avoidance = 6), but a higher score than brief avoidance or persistent low-keyedness (Avoidance = 4). Thus, though rather different, they are all assigned scores of 5.

This kind of detail and grounding in actual behavior enables coders to make sense out of what, otherwise, seem to be overwhelmingly diverse responses. It is also endlessly interesting, as if someone had given you the key to unlocking infant behavior. At the same time, scoring interactive behavior, especially in the reunion episodes, is slow work and takes time. It is not simply a matter of viewing the episode and assigning scores. Coders routinely scroll back and forth over brief bits of video, making sure of the order in which things occurred, determining whether a maternal vocalization occurred before or after the child looked at her, and on and on. This was difficult in Ainsworth's initial work, when coders had to rely on typed transcripts of two simultaneous verbal descriptions. Video recording is a tremendous help. Still, this level of analysis is largely out of reach if you have viewed a single episode without pausing or reviewing the recording. All the more so if you watch all eight episodes straight through on videotape, much less if you only observe the SSP live.

A few infants show such strong positive responses on reunion, or such clear-cut and persistent avoidance throughout, or anger, such as slapping at toys the mother offers without following up with efforts to seek contact, that their classification is obvious. But the majority require the kind of close analysis ensured by scoring the interactive behavior scales. It is also useful to have the interactive behavior scores when investigating classification disagreements. In brief, we have never reported SSP classifications that were not built on scoring the interactive behaviors and crying in all eight episodes.

22 Why am I not finding as many B_3 infants as Mary Ainsworth did? In Ainsworth's Baltimore study, nearly half of the infants (45/106 = 42%) were classified B_3. Only a quarter as many (11/106 = 10%) were classified B_2 (Ainsworth et al., 1978/2015, p. 230). Today, B_2 classifications often equal or outnumber B_3, sometimes by as much as three to one. This is not to say that infants today are less secure, only that the strong proximity seeking and contact maintaining in response to brief separations, characteristic of infants classified B_3, occur less often.

There are several common themes in the B (secure) classification. The infants show strong interest in exploring the room and the toys, often with clear indications that this is facilitated by their mother's presence. They may or may not cry or search when the mother leaves the room. But when she returns, they show more than a casual greeting and no significant avoidance or resistance. The primary difference between infants classified B_3 versus B_2 is in the degree of separation distress and the level of contact they seek in the reunion episodes. Infants classified B_2 rarely cry in response to separation. They greet mother when she returns and accept contact if picked up, but they are less active in seeking contact and clinging, and are less likely to resist being put down. Like infants classified B_3, they show little if any avoidance or resistance, especially in the second reunion. One might say that they are simply confident that the mother will return.

Several possible explanations for the higher rate of B_2 classifications occur to us: (1) narrative records are less detailed than video recording—today's coders may see finer gradations in the timing and manner of proximity seeking and contact maintaining than when SSPs were scored from narrative records, or (2) infants in the Baltimore sample were home-reared; infants today are more likely to have experienced out-of-home care and might therefore be more acclimated to brief separations. It is also the case that attachment research has branched out from the early focus on healthy, middle-class, home-reared infant to include a wider range of caregiving practices and risk status. If you are seeing not only a change in the ratio of B_3 to B_2 classifications but also a shift in the entire distribution away from the B group, it is possible that there actually is a shift toward more insecure–avoidant behavior in your sample, and some of the excess B_2 infants might be candidates for reclassification as B_1 or even A_1. Another possibility is that infants showing considerable avoidance in the first reunion, then a marked decline in the second, might be considered for a new classification (B_0 or A_3, depending on the antecedents and correlates). Such issues are best resolved collaboratively, by sharing video records and data across projects.

23 What is a satisfactory level of agreement with expert scorers after training and for reporting research results? Establishing agreement with expert coders in an important part of SSP training. New scorers should ordinarily agree on all of the cases in the set of expertly scored SSPs available from the Minnesota training group. Subsequently, it is reasonable to expect coders to agree with the most experienced coder in their laboratory 90% of the time on A, B, C, and perhaps 80% of the time on D classifications. Disagreements with these criterion cases should be discussed and clarified. It is also important to keep in mind that coding skill depends on continuing practice. Skilled coders who have not been scoring SSP data for several years should reevaluate their own agreement with expertly scored SSPs before teaching or serving as an agreement criterion for less experienced coders. Finally, when the SSP is used in very large studies, scoring can be spread over long periods. It is important to conduct blind checks on scoring agreement throughout the course of the study.

24 **Can I obtain SSP classifications from AQS data?** The AQS was designed to assess secure base behavior at home and other places in which an infant or toddler has some range to explore. Group B infants consistently score higher than non-B or A or C infants. However, we have not found a pattern of AQS items that consistently distinguishes group A from group C. Nor does attachment theory predict or require such differences. As mentioned earlier (FAQ 16), the two insecure SSP groups seem similarly, diversely inconsistent and ineffective at using the mother as a secure base at home.

Regarding the D group, several small studies have reported very low AQS security scores (see Posada, Waters, Vaughn, Pederson, & Moran, Chapter 1, this volume). This is important evidence for the attachment-relatedness of the D classification. SSP behavior that does not fall neatly into one of the ABC classifications cannot be taken as indicative of insecure attachment without validation against secure base use at home. To date, there have been too few AQS-SSP studies, and sample sizes have been too small so far, to explore item-level differences between infants classified D versus non-D and secure-D versus insecure-D. Research on diversity in the D group deserves high priority in new research. Work on behavioral diversity within the SSP can be useful here but ultimately it should be anchored in behavior in naturalistic settings.

25 **Is the SSP useful in applied settings such as child custody decisions?** Attachment theory and measures have considerable potential to inform psychological work in applied contexts. At the same time, applied contexts are usually complex, and an attachment perspective or assessment alone does not provide a simple solution for a complex, changing situation. Moreover, the best solution for a child or a family at a given point in time may not be the best solution later on. Experienced clinicians are aware of the limitations of their skills and tools, the frailty (as well as resiliency) of individuals, and the uncertainty inherent in the way family life unfolds.

Two concerns in the use of attachment theory in general and the SSP in particular, are that (1) like any tools, attachment theory and assessments can be misunderstood and misused (see Byrne, O'Connor, Marvin, & Whelan, 2005) and (2) attachment assessments can be given undue weight in reports and in judges' decisions. The latter can happen simply because a measure such as the SSP has a scientific pedigree or seems more objective than other sources of information that are more complex, depend on a clinician's experience to integrate and interpret, or seem to complicate rather than simplify the decisions that need to be made. It is also important to keep in mind that validity data based on groups are true on average but do not necessarily apply to every individual.[6]

[6]Some have suggested that atypical attachment behavior in the SSP is understandable or even adaptive in light of their circumstances. This may be an important insight or an instance of what biologists refer to as the adaptationist fallacy. Whether such behavior promises good adjustment or later difficulties should be an empirical question addressed in concurrent and longitudinal research.

In brief, the SSP can play a useful role as a component of a multifaceted assessment that includes parental interviews and mental health assessments, parent–child observations, assessments of the family environment, child health records, review of documents provided by Social Services, and so forth. SSP data *should not be privileged over other sources of information.* Unfortunately, aside from the domains to be assessed, there seems little consensus or standardization of what such assessments should include (Bow & Quinnell, 2002). Thus, it is hard to know the context of other information in which SSP data will be interpreted. Properly used and skillfully explained, the SSP can be a useful window on the extent to which a wide range of influences have impacted primary caregivers and on the coherence of the child's early relationships.

REFERENCES

Ainsworth, M. D. S. (1967). *Infancy in Uganda: Infant care and the growth of love.* Baltimore: Johns Hopkins University Press.

Ainsworth, M. D. S., Blehar, M., Waters, E., & Wall, S. (2015). *Patterns of attachment: A psychological study of the Strange Situation.* New York: Taylor & Francis (Psychology Press). (Original work published 1978)

Ainsworth, M. D. S., & Bowlby, J. (1991). An ethological approach to personality development. *American Psychologist, 46*(4), 333–341.

Attri, R. K. (2018). *The models of skill acquisition and expertise development.* Singapore: Speed to Proficiency Research.

Bow, J. N., & Quinnell, F. A. (2002). A critical review of custody evaluation reports. *Family Court Review, 40*(2), 164–176.

Bowlby, J. (1957). An ethological approach to research on child development. *British Journal of Medical Psychology, 30*(4), 230–240.

Bowlby, J. (1958). The nature of the child's tie to his mother. *International Journal of Psychoanalysis, 39,* 350–373.

Bowlby, J. (1969). *Attachment and loss: Vol. 1. Attachment.* New York: Basic Books.

Bowlby, R. (2006). *John Bowlby and attachment theory: An interview with Sir Richard Bowlby* (25 min.). Interviewer: E. Waters. Retrieved from *www.youtube.com/watch?v=Exf_rR1NnNs.*

Byrne, J. G., O'Connor, T. G., Marvin, R. S., & Whelan, W. F. (2005). Practitioner review: The contribution of attachment theory to child custody assessments. *Journal of Child Psychology and Psychiatry, 46*(2), 115–127.

Chess, S., & Thomas, A. (1982). Infant bonding: Mystique and reality. *American Journal of Orthopsychiatry, 52,* 213–222.

Cicchetti, D., & Serafica, F. C. (1981). The interplay among behavioral systems: Illustrations from the study of attachment, affiliation, and wariness in young Down's syndrome children. *Developmental Psychology, 17,* 36–49.

Crowell, J. A., Treboux, D., Gao, Y., Fyffe, C., Pan, H., & Waters, E. (2002). Secure base behavior in adulthood: Measurement, links to adult attachment representations, and relations to couples' communication and self-reports. *Developmental Psychology, 38,* 679–693.

Darwin, C. (1877). A biographical sketch of an infant. *Mind, 2,* 285–294.

DeVore, I. (1963). Mother–infant relations in free-ranging baboons. In H. Rheingold (Ed.), *Maternal behavior in mammals* (pp. 305–335). New York: Wiley.

DeVore, I. (Ed.). (1965). *Primate behavior: Field studies of monkeys and apes.* New York: Holt, Rinehart & Winston.

Doyle, A. C., & Klinger, L. S. (2007). A scandal in Bohemia. In *The new annotated Sherlock Holmes: Vol. 1. The adventures of Sherlock Holmes* and *The memoirs of Sherlock Holmes.* New York: Norton. Retrieved from *www.gutenberg.org/files/1661/1661-h/1661-h.htm#chap01.*

Dozier, M., & Bernard, K. (2019). *Coaching parents of vulnerable infants: The Attachment and Biobehavioral Catch-Up Approach.* New York: Guilford Press.

Drummond, H. (2012). The nature and description of behavior patterns. In P. P. G. Bateson & P. Klopfer (Eds.), *Perspectives in ethology* (Vol. 4, pp. 1–34). New York: Springer. (Original work published 1981)

Duschinsky, R. (2020). *Cornerstones of attachment research.* Oxford, UK: Oxford University Press. Available as an open-access document at *http://fdslive.oup.com/www.oup.com/academic/pdf/openaccess/9780198842064.pdf.*

Fraley, R. C. (2002). Attachment stability from infancy to adulthood: Meta-analysis and dynamic modeling of developmental mechanisms. *Personality and Social Psychology Review,* 6(2), 123–151.

Fraley, R. C., & Roisman, G. I. (2014). Categories or dimensions?: A taxometric analysis of the Adult Attachment Interview. In C. Booth-LaForce & G. I. Roisman (Eds.), The Adult Attachment Interview: Psychometrics, stability and change from infancy, and developmental origins. *Monographs of the Society for Research in Child Development, 79,* 36–50.

Fraley, R. C., & Spieker, S. J. (2003a). Are infant attachment patterns continuously or categorically distributed?: A taxometric analysis of Strange Situation behavior. *Developmental Psychology, 39,* 387–404.

Fraley, R. C., & Spieker, S. (2003b). What are the differences between dimensional and categorical models of individual differences in attachment?: Reply to Cassidy (2003), Cummings (2003), Sroufe (2003), and Waters and Beauchaine (2003). *Developmental Psychology, 39,* 423–429.

Frege, G. (1884). *The foundations of arithmetic: A logico-mathematical enquiry into the concept of number* (D. Jacquette, trans.). New York: Taylor & Francis. (English trans. 2007)

Fridland, E., & Pavese, C. (Eds.). (2020). *The Routledge handbook of philosophy of skill and expertise.* New York: Routledge.

Grossmann, K., & Grossmann, K. E. (2017). *Bindungen—Das Gefuge psychischer Sicherheit* [*Attachment the construction of psychological security*] (7th ed.). Stuttgart: Klett-Cotta. (First ed., 2004; revised ed., 2012)

Grossman, K. E., Grossman, K., Huber, F., & Wartner, U. (1981). German children's behavior toward their mothers at 12 months and their fathers at 18 months in Ainsworth's Strange Situation. *International Journal of Behavioral Development, 4,* 157–181.

Hinde, R. A. (1959). Some recent trends in ethology. In S. Koch (Ed.), *Psychology: A study of a science* (Vol. 2, pp. 561–610). New York: McGraw-Hill.

Hinde, R. A. (1966). *Animal behaviour: A synthesis of ethology and comparative psychology.* New York: McGraw-Hill.

Hoffman, K., Marvin, R., Cooper, G., & Powell, B. (2006). Changing toddlers' and preschoolers' attachment classifications: The Circle of Security Intervention. *Journal of Consulting and Clinical Psychology, 74,* 1017–1026.

Huxley, J. (1914). The courtship habits of the great crested grebe. *Proceedings of the Zoological Society of London, 84*(3), 491–562.

Kagan, J. (1982). *Psychological research on the human infant: An evaluative summary.* New York: W. T. Grant Foundation.

Kuhn, T. S. (2012). *The structure of scientific revolutions* (4th ed.). Chicago: University of Chicago Press. (Original work published 1962)

Lorenz, K. (1935). Der Kumpan in der Umwelt des Vogels (Der Artgenosse als auslösendes Moment sozialer Verhaltungsweisen) [The companion in the bird's world: The fellow-member of the species as a releasing factor of social behavior]. *Journal of Ornithology, 83,* (Pt. 2–3), 137–213. [English summary (1937) in *The Auk, 54,* 245–273.]

Maccoby, E., & Masters, J. C. (1970). Attachment and dependency. In P. H. Mussen (Ed.), *Carmichael's manual of child psychology* (Vol. 2, pp. 73–159). New York: Wiley.

Main, M., & Solomon, J. (1986). Discovery of a new, insecure–disorganized/disoriented attachment pattern. In M. Yogman & T. B. Brazelton (Eds.), *Affective development in infancy* (pp. 195–124). Norwood, NJ: Ablex.

Main, M., & Solomon, J. (1990). Procedures for identifying infants as disorganised/disoriented during the Ainsworth Strange Situation. In M. T. Greenberg, D. Cicchetti, & E. M. Cummings (Eds.), *Attachment in the preschool years* (pp. 121–160). Chicago: University of Chicago Press.

Main, M., & Weston, D. (1981). The quality of the toddler's relationship to mother and father. *Child Development, 52,* 932–940.

Martin, P., & Bateson, P. P. G. (2007). *Measuring behaviour: An introductory guide.* Cambridge, UK: Cambridge University Press.

Masterman, M. (1970). The nature of a paradigm. In I. Lakatos & A. Musgrave (Eds.), *Criticism and the growth of knowledge* (pp. 59–89). London: Cambridge University Press.

Masters, J. C., & Wellman, H. M. (1974). The study of human infant attachment: A procedural critique. *Psychological Bulletin, 81*(4), 218–237.

Meehan, C. L., & Hawkes, S. (2013). Cooperative breeding and attachment among the Aka foragers. In N. Quinn & J. M. Mageo (Eds.), *Attachment reconsidered: Cultural perspectives on a western theory* (pp. 85–113). New York: Palgrave Macmillan.

Meehl, P. E. (1965). *Detecting latent clinical taxa by fallible quantitative indicators lacking an accepted criterion* (Report No. PR-65-2). Minneapolis: University of Minnesota, Research Laboratories of the Department of Psychiatry.

Melville, H. (1851). *Moby Dick.* London: Richard Bentley.

Mischel, W. (1968). *Personality and assessment.* New York: Wiley.

Petters, D. (2019). The attachment control system and computational modeling: Origins and prospects. *Developmental Psychology, 55*(2), 227–239.

Petters, D., & Beaudoin, L. (2017). Attachment modelling: From observation to scenario to design. In P. Erdi, B. Bhattacharya, & A. Cochran (Eds.), *Computational neurology and psychiatry* (pp. 227–271). London: Springer.

Piaget, J. (1936). *The origins of intelligence in children.* New York: International Universities Press. (English trans. 1952)

Posada, G. (2006). Assessing attachment security at age three: Q-sort observations and the MacArthur Strange Situation adaptation. *Social Development, 15*(4), 644–658.

Posada, G., & Waters, H. (2018). The co-construction of mother–child attachment relationships in early childhood. In G. Posada & H. Waters (Eds.), The mother–child attachment partnership in early childhood: Secure base behavioral and representational processes. *Monographs of the Society for Research in Child Development, 83*(4), 7–21.

Richters, J. E., Waters, E., & Vaughn, B. (1988). An empirical classification system for the Strange Situation. *Child Development, 59,* 512–522.

Ruscio, J., Haslam, N., & Ruscio, A. M. (2013). *Introduction to the taxometric method: A practical guide.* New York: Routledge.

Sroufe, L. A. (1985). Attachment classification from the perspective of infant–caregiver relationships and infant temperament. *Child Development, 56,* 1–14

Sroufe, L. A., & Waters, E. (1977). Attachment as an organizational construct. *Child Development, 48,* 1184–1189.

Tinbergen, N. (1951). *The study of instinct.* London: Oxford University Press.

Tinbergen, N. (1963). On aims and methods of ethology. *Zeitschrift für Tierpsychologie, 20,* 410–433.

van der Horst, F. C. P. (2011). *John Bowlby—From psychoanalysis to ethology: Unraveling the roots of attachment theory.* Malden, MA: Wiley-Blackwell.

van Rosmalen, L., van der Veer, R., & van der Horst, F. (2015). Ainsworth's Strange Situation Procedure: The origin of an instrument. *Journal of the History of the Behavioral Sciences, 51*(3), 261–284.

Vaughn, B. E., Bost, K. K., & van IJzendoorn, M. H. (2008). Attachment and temperament: Additive and interactive influences on behavior, affect, and cognition during infancy and childhood. In J. Cassidy & P. Shaver (Eds.), *Handbook of attachment: Theory, research, and clinical applications* (pp. 192–216). New York: Guilford Press.

Vaughn, B. E., & Shin, N. (2011). Attachment, temperament, and adaptation: One long argument. In D. Cicchetti & G. I. Roisman (Eds.), *Minnesota Symposia on Child Psychology: Vol. 36. The origins and organization of adaptation and maladaptation* (pp. 55–107). New York: Wiley.

Vaughn, B., & Waters, E. (1990). Attachment behavior at home and in the laboratory: Q-sort observations and Strange Situation classifications of one-year-olds. *Child Development, 61,* 1965–1973.

Waller, N. G., & Meehl, P. E. (1997). *Multivariate taxonomic procedures: Distinguishing types from continua.* Thousand Oaks, CA: SAGE.

Waters, E. (1978). The reliability and stability of individual differences in infant–mother attachment. *Child Development, 49,* 483–494.

Waters, E. (2008). Live long and prosper: A note on attachment and evolution (Original work published 2002). Retrieved January 28, 2020, from *www.psychology.sunysb.edu/attachment/gallery/live_long/live_long.html.*

Waters, E., & Beauchaine, T. (2003). Are there really patterns of attachment?: Theoretical and empirical perspectives. *Developmental Psychology, 39,* 417–432.

Waters, E., Bretherton, I., & Vaughn, B. E. (2015). New Preface to *Patterns of attachment* (2015). In M. Ainsworth, M. Blehar, E. Waters, & S. Wall (Eds.), *Patterns of attachment* (pp. x–xxxvi). New York: Taylor & Francis (Psychology Press).

Waters, E., & Cummings, M. (2000). A secure base from which to explore close relationships. *Child Development, 71,* 164–172.

Waters, E., & Deane, K. (1985). Defining and assessing individual differences in attachment relationships: Q-methodology and the organization of behavior in infancy and early childhood. In I. Bretherton & E. Waters (Eds.), Growing points of attachment theory and research. *Monographs of the Society for Research in Child Development, 50*(1–2), 41–65.

Waters, E., & Valenzuela, M. (2000). Explaining disorganized attachment: Clues from research on mild-to-moderately undernourished children in Chile. In J. Solomon & C. George (Eds.), *Attachment disorganization* (pp. 265–287). New York: Guilford Press.

Waters, H., Steiner, M. A., Zaman, W., Apetroaia, A., & Crowell, J. A. (2018). Co-construction of attachment representations and affect regulating cognitions: The role of maternal attachment security. In G. Posada & H. Waters (Eds.), The mother–child attachment partnership in early childhood: Secure base behavioral and representational processes. *Monographs of the Society for Research in Child Development, 83*(4), 60–73.

Waters, H., & Waters, E. (2006). The attachment working models concept: Among other things, we build script-like representations of secure base experiences. *Attachment and Human Development, 8,* 185–197.

Waters, H., Waters, T. E. A., & Waters, E. (2021). From internal working models to script-like attachment representations. In R. A. Thompson, J. A. Simpson, & L. Berlin (Eds.), *Attachment: The fundamental questions* (pp. 111–119). New York: Guilford Press.

Waters, T. E. A., Facompre, C. R., Dujardin, A., van de Walle, M., Verhees, M., Bodner, N., . . . Bosmans, G. (2019). Taxometric analysis of secure base script knowledge in middle childhood reveals categorical latent structure. *Child Development, 90*(3), 694–707.

Waters, T. E. A., Fraley, R. C., Groh, A. M., Steele, R. D., Vaughn, B. E., Boost, K. K., . . . Coppola, G. (2015). *The latent structure of secure base script knowledge. Developmental Psychology, 51,* 823–830.

CHAPTER 4

Attachment Disturbance

Disorganization and Disorder

Elizabeth A. Carlson

Attachment disturbances of disorganization and disorder highlight the complex, dynamic nature of behavioral systems and the importance of an organizational framework for understanding relational experiences in the early years. Consider the behavior of three 12-month-old infants in a laboratory attachment assessment.

> In the first assessment, Ana and her primary caregiver enter a laboratory playroom. Ana begins to explore the toys in the center of the floor with her caregiver nearby. An unfamiliar adult enters and interacts first with the caregiver, then with the infant. With a wary look to the stranger, Ana moves closer to her caregiver and continues to explore. Two caregiver-infant separations and reunions follow. Ana cries and searches at the door during the separations, and on reunion, approaches and reaches to her caregiver. When picked up, Ana settles readily and returns to explore when released on the floor.
>
> In a second assessment, Tony and his caregiver reproduce the same sequence of events. Tony explores in the presence of his caregiver, and cries and searches for the caregiver during separations. However, on each reunion with his caregiver, Tony interrupts his distress and approach to the caregiver with a wary expression and a sudden step back. He turns away, waits near the wall, then returns to the toys to explore independently.
>
> In a third assessment, Alex engages in minimal exploration and interaction in the presence of her caregiver. When the stranger enters, Alex spontaneously approaches the unfamiliar adult with a reach (despite the

presence of her caregiver). During separations from her caregiver, Alex cries and rocks back and forth. On reunions, Alex approaches each adult (stranger and caregiver) with a reach for physical contact.

The infants in these observational scenarios exhibit common attachment-related behaviors of crying, reaching, and approaching, as well as variations in expressions of wariness and exploration. What significantly differ are the conditions that elicit the attachment behaviors, the objects or targets of the behaviors, and the completeness of the behavioral sequences, in other words, their organization. Understanding differences in behavioral organization and relations among the associated behavioral systems is central to understanding and identifying disturbances in attachment, the distinctions between effective, interpretable responses to distress, inconsistent ineffective responses, and signs of disorder.

Preceding chapters in this volume have identified central themes in attachment theory and measurement, especially with reference to secure base phenomena and the role of caregiving relationships in development. Grounded in an organizational developmental perspective, this chapter extends the discussion of attachment development and organization from normative or expectable expressions of relational experience to patterns of disturbance and pathology reflected in attachment disorganization and disorder.

AN ORGANIZATIONAL DEVELOPMENTAL PERSPECTIVE

In natural environments, ground-living primates when frightened or threatened seek a caregiving figure rather than a place or dwelling (Bowlby, 1969/1982). This person is the attachment figure. In humans, parents or caregivers are motivated (for survival-based biological reasons) to promote the safety and health of their offspring. Bowlby pointed out that over time, infants, too, are motivated to pursue their own safety through caregiving relationships. Organisms with prolonged juvenile periods require complementary behavioral systems to maintain proximity between the vulnerable infant and the protective caregiver (Bowlby 1969/1982). Seeking physical closeness to a caregiver ensures that infants not only are not injured, lost, or abandoned, but that they also explore and learn from adult behavior and the immediate surround until maturity.

An evolutionary perspective suggests that there is a species-specific range of expectable environmental conditions (including a protective, nurturing caregiver for infants) that elicit normative developmental processes (Bowlby, 1969/1982; Hartman, 1958). When environments fall outside the expectable range, normal development is impeded. For human infants, such adverse caregiving environments (e.g., maltreatment, institutionalization) disrupt or fail to support the typical development of critical relational mechanisms related to attachment, fear/wariness, and related systems. Distinguishing disturbance in these systems is challenging. Human functioning is complex, and guidance from developmental theory and research is required to discern meaningful patterns from the infinite variations in infant behavior and experience.

Although there is no single theory of development, core assumptions and regulatory principles from organizational models provide a starting point for understanding the nature of both infant–caregiver disturbance and normative functioning (Bowlby, 1973; Cicchetti & Sroufe, 1978; Santostefano, 1978; Sroufe & Rutter, 1984; Werner, 1957). Derived from the study of embryology and evolution, these assumptions reflect qualities and processes common to both biological and psychological development (Sameroff, 1983).

Critical organizational propositions include the view that the individual develops and functions as a unified whole (Block, 1971; Fogel & Thelen, 1987; Gottlieb, 1991; Sameroff, 1983; Santostefano, 1978; Schore, 1994; Sroufe & Rutter, 1984; Werner, 1948). Biological and psychological systems and processes function in relation to each other such that no single system causes development. Rather, it is the complex relations among systems that bring about development. Conceptualizations of relations among attachment-related systems illustrate this principle of interaction and mutual relevance (Ainsworth, 1973; Ainsworth & Wittig, 1969; Bischof, 1975; Bretherton & Ainsworth, 1974).

Within and across systems, organization of experience is a central motive. The patterning or organization of behavior (as well as attention, emotion, and cognition) distinguishes individual functioning, with development conceived as a series of adaptations and qualitative reorganizations over time. From this perspective, social and emotional development in infancy is characterized by an increasing ability to maintain organization under stress (Sroufe & Waters, 1977). Disturbances in functioning may evolve from experiences of extreme arousal that distort, overwhelm, or defeat these developing capacities.

Another critical organizational proposition suggests that across the lifespan, development is characterized by increasing complexity and self-organization. Diverse and complex modes of functioning evolve from relatively diffuse and undifferentiated states through iterative cycles of differentiation and coordination (Cicchetti, 1984; Sroufe & Rutter, 1984; Werner, 1948). Typically, with experience, organization within the individual and within relationships progresses toward increasing levels of complexity and integration. In contrast, pathological processes may be characterized by rigid deviation, distortion, and compartmentalization of experience that compromise immediate and subsequent development, or increasing differentiation with a lack of integration (Carlson, Yates, & Sroufe, 2009; Cicchetti, 1984; Waters & Sroufe, 1983).

From this organizational developmental perspective, systems and system components (e.g., individual behaviors) are best understood with respect to the ways they serve to organize and integrate experience. Focus is on the meaning and function of behavior within developing systems rather than exclusively on form. Thus, morphologically similar behaviors may serve different behavioral systems and may have different meanings and functions in different contexts or at different points in development (Sameroff & Chandler, 1975; Sroufe & Waters, 1977; Waddington, 1957). For example, the same infant behavior of falling prone and remaining silent may be viewed as adaptive in one context (e.g., in the absence of a caregiver) and maladaptive in another (e.g., in the presence of the primary caregiver). Separated from the caregiver, a prone or still posture may divert attention from predators; in the presence of the caregiver, the same posture prevents protective closeness. The meaning of behavior derives from an understanding of the developing capacities of the individual child within a context of environmental resources and demands.

Finally, within an organizational framework and consistent with a view of pathology as developmental deviation, understanding disturbance requires first an understanding of normative development (Cicchetti, 1984; Sroufe, 1990; Sroufe & Rutter, 1984; Werner, 1948, 1957). Through the study of normative functioning, salient patterns of adaptation (e.g., attachment in infancy) are identified, and pathways of disturbance or repeated failure of positive adaptation related to these issues, may be distinguished. Moreover, the aberrations or deficits within and among systems that define disorder may contribute to an understanding of the underlying structure, development, and interdependence of areas of functioning not readily apparent under normal conditions (Cicchetti & Sroufe, 1978, Labella & Cicchetti, 2017).

ATTACHMENT DEVELOPMENT

Attachment, from an organizational framework, is conceived as one of several biologically based interactive behavioral systems with activations, functions, and outcomes that emerge at different times in early development (Bowlby, 1969/1982, 1973; Emde & Harmon, 1978). Selected for its effect on reproductive success, the attachment system functions to promote survival of the young (through access to a caregiver) and integration of information regarding caregiver whereabouts and cues to danger (e.g., darkness, unfamiliar settings, separation from adults) as the basis for response selection.

Infants enter the world with a biologically based propensity for interaction (Bowlby, 1969/1982), initiating, maintaining, and terminating interactions reflexively and without intention through behaviors such as orienting, smiling, crying, and clinging that promote infant–caregiver proximity (Ainsworth, Bell, & Stayton, 1974). However, the initial repertoire of infant behavior or early development of perceptual and motor systems does not provide for the capacity to adapt or survive alone. The emergence of an organized system of attachment behavior requires reasonable access to adult caregiving coadapted to the attachment behavioral system, an average expectable environment (Bowlby, 1969/1982; Waters, Kondo-Ikemura, Posada, & Richters,

1991). Access to and stability in this organizing caregiving environment are critical to the development of infant physiological, perceptual, and behavioral control systems.

During the first year, the caregiver reads, interprets, and responds to infant affective communications, especially signs of distress. In the course of interaction and routine care, sensorimotor anticipations become predictable, and from predictability evolve preference and an emotional bond (Waters et al., 1991). Typically, based on experience of responsive caregiver-orchestrated interactions, the infant increasingly directs intentional communications to the caregiver, takes purposive action to achieve contact, and flexibly selects and alters behaviors from an expanded repertoire until the goal of proximity and stabilization is achieved (Sroufe & Waters, 1977). Consistent with a developmental framework, attachment is defined not by the presence, intensity, or frequency of these behaviors but by their organization in a particular context to promote survival. *Organization,* or the formation of links between isolated repeated experiences and the extraction of invariants in relationship interactions, is not consciously imposed, but forged in caregiving experiences.

If the attachment system depends on organized and organizing experiences of supportive caregiving, it follows that the system will not function properly if such support is disorganized, markedly discrepant, or absent from the species typical caregiving environment (Cicchetti & Valentino, 2006; Waters et al., 1991). When caregiving aspects of the attachment system responsible for this integration emit conflicting signals or fail to pass along a signal strong enough to activate and maintain a consistent predominant response, disturbances of attachment may result. Possible outcomes range from the simultaneous activation of more than one response to alternating or interrupted responses to no response. With development, children may be better equipped to detect weak or inconsistent caregiving behavior and to actively elicit organized care; however, in infancy, organization depends on the caregiving environment.

ATTACHMENT ORGANIZATION

Attachment organization observed in the home and under stress in the laboratory environment is reflected in secure, anxious–avoidant, and anxious–resistant behavioral patterns (Ainsworth, Blehar, Waters, & Wall, 1978/2015). Derived from the history of caregiver–infant interactions, these patterns represent expectable sequences of infant behavior and attention in relation to the caregiver when under stress. For infants classified as secure, attachment behavior and attention are flexibly modified to serve the goals of proximity to the caregiver and exploration. The infant is able to engage in exploration but readily employs attachment-seeking behaviors when overly aroused or frightened. Less flexible and effective patterns of avoidance and resistance reflect acquired reactions ("conditional behavioral strategies") for maintaining proximity with the caregiver in the context of unresponsive or inconsistent caregiving (Main & Hesse, 1990). For some infants (in anxious–avoidant, avoidant relationships), minimizing expression of attachment behavior or shifting of attention away from the caregiver permits the organism to resolve conflicting behavioral tendencies and, even though not completely effective, to modulate arousal to some degree. For others (in anxious–resistant relationships), maximizing displays of anger support oscillating dyadic engagement. Whether flexible or inflexible in organization, the three forms (secure, anxious–avoidant, anxious–resistant) represent relational patterns of maintaining proximity and regulating arousal, and are within the normal range of attachment resolutions to stressful conditions (Ainsworth et al., 1978/2015; Main & Hesse, 1990; Sroufe & Waters, 1977). Thus, in the face of external threat or internal arousal, in these dyads, organization is maintained within the caregiving relationship, and infant cognitive and affective regulatory capabilities are not overly taxed despite caregiving limitations.

ATTACHMENT DISORGANIZATION

In response to extreme emotionally arousing experience, the normally developing organized attachment system mobilizes the child to flee *from* external threat and *toward* an attachment figure for protection and security (Bowlby, 1969/1982). However, when caregiving behavior is threatening or unusual in ways that may be frightening or overwhelming to an infant (e.g., lapses in monitoring), the young child is confronted with a biologically-based paradox: the simultaneous need to *approach* and *flee* from the same caregiver (Hesse & Main, 2000). The maintenance of an organized attachment strategy becomes difficult or impossible. Strong contradictory behavioral tendencies inhibit the employment of relational strategies typically used by alarmed infants, such as seeking comfort and support from the caregiver, shifting attention to the environment while maintaining proximity, or signaling the caregiver via heightened distress. Repeated experiences of dramatically contradictory or fluctuating cues from the caregiver may overwhelm immature cognitive and emotional processing, and contribute to a lapse or collapse in attentional and behavioral strategies for coping with distress within the relationship (Hesse & Main, 2000; Main & Solomon, 1990).

As noted by ethologists, antagonistic motivations may be manifested in a range of compromise behaviors. For example, without sufficient protection, frightened animals may run around frantically to escape or may freeze and limit their movement. Similarly, in human infants, opposing tendencies may be manifested in the simultaneous activation of contradictory behaviors and attentional patterns (e.g., approach and avoidance) or in their mutual inhibition (e.g., freezing, stilling). In each of these conditions, the infant is challenged to manage extreme arousal independently at a time when infant capabilities are insufficient to ensure self-regulation.

The attachment disorganization/disorientation classification refers to this diverse array of odd, fearful, disjointed, contradictory, and seemingly inexplicable behavioral responses exhibited by some infants in relation to the caregiver in the attachment assessment (Main & Solomon, 1990). The term *disorganization* refers to observed contradictions and inconsistencies in expected attachment-related behavioral sequences or movement patterns (e.g., creeping sideways toward the parent with head averted) that may reflect contradictions in intentions. *Disorientation* refers to behaviors that indicate a lack of orientation to the present environment (e.g., immobilized behavior accompanied by dazed expression in the presence of the caregiver). With development, increasingly complex behavioral strategies for coping with stress, fear, or incomprehensible caregiving are likely to emerge and reflect the evolving capacities of the child.

Attachment Disorganization: Classification

Classification History

The classification of attachment disorganization/disorientation evolved from efforts to explain exceptional attachment patterns of infants in both high- and low-risk samples who, for a time, appeared to lack coherent behavior consistent with the tripartite system described by Ainsworth (Ainsworth et al., 1978/2015; Main & Solomon, 1990). For example, an unclassifiable mix of avoidant and resistant behaviors was frequently observed in maltreatment samples (Crittenden, 1981; Radke-Yarrow, Cummings, Kuczinski, & Chapman, 1985; Main & Solomon, 1990). Contrary to expectations, new response patterns comparable in coherence to those identified by Ainsworth were not identified. Rather, what the unclassifiable cases had in common were infant displays of inexplicable disorganized, disoriented, or overtly conflicted behaviors in the presence of the caregiver. Many of the behaviors were suggestive of an underlying experience of apprehension or overwhelming distress. Through the review of these cases, common characteristics and strong indicators were discerned, classification guidelines were developed, and with the newly devised protocol, classifiable cases were reviewed for the absence of indicators. (For a complete description of category development, see Main & Solomon, 1990.)

Classification System

The attachment disorganization/disorientation classification system, including behavioral indices that provide the foundation for determining category placement, are intended for use with infants with no evidence of neurological difficulty who range in age from 12 to 18 months. Markers of disorganization include individual behaviors and behavioral sequences representing acts of commission and omission (e.g., signs of inhibition, contradiction, and apprehension; see Table 4.1 for examples). By definition, and consistent with an organizational perspective (Sroufe & Waters, 1977), there is no exhaustive list of behaviors, and no single behavior indicates disorganization. Markers of disorganization may be extensive and pronounced or fleeting and difficult to detect. Common infant behaviors may indicate disorganization depending upon the timing and context of their expression. Moreover, most infants exhibit variations of these behaviors at times.

As Bowlby (1969/1982) noted, all behavior patterns are rational or meaningful in terms of individual experience but may be incoherent or paradoxical within a particular context. For example, behaviors reflecting moderate apprehension or avoidance of the caregiver may be expectable infant responses to a playful "chase" game but contradictory and incomprehensible responses to distress in the presence of the caregiver. Similarly, low-level repetitive stress behaviors (e.g., rocking) commonly observed in infants in the absence of the caregiver are expected to diminish in the presence of an expectable source of comfort and reassurance. As markers of disorganization, behaviors represent unexpected, often extreme, displays of contradictory behavior and affect with

TABLE 4.1. Markers of Disorganization/Disorientation
I. Sequential display of contradictory behaviors *Example:* Strong display of attachment behavior suddenly followed by avoidance, freezing, or dazed behavior.
II. Simultaneous display of contradictory behaviors *Example:* Strong display of avoidance accompanied by contact-seeking behavior, anger, or distress.
III. Undirected, misdirected, incomplete movements and expressions *Example:* Extensive expressions of distress with no movement or look to the caregiver.
IV. Stereotypies, asymmetrical, mistimed movements, anomalous postures *Example:* Extended or repeated rhythmical movements or assumption of huddled, prone postures in the presence of the caregiver.
V. Freezing, stilling, and maintenance of slowed movements and expressions *Example:* Behavior or attention that represents more than a momentary interruption of activity.
VI. Direct indices of apprehension regarding the parent *Example:* Fearful facial expressions toward or rapid movements away from the caregiver.
VII. Direct indices of disorganization or disorientation *Example:* Disoriented wandering, or rapid changes in affect and behavior in relation to the caregiver.
Data from Main and Solomon (1990).

respect to the goal of maintaining proximity to the caregiver and organization under stress.

Classification Procedure

Attachment disorganization classification requires the researcher first to discern the pattern of relationship organization exhibited by the infant and caregiver in the laboratory attachment assessment based on Ainsworth's system of interactive behavioral rating and classification (Ainsworth et al., 1978/2015; Main & Solomon, 1990). Thus, assessment standardization and experience recognizing organized patterns of security, anxious avoidance, and anxious resistance are critical aspects of the classification process. A subsequent review of the assessment focuses on the presence of anomalous behaviors or behavioral sequences that fail to align with or promote coherent organization of behavior. Special attention is paid to lapses or pronounced deviations in attachment behavior (e.g., proximity-seeking, avoidance, resistance) with consideration of alternative explanations. Coders are challenged to determine whether behavior is *inexplicable* (no evidence of immediate goal or rationale in relation to attachment or exploration) or explicable in terms of expressed or inferred fear (e.g., fearful facial expression directed toward the caregiver, startle and darting away from the caregiver, or inhibited, interrupted approach to the caregiver; Main & Solomon, 1990).

Attachment disorganization coding considers behavioral indices observed in the presence of the caregiver throughout the laboratory assessment, taking into account behaviors not captured in the Ainsworth rating system (e.g., extreme avoidance beyond the first moments of reunion, simultaneous displays of extreme distress and avoidance). However, timing of the appearance of behaviors indicative of disorganization is also considered. Infant behaviors that occur immediately on reunion with the caregiver represent stronger indices of organizational lapse, whereas behaviors followed by an immediate approach to the caregiver (i.e., reorganization) represent weaker indices. Single temporary lapses in organization are viewed as distinct from prolonged or repeated signs of inhibition or disturbance.

In the classification process, observed markers of disorganization are reviewed in relation to behavioral themes or subtypes and assigned ratings (1–9) representing the degree of disruption in the behavioral pattern. Disorganization ratings may range from low (1–3), indicating no or slight lapse in organization to high (7–9), indicating clear or extreme lapse or collapse of an expected behavioral pattern. Indicators of disorganization may occur in conjunction with otherwise well-organized attachment behavior. Conversely, not all infants in relationships that are dysregulated or "difficult to classify" exhibit disorganized behaviors or lapses in an attachment strategy. Assignment of the attachment disorganization classification is based on high overall summary ratings that typically reflect strong or repeated behaviors fitting one or more thematic subtypes of disorganization or disorientation.

Patterns of attachment disorganization/disorientation are distinguished from organized patterns of security and insecurity by the inability of infants to maintain behavioral organization and attention within the caregiving relationship. Even so, in research, the disorganized classification is generally accompanied by a secondary assignment to an organized category (secure, anxious–avoidant, anxious–resistant) reflecting the best fitting underlying relational pattern. In the case of a pervasive collapse or lack of a consistent infant–caregiver relational strategy, no secondary classification is assigned.

Adequate interrater reliability in classification of attachment disorganization/disorientation is well-documented (e.g., van IJzendoorn, Schuengel, & Bakermans-Kranenberg, 1999). See Appendix 4.1 for guidelines regarding training and reliability.

Attachment Disorganization: Prevalence, Antecedents, Developmental Sequelae

Prevalence and Stability

Infant–caregiver relationships classified as disorganized have been found in low and high socioeconomic samples, clinical and nonclinical groups, and across cultures and childrearing contexts, although in varying rates (e.g., range = 4% to 77%; van IJzendoorn et al., 1999; Mesman, van IJzendoorn, & Sagi-Schwartz, 2016). Attachment disorganization subtypes may be differentially distributed in low- and high-risk samples, with a secondary classification of secure more common in low-risk samples and a secondary classification of insecure predominant in higher risk samples (Lyons-Ruth & Jacobvitz, 2016). Based on meta-analytic review, short-term stability of attachment disorganization assessed with the Main and Solomon (1990) coding system has been found to be modest ($r = .35$, $N = 286$; van IJzendoorn et al., 1999). As with organized attachment categories (Vaughn, Egeland, Sroufe, & Waters, 1979), the stability of infant attachment disorganization may be related to contextual stability in the early years of life (e.g., van IJzendoorn et al., 1999).

Antecedent Environmental Factors

Systematic home observations linking proximal environmental factors to attachment disorganization are relatively rare (Jacobvitz, Hazen, Zaccagnino, Messnia, & Beverung, 2011; Schuengel, Bakermans-Kranenburg, van IJzendoorn, & Blom, 1999). However, from its introduction, and consistent with theoretical formulations, the disorganized classification has been linked to alarming caregiving behavior (Hesse & Main, 2006; Madigan et al., 2006), maltreatment (e.g., E. Carlson, 1998; V. Carlson, Cicchetti, Barnett, & Braunwald, 1989; George & Main, 1979) and caregiver hostility and withdrawal (Lyons-Ruth, Lyubchik, Wolfe, & Bronfman, 2002). Especially high rates of disorganization (80–90%) have been found in maltreatment samples in which caregiving is characterized as explicitly frightening or incomprehensible (V. Carlson et al., 1989; Cicchetti, Rogosch, & Toth, 2006). Attachment disorganization in infancy has also been linked to caregiving compromised by psychopathology (e.g., Hobson, Patrick, Crandell, Garcia-Pérez, & Lee, 2005; Lyons-Ruth, Connell, Grunebaum, & Botein, 1990; Martins & Gaffan, 2000; Tomlinson, Cooper, & Murray, 2005; van IJzendoorn et al., 1999), substance use (e.g., Melnick, Finger, Hans, Patrick, & Lyons-Ruth, 2008; O'Connor, Sigman, & Brill, 1987; Rodning, Beckwith, & Howard, 1991), and significant parent–child separations (Solomon & George, 2011). Predictors of attachment disorganization also include infant nutritional status (e.g., Valenzuela, 1997) and cumulative socioeconomic risk (e.g., Cyr, Euser, Bakermans-Kranenburg, & van IJzendoorn, 2010). However, in general, conditions of family risk most generative of disorganization are those that directly relate to or impact the infant–parent interaction and child emotional well-being (e.g., Barnett, Ganiban, & Cicchetti, 1999; Carlson, 1998; van IJzendoorn et al., 1999; Valenzuela, 1997; Zevalkink, Riksen-Walraven, & van Lieshout, 1999).

Of particular theoretical and clinical interest are the links between caregiver state of mind with respect to attachment experience (i.e., unresolved loss and trauma), frightening or incomprehensible caregiving behavior, and infant attachment disorganization. Support for these associations has been demonstrated in a meta-analytic review ($r = .31$; $N = 548$; effect size = 0.65; van IJzendoorn, 1995) and in studies of mediation of intergenerational transmission via maternal frightening behavior (e.g., Jacobvitz et al., 2011) and disrupted communication (Madigan et al., 2006).

Overall, findings related to environmental antecedents suggest that attachment disorganization emerges as a function of both the intensity and frequency of fear-producing experience and the adequacy of the caregiving relationship (Solomon & George, 1999; Waters & Valenzuela, 1999). Frightening caregiving may be sufficient to disorganize (create lapses in) the attachment system of a child who otherwise has developed an adequate relationship with the caregiver. However, normative stress-producing experiences of infancy that remain unbuffered (e.g., emotionally unavailable caregiving) may also lead to disorganized attachment responses. Further research is needed to fully elucidate the meaning of the pattern (Duschinsky & Solomon, 2017; Rutter, Kreppner, & Sonuga-Barke, 2009) and the multiple pathways to disturbance within the infant–caregiver relationship (e.g., Padrón, Carlson, & Sroufe, 2014).

Antecedent Endogenous Factors

Given the heterogeneous nature of attachment disorganization as a classification category, the contributions of child factors (e.g., neonatal behavioral organization and neurological impairment) to attachment disorganization have been of great interest. In general, however, there is little evidence that constitutional factors or inborn traits account for the attachment phenomenon. A meta-analytic study and related research have revealed non-significant associations between behavioral assessments of infant temperament and attachment disorganization (Barnett, Ganiban, et al., 1999; Carlson, 1998; van IJzendoorn et al., 1999; also see Vaughn & Bost, 2016). Furthermore, ratings of disorganization were not related to maternal histories of serious medical or psychological problems, pre- and perinatal medical complications, or infant anomalies in a risk sample (Carlson, 1998). In addition to direct evidence, studies examining concordance across caregivers suggest that infants are unlikely to be classified as disorganized with multiple caregivers (e.g., mother and a second caregiver or day care provider; Krentz, 1982; Main & Solomon, 1990; Steele, Steele, & Fonagy, 1996; van IJzendoorn et al., 1999).

Although a phenotypic resemblance between disorganized behavioral markers (e.g., stereotypies) and indices of neurological dysfunction also suggests a link between attachment disorganization and organic impairment, there has been little empirical support for this relation (van IJzendoorn et al., 1999). Barnett, Hunt, et al. (1999) noted that attachment insecurity in children with neurological disorders, as well as other medical conditions, may be attributable to challenges that special needs pose for otherwise sensitive parents. Furthermore, despite the measurement similarities (e.g., overlap in indices), neurological symptoms and signs of relationship disorganization may be distinguished reliably (e.g., Barnett, Hunt, et al., 1999; Pipp-Siegel, Siegel, & Dean, 1999).

Consistent with the view that attachment disorganization reflects a breakdown of a strategy to cope with stress (Main & Solomon, 1990), the pattern has been related to infant stress reactivity (as indexed by high levels of salivary cortisol) in response to brief separations (e.g., Bernard & Dozier, 2010; Hertsgaard, Gunnar, Erickson, & Nachmias, 1995; Spangler & Grossmann, 1993). In animal models, elevated cortisol secretion has been related to an inability of the organism to mobilize an effective strategy to cope with a stressor (e.g., Levine, Wiener, & Coe, 1993). Attachment disorganization has also been associated with atypical patterns of diurnal cortisol secretion (e.g., flattened slope of cortisol levels over the course of the day; Luijk et al., 2010). Similar atypical rates of change have been observed in maltreated infants (Dozier et al., 2006), suggesting that the flattened pattern may be an indicator of caregiving disturbance.

Recent studies have examined the role of genetic factors in the etiology of attachment disorganization. Based on behavioral genetics methods, only nonshared environmental factors have been found to contribute to twin concordances in attachment disorganization, suggesting the primary influence of nonshared environmental factors (Bokhorst et al., 2003).

In the area of molecular genetics, study has focused on dopamine and serotonin pathways, specifically, the dopamine receptor gene (*DRD4*) associated with reward mechanisms involved in social interactions (including mother–infant attachment; Insel, 2003) and the serotonin transporter gene (*5-HTTLPR*) associated with increased negative emotion (Canli & Lesch,

2007). In low-risk samples, research has yielded inconsistent results regarding the link between a *DRD4* allele and increased risk for disorganized attachment (e.g., Bakermans-Kranenburg & van IJzendoorn, 2007, 2016; Lakatos et al., 2000). However, in a low socioeconomic sample, polymorphisms of *DRD4* and *5-HTTLPR* genes differentially influenced the development of attachment disorganization in nonmaltreated and maltreated children (Cicchetti, Rogosch, & Toth, 2011). In this study, nonmaltreated children with the alleles more likely to be classified as disorganized. The authors speculated that whereas low-stress environments may enable the manifestation of genetic variation, the impact of genetic contributions in the evolution of disorganization may be reduced in the context of environmental stress or adversity (e.g., anomalous parenting).

Overall, research regarding genetic variation and attachment disorganization suggests that genes alone or separate measures of environmental and genetic influence may not account for the formation of this phenomenon. Furthermore, while correlational and experimental studies have documented the importance of considering gene–environment interactions in explaining development, investigations related to attachment disorganization have produced conflicting results (Gervai et al., 2007; Luijk et al., 2011). The differential susceptibility or developmental plasticity hypothesis (e.g., sensitivity to positive and negative parenting influences; Belsky, 1997) may provide a useful approach to understanding the relations (Belsky, Bakermans-Kranenburg, & van IJzendoorn, 2007). (For a review of the study on behavioral and molecular genetics and attachment, see Bakermans-Kranenburg & van IJzendoorn, 2016.)

The neuroscience of attachment, including the study of neural mechanisms underlying attachment disorganization and disturbance, is an emerging area of research (Coan, 2016; Schore, 2013). Current knowledge is informed primarily by nonhuman animal work on neural mechanisms related to social bonding and caregiving, as well as preliminary investigations of the neurobiology of normative and disturbed attachment in humans (e.g., Tharner et al., 2013). The work challenges researchers to differentiate behavioral and underlying neural systems given that direct correspondence or alignment is unlikely (e.g., similar behaviors may be caused by dissimilar neural systems, and similar neural activations may result in distinct behavioral manifestations). Integrating what is known about the social brain and affect regulation with attachment theory and research, especially related to disorganization, will require longitudinal, multidisciplinary collaborative approaches (Coan, 2016).

Developmental Sequelae

Internalized regulatory patterns and relational expectations derived from a history of caregiver–infant interaction are thought to guide developmental trajectories of behavioral and emotional organization and expression (Kobak

& Shaver, 1987; Main & Hesse, 1990; Sroufe, 1996; Sroufe & Waters, 1977). Consistent with this view, disrupted attachment relationships have been linked to later psychopathology, not as early disorders of the infant but as markers of beginning pathological processes in the context of interactive biological and environmental influences (Cicchetti, Toth, & Bush, 1988; Sameroff & Emde, 1989; Sroufe, 1997; Sroufe, Egeland, Carlson, & Collins, 2005).

Attachment disorganization/disorientation has been associated with a range of negative outcomes, including externalizing behavior (e.g., Fearon, Bakermans-Kranenburg, van IJzendoorn, Lapsley, & Roisman, 2010; Lyons-Ruth, Alpern, & Repacholi, 1993; Shaw, Owens, Vondra, Keenan, & Winslow, 1996), internalizing symptoms (e.g., Carlson, 1998; Shaw, Keenan, Vondra, Delliquadri, & Giovanelli, 1997), poor attentional performance (Fearon & Belsky, 2004), and global indices of psychopathology (Carlson, 1998). In predictive statistical models including attachment disorganization and risk factors common to both disorganization and psychopathology (e.g., maternal psychosocial problems, depression, family stress), disorganized attachment and related family risks combine to predict later psychopathology (Carlson, 1998; Lyons-Ruth et al., 1993; Shaw et al., 1997). These findings align with a developmental psychopathology perspective wherein early risk, or compromised experience, initiates a cumulative developmental process of child–environment transactions that may lead to disturbance. Whereas the attachment patterns of avoidance and resistance pose risks for later disturbance with some specificity (antisocial behavior and anxiety, respectively), trajectories associated with disorganization reflect more serious overall psychiatric profiles (Sroufe et al., 2005).

Drawing on the notion of a developmental prototype (Spitz, Emde, & Metcalf, 1970) in which a precursor root form is elaborated into more complex phenomena, attachment theorists suggest that disorganization may be one mechanism by which traumatic experience in the caregiving environment is translated into adaptational vulnerabilities, such as dissociative phenomena (e.g., Liotti, 1992, 1999). Noting the resemblance of disorganization behaviors (e.g., stilling) to lapses in orientation and control associated with dissociative disorders (Putnam, 1985, 1994; Hilgard, 1986), Liotti (1992, 1999) and others have suggested that the lack of integration of early caregiving experience (e.g., extreme threat without reparation) may leave infants vulnerable to developing enduring altered forms of processing and encoding information. Preliminary support for this hypothesis has been demonstrated in relations between attachment disorganization measured in infancy and dissociative behaviors and experiences assessed from middle childhood through adulthood (Carlson, 1998; Dutra, Bureau, Holmes, Lyubchik, & Lyons-Ruth, 2009; Ogawa, Sroufe, Weinfield, Carlson, & Egeland, 1997; Smeekens, Riksen-Walraven, & van Bakel, 2009). Research is needed to clarify and confirm these relations across varied samples (e.g., Haltigan & Roisman, 2015) and to identify factors and processes that may shape (e.g., maintain or deflect individuals from) dissociative developmental trajectories.

Attachment Disorganization Summary

Understanding attachment disorganization requires a fundamental knowledge of attachment organization and an awareness of the complex relations within and among developing behavioral systems. However, understanding the meaning of any behavioral pattern related to attachment also involves a process of (1) identification, or description of the pattern; (2) validation, or demonstration that the pattern reflects individual differences in secure base behavior, not other behavioral or psychological constructs; and (3) explanation, or developing and testing hypotheses regarding mechanisms underlying the attachment pattern (Waters & Valenzuela, 1999).

Although the breakdown in attachment relationship organization manifested in disorganization/disorientation has been identified and reliably linked to predictable correlates, explanation of developmental processes and cultural influences lags behind that available for differences in attachment organization. For example, little is known about the etiologies of differing manifestations of disorganization, how endogenous and environmental factors interact to yield variations in disturbance, or whether, for some infants, the disturbance represents a delay in the consolidation of attachment organization (e.g., Rutter et al., 2009; Waters et al., 1991). Research is also required to better understand the developmental sequelae of attachment disorganization, specifically, the level of risk posed by different forms of disturbance, the mechanisms that link disorganization and later psychopathology, and the developmental processes or intervention approaches required to support the repair of early relationships (Duschinsky & Solomon, 2017). See Solomon, Duschinsky, Bakkum, and Schuengel (Chapter 5, this volume) for discussion of future directions.

DISORDERED AND ATYPICAL ATTACHMENTS

From an evolutionary perspective, the attachment system is highly canalized. Even in aberrant and abusive conditions of care, such as neglectful institutional care, the majority of children create attachments to new caregivers, often long after the normative developmental period for creating first relationships. Despite this apparent resilience and flexibility, social attachments in animals that do not receive the normal or expected environmental input early exhibit fundamental developmental deviations (e.g., Suomi, 2000, 2016). Disturbed early relationships in nonhuman primates (e.g., peer rearing in the absence of consistent adult caregiving) predict disordered behavior (e.g., excessive reactivity and impulsivity) that is both lifelong and cross-generational (Suomi, 2016). Similarly, in humans, atypical social relationships associated with extreme deprivation may reflect fundamental and enduring disturbances in individual and relationship functioning. In contrast to the often episodic lapses in behavioral coherence associated with attachment disorganization, attachment disturbances associated with early deprivation and chronic disruption of early relationship experience may represent more pervasive deficits or lack of organization within and across multiple developing systems.

Description

Fundamental deviations and delays in early functioning, including the development of attachment, have been well-documented in infants exposed to experiences of extreme neglect and separation (e.g., Ames & Chisholm, 2001; Chisholm, 1998; MacLean, 2003; Rutter & the ERA Study Team, 1998). Notable attachment-related disturbances have included marked displays of isolated attachment behaviors (e.g., excessive clinging), contradictory behavioral sequences directed toward unfamiliar adults (e.g., immediate sociability followed by wariness), and the failure to reference appropriate caregivers in new and threatening situations (e.g., Bruce, Tarullo, & Gunnar, 2009; Chisholm, 1998; O'Connor, Bredenkamp, Rutter, & the ERA Study Team, 1999). These behavioral markers are consistent with those identified in early clinical observations of institutionalized children (Freud & Burlingham, 1973; Goldfarb, 1955; Provence & Lipton, 1962; Tizard, 1977; Tizard & Rees, 1975). Aberrant, deprivation-specific behaviors also include autistic-like behaviors (e.g., rocking and self-hitting) and atypical reactions to environmental stimuli (e.g., extreme fear and anxiety, overarousal and hyperactivity; e.g., Beckett et al., 2002; MacLean, 2003; Rutter et al., 2010; Verhulst, Althaus, & Versluis-Den Bieman, 1990; Zeanah, Smyke, & Dumitrescu, 2002).

Classification/Diagnosis

Clinically, early relational disorders have been conceptualized as disorders of reactive attachment and disinhibited social engagement. These conditions (along with other disorders related to stress and trauma) are described in the *Diagnostic Classification of Mental Health and Developmental Disorders of Infancy and Early Childhood* (ZERO TO THREE, 2016), the fifth edition of the *Diagnostic and Statistical Manual of Mental Disorders* (American Psychiatric Association, 2013), and the 10th revision of the *International Classification of Diseases* (World Health Organization, 1992). Manifestations of reactive attachment disorder include extreme emotional withdrawal, absence or minimal developmentally appropriate comfort-seeking behavior (or response to comfort) when distressed, and minimal social reciprocity with adult caregivers. Disinhibited social engagement disorder is characterized by indiscriminate sociability (e.g., excessive familiarity with unfamiliar adults) and risk-taking behavior (e.g., not checking back with adult caregivers).

Patterns of extreme withdrawal and disinhibited social engagement have been observed in both institutionalized (e.g., Chisholm, Carter, Ames, & Morison, 1995; O'Connor et al., 2003; Tizard & Rees, 1975; Zeanah, 2000) and maltreated children (Albus & Dozier, 1999; Boris et al., 2004; Lyons-Ruth, Bureau, Riley, & Atlas-Corbett, 2009; Zeanah et al., 2004). However, evidence from the study of postinstitutionalized and severe maltreatment samples suggests that patterns of extreme withdrawal or inhibition may be relatively rare and short lived, reflecting developmental delays and deficits in signaling behavior that resolve in the context of subsequent consistently available care (Zeanah, Smyke, Koga, Carlson, & the BEIP Core Group, 2005). In contrast, the disinhibited pattern of social engagement may be a more enduring abnormality, persisting even as attachment security develops and challenging conceptualizations of the disorder as attachment-based (Chisholm, 1998; Zeanah et al., 2002). In addition to diagnosable disorders, children exposed to severe and prolonged early deprivation may exhibit enduring deficits in social communication (e.g., reciprocal interaction), emotional expression (e.g., empathy), and behavioral regulation (e.g., hyperactivity) that impact the formation of early attachment relationships, as well as interpersonal functioning (e.g., peer relationships) across development (Rutter et al., 2010).

Organizational Developmental Perspective

An organizational developmental perspective provides a useful framework for understanding extreme patterns of social relatedness (e.g., inhibition, disinhibition) attributed to disturbances in attachment. As noted, in evolutionary terms, in the absence of an expectable caregiving environment, normative systems processes may become misdirected, distorted, or diminished. Moreover, related systems, typically coordinated within the caregiving relationship experience, may develop unevenly or be decoupled, resulting in persistently impaired functioning. Thus, exceptional adverse caregiving circumstances (e.g., institutionalization) may result in significant delays and distortions within and among developing behavioral and biological systems.

Attachment relationship phenomena observed among institutionalized infants are consistent with this perspective (Vorria et al., 2003; Zeanah et al., 2005). Patterns of fragmented behavioral sequences, indiscriminate social engagement, and emotional dysregulation related to early deprivation reflect descriptions of undeveloped systems of attachment described by ethologists (Hinde, 2005), as well as stages in attachment formation described by Ainsworth (1967, 1973, 1990). Variations in relationship formation among infants with histories of social deprivation have been documented in studies of institutionalized and postinstitutionalized infants (Carlson, Hostinar, Mliner, & Gunnar, 2014; Zeanah et al., 2005) using a measure of attachment formation (derived from the naturalistic observations of attachment development; Ainsworth, 1967). Rating indices included signs of minimal or no attachment (e.g., lack of separation-related distress and response to the caregiver, minimal exploratory behavior), evidence of a preferred caregiver (e.g., differential distress, visual–postural orientation, and following), and infant initiatives in interaction and exploration in relation to a preferred caregiver (e.g., distress and search behavior during separations, active proximity seeking on reunion). The research highlights attachment formation and organization (e.g., security, disorganization) as differentiable constructs, and the importance of both stability and quality of caregiving in attachment development, organization, and repair (Carlson et al., 2014; Zeanah et al., 2005).

Atypical and Disordered Attachment Summary

Studies of atypical social behavior of institutionalized and postinstitutionalized infants illustrate the complexity of relations within and among systems involved in attachment organization and disturbance. Understanding the sequelae of early deprivation and aberrant caregiving requires extensive observational and longitudinal study similar to that available in the early evolution of attachment theory and the study of normative individual differences (e.g., Humphreys, Nelson, Fox, & Zeanah, 2017; Rutter et al., 2010). Systematic research is needed to understand the origins and course of enduring atypical patterns of social relatedness, the extent to which deprivation-specific patterns may be related to attachment or other developing systems, and the roles of genetic variation and environmental experience in shaping trajectories of disturbance (e.g., Humphreys et al., 2017; Rutter et al., 2009, 2010). Clinically, naturalistic observation and rigorous empirical study may inform the development of effective intervention strategies, specifically, the environmental input required and processes involved in the organization of attachment beyond infancy (Solomon & George, 1999; Rutter et al., 2009; Thompson & Raikes, 2003; Zeanah & Boris, 2018).

CONCLUSION

Returning to the observational assessments of three young infants (Ana, Tony, and Alex) and their caregivers, the brief case descriptions illustrate the importance of an organizational developmental perspective in understanding attachment experience in the early years. Highlighted in these accounts are fundamental differences in the organization of behavior (e.g., integrative, contradictory, and indiscriminate displays of attachment behavior) and related systems (e.g., fear/wariness, attachment, exploration). Although represented in classification schemas related to attachment organization, disorganization, and disorder, the behavioral examples reflect a complexity of relations within and among developing systems not fully explained by current theory and research. Careful observation and description of basic phenomena from an organizational framework may generate useful hypotheses regarding both the nature of and processes that lead to early relationship disturbance. At the same time, understanding the origin and course of disturbance (e.g., delays, lack of coordination in developing systems) may advance our understanding of the mechanisms that underlie organization and integration of early development under normative conditions.

REFERENCES

Ainsworth, M. D. S. (1967). *Infancy in Uganda: Infant care and the growth of love.* Baltimore: Johns Hopkins University Press.

Ainsworth, M. D. S. (1973). The development of infant–mother attachment. In B. Caldwell & H. Ricciuti (Eds.), *Review of child development research* (Vol. 3, pp. 1–94). Chicago: University of Chicago Press.

Ainsworth, M. D. S. (1990). Some considerations regarding theory and assessment relevant to attachments beyond infancy. In M. T. Greenberg, D. Cicchetti, & E. M. Cummings (Eds.), *Attachment in the preschool years: Theory, research, and intervention* (pp. 463–488). Chicago: University of Chicago Press.

Ainsworth, M. D. S., Bell, S. M., & Stayton, D. J. (1974). Infant–mother attachment and social development: "Socialization" as a product of reciprocal responsiveness to signals. In M. P. Richards (Ed.), *The integration of the child into a social world* (pp. 99–135). London: Cambridge University Press.

Ainsworth, M. D. S., Blehar, M. C., Waters, E., & Wall, S. (2015). *Patterns of attachment: A psychological study of the Strange Situation.* New York: Taylor & Francis (Psychology Press). (Original work published 1978)

Ainsworth, M. D. S., & Wittig, B. A. (1969). Attachment and exploratory behavior of one-year-olds in a Strange Situation. In B. M. Foss (Ed.), *Determinants of infant behavior* (Vol. 4, pp. 111–136). London: Methuen.

Albus, K. E., & Dozier, M. (1999). Indiscriminate friendliness and terror of strangers in infancy: Contributions from the study of infants in foster care. *Infant Mental Health Journal, 20*(1), 30–41.

American Psychiatric Association. (2013). *Diagnostic and statistical manual of mental disorders* (5th ed.). Arlington, VA: Author.

Ames, E. W., & Chisholm, K. (2001). Social and emotional development in children adopted from institutions. In D. B. Bailey, Jr., J. T. Bruer, F. J. Symons, & J. W. Lichtman (Eds.), *Critical thinking about critical periods* (pp. 129–148). Baltimore: Brookes.

Bakermans-Kranenburg, M. J., & van IJzendoorn, M. H. (2007). Genetic vulnerability or differential susceptibility in child development?: The case of attachment. *Journal of Child Psychology and Psychiatry, 48,* 1160–1173.

Bakermans-Kranenburg, M. J., & van IJzendoorn, M. H. (2016). Attachment, parenting, and genetics. In J. Cassidy & P. R. Shaver (Eds.), *Handbook of attachment: Theory, research, and clinical applications* (3rd ed., pp. 155–179). New York: Guilford Press.

Barnett, D., Ganiban, J., & Cicchetti, D. (1999). Maltreatment, negative expressivity, and the development of Type D attachment from 12 to 24 months of age. *Society for Research in Child Development Monograph, 64,* 97–118.

Barnett, D., Hunt, K. H., Butler, C. M., McCaskill, J. W., Kaplan-Estrin, M., & Pipp-Siegel, S. (1999). Indices of attachment disorganization among toddlers with neurological and non-neurological problems. In J. Solomon & C. George (Eds.), *Attachment disorganization* (pp. 189–212). New York: Guilford Press.

Beckett, C., Bredenkamp, D., Castle, J., Groothues, C., O'Connor, T. G. Rutter, M., & the ERA Study Team. (2002). Behavior problems associated with institutionalized deprivation: A study of children adopted from Romania. *Journal of Developmental and Behavioral Pediatrics, 23,* 297–303.

Belsky, J. (1997). Variation in susceptibility to environmental influence: An evolutionary argument. *Psychological Inquiry, 8,* 182–186.

Belsky, J., Bakermans-Kranenburg, M. J., & van IJzendoorn, M. H. (2007). For better and worse: Differential susceptibility to environmental influences. *Current Directions in Psychological Science, 16*(6), 300–304.

Bernard, K., & Dozier, M. (2010). Examining infants' cortisol responses to laboratory tasks among children varying in attachment disorganization: Stress reactivity or return to baseline? *Developmental Psychology, 46,* 1771–1778.

Bischof, N. (1975). A systems approach toward the functional connections of attachment and fear. *Child Development, 46,* 801–817.

Block, J. (1971). *Lives through time.* Berkeley, CA: Bancroft Books.

Bokhorst, C., Bakermans-Kranenburg, M., Fearon, R., van IJzendoorn, M., Fonagy, P., & Schuengel, C. (2003). The importance of shared environment in mother–infant attachment security: A behavioral genetic study. *Child Development, 74,* 1769–1782.

Boris, N. W., Hinshaw-Fuselier, S. S., Smyke, A. T., Scheeringa, M., Heller, S. S., & Zeanah, C. H. (2004). Comparing criteria for attachment disorders: Establishing reliability and validity in high-risk samples. *Journal of the American Academy of Child and Adolescent Psychiatry, 43*(5), 568–577.

Bowlby, J. (1973). *Separation.* New York: Basic Books.

Bowlby, J. (1982). *Attachment and loss: Vol. 1. Attachment.* New York: Basic Books. (Original work published 1969)

Bretherton, I., & Ainsworth, M. D. S. (1974). One-year-olds in the Strange Situation. In M. Lewis & L. Rosenblum (Eds.), *The origins of fear* (pp. 134–164). New York: Wiley.

Bruce, J., Tarullo, A. R., & Gunnar, M. R. (2009). Disinhibited social behavior among internationally adopted children. *Development and Psychopathology, 21,* 157–171.

Canli, T., & Lesch, K. (2007). Long story short: Serotonin transporter in emotion regulation and social cognition. *Nature Neuroscience, 10,* 1103–1109.

Carlson, E. A. (1998). A prospective longitudinal study of disorganized/disoriented attachment. *Child Development, 69,* 1107–1128.

Carlson, E. A., Hostinar, C. E., Mliner, S. B., & Gunnar, M. R. (2014). The emergence of attachment following early social deprivation. *Development and Psychopathology, 26*(2), 479–489.

Carlson, E. A., Yates, T. M., & Sroufe, L. A. (2009). Dissociation and development of the self. In P. F. Dell, J. O'Neil, & E. Somer (Eds.), *Dissociation and the dissociative disorders: DSM V and beyond* (pp. 39–52). New York: Routledge.

Carlson, V., Cicchetti, D., Barnett, D., & Braunwald, K. (1989). Finding order in disorganization: Lessons from research on maltreated infants' attachments to their caregivers. In D. Cicchetti & V. Carlson (Eds.), *Child maltreatment: Theory and research on the causes and consequences of child abuse and neglect* (pp. 494–528). New York: Cambridge University Press.

Chisholm, K. (1998). A three-year follow-up of attachment and indiscriminate friendliness in children adopted from Romanian orphanages. *Child Development, 69,* 1092–1106.

Chisholm, K., Carter, M. C., Ames, E. W., & Morison, S. J. (1995). Attachment security and indiscriminately friendly behavior in children adopted from Romanian orphanages. *Development and Psychopathology, 7,* 283–294.

Cicchetti, D. (1984). The emergence of developmental psychopathology. *Child Development, 55,* 1–7.

Cicchetti, D., Rogosch, F. A., & Toth, S. (2006). Fostering secure attachment in infants in maltreating families through preventative interventions. *Development and Psychopathology, 18,* 623–649.

Cicchetti, D., Rogosch, F., & Toth, S. (2011). The effects of child maltreatment and polymorphisms of the serotonin transporter and dopamine D4 receptor genes on infant attachment and intervention efficacy. *Development and Psychopathology, 23,* 357–372.

Cicchetti, D., & Sroufe, L. A. (1978). An organizational view of affect: Illustration from the study of Down's syndrome infants. In M. Lewis & L. Rosenblum (Eds.), *The development of affect* (pp. 309–350). New York: Plenum Press.

Cicchetti, D., Toth, S., & Bush, M. (1988). Developmental psychopathology and incompetence in childhood: Suggestions for intervention. In B. Lahey & A. Kazdin (Eds.), *Advances in clinical child psychology* (Vol. 11, pp. 1–71). New York: Plenum Press.

Cicchetti, D., & Valentino, K. (2006). An ecological transactional perspective on child maltreatment: Failure of the average expectable environment and its influence upon child development. In D. Cicchetti & D. J. Cohen (Eds.), *Developmental psychopathology: Risk, disorder, and adaptation* (2nd ed., Vol. 3, pp. 129–201). Hoboken, NJ: Wiley.

Coan, J. A. (2016). Toward a neuroscience of attachment. In J. Cassidy & P. R. Shaver (Eds.), *Handbook of attachment: Theory, research, and clinical applications* (3rd ed., pp. 242–269). New York: Guilford Press.

Crittenden, P. M. (1981). Abusing, neglecting, problematic, and adequate dyads: Differentiating by patterns of interaction. *Merrill–Palmer Quarterly, 27,* 201–208.

Cyr, C., Euser, E. M., Bakermans-Kranenburg, M., & van IJzendoorn, M. (2010). Attachment security and disorganization in maltreating and high-risk families: A series of meta-analyses. *Development and Psychopathology, 22*(1), 87–108.

Dozier, M., Manni, M., Gordon, M., Peloso, E., Gunnar, M., Stovall-McClough, K., . . . Levine, S. (2006). Foster children's diurnal production of cortisol: An exploratory study. *Child Maltreatment, 2,* 189–197.

Duschinsky, R., & Solomon, J. (2017). Infant disorganized attachment: Clarifying levels of analysis. *Clinical Child Psychology and Psychiatry, 22,* 524–538.

Dutra, L., Bureau, J.-F., Holmes, B., Lyubchik, A., & Lyons-Ruth, K. (2009). Quality of early care and childhood trauma: A prospective study of developmental pathways to dissociation. *Journal of Nervous and Mental Disease, 197,* 383–390.

Emde, R. N., & Harmon, R. J. (1978). *The development of attachment and affiliative systems.* New York: Plenum Press.

Fearon, R. M. P., Bakermans-Kranenburg, M. J., van IJzendoorn, M. H., Lapsley, A., & Roisman, G. I. (2010). The significance of insecure attachment and disorganization in the development of children's externalizing behavior: A meta-analytic study. *Child Development, 81,* 435–456.

Fearon, R. M. P., & Belsky, J. (2004). Attachment and attention: Protection in relation to gender and cumulative social-contextual adversity. *Child Development, 75*(6), 1677–1693.

Fogel, A., & Thelen, E. (1987). The development of expressive and communicative action in the first year: Reinterpreting the evidence from dynamic systems perspective. *Developmental Psychology, 23,* 747–761.

Freud, A., & Burlingham, D. (1973). *The writings of Anna Freud: Vol. 2. Infants without families 1939–1945*. Madison, CT: International Universities Press.

George, C., & Main, M. (1979). Social interaction of young abused children: Approach, avoidance, and aggression. *Child Development, 50*, 306–318.

Gervai, J., Novak, A., Lakatos, K., Toth, I., Danis, I., Ronai, Z., . . . Lyons-Ruth, K. (2007). Infant genotype may moderate sensitivity to maternal affective communications: Attachment disorganization, quality of care, and *DRD4* polymorphism. *Social Neuroscience, 2*, 1–13.

Goldfarb, W. (1955). Emotional and intellectual consequences of psychologic deprivation in infancy: A re-evaluation. In P. Hoch & J. Zubin (Eds.), *Psychopathology of childhood* (pp. 105–119). New York: Guilford Press.

Gottlieb, G. (1991). Experiential canalization of behavioral development. *Developmental Psychology, 27*, 4–13.

Haltigan, J. D., & Roisman, G. I. (2015). Infant attachment insecurity and dissociative symptomatology: Findings from the NICHD Study of Early Care and Youth Development. *Infant Mental Health Journal, 36*(1), 30–41.

Hartman, H. (1958). *Ego psychology and the problem of adaptation*. New York: International Universities Press.

Hertsgaard, L., Gunnar, M., Erickson, M. F., & Nachmias, M. (1995). Adrenocortical responses to the Strange Situation in infants with disorganized/disoriented attachment relationships. *Child Development, 66*, 1100–1106.

Hesse, E., & Main, M. (2000). Disorganized infant, child, and adult attachment: Collapse in behavioral and attentional strategies. *Journal of the American Psychoanalytic Association, 48*(4), 1097–1127.

Hesse, E., & Main, M. (2006). Frightening, threatening and dissociative parental behavior in low-risk samples: Description, discussion, and interpretations. *Development and Psychopathology, 18*(2), 309–343.

Hilgard, E. R. (1986). *Divided consciousness: Multiple controls in human thought and action*. New York: Wiley.

Hinde, R. A. (2005). Ethology and attachment theory. In K. Grossmann, K. E. Grossmann, & E. Waters (Eds.), *Attachment from infancy to adulthood: The major longitudinal studies* (pp. 1–12). New York: Guilford Press.

Hobson, R. P., Patrick, M., Crandell, L., García-Pérez, R., & Lee, A. (2005). Personal relatedness and attachment in infants of mothers with borderline personality disorder. *Development and Psychopathology, 17*, 329–347.

Humphreys, K. L., Nelson, C. A., Fox, N. A., & Zeanah, C. H. (2017). Signs of reactive attachment disorder and disinhibited social engagement disorder at age 12 years: Effects of institutional care history and high-quality foster care. *Development and Psychopathology, 29*(2), 675–684.

Insel, T. (2003). Is social attachment an addictive disorder? *Physiology and Behavior, 79*, 351–357.

Jacobvitz, D., Hazen, N., Zaccagnino, M., Messina, S., & Beverung, L. (2011). Frightening maternal behavior, infant disorganization, and risks for psychopathology. In D. Cicchetti & G. Roisman (Eds.), *Minnesota Symposium on Child Psychology: The origins and organization of adaptation and maladaptation* (Vol. 36, pp. 283–322). New York: Wiley.

Kobak, R. R., & Shaver, P. (1987, June). *Strategies for maintaining felt security: A theoretical analysis of continuity and change in styles of social adaptation*. Paper presented at the conference honoring John Bowlby's 80th birthday, London, UK.

Krentz, M. S. (1982). *Qualitative differences between mother–child and caregiver–child attachments in family daycare.* Unpublished doctoral dissertation, California School of Professional Psychology, Berkeley, CA.

Labella, M., & Cicchetti, D. (2017). Developmental psychopathology. In *The SAGE Encyclopedia of abnormal and clinical psychology* (pp. 1075–1078). Thousand Oaks, CA: SAGE.

Lakatos, K., Toth, I., Nemoda, Z., Ney, K., Sasvari-Szekely, M., & Gervai, J. (2000). Dopamine D4 receptor (DRD4) gene polymorphism is associated with attachment disorganization in infants. *Molecular Psychiatry, 5,* 633–637.

Levine, S., Wiener, S. G., & Coe, C. L. (1993). Temporal and social factors influencing behavioral and hormonal responses to separation in mother and infant squirrel monkeys. *Psychoneuroendocrinology, 18,* 297–306.

Liotti, G. (1992). Disorganized/disoriented attachment in the etiology of the dissociative disorders. *Dissociation, 4,* 196–204.

Liotti, G. (1999). Understanding the dissociative processes: The contribution of attachment theory. *Psychoanalytic Inquiry, 19,* 757–783.

Luijk, M., Roisman, G., Haltigan, J., Tiemeier, H., Booth-LaForce, C., van IJzendoorn, M., . . . Bakermans-Kranenburg, M. J. (2011). Dopaminergic, serotonergic, and oxytonergic candidate genes associated with infant attachment security and disorganization?: In search of main and interaction effects. *Journal of Child Psychology and Psychiatry, 52,* 1295–1307.

Luijk, M. P., Saridjan, N., Tharner, A., van IJzendoorn, M. H., Bakermans-Kranenburg, M. J., Jaddoe,V. W., . . . Tiemeier, H. (2010). Attachment, depression, and cortisol: Deviant patterns in insecure–resistant and disorganized infants. *Developmental Psychobiology, 52*(5), 441–452.

Lyons-Ruth, K., Alpern, L., & Repacholi, B. (1993). Disorganized infant attachment classification and maternal psychosocial problems as predictors of hostile–aggressive behavior in the preschool classroom. *Child Development, 64,* 572–585.

Lyons-Ruth, K., Bureau, J.-F., Riley, C., & Atlas-Corbett, A. (2009). Socially indiscriminate attachment behavior in the Strange Situation: Convergent and discriminant validity in relation to caregiving risk, later behavior problems, and attachment insecurity. *Development and Psychopathology, 21,* 355–372.

Lyons-Ruth, K., Connell, D., Grunebaum, H., & Botein, S. (1990). Infants at social risk: Maternal depression and family support services as mediators of infant development and security of attachment. *Child Development, 61,* 85–98.

Lyons-Ruth, K., & Jacobvitz, D. (2016). Attachment disorganization from infancy to adulthood: Neurobiological correlates, parenting contexts, and pathways to disorder. In J. Cassidy & P. R. Shaver (Eds.), *Handbook of attachment: Theory, research, and clinical applications* (3rd ed., pp. 667–695). New York: Guilford Press.

Lyons-Ruth, K., Lyubchik, A., Wolfe, R., & Bronfman, E. (2002). Parental depression and child attachment: Hostile and helpless profiles of parent and child behavior among families at risk. In S. Goodman & I. Gottlieb (Eds.), *Children of depressed parents: Alternative pathways to risk for psychopathology* (pp. 89–121). Washington, DC: American Psychological Association.

MacLean, K. (2003). The impact of institutionalization on child development. *Development and Psychopathology, 15,* 853–884.

Madigan, S., Bakermans-Kranenburg, M. J., van IJzendoorn, M. H., Moran, G.,

Pederson, D. R., & Benoit, D. (2006). Unresolved states of mind, anomalous parental behavior, and disorganized attachment: A review and meta-analysis of a transmission gap. *Attachment and Human Development, 8,* 89–111.

Main, M., & Hesse, E. (1990). Parents' unresolved traumatic experiences are related to infant disorganized attachment status: Is frightened and/or frightening parental behavior the linking mechanism? In M. T. Greenberg, D. Cicchetti, & E. M. Cummings (Eds.), *Attachment in the preschool years* (pp. 161–182). Chicago: University of Chicago Press.

Main, M., & Solomon, J. (1990). Procedures for identifying infants as disorganized/disoriented during the Ainsworth Strange Situation. In M. T. Greenberg, D. Cicchetti, & E. M. Cummings (Eds.), *Attachment in the preschool years* (pp. 121–160). Chicago: University of Chicago Press.

Martins, C., & Gaffan, E. A. (2000). Effects of early maternal depression on patterns of infant–mother attachment: A meta-analytic investigation. *Journal of Child Psychology and Psychiatry, 41*(6), 737–746.

Melnick, S. M., Finger, B., Hans, S., Patrick, M., & Lyons-Ruth, K. (2008). Hostile–helpless states of mind in the Adult Attachment Interview (AAI): A proposed additional AAI category with implications for identifying disorganized infant attachment in high-risk samples. In H. Steele & M. Steele (Eds.), *Clinical applications of the Adult Attachment Interview* (pp. 399–423). New York: Guilford Press.

Mesman, J., van IJzendoorn, M. H., & Sagi-Schwartz, A. (2016). Cross-cultural patterns of attachment: Universal and contextual dimensions. In J. Cassidy & P. R. Shaver (Eds.), *Handbook of attachment: Theory, research, and clinical applications* (3rd ed., pp. 852–877). New York: Guilford Press.

O'Connor, M. J., Sigman, M., & Brill, N. (1987). Disorganization of attachment in relation to maternal alcohol consumption. *Journal of Consulting and Clinical Psychology, 55,* 831–836.

O'Connor, T. G., Bredenkamp, D., Rutter, M., & the ERA Study Team. (1999). Attachment disturbances and disorders in children exposed to early severe deprivation. *Infant Mental Health Journal, 20,* 10–29.

O'Connor, T. G., Marvin, R. S., Rutter, M., Olrick, J. T., Britner, P. A., & the ERA Study Team. (2003). Attachment following early institutional deprivation. *Development and Psychopathology, 15,* 19–38.

Ogawa, J. R., Sroufe, L. A., Weinfield, N. S., Carlson, E. A., & Egeland, B. (1997). Development and the fragmented self: Longitudinal study of dissociative symptomatology in a nonclinical sample. *Development and Psychopathology, 9,* 855–879.

Padrón, E., Carlson, E., & Sroufe, L. A. (2014). Frightened versus not frightened disorganized infant attachment: Newborn characteristics and maternal caregiving, *American Journal of Orthopsychiatry, 84,* 201–208.

Pipp-Siegel, S., Siegel, C. H., & Dean, J. (1999). Neurological aspects of the disorganized/disoriented attachment classification system: Differentiating quality of the attachment relationship from neurological impairment. In J. I. Vondra & D. Barnett (Eds.), Atypical attachment in infancy and early childhood among children at developmental risk. *Monographs of the Society for Research in Child Development, 64,* 25–44.

Provence, S., & Lipton, R. C. (1962). *Infants in institutions: A comparison of their development with family-reared infants during the first year of life.* New York: International Universities Press.

Putnam, F. W. (1985). Dissociation as a response to extreme trauma. In R. P. Kluft (Ed.), *The childhood antecedents of multiple personality* (pp. 65–98). Washington, DC: American Psychiatric Press.

Putnam, F. W. (1994). Dissociation and disturbances of self. In D. Cicchetti & S. Toth (Eds.), *Rochester Symposium on Developmental Psychopathology: Vol. 5. Disorders and dysfunctions of the self* (pp. 251–265). Rochester, NY: University of Rochester Press.

Radke-Yarrow, M., Cummings, E. M., Kuczynski, L., & Chapman, M. (1985). Patterns of attachment in 2- and 3-year-olds in normal families with parental depression. *Child Development, 56,* 884–893.

Rodning, C., Beckwith, L., & Howard, J. (1991). Quality of attachment and home environments in children prenatally exposed to PCP and cocaine. *Development and Psychopathology, 3,* 351–366.

Rutter, M., & the ERA Study Team. (1998). Developmental catch-up and deficit, following adoption after severe global early privation. *Journal of Child Psychology and Psychiatry and Allied Disciplines, 39,* 465–476.

Rutter, M., Kreppner, J., & Sonuga-Barke, E. (2009). Emanuel Miller Lecture: Attachment insecurity, disinhibited attachment, and attachment disorders: Where do research findings leave the concepts? *Journal of Child Psychology and Psychiatry, 50*(5), 529–543.

Rutter, M., Sonuga-Barke, E. J., Beckett, C., Bell, C. A., Kreppner, J., Kumsta, R., . . . Stevens, S. (2010). Deprivation-specific psychological patterns: Effects of institutional deprivation by the English and Romanian Adoptee Study Team. *Monographs of the Society for Research in Child Development, 75*(Serial No. 1), 1–252.

Sameroff, A. (1983). Developmental systems: Context and evolution. In W. Kessen (Ed.), *Handbook of child psychology: Vol. 1. History, theories, and methods* (pp. 327–394). New York: Wiley.

Sameroff, A. J., & Chandler, M. J. (1975). Reproductive risk and the continuum of caretaking casualty. In F. D. Horowitz, M. Hetherington, S. Scarr-Salapatek, & G. Siegel (Eds.), *Review of child development research* (Vol. 4, pp. 187–243). Chicago: University of Chicago Press.

Sameroff, A., & Emde, R. (1989). *Relationship disturbances in early childhood.* New York: Basic Books.

Santostefano, S. (1978). *A biodevelopmental approach to clinical child psychology.* New York: Wiley.

Schore, A. N. (1994). *Affect regulation and the origin of the self: The neurobiology of emotional development.* Hillsdale, NJ: Erlbaum.

Schore, A. N. (2013). Bowlby's "environment of evolutionary adaptedness": Recent studies on the interpersonal neurobiology of attachment and emotional development. In D. Narvaez, J. Panksepp, A. N. Schore, & T. R. Gleason (Eds.), *Evolution, early experience and human development: From research to practice and policy* (pp. 31–67). New York: Oxford University Press.

Schuengel, C., Bakermans-Kranenburg, M., van IJzendoorn, M., & Blom, M. (1999). Unresolved loss and infant disorganization: Links to frightening maternal behavior In J. Solomon & C. George (Eds.), *Attachment disorganization* (pp. 71–94). New York: Guilford Press.

Shaw, D. S., Keenan, K., Vondra, V., Delliquadri, E., & Giovannelli, J. (1997). Antecedents of preschoolers' internalizing problems: A longitudinal study of low-income families. *Journal of the American Academy of Child and Adolescent Psychiatry, 36,* 1760–1767.

Shaw, D. S., Owens, E., Vondra, I. J., Keenan, K., & Winslow, E. (1996). Early risk factors and pathways in the development of early disruptive behavior problems. *Development and Psychopathology, 8,* 679–699.

Smeekens, S., Riksen-Walraven, J., & van Bakel, H. (2009). The predictive value of different infant attachment measures for socioemotional development at age five. *Infant Mental Health Journal, 30,* 366–383.

Solomon, J., & George, C. (1999). The place of disorganization in attachment theory: Linking classic observations with contemporary findings. In J. Solomon & C. George (Eds.), *Attachment disorganization* (pp. 3–32). New York: Guilford Press.

Solomon, J., & George, C. (2011). The disorganized attachment–caregiving system: Dysregulation of adaptive processes at multiple levels. In J. Solomon & C. George (Eds.), *Disorganized attachment and caregiving* (pp. 3–24). New York: Guilford Press.

Spangler, G., & Grossmann, K. E. (1993). Biobehavioral organization in securely and insecurely attached infants. *Child Development, 64,* 1439–1450.

Spitz, R., Emde, R., & Metcalf, D. (1970). Further prototypes of ego formation. *Psychoanalytic Study of the Child, 25,* 417–444.

Sroufe, L. A. (1990). An organizational perspective on the self. In D. Cicchetti & M. Beeghly (Eds.), *The self in transition: Infancy to childhood* (pp. 281–307). Chicago: University of Chicago Press.

Sroufe, L. A. (1996). *Emotional development: The organization of emotional life in the early years.* New York: Cambridge University Press.

Sroufe, L. A. (1997). Psychopathology as an outcome of development. *Development and Psychopathology, 9,* 251–268.

Sroufe, L. A., Egeland, B., Carlson, E., & Collins, W. A. (2005). *The development of the person: The Minnesota Study of Risk and Adaptation from Birth to Adulthood.* New York: Guilford Press.

Sroufe, L. A., & Rutter, M. (1984). The domain of developmental psychopathology. *Child Development, 55,* 17–29.

Sroufe, L. A., & Waters, E. (1977). Attachment as an organizational construct. *Child Development, 48,* 1184–1199.

Steele, H., Steele, M., & Fonagy, P. (1996). Associations among attachment classifications of mothers, fathers, and their infants: Evidence for a relationship-specific perspective. *Child Development, 67,* 541–555.

Suomi, S. J. (2000). A biobehavioral perspective on developmental psychopathology: Excessive aggression and serotonergic dysfunction in monkeys. In A. J. Sameroff, M. Lewis, & S. M. Miller (Eds.), *Handbook of developmental psychopathology* (2nd ed., pp. 237–256). Dordrecht, the Netherlands: Kluwer Academic.

Suomi, S. J. (2016). Attachment in rhesus monkeys. In J. Cassidy & J. Shaver (Eds.), *Handbook of attachment: Theory, research, and clinical applications* (pp. 133–154). New York: Guilford Press.

Tharner, A., Dierckx, B., Luijk, M., van IJzendoorn, M., Bakermans-Kranenburg, M., Ginkel, J. R., . . . Tiemeier, H. (2013). Attachment disorganization moderates the effect of maternal postnatal depressive symptoms on infant autonomic functioning. *Psychophysiology, 50*, 195–203.

Thompson, R. A., & Raikes, H. A. (2003). Toward the next quarter-century: Conceptual and methodological challenges for attachment theory. *Development and Psychopathology, 15*, 691–718.

Tizard, B. (1977). *Adoption: A second chance*. London: Open Books.

Tizard, B., & Rees, J. (1975). The effect of early institutional rearing on the behavior problems and affectional relationships of 4-year-old children. *Journal of Child Psychology and Psychiatry, 27*, 61–73.

Tomlinson, M., Cooper, P., & Murray, L. (2005). The mother–infant relationship and infant attachment in a South African peri-urban settlement. *Child Development, 7*, 1044–1054.

Valenzuela, M. (1997). Maternal sensitivity in a developing society: The context of urban poverty and infant chronic malnutrition. *Developmental Psychology, 33*, 845–855.

van IJzendoorn, M. (1995). Adult attachment representations, parental responsiveness, and infant attachment: A meta-analysis on the predictive validity of the Adult Attachment Interview. *Psychological Bulletin, 117*, 387–403.

van IJzendoorn, M. H., Schuengel, C., & Bakermans-Kranenburg, M. J. (1999). Disorganized attachment in early childhood: A meta-analysis of precursors, concomitants, and sequelae. *Development and Psychopathology, 11*, 225–249.

Vaughn, B. E., & Bost, K. K. (2016). Attachment and temperament as intersecting developmental products and interacting developmental contexts throughout infancy and childhood. In J. Cassidy & J. Shaver (Eds.), *Handbook of attachment: Theory, research, and clinical applications* (pp. 202–222). New York: Guilford Press.

Vaughn, B. E., Egeland, B., Sroufe, L. A., & Waters, E. (1979). Individual differences in infant–mother attachment at twelve and eighteen months: Stability and change in families under stress. *Child Development, 50*, 971–975.

Verhulst, F., Althaus, M., & Versluis-Den Bieman, H. J. (1990). Problem behavior in international adoptees: I. An epidemiological study. *Journal of the American Academy of Child and Adolescent Psychology, 29*, 94–103.

Vorria, P., Papaligoura, Z., Dunn, J., van IJzendoorn, M. H., Steele, H., Kontopoulou, A., & Sarafidou, Y. (2003). Early experiences and attachment relationships of Greek infants raised in residential group care. *Journal of Child Psychology, Psychiatry, and Allied Disciplines, 44*, 1208–1220.

Waddington, C. H. (1957). *The strategy of the genes*. London: Allen & Unwin.

Waters, E., Kondo-Ikemura, K., Posada, G., & Richters, J. (1991). Learning to love: Mechanisms and milestones. In M. Gunnar & L. A. Sroufe (Eds.), *Minnesota Symposium on Child Psychology: Vol. 23. Self processes and development* (pp. 217–255). Hillsdale, NJ: Erlbaum.

Waters, E., & Sroufe, L. (1983). Social competence as a developmental construct. *Developmental Review, 3*, 79–97.

Waters, E., & Valenzuela, M. (1999). Explaining disorganized attachment: Clues from research on mild-to-moderately undernourished children in Chile. In J. Solomon & C. George (Eds.), *Attachment disorganization* (pp. 265–290). New York: Guilford Press.

Werner, H. (1948). *The comparative psychology of mental development*. New York: International Universities Press.

Werner, H. (1957). The concept of development from a comparative and organismic point of view. In D. Harris (Ed.), *The concept of development* (pp. 125–148). Minneapolis: University of Minnesota Press.

World Health Organization. (1992). *The ICD-10 classification of mental and behavioral disorders: Clinical descriptions and diagnostic guidelines.* Geneva, Switzerland: Author.

Zeanah, C. H. (2000). Disturbances of attachment in young children adopted from institutions. *Journal of Developmental and Behavioral Pediatrics, 21,* 230–236.

Zeanah, C. H., & Boris, N. W. (2018). Attachment disorders in early childhood. In C. H. Zeanah (Ed.), *Handbook of infant mental health* (4th ed., pp. 452–466). New York: Guilford Press.

Zeanah, C. H., Scheeringa, M., Boris, N. W., Heller, S. S., Smyke, A. T., & Trapani, J. (2004). Reactive attachment disorder in maltreated toddlers. *Child Abuse and Neglect, 28,* 877–888.

Zeanah, C. H., Smyke, A. T., Dumitrescu, B. A. (2002). Attachment disturbances in young children: Indiscriminate behavior and institutional care. *Journal of the American Academy of Child and Adolescent Psychiatry, 41*(8), 983–989.

Zeanah, C. H., Smyke, A. T., Koga, S., Carlson, E. A., & the BEIP Core Group. (2005). Attachment in institutionalized and community children in Romania. *Child Development, 76*(5), 1015–1028.

ZERO TO THREE. (2016). *DC:0–5, Diagnostic classification of mental health and developmental disorders of infancy and childhood.* Washington, DC: Author.

Zevalkink, J., Riksen-Walraven, J. M., & van Lieshout, C. F. M. (1999). Attachment in the Indonesian caregiving context. *Social Development, 8,* 21–40.

APPENDIX 4.1. Attachment Classification Training, Practice, and Reliability

Reliable classification of infant attachment relationships based on the Strange Situation laboratory procedure (Ainsworth et al., 1978/2015) requires training, extensive coding practice, and completion of a reliability test. Introductory assessment and classification training is available at the University of Minnesota (United States), as well as through individual research laboratories.

An infant attachment reliability test is available at the University of Minnesota. The reliability test consists of 35 Strange Situation assessments coded for ABCD by expert coders. Coders of the original set of reliability videos included Mary Ainsworth, Mary Main, Alan Sroufe, Brian Vaughn, Everett Waters, and others with extensive training in administration and classification of the laboratory attachment assessment traced to Mary Ainsworth. All current judges are reliable, experienced coders, having collectively coded more than 5,000 cases representing diverse ethnic, socioeconomic, and risk (e.g., prematurity, maltreatment) categories.

The attachment reliability assessments are drawn from multiple research laboratories, and the set of videos is updated every 3–5 years. The assessments represent the range of infant attachment classification categories (e.g., secure, insecure, and disorganization classifications and subcategories) and difficulty levels. All reliability classifications reflect agreement of at least two expert coders, and no cases are considered unclassifiable. All videos are confidential research material to be used individually by researchers for reliability purposes only.

The University of Minnesota attachment reliability test may be completed at any time by any researcher trained in the coding and classification of infant–caregiver dyads. Researchers may code the assessments to establish reliability across three (ABC, or secure, anxious–avoidant, anxious–resistant) or four (ABCD, or secure, anxious–avoidant, anxious–resistant, disorganized) categories or at the level of security (secure, insecure). Reliability coding must be completed individually without consultation.

In order to protect the integrity of the test, specific feedback is limited. Coders are informed of reliability agreement (e.g., percent agreement), general coding errors (e.g., under- or overcoding of behavioral or disorganization ratings) and, if needed, training recommendations. The test may be repeated, if needed. Once certified as reliable, training, practice, and a reliability check are recommended following a lapse in coding experience.

CHAPTER 5

Issues of Method in the Assessment of Disorganized Attachment

Judith Solomon, Robbie Duschinsky, Lianne Bakkum, and Carlo Schuengel

The disorganized/disoriented (D) infant attachment classification was introduced by Main and Solomon (1986, 1990) to capture infant behavior in the Strange Situation (Ainsworth & Wittig, 1969) that appears strongly contradictory or inexplicable with respect to the well-established Ainsworth secure and insecure patterns. The particular indices of these qualities are very diverse. For instance, some infants display behavior exhibiting a simultaneous contradiction between approach to the caregiver and avoidance of the caregiver, such as approaching the caregiver with their head awkwardly averted. Other infants fall to the floor on reunion with their caregiver, appearing confused or frightened. Or to give another example, some infants greet their caregiver with a smile that also contains elements of fear or apprehension. Main and Solomon reviewed 200 "unclassifiable" Strange Situation videos drawn from both normative and high-risk samples. They did not find one or more coherent sets or patterns of behaviors to be characteristic of the these infants; rather, they were struck by what appeared to be a unifying theme of *disruption* of the attachment system or strong conflict between the behavioral tendencies of approach, avoidance, or resistantance. Since its introduction, the disorganized classification has been found to be associated with proximal precursors such as alarming caregiver behavior (Hesse & Main, 2006; Madigan et al., 2006), long-term caregiver–child separations (Solomon & George, 2011), caregiver withdrawing behaviors (Lyons-Ruth et al., 2013), as well as more distal factors such as cumulative socioeconomic risk (Cyr, Euser, Bakermans-Kranenburg, & van IJzendoorn, 2010). The disorganized classification is also associated with various negative outcomes, most prominently, later externalizing disorders (Fearon, Bakermans-Kranenburg, van IJzendoorn, Lapsley, & Roisman, 2010). Significant gaps in our knowledge remain, however. The disorganized classification "undoubtedly identifies behavioral features of considerable theoretical and clinical significance, but the meaning of the pattern remains rather unclear" (Rutter, Kreppner, & Sonuga-Barke, 2009, p. 532). This ambiguity is due, in part, to the fact that the classification was created before any detailed observations of parent–infant interaction were available for this group beyond the Strange Situation. It was not the operationalization of a preexisting concept; rather, the term *disorganization* was allocated to a heterogenous group of behaviors, with expectation that a good number related to one another in some way, but without expectation that they all meant the same thing (Duschinsky, 2015; Duschinsky, 2020). Subsequent researchers have used the term *disorganization* to refer variously to the category, to a psychological process imputed by the category, and to the behaviors identified by Main and Solomon, on the assumption that these all align (Duschinsky & Solomon, 2017). This assumption has left the concept of disorganization *underspecified,* producing a number of theoretical and psychometric questions that have been elided by confusion about the nature of the construct and too rarely discussed explicitly.

Our primary focus in this chapter is to raise the question and offer some speculations regarding whether all of the behavior indices currently used to identify disorganization reflect similar etiologies and equivalent levels of risk. To address this question we mine one important, largely unknown source of theory relevant to disorganized attachment: Bowlby's discussions of conflict and disorganization, contained in his unpublished texts housed at the Wellcome Trust Library Archive in London. On the basis of the unpublished texts, Bowlby's rigorous and systematic approach to thinking about conflict can be brought into focus, permitting distinctions to be drawn where to date there has been largely the assumption that the indices are inherently meaningless or chaotic products of disorganized processes. We propose that this new lens points to a more differentiated picture of the indices, wherein behaviors that are manifestly indicative of fear and dissociative processes may be hypothesized to represent the highest developmental risk; not incidentally, these are also the processes most closely aligned with the dominant theories of etiology. These theories all point to experiences of fear or alarm, either as a direct product of the cargiver's behavior or due to other events that lead to what Bowlby termed "activation without assuagement" such as major separation or chronic caregiver withdrawal. We suggest that the remainder of the indices may originate from other causes, including, for example, aversive but not necessarily alarming caregiver behavior, developmental vulnerabilities in the child, and even, situationally induced alarm and anxiety. We begin the chapter, however, with additional background for readers who are unfamiliar with the disorganized classification and consideration of additional questions of both psychometric and theoretical interest that may be illuminated by this revised perspective on the indices.

DISORGANIZED ATTACHMENT: SOME BACKGROUND

In our thinking leading up to the introduction of a new disorganized/disoriented (D) attachment classification for the Ainsworth Strange Situation, Main and Solomon were heavily influenced by the ideas of ethologist Robert Hinde (1970), an expert in animal behavior and a friend of John Bowlby. In the mid-1960s, one of Hinde's major areas of research was to conceptualize and systemize the observations of conflict behavior seen across dozens of species in his own research and reported by other ethologists and psychologists. In his book *Animal Behaviour* (1970), Hinde describes several forms of conflict behavior in animals: sequential contradiction (sequential display of two tendencies); simultaneous "compromise" contradiction (simultaneous expression of two tendencies in one action); poorly coordinated forms of simultaneous or sequential contradiction; immobility or freezing; and seemingly irrelevant, stereotypical behavior. Hinde's ideas helped Main and Solomon to identify the behaviors used to index disorganized attachment and to conceptualize them, to varying degrees, as having something in common in a child's experience of conflict in relation to approaching and proximity to the caregiver in the Strange Situation. To the list of conflict behaviors described by Hinde, Main and Solomon added headings for displays of disoriented behavior and directly apprehensive behavior toward the caregiver, since in both cases it was assumed that this would require conflict at the level of the attachment system in some way. Based on and developing Hinde's description of forms of conflict behavior, Main and Solomon therefore clustered their observations into seven classes:

I. Sequential display of contradictory behavior
II. Simultaneous display of contradictory behavior
III. Undirected, misdirected, or incomplete movements
IV. Stereotypies, mistimed movements, and anomalous postures
V. Freezing or stilling
VI. Display of apprehension of the caregiver
VII. Overt signs of disorientation

Under these headings, Main and Solomon presented over 50 exemplars, all based on actual observations of Strange Situation behavior. Coders who investigate disorganized attachment in their own studies obtain training to match exemplars of the seven clusters to their own observations of children's responses to the Strange Situation Procedure. These matches are then taken into consideration when the coder chooses a score on a 9-point rating scale. At a score of 5 or higher, the attachment relationship is classified as disorganized. Strong exemplars, to be more heavily weighted by coders, are marked in *italics* in the table of indices devised by the authors. Scores also reflect the frequency of a behavior, its pervasiveness or duration, its abruptness in behavioral sequence, the extent to which it occurs either close to reunion or in physical proximity with the caregiver, and whether the behavior can be better explained as a reaction to the immediate environment. It should be noted that an infant may be placed into the D group based on relatively brief disruptions in behavior, a point that is often misunderstood by those who are unfamiliar with the coding process.

Attempting to be cautious, Main and Solomon (1990) clustered the behaviors suggestive of disorganization based on morphology (i.e., their appearance alone). The introduction of the classification in such a state of "theory neutrality" reflected the general assumption that the behaviors are essentially interchangeable as expressions of disruption of the attachment system. Main and Solomon selected the label "disorganized," also based on Ainsworth's (1972) usage of the construct of "organization." For Ainsworth, organization referred to the way the infant's attention and behaviors were brought together to form a coherent pattern that functioned smoothly as a whole to maintain the availability of the caregiver in the Strange Situation. The term *disorganization,* then, was intended to represent discrepant infant behaviors observed in the Strange Situation. In most cases, the behavior of the infants placed into the D classification appeared to be distortions to greater or lesser degree of the secure, avoidant, and ambivalent patterns, such as when a child approaches with head averted or shows direct displays of fear or apprehension upon reunion.

QUESTIONS RAISED BY THE CURRENT STATUS OF DEVELOPMENT OF THE MAIN AND SOLOMON CODING SYSTEM

Below we discuss some of the outstanding questions pertaining to the disorganized classification. Some are of more psychometric interest, others are more theoretical, although these areas are necessarily closely interrelated.

Should Disorganization Be Reported as a Category?

Against the background of the almost uniform reliance at that time on Ainsworth, Blehar, Waters, and Wall's (1978) categorical system for coding quality of attachment relationships, Main and Solomon introduced disorganized attachment as a category (Duschinsky, 2015). However the coding protocols also indicate that other information on disorganized attachment should be collected as well. Consistent with their notion that disorganization reflects disruption of an underlying organized attachment pattern, Main and Solomon recommended that coders also attempt to force a secondary classification as avoidant, secure, or resistant in cases classified as disorganized. In addition, as already noted, Main and Solomon devised a 9-point scale to represent, "how much" disorganization is evident, which requires the rater to consider a number of criteria, as well as whether that amount is sufficient to place the case in the disorganized group. Researchers are thus provided with multiple options when they formulate their hypotheses and design their statistical analysis plans. They may elect to operationalize disorganization as (1) a single ordinal rating score; (2) a dichotomy (organized vs. disorganized); or (3) a fourth category in a nominal variable together with avoidant, secure, and resistant attachment. Variation in these practices complicate the synthesis of findings across studies and facilitates selective reporting, reducing the replicability of findings (Duschinsky, 2020).

It may strike one as odd that three decades after the discovery of disorganized attachment researchers still vary in how they define attachment variables. Observational attachment data are relatively time-consuming and expensive to collect, with the result that sample sizes are generally not large (cf. Verhage et al., 2016). This limits the possibility for running sensitivity analyses to test how arbitrary decisions in defining variables and analyzing categories may impact findings, and it limits the possibility for testing differences among categorical and dimensional operationalizations in construct validity. This situation is now starting to change, not only with the large National Institute of Child Health and Human Development (NICHD) study (NICHD Early Child Care Research Network, 1997), but also with several other datasets in which Strange Situations are of sufficient size for structural equation modeling. In addition, attachment researchers collaborate to curate and combine their existing datasets, making possible large-scale individual participant data (IPD) meta-analyses (Riley, Lambert, & Abo-Zaid, 2010), which also can be used to settle psychometric hypotheses (Verhage et al., 2020). The day has not yet arrived when the results of this new methodological phase permit firm guidelines with respect to reporting disorganized phenomena.

Regardless of How One Measures It, Is There An Underlying Process of Disorganization?

For some researchers, the decision between different ways of defining and reporting disorganized attachment is solely pragmatic. Despite the fact that coders get certified in reliability on the category—not the scale—reporting of the 1- to 9-point scale is nonetheless preferred by some groups, for example, as "a continuous measure of extent of disorganization" in order "to maximize the power of the analyses" (Bureau, Easterbrooks, & Lyons-Ruth, 2009, p. 270). However, for other researchers, also at stake here is the fundamental nature of the construct of disorganization. The stakes raised by this question are high, as Main and Cassidy (1988) observe. By definition, the D group is not characterized by a fixed assemblage of behaviors. Nevertheless, whether understood as a category or a dimension, the construct requires the assumption of a common underlying mechanism or process that produces these behaviors. Main and Cassidy suggested that "disorganization operates as a category only in extreme cases, being otherwise a response to stressful conditions which may disappear under less stressful situations, that is, in other cases, operating as a dimension" (pp. 423–424). They suggested that the parent's experience of severe trauma might be more likely to dominate caregiving, whereas less severe trauma or trauma that is partially resolved might produce infrequent disruption in the the attachment–caregiver relationship. They also offered that lower frequencies of disorganized behaviors or lower ratings may result from temporary stress among parents and children.

Parents' and children's experiences of fear have played a large role in Main's thinking about attachment. Specifically, Main and Hesse (1990) predicted that caregivers' frightened or frightening behavior was likely to be a key causal agent for disorganized behavior, because these affects would be likely both to activate the infant's attachment and fear systems, confronting the infant with the paradoxical dispositions to approach as well as to flee the attachment figure. Empirical evidence that the infant is experiencing fear (or has at some time experienced fear) in interaction with the attachment figure is, largely, an open question and at this time has only been inferred from the observation of parental behaviors that appear likely to engender fear or wariness in an infant (e.g., Schuengel, Bakermans-Kranenburg, & van IJzendoorn, 1999).

One widespread, alternative stance, associated particularly with Mikulincer and Shaver (2016), has been to conceptualize attachment disorganization as a general dimension, the product of the combination of the two insecure attachment styles: avoidance and anxiety. Yet it may well be a mistake to conflate disorganized attachment and the combination of avoidance and anxiety. There may be aspects of disorganized attachment irreducible to avoidance and anxiety, such as dissociative phenomena or outright fright; there may also be aspects of the combination of avoidance and anxiety that are irreducible to disorganized attachment. A second stance implies that disorganization is more parsimoniously included as a part of a broader dimension of angry and resistant strategies (e.g., Fraley, Roisman, Booth-LaForce, Owen, & Holland, 2013, Web-based supplement C). In contrast to Mikulincer and Shaver (2016), Fraley and colleagues see disorganization as not or as only weakly associated with avoidant strategies. A counterpoint to the discussion would be to sidestep the essentialistic debate on the categorical or dimensional nature of individual differences in attachment altogether given the lack of external criteria for deciding which of the two models is more true to nature. In the context of the debate on the continuous or categorical nature of individual differences in adult attachment representations, van IJzendoorn and Bakermans-Kranenburg (2014) have argued that even factor-analytic and taxometric analyses may be insufficient for settling the issue, because these analyses are based on rating scale data produced by coders who may base their scoring partly on their conception of attachment quality as a quantitatively or qualitatively distributed phenomenon. This is particularly relevant for the disorganization scale, where a score of 5 still leaves the decision up to the coder to classify the relationship as disorganized or nondisorganized. van IJzendoorn and Bakermans-Kranenburg proposed to consider the incremental validity of coding systems with respect to each other, in pursuit of improving the field's prediction of phenomena of interest.

Efforts to determine the true form of the disorganization construct (rather than optimizing prediction) through factor analysis of currently existing scale data may be premature given the underspecification of the construct in question, with the single scale preventing any test of structural invariance. For example, in low-risk populations, disorganized behaviors that belong in the category "direct indices of apprehension of the caregiver," may be relatively infrequent, as Padrón, Carlson, and Sroufe (2014) suggest. Exploratory factor analyses of interactive attachment behavior scales including disorganized attachment in low-risk samples—but not in high-risk samples—may then find that disorganization scores covary with resistant behavior, as indicative of high distress. Indeed, in the general population sample for the NICHD Study of Early Child Care, Fraley and Spieker (2003) found that disorganization scores loaded moderately on a factor that represented resistant interactive behavior in the Strange Situation episodes and not on the factor that included avoidance, contact maintenance, and proximity seeking.

How Does Infant Disorganized Attachment Relate to Later Atypical Attachment Forms?

There has been inadequate attention to how disorganization relates to later maturation. Famously, Main and Cassidy (1988) reported that infant disorganized attachment predicted controlling–caregiving and controlling–punitive behaviors in later childhood. Yet, in their unpublished coding system (Main & Cassidy, 1986), they noted that among the children showing controlling behavior, "there still may be some direct though subtle signs of behavioral disorganization" (p. 342). In addition, they described a child with disordering of expected temporal sequence in approach and avoidance and another child showing apprehension directly by putting hand to mouth on reunion. Nevertheless, the disorganization rating scale for 6-year-olds' reunion behavior has not been published, and the number of researchers trained in the classification system has remained extremely limited. Thus, while reunion behaviors at age 6 may include behaviors morphologically similar to those in the infant disorganized attachment coding system, it is yet unclear how the diverse D behaviors shown by infants relate to the same behaviors shown by older children and to the controlling patterns that Main and Cassidy found to predominate among formerly disorganized children when seen at age 6. Main and Cassidy proposed that the controlling patterns reflected the ability of older children to manage and contain the frightening and frightened behavior of their caregivers, as well as their own experience of fear. In support of this hypothesis, assessments of children's symbolic representation of attachment provide direct evidence that their subjective experience of their relationships is characterized by fear. The stories created by controlling–punitive children depict frightening events, such as death of the family, destruction of the family home, and unpredictably frightening elements such as ghosts and animated machines. Controlling–caregiving children, on the other hand, tend to be almost entirely silent and constricted when asked to create attachment stories. Yet repeated questioning or accidental cues result in the children creating stories very similar to those of the controlling–punitive children, suggesting that the attachment stories also evoked fear (Solomon, George, & De Jong, 1995). Mother–child interaction of controlling–punitive dyads is more negative than than that of the controlling–caregiving group (George & Solomon, 2016; Lecompte & Moss, 2014). The mothers in the former group also had more negative representations of the relationship with the child. Little else is known about differences between these dyads. One approach to better understanding the emergence of these subgroups may be to investigate their differential linkages to indices of disorganized attachment in infancy.

Do All the Behaviors Point to the Same Process?

As the previous remarks demonstrate, we are concerned that debates about disorganized attachment have been hindered by inadequate attention to the question of whether all parties are talking about the same thing. It could be that there are forms of behavior and/or psychological processes currently included within the construct of disorganized attachment that only gesture weakly in the same direction. However, until recently, the very question of whether all the behaviors reflect the same process has been powerfully obscured by the widely held assumption that *disorganization* means simply "chaos." Use of the term *disorganized* likely helped this assumption along, since in ordinary language the term means "randomness" or "chaos" (Duschinsky & Solomon, 2017). Similarly, the dominant theoretical framework used in thinking about the causes of disorganized attachment has been Main and Hesse's (1990) proposal that the behaviors represent experiences by the child of being afraid of or for their caregiver; yet this has also been a source of ambiguity, as the idea of "fear" was underspecified by the authors, and the way that it was used supported the idea that a single causal process—fear—was disrupting the infant's behavior. Yet there are clear differences in the appearance of behaviors, many of which are suggestive of different psychological processes and, perhaps, etiology. As Main and Hesse (1992) later observed, whereas some appear dissociative, others appear to reflect fear of the parent. Yet other behaviors suggest a conflict about approaching the parent, but without the child appearing evidently fearful. Hesse and Main (2006) went on to argue that studying different caregiving contexts and "comparing these to the forms of D behavior exhibited by infants" would therefore be a "worthwhile endeavor for developmental psychopathology" (p. 335). Similar calls have been made by other researchers (e.g., Beebe & Lachmann, 2014; Crittenden, 2016; Lyons-Ruth et al., 2013; Paetzold, Rholes, & Kohn, 2015; Slade, 2014; Solomon & George, 2016; Waters & Crowell, 1999; Zeanah & Gleason, 2010). For example, Padrón et al. (2014)

have expressed concern about the assumption that disorganized/disoriented attachment represents an undifferentiated category, calling this a misapprehension that "has moved researchers away from attempting to examine patterns in the attachment behavior of disorganized infants" (p. 202). Demonstrating the fruitfulness of this approach, these researchers divided infants placed in the D category into two groups. The first group either showed fear (Index VI) or disorientation (Index VII) in the Strange Situation. The other group did not show characteristics of either index. The investigators then compared the two groups with respect to affect regulation and orientation as newborns. They found that the group that displayed Index I through Index V behaviors had been lower in affect regulation than infants who displayed Index VI and Index VII behaviors, suggesting that the former may be predisposed by neurological difficulties. The authors concluded that Index VI and Index VII may be more closely related to experiences of fear in relation to the caregiver, and so represent more closely the essence of the classification as a whole.

THE NEED FOR THEORY

As we have seen, there are a variety of psychometric challenges facing the construct of disorganized attachment. One solution, offered by Lyons-Ruth and Jacobvitz (2016) in the chapter on disorganization in the *Handbook of Attachment,* has been that data on prediction of developmental outcomes should be used to decide which of the exemplars are indicative of "true" attachment disorganization. Lyons-Ruth and Jacobvitz therefore offer a solution to the dilemma inevitably brought about when Main and Solomon (1986) first used "disorganization" as a label for a heterogenous group of behaviors. For Lyons-Ruth and Jacobvitz, the true nature of disorganization is simply those behaviors that predict later pathology. Another approach to understand the potential heterogeneity of disorganization and the relationship with avoidance and resistance would be to examine the underlying psychometric structure of the "D" coding system itself, of which the D score and classification are the final product. This work may use techniques such as factor analysis and data mining on large datasets. Such work is presently being undertaken by several groups, including efforts by the authors of this chapter. However, whichever path is pursued, it is notable that there is relatively little framework or theory for conceptualizing qualitative differences among the indices of disorganized attachment, and their relationship with conflict and with fear (exceptions include Crittenden, 1999; Padrón et al., 2014). This is likely to hamper the judicious interpretation of findings; the design of future studies of the relationship among caregiving, attachment, and later outcomes; and the flow of insights between clinical practice and basic research. In the second half of the chapter, we therefore turn to a previously unrecognized source of theory regarding potential differences among the indices of disorganized attachment: the unpublished reflections of John Bowlby. As mentioned earlier, Main and

Solomon were deeply influenced by the ideas of the ethologist Robert Hinde, in their thinking leading to the introduction of the disorganized classification. Main's introduction to Hinde had been at John Bowlby's urging, and Bowlby, too, developed reflections on this subject. Yet many of Bowlby's ideas about fear and conflict have remained unpublished. Crucially, Main and Solomon, and other attachment researchers, have not been aware of these texts in work to date on disorganized attachment. As a result of this missing wider context, the considerations that Bowlby did publish—for instance, a whole chapter on conflict and motor breakdown in *Attachment* (1969a, Chapter 6)—have been difficult for readers to interpret effectively, consider clinically, or link to developments in the classification of infant attachment in the Strange Situation.

THE LOGIC WITHIN CONFLICT

In May 1963, John Bowlby organized a conference funded by the Medical Research Council on the nature of conflict behaviors. Following the keynote speakers, Tinbergen and Hinde, Bowlby presented his own considerations about this subject. He argued that lines of determinate difference among conflict behaviors are difficult but not impossible to discern. In this proposal, Bowlby was aligning himself with a consensus position in the ethological community—that different psychological processes likely underlie different forms of conflict behaviors, and that they are *not* inexplicable or interchangeable (e.g., Hinde, 1954; McFarland, 1966; Tinbergen, 1952). Based on behaviors observed by ethologists and psychoanalysts, Bowlby characterized five kinds of conflict behaviors, which he wrote down in the conference paper (PP/Bow/D.6/5, unpublished text housed at the Wellcome Trust Library Archive in London):

- Alternation between behavioral tendencies
- Simultaneous contradiction between behavioral tendencies
- A simultaneous contradiction in which some compromise is reached between the tendencies in behavior that expresses both
- The redirection or misdirection of a tendency
- Displacement or stereotypic behaviors

Clearly, these forms of behavior correspond to some of the indices for the disorganized attachment classification listed by Main and Solomon (1990). Indeed, they are even placed in the same order. This is surely due to both Bowlby and Main and Solomon being indebted to the essential groundwork provided by Hinde.

From the 1950s on, Bowlby's reflections on the disruption of the attachment system resulted in many unpublished texts and notes about different forms of conflict behavior, available in the Wellcome Library Archive.

Bowlby's reflections suggest that the behaviors that would later form the Main and Solomon indices can be categorized into four clusters, and arranged in order as a hierarchy of risk:

- Cluster 1: Direct expressions of the fear behavioral system
- Cluster 2: Disorientation
- Cluster 3: Conflict behavior without overt fear
- Cluster 4: Stereotypies

Bowlby discussed Clusters 1 and 2 as more directly associated with contexts of maltreatment or trauma, whereas Clusters 3 and 4 had weaker links to such experiences and could have a variety of causes associated with stress in the child–caregiver relationship or child neurological difficulties. We are struck by the alignment of Bowlby's reflections with the general conclusions of Padrón et al. (2014), who also distinguish fear and disorientation from other forms of disorganization, and with Main and Cassidy's (1988) position that disorganization may in severe cases behave as a category and under less stressful conditions as a dimension.

Chronologically, it was Clusters 3 and 4 that first came into explicit view in Bowlby's theorizing. As we have seen, they were addressed in Bowlby's 1963 Medical Research Council conference. They receive substantial discussion in *Attachment* (1969a) in the section "Incompatible behavioural systems: Results of simultaneous activation." In the Strange Situation, a distressed child will be impelled by the attachment system to seek the availability of their caregiver. However, children who have had aversive or confusing interactions with the caregiver may experience and display conflict in the context of approach. The classic form of such a conflict is the simultaneous display of approach and avoidance, which would later be described by Main and Solomon in Index II.

Clusters 1 and 2 became subject to sustained attention from 1968, provoked by dialogue with Gordon Bronson about the relationship between attachment and the fear system. Key texts on these clusters include "Types of fear response" from 1968 (PP/Bow/H.209, unpublished text housed at the Wellcome Trust Library Archive in London), the chapter "Forms of Behaviour Indicative of Fear" published in *Separation* (1973), and the letter to Gordon Bronson of April 11, 1974 (PP/BOW/J.9/40, unpublished text housed at the Wellcome Trust Library Archive in London). For Bowlby, the fear system is a behavioral system adapted to ensure distance from danger or cues for danger, and when directly expressed at a behavioral level its outputs are fleeing or freezing, as well as characteristic facial expressions. Bowlby also theorized disorientation in attachment contexts as a response linked to chronic experiences of threat, loss, or trauma. However, he left open the prospect that there could be other causes of disorientation in attachment contexts as well. In their coding system, Main and Solomon italicized the behaviors that were associated most reliably with D classification. Descending through Indices 1–4, these italicizations become less frequent; their frequency increases again in Indices 5, 6, and 7. Similarly, Bowlby considered a hierarchy of risk regarding the conflict behaviors he discussed in his writings. He expected direct "apprehension of the caregiver" and "disorientation" to be associated with greater risk, whereas he suggested that stereotypic behaviors are mostly nonspecific indicators of tension. It is striking the degree to which the hierarchy of risk in Bowlby's thinking matches the distribution of italicized exemplars in Main and Solomon. This distribution is skewed firmly toward behaviors that indicate apprehension or disorientation, whereas stereotypic behaviors are never italicized. Table 5.1 presents a crosswalk between Bowlby's "clusters" of conflict behavior and the Main and Solomon indices used to code disorganized attachment, identifying the primary location in which the Bowlby "cluster" would fall in Main and Solomon's coding system.

With Hinde's ethological theory of conflict at the heart of both accounts, Bowlby's "clusters" align closely with Main and Solomon's behavioral indices. Cluster 1 parallels "direct indices of apprehension" in Main and Solomon (Index VI). Cluster 2 parallels "direct indices of disorientation" (Index VII). Cluster 3 parallels "sequential" and "simultaneous" contradiction without overt fear (Indices I and II). Cluster 4 corresponds to Main and Solomon's identification of "stereotypies" (IV). What is crucial for our concerns is that, for Bowlby, differences among these behaviors likely indicate qualitative differences in parent–child interaction or in the child's processing of experiences with the parent. Of course, a single child may display more than one cluster of behavior in the Strange Situation. This was part of the reason that "disorganization" was originally formed without subdivisions by Main and Solomon (1990). However, the display of behaviors in more than one cluster by a single

TABLE 5.1. Crosswalk between Bowlby and Main and Solomon

Bowlby	Primary location(s) in Main and Solomon[a]
Cluster 1. Direct expressions of the fear behavioral system	Index VI (direct indices of apprehension)
Cluster 2. Disorientation	Index VII (direct indices of disorientation) Index V (freezing and stilling) where this occurs without signs of vigilance
Cluster 3. Conflict behaviors without overt fear	Indices I and II (sequential or simultaneous contradiction) Index III (undirected/misdirected) where these are without signs of fear or disorientation
Cluster 4. Stereotypies	Index IV (stereotypies and anomalous postures)

Note. From Solomon et al. (2017). Reprinted by permission.
[a]Roman numerals refer to the category of disorganized behavior in Main and Solomon (1990).

child was not considered by Bowlby to invalidate the qualitative distinctions between them. It just meant that the distinctions were both real and fuzzy-boundaried (cf. Rosch, 1987).

Each of the four clusters is discussed in turn, drawing together history, theory, and observation. This discussion is taken in condensed form from Solomon, Duschinsky, Bakkum, and Schuengel (2017).

Cluster 1: Fear

The first of Bowlby's "clusters" comprises *direct* expressions of the fear behavioral system. Bowlby theorized that even children who get threatened or maltreated by their caregiver display attachment behavior to the caregiver when facing threat or danger:

> A special but not unusual situation in which there is conflict between attachment behaviour and withdrawal is when the attachment figure is also the one who elicits fear, perhaps by threats or violence. In such conditions young creatures, whether human or non-human, are likely to cling to the threatening or hostile figure rather than run away from him or her. (1973, p. 117). Following this line of reasoning, Main and Hesse (1990) stated that the attachment behavioral system "paradoxically" predisposes children who are afraid of or for their caregivers to still approach these caregivers in times of danger. However, Main and Hesse's (1990) chapter fell subject to a danger identified by Bowlby (1960, p. 110):
>
> unfortunately in colloquial English the word "fear" is used in many senses, often being synonymous with expectant anxiety and sometimes with fright: with fear, we are dealing, not with some single comprehensive form of behavior, but with a heterogeneous collection of interrelated forms, each elicited by a slightly different set of causal conditions and each having a distinctive outcome" (Bowlby, 1973, p. 114)

As Main and Hesse subsequently acknowledged, their use of the term *fear* in the chapter was underspecified, varying between (1) the idea of the infant being directly scared of the caregiver and (2) the idea of the caregiver as a source of alarm for any number of possible reasons.

Bowlby's notes, based on ethological observations, suggest that the fear behavioral system is able to override other systems of behavior, without the emergence of conflict (PP/Bow/H.65, unpublished text housed at the Wellcome Trust Library Archive in London). This may be an explanation for Main and Solomon's (1990) observations of children who displayed a coherent fleeing response during the Strange Situation, without showing conflict behavior. Bowlby further highlighted that "it is now known that young creatures show fear and take avoiding action without pain having played any part whatsoever" (1969b, p. 321). This is an important point for clinicians—disorganization in the Strange Situation does not specifically indicate maltreatment by the caregiver (see also Granqvist et al., 2016).

Bowlby described fleeing and freezing as two possible outputs of the fear behavioral system (1960, p. 96). In his notes on "Types of fear response" from 1968 (PP/Bow/H.209, unpublished text housed at the Wellcome Trust Library Archive in London) and in his book *Separation* (1973, p. 133), he theorized about differences between the two responses. He associated fleeing with avoiding threat by displaying a "frightened facial expression accompanied perhaps by trembling or crying, cowering, hiding, running away," whereas freezing might be associated with anxious, tense vigilance and perhaps the startle reflex. He further reasoned that "the conditions that elicit one form of fear behavior may differ in certain regards from those that elicit another form" (Bowlby, 1973, p. 113). These reflections can help clarify an ambiguity with the phrase "freezing behavior," often used in discussions of disorganized attachment. Strange Situation behavior matching Bowlby's definition of "freezing" is placed in Main and Solomons's Index VI (direct indices of apprehension), that is, "Highly vigilant posture or appearance when in presence of parent. Movements or posture tense, infant gives the impression of being hyperalert to parent even or especially when parent is positioned behind her" (1990, p. 139). Behaviors categorized under Main and Solomon's Index V (freezing and stilling) are not defined as vigilant or tense: "the holding of movements, gestures, or positions in a posture that involves active resistance to gravity," for example, "infant sits or stands with arms held out waist high and to sides." These latter behaviors are perhaps closer to "tonic immobility," a phylogenetically more ancient defense strategy that "appears to activate only when newer structures such as the amygdala are deactivated and when freezing and flight or fight are switched off" (Kozlowska, Walker, McLean, & Carrive, 2015, p. 9). In contrast to freezing in fear, where the function is to gather more information, "playing dead," the common name for tonic immobility, has the function of suppression of fear and movement. Its evolutionary origins may lie in the fact that an immobile organism is more likely to be ignored by predators (Porges, 2007). Kozlowska and colleagues (2015) regard tonic immobility as expressing dissociative states such as derealization and depersonalization. This leads us now on to Bowlby's attention to disorientation and dissociative processes.

Cluster 2: Disorientation

During his time as a military psychiatrist, Bowlby had observed signs of disorientation in combat veterans. He wrote about these observations in the 1940 "War Neurosis Memorandum, British Army" together with Kenneth Soddy (Unpublished Wellcome Trust Memorandum, PB/BOW/C.5/1). They proposed that the disorientation in these soldiers emerged from conflict arising from the equal combination of a chronically activated fear behavioral system and a chronic frustration of their desire to escape from battle (PP/Bow/C.5/1). In his later reflections on disorientation among children, Bowlby predicted that a child would be predisposed to disorientation when facing a threat if his or her caregiver had not served as "the psychic organizer . . . the one who orients him [the child] in space and time" (1951, p. 53). The paradigmatic case to which Bowlby always returned was Laura—the girl seen in Robertson's famous film *A Two-Year-Old Goes to Hospital.* Bowlby, Robertson, and Rosenbluth (1952) reported that during the hospitalization, Laura would initially appear not to recognize her mother, but that "after a few minutes of blankness she 'came to' and responded to her real mother" (p. 86). Bowlby et al. also document Laura's return home. They reported that she continued expressing her desire for reunion in a fixed way, even after her mother was in the room: "when her mother opened the door, Laura looked at her blankly and said, 'But I want my Mummy' " (p. 86).

Melanie Klein (1957, p. 12) had written of disorientation and confusion as a defense used in the transference to respond to a therapist perceived as potentially bad and threatening. Bowlby annotated this passage in his personal copy of Klein's work (now held by Human Development Scotland, in Glasgow) as being of particular interest. Unpublished manuscripts from the years after Klein's death in 1960, such as "Defenses that Follow Loss: Causation and Function" (PP/Bow/D.3/78, unpublished text housed at the Wellcome Trust Library Archive in London), reflect Bowlby's attempt to pin down more precisely the relationship between disorientation and defense. In these works, forms of splitting—or what Bowlby called the "segregation" of mental processes—permit resilience in the face of disintegrative threats precisely by accepting some determinate and limited degree of segregation, though they do disadvantage the organism in certain ways in the long run. Avoidance, for instance, achieves a limited segregation by diverting attention away from attachment cues and toward, for example, the world of physical objects. It rigidifies but does not in itself undermine organization. In contrast to avoidance, dissociation is a more emergency measure for Bowlby, enacting a greater segregation in response to a higher intensity of threat of danger or loss of an attachment figure.

Main and Solomon's Index VII comprises "direct indices of disorientation." However, as noted by Main and Morgan (1996, p. 108) and Carlson, Yates, and Sroufe (2008, p. 44), behaviors that indirectly indicate disorientation also are placed into other indices (e.g., Index III misdirected behaviors, where an infant seems confused). Main proposed that dissociation could play a possible role in such behaviors, which is similar to Bowlby's ideas. For Main, some forms of disorganization do not involve dissociation, whereas others may:

> One candidate for dissociated action consists in an episode of distress or angry behavior which appears without explanation or warning . . . in addition, some infants have been observed raising arms to the stranger (with whom they have already spent several minutes) with a bright greeting as the parent enters the room (Main & Morgan, 1996, p. 125).

Developing this discussion, Main and Hesse make a similar distinction to Bowlby in identifying a disoriented cluster of behaviors as qualitatively distinct from others in terms of their links to a dissociative psychological process: "While many D behaviors identified as disorganized are unlikely dissociative, as hiding under the chair at the entrance of a clearly frightening mother, some D behaviors (chiefly trance-like behaviors and seemingly dissociated actions") do seem to fit a dissociative model" (Hesse & Main, 2006, p. 334).

Bowlby considered disoriented–dissociative forms of child behavior toward their caregiver as especially worrying, high on the "hierarchy of risk." This conclusion has significant interest today for understanding an apparent contradiction in the research literature on disorganized attachment. Carlson et al. (2008) reported empirical findings on the risk of dissociation: "Prospectively, most infant disorganization is not related to manifest pathological dissociation, but, retrospectively, most dissociation in later development can be traced to attachment disorganization in infancy" (p. 45). These findings, based on the sample of the Minnesota Longitudinal Study of Risk and Adaptation, were not replicated in the NICHD sample (Haltigan & Roisman, 2015). However, the NICHD sample was a normative cohort. Families within the Minnesota sample, by contrast, were recruited on the basis of extensive adversity. Arguing from Bowlby's perspective, it is not clear that dissociative forms of disorganization occurred frequently enough in the NICHD sample to lead to prediction.

Cluster 3: Conflict Behaviors without Overt Fear

A third cluster of infant behaviors, discussed by Bowlby with particular attention in the 1960s, is conflict behaviors toward the caregiver shown without overt fear. This cluster parallels Main and Solomon's categories I (sequential contradiction, such as "strong proximity seeking immediately followed by strong avoidance"), II (simultaneous contradiction, such as "approach to parent with head sharply averted"), and III (misdirected, interrupted, and incomplete behaviors, such as failure to approach the parent when frightened or distressed). These categories are coded independently of direct signs of fear or disorientation for the purposes of D classification and usually occur in their absence.

Bowlby proposed that the intensity and nature of emotional conflict will be substantially shaped by an individual's attachment experiences. So long as the motivational responses in conflict were not too strong, Bowlby argued, conflict behavior could still be regulated. In a seminar delivered at the Tavistock in 1958, he emphasized that

> conflicts can vary in their intensity, i.e. in the amount of energy spent by conflicting forces, the importance attached by these forces to certain issues, the "cost" of victory or defeat. Conflicts can also vary in their violence of expression, i.e.

> in the militancy of the means chosen for expressing conflict. It is important to clearly distinguish between these two. (PP/Bow/H.67, unpublished text housed at the Wellcome Trust Library Archive in London)

A regulated form of motivational conflict can be seen in the Ainsworth's insecure–avoidant and insecure–resistant categories (Ainsworth et al., 1978/2015). Infants classified as avoidant regulate their distress through directing their attention away from the caregiver, whereas resistant infant behavior alternates between anger and attachment. Compared to secure attachment, the avoidant and resistant classifications are associated with less desirable outcomes (Groh, Fearon, van IJzendoorn, Bakermans-Kranenburg, & Roisman, 2017; Sroufe, Egeland, Carlson, & Collins, 2009).

In contrast, when conflicting tendencies are activated very strongly, behavioral output "may be unstable or inefficient and the result may be alternating behaviour of a non-functional kind" (Bowlby, 1969a, p. 100). Whereas resistant behavior is a clear expression of conflict, for Bowlby, it is distinguished by retaining environmental responsiveness in compelling the attention of the caregiver. However, even when a caregiver has not been frightened of or frightening for his or her infant, if the caregiver is associated with alarm for the child, the resulting conflict may become disruptively intense. Based on this reasoning, it may be speculated that *alarming but not frightening* caregiver behavior—such as dissociative, timid/deferential (Hesse & Main, 2006), grossly aversive or hostile behaviors (Main & Stadtman, 1981), or other caregiver behaviors that leave the child without support for organizing a response to distress (Waters & Valenzuela 1999)—might therefore lead to a child's expression of conflict behavior without manifest fear, such as forms of approach–avoidance behavior (Duschinsky, 2018).

Cluster 4: Stereotypies

Bowlby's fourth cluster comprises stereotypies and other behavior fragments. It is represented by Index IV in the Main and Solomon (1990) coding system. In his observations of traumatized soldiers returning from World War II, Bowlby had first noticed stereotypic behaviors as accompaniments to severe conflict and other worrisome psychological states: "amnesias, confusional states, transient psychoses, anxieties, depressions, dreams and panic states, trance states, severe tics" (PP/Bow/C.5/1, unpublished text housed at the Wellcome Trust Library Archive in London). In his 1940 essay, "The Influence of Early Environment in the Development of Neurosis and Neurotic Character," Bowlby gives a case study of a young boy with a severe tic and obsessional symptoms that occurred especially around expressions of desire or anger. In line with wider psychoanalytic thinking about stereotypies and tics (e.g., Ferenczi, 1921), Bowlby interpreted the tic and obsessional symptoms as expressions of psychological conflict between prohibitions held in place by the mother's anxiety about the boy and his anger at the demands she made on him (1940, p. 168). In his literature review of the effects of institutionalization on children—written for the World Health Organization—Bowlby also noted a variety of sensory and motor stereotypies in institutionalized children (Bowlby, 1951, p. 17).

Bowlby's position was that stereotypic behavior is a more general indicator of tension or stress, rather than being indicative of disruption of the attachment system. He was fascinated with Ainsworth's findings on repeating the Strange Situation 2 weeks later with her original sample, at which time infants who showed signs of avoidance in the first assessment now showed both more distress and more stereotypic behavior (Mary Main, personal communication, March 5, 2013). In this regard, it is worth highlighting that in the Main and Solomon coding system, stereotypies are not italicized. Main and Solomon already considered these behaviors weak indices of disorganization. Given that stereotypies are also typical of autism spectrum and other developmental disorders, several early childhood specialists have questioned their discriminant validity as indices of disorganized attachment (Pipp-Siegel, Siegel, & Dean, 1999; Willemsen-Swinkels, Bakermans-Kranenburg, Buitelaar, & van IJzendoorn, 2000; Rozga et al., 2018).

CONCLUDING REFLECTIONS

The disorganized attachment classification has been validated as an aggregate, and has been found to have a number of concerning antecedents and sequelae. However, there remain significant outstanding conceptual and psychometric questions, and a need for renewed theoretical discussion of the meaning and use of the disorganized classification. Such work will also require greater conceptual precision than has generally been the norm, particularly in the use of the concept of "fear." We agree with Bowlby (1973, p. 114), as cited earlier, that with fear, "we are dealing, not with some single comprehensive form of behavior, but with a heterogeneous collection of interrelated forms, each elicited by a slightly different set of causal conditions and each having a distinctive outcome." The work of Padrón et al. (2014), as well as remarks by Hesse and Main (2006), raise the prospect that the kind of fear associated with maltreating caregivers is both qualitatively and quantitatively distinct, and associated with different kinds of behavior in the Strange Situation. We can speculate along with Bowlby that major separation experiences may be associated with yet different types or constellations of disorganized behaviors. Based on classic descriptions of their reunion behavior, disorientation, unpredictable anger and distress, and forms of approach–avoidance behavior are likely to be salient features (Bowlby, 1973; Heinicke & Westheimer, 1965).

Though infants with a "D" classification may show more than one form of conflict behavior during the Strange Situation, it may still be meaningful to differentiate clusters of behavior. Bowlby's unpublished writings offer a possible logic and conceptualization to the construct of attachment disorganization—which, to date, has often been seen as undifferentiated or chaotic. Consideration of the Main and Solomon indices in light of Bowlby's reflections draws attention to the differences between stereotypies, nonfearful conflict, disorientation, and apprehensive behavior toward the caregiver. Bowlby's writings about these behaviors also suggest a hierarchy of risk. Direct apprehension of the caregiver, dissociation, conflict without overt fear, and stereotypies all *can* be provoked by fear of caregivers or wariness in their presence (Main & Hesse, 1990), but not all these indices reflect fear of physical harm on the part of the infant. Some behaviors, like stereotypies and conflict behavior without manifest fear, may also have many other, less concerning proximal causes.

Such hypotheses immediately raise a fundamental methodological issue. Coders already struggle to become reliable on the disorganized classification as a whole. It might then appear that differentiating subtypes of disorganized attachment would be a fiendish undertaking, with low chances of success. We suspect, however, that a good part of the reason why reliability is difficult to achieve is that the disorganization rating scale requires coders to mentally summarize across several indices, while balancing considerations such as frequency, intensity, and timing of the behavior. Furthermore, apart from the italicization of some indicators, coders have limited guidance about how to weight the implications of these variables either for making a classification decision or for imputing disruption of the underlying attachment system. Scales that focus separately on Bowlby's behavior clusters are likely to be easier to code, while the hierarchy of risk suggested by Bowlby's writing indicates how observed indices should be weighted in arriving at a summary score for disorganization.

Further research must therefore pursue psychometric inquiry *and* theory to the point that we have a sense of what coders might be asked to agree upon. Should this prove fruitful (i.e., theoretically meaningful factors identified in the data), then scales might be developed for different clusters hitherto subsumed within the disorganized construct. The reliability of using these scales as guideposts to a summary scale of disorganization "risk" can be compared to the original Main and Solomon scale and, even more importantly, can be used to predict maladaptive behavioral outcomes within and across study samples.

Long-standing questions can now be asked of such data. For instance, factor-analytic and taxometric work may be conducted to describe the ordered structure of disorganized attachment, its independence from other attachment dimensions, and the invariance of this structure across populations. As another avenue for research, the development of attachment disorganization beyond infancy may be examined afresh, with potentially important implications for the current coding systems for attachment relationships of preschoolers and children at age 6. The latter question already illustrates the interplay between psychometric and developmental questions. Rather than needing to combine controlling attachment and disorganized behavior in an overarching disorganized category in middle childhood, investigators may test in data from multiple samples Main and Cassidy's hypothesis that controlling attachment brings relief from a parent who otherwise behaves in frightening or alarming ways (cf. Moss, Cyr, & Dubois-Comtois, 2004; Lecompte & Moss, 2014). It would also be of clinical interest to examine whether particular clusters of of the indices relate differentially to later controlling attachment and disorganized behaviors, and whether clusters of infant behavior have different implications for how and whether fear plays a role in later representations regarding attachment relationships. Such inquiry would also significantly further our understanding of the proximal factors that elicit disorganized behavior and the behavioral systems that are involved.

Over the years, various calls have been made to further develop the conceptualization and operationalization of disorganized attachment in infancy and beyond. Waters and Valenzuela (1999) some time ago stressed the importance of discovering and describing the different ways in which attachment can be disorganized. This type of work would then need to be followed by formulating testable hypotheses ragarding the ways in which the input, integrative, and output functions of the attachment control systems are negatively affected. Through his notes and reflections on the phenomenon of disorganization, Bowlby once again is surprising modern researchers with a compelling direction for this program of research.

REFERENCES

Ainsworth, M. (1972). Attachment and dependency: A comparison. In J. Gewirtz (Ed.), *Attachment and dependency* (pp. 97–137). Washington, DC: Winston.

Ainsworth, M. D. S., Blehar, M., Waters, E., & Wall, S. (2015). *Patterns of attachment: A psychological study of the Strange Situation*. New York: Taylor & Francis (Psychology Press). (Original work published 1978)

Ainsworth, M., & Wittig, B. (1969). Attachment and exploratory behaviour of one-year-olds in a Strange Situation. In B. M. Foss (Ed.), *Determinants of infant behaviour* (Vol. 4, pp. 111–136). London: Methuen.

Beebe, B., & Lachmann, F. M. (2014). *The origins of attachment: Infant research and adult treatment*. London: Routledge.

Bowlby, J. (1940). The influence of early environment in the development of neurosis and neurotic character. *International Journal of Psychoanalysis*, *21*, 154–178.

Bowlby, J. (1951). *Maternal care and mental health*. Geneva, Swizerland: World Health Organization.

Bowlby, J. (1960). Separation anxiety. *International Journal of Psychoanalysis*, *41*, 89–113.

Bowlby, J. (1969a). *Attachment*. London: Penguin.

Bowlby, J. (1969b). Affectional bonds: Their nature and origin. In H. Freeman (Ed.), *Progress in mental health* (pp. 319–327). London: Churchill.

Bowlby, J. (1973). *Separation: Anxiety and anger*. New York: Basic Books.

Bowlby, J., Robertson, J., & Rosenbluth, D. (1952). A two-year-old goes to hospital. *Psychoanalytic Study of the Child*, *7*, 82–94.

Bowlby, J., & Soddy, K. (1940). *War Neurosis Memorandum, British Army*. Unpublished Wellcome Trust Memorandum PB/BOW/C.5/1.

Bureau, J. F., Easlerbrooks, M. A., & Lyons-Ruth, K. (2009). Attachment disorganization and controlling behavior in middle childhood: Maternal and child precursors and correlates. *Attachment and Human Development, 11*(3), 265–284.

Carlson, E., Yates, T., & Sroufe, L. A. (2008). Development of dissociation and development of the self. In P. Dell, J. O'Neil, & E. Somer (Eds.), *Dissociation and dissociative disorders* (pp. 39–52). New York: Routledge.

Crittenden, P. M. (1999). Danger and development: The organisation of self-protective strategies. In J. I. Vondra & D. Barnett (Eds.), *Atypical attachment in infancy and early childhood among children at developmental risk* (pp. 145–171). Oxford, UK: Blackwell.

Crittenden, P. (2016). *Raising parents* (2nd ed.). London: Routledge.

Cyr, C., Euser, E. M., Bakermans-Kranenburg, M. J., & van IJzendoorn, M. H. (2010). Attachment security and disorganization in maltreating and high-risk families: A series of meta-analyses. *Development and Psychopathology, 22*(1), 87–108.

Duschinsky, R. (2015). The emergence of the disorganized/disoriented (D) attachment classification, 1979–1982. *History of Psychology, 18*(1), 32–46.

Duschinsky, R. (2018). Disorganization, fear and attachment: Working towards clarification. *Infant Mental Health Journal, 39*(1), 17–29.

Duschinsky, R. (2020). *Cornerstones of attachment research*. New York: Oxford University Press.

Duschinsky, R., & Solomon, J. (2017). Infant disorganized attachment: Clarifying levels of analysis. *Clinical Child Psychology and Psychiatry, 22*, 524–538.

Fearon, P., Bakermans-Kranenburg, M. J., van IJzendoorn, M. H., Lapsley, A.-M., & Roisman, G. (2010). The significance of insecure attachment and disorganization in the development of children's externalizing behavior. *Child Development, 81*(2), 435–456.

Ferenczi, S. (1921). Psycho-analytical observations on tics. *International Journal of PsychoAnalysis, 2*, 1–30.

Fraley, R. C., Roisman, G. I., Booth-LaForce, C., Owen, M. T., & Holland, A. S. (2013). Interpersonal and genetic origins of adult attachment styles: A longitudinal study from infancy to early adulthood. *Journal of Personality and Social Psychology, 104*(5), 817–838.

Fraley, R. C., & Spieker, S. J. (2003). Are infant attachment patterns continuously or categorically distributed?: A taxometric analysis of Strange Situation behavior. *Developmental Psychology, 39*(3), 387–404.

George, C., & Solomon, J. (2016). The Attachment Doll Play Assessment: Predictive validity with concurrent mother–child interaction and maternal caregiving representations. *Frontiers in Psychology, 7*, 1594.

Granqvist, P., Hesse, E., Fransson, M., Main, M., Hagekull, B., & Bohlin, G. (2016). Prior participation in the Strange Situation and overstress jointly facilitate disorganized behaviours: Implications for theory, research and practice. *Attachment and Human Development, 18*(3), 235–249.

Groh, A. M., Fearon, R. M., van IJzendoorn, M. H., Bakermans-Kranenburg, M. J., & Roisman, G. I. (2017). Attachment in the early life course: Meta-analytic evidence for its role in socioemotional development. *Child Development Perspectives, 11*(1), 70–76.

Haltigan, J. D., & Roisman, G. I. (2015). Infant attachment insecurity and dissociative symptomatology: Findings from the NICHD Study of Early Child Care and Youth Development. *Infant Mental Health Journal, 36*(1), 30–41.

Heinicke, C. M., & Westheimer, I. (1965). *Brief separations.* New York: International Universities Press.

Hesse, E., & Main, M. (2006). Frightened, threatening, and dissociative parental behavior. *Development and Psychopathology, 18*(2), 309–343.

Hinde, R. (1954). Factors governing the changes in strength of a partially inborn response. *Proceedings of the Royal Society B: Biological Sciences, 142*(908), 306–330.

Hinde, R. (1970). *Animal behaviour* (2nd ed.). New York: McGraw-Hill.

Klein, M. (1957). *Envy and gratitude: A study of unconscious sources.* London: Tavistock Press.

Kozlowska, K., Walker, P., McLean, L., & Carrive, P. (2015). Fear and the defense cascade: Clinical implications and management. *Harvard Review of Psychiatry, 23*(4), 1–25.

Lecompte, V., & Moss, E. (2014). Disorganized and controlling patterns of attachment, role reversal, and caregiving helplessness: Links to adolescents' externalizing problems. *American Journal of Orthopsychiatry, 84*(5), 581–589.

Lyons-Ruth, K., Bureau, J.-F., Easterbrooks, M., Obsuth, I., Hennighausen, K., & Vulliez-Coady, L. (2013). Parsing the construct of maternal insensitivity: Distinct longitudinal pathways associated with early maternal withdrawal. *Attachment and Human Development, 15*(5–6), 562–582.

Lyons-Ruth, K., & Jacobvitz, D. (2016). Attachment disorganization from infancy to adulthood. In J. Cassidy & P. Shaver (Eds.), *Handbook of attachment: Theory, research, and clinical applications* (3rd ed., pp. 667–695). New York: Guilford Press.

Madigan, S., Bakermans-Kranenburg, M. J., van IJzendoorn, M. H., Moran, G., Pederson, D. R., & Benoit, D. (2006). Unresolved states of mind, anomalous parental behavior, and disorganized attachment. *Attachment and Human Development, 8*(2), 89–111.

Main, M., & Cassidy, J. (1986). *Assessments of child–parent attachment at six years of age.* Unpublished manuscript, University of California, Berkeley, Berkeley, CA.

Main, M., & Cassidy, J. (1988). Categories of response to reunion with the parent at age six: Predicted from infant attachment classifications and stable over a one-month period. *Developmental Psychology, 24*(3), 415–426.

Main, M., & Hesse, E. (1990). Parents' unresolved traumatic experiences are related to infant disorganized attachment status. In M. T. Greenberg, D. Cicchetti, & E. M. Cummings (Eds.), *Attachment in the preschool years* (pp. 161–181). Chicago: University of Chicago Press.

Main, M., & Hesse, E. D. (1992). Disorganized/disoriented infant behavior in the Strange Situation, lapses in the monitoring of reasoning and discourse during the parent's Adult Attachment Interview, and dissociative states. In M. Ammaniti & D. Stern (Eds.), *Attachment and psychoanalysis* (pp. 86–140). Rome: Gius.

Main, M., & Morgan, H. (1996). Disorganization and disorientation in infant Strange Situation behavior. In L. K. Michelson & W. J. Ray (Eds.), *Handbook of dissociation: Theoretical, empirical, and clinical perspectives* (pp. 107–138). New York: Springer.

Main, M., & Solomon, J. (1986). Discovery of a new, insecure-disorganized/

disoriented attachment pattern. In M. Yogman & T. B. Brazelton (Eds.), *Affective development in infancy* (pp. 195–124). Norwood, NJ: Ablex.

Main, M., & Solomon, J. (1990). Procedures for identifying infants as disorganised/disoriented during the Ainsworth Strange Situation. In M. T. Greenberg, D. Cicchetti, & E. M. Cummings (Eds.), *Attachment in the preschool years: Theory, research, and intervention* (pp. 121–160). Chicago: University of Chicago Press.

Main, M., & Stadtman, J. (1981). Infant response to rejection of physical contact by the mother. *Journal of the American Academy of Child Psychiatry, 20*(2), 292–307.

McFarland, D. J. (1966). On the causal and functional significance of displacement activities. *Ethology, 23*(2), 217–235.

Mikulincer, M., & Shaver, P. R. (2016). *Attachment in adulthood: Structure, dynamics, and change* (2nd ed.). New York: Guilford Press.

Moss, E., Cyr, C., & Dubois-Comtois, K. (2004). Attachment at early school age and developmental risk: Examining family contexts and behavior problems of controlling–caregiving, controlling–punitive, and behaviorally disorganized children. *Developmental Psychology, 40*(4), 519–531.

NICHD Early Child Care Research Network. (1997). The effects of infant child care on infant–mother attachment security: Results of the NICHD Study of Early Child Care. *Child Development, 68,* 860–879.

Padrón, E., Carlson, E. A., & Sroufe, L. A. (2014). Frightened versus not frightened disorganized infant attachment. *American Journal of Orthopsychiatry, 84*(2), 201–208.

Paetzold, R. L., Rholes, W. S., & Kohn, J. L. (2015). Disorganized attachment in adulthood: Theory, measurement, and implications for romantic relationships. *Review of General Psychology, 19*(2), 146–156.

Pipp-Siegel, S., Siegel, C. H., & Dean, J. (1999). Neurological aspects of the disorganized/disoriented attachment classification system: Differentiating quality of the attachment relationship from neurological impairment. *Monographs of the Society for Research in Child Development, 64,* 25–44.

Porges, S. W. (2007). The polyvagal perspective. *Biological Psychology, 74*(2), 116–143.

Riley, R. D., Lambert, P. C., & Abo-Zaid, G. (2010). Meta-analysis of individual participant data: Rationale, conduct, and reporting. *British Medical Journal, 340,* c221.

Rosch, E. (1987). Wittgenstein and categorization research in cognitive psychology. In M. Chapman & R. A. Dixon (Eds.), *Meaning and the growth of understanding* (pp. 151–166). New York: Springer.

Rozga, A., Hesse, E., Main, M., Duschinsky, R., Beckwith, L., & Sigman, M. (2018). A short-term longitudinal study of correlates and sequelae of attachment security in autism. *Attachment and Human Development, 20*(2), 160–180.

Rutter, M., Kreppner, J., & Sonuga-Barke, E. (2009). Emanuel Miller Lecture: Attachment insecurity, disinhibited attachment, and attachment disorders: Where do research findings leave the concepts? *Journal of Child Psychology and Psychiatry, 50,* 529–543.

Schuengel, C., Bakermans-Kranenburg, M. J., & van IJzendoorn, M. H. (1999). Frightening maternal behavior linking unresolved loss and disorganized infant attachment. *Journal of Consulting and Clinical Psychology, 67,* 54–63.

Slade, A. (2014). Imagining fear: Attachment, threat, and psychic experience. *Psychoanalytic Dialogues, 24*(3), 253–266.

Solomon, J., Duschinsky, R., Bakkum, L., & Schuengel, C. (2017). Toward an architecture of attachment disorganization: John Bowlby's published and unpublished reflections. *Clinical Child Psychology and Psychiatry, 22*(4), 539–560.

Solomon, J., & George, C. (2011). Disorganization of maternal caregiving across two generations. In J. Solomon & C. George (Eds.), *Disorganized attachment and caregiving* (pp. 25–51). New York: Guilford Press.

Solomon, J., & George, C. (2016). The measurement of attachment security and related constructs. In J. Cassidy & P. R. Shaver (Eds.), *Handbook of attachment: Theory, research, and clinical applications* (3rd ed., pp. 366–398). New York: Guilford Press.

Solomon, J., George, C., & De Jong, A. (1995). Children classified as controlling at age six: Evidence of disorganized representational strategies and aggression at home and at school. *Development and Psychopathology, 7*(3), 447–463.

Sroufe, L. A., Egeland, B., Carlson, E. A., & Collins, W. A. (2009). *The development of the person: The Minnesota Study of Risk and Adaptation from Birth to Adulthood.* New York: Guilford Press.

Tinbergen, N. (1952). "Derived" activities: Their causation, biological significance, origin, and emancipation during evolution. *Quarterly Review of Biology, 27*(1), 1–32.

van IJzendoorn, M. H., & Bakermans-Kranenburg, M. J. (2014). Confined quest for continuity: The categorical versus continuous nature of attachment. *Monographs of the Society for Research in Child Development, 79*(3), 157–167.

Verhage, M. L., Schuengel, C., Duschinsky, R., van IJzendoorn, M. H., Fearon, R. M. P., Madigan, S., . . . Collaboration of Attachment Transmission Synthesis. (2020). The Collaboration on Attachment Transmission Synthesis (CATS): A move to the level of individual-participant-data meta-analysis. *Current Directions in Psychological Science, 29*(2), 199–206.

Verhage, M. L., Schuengel, C., Madigan, S., Fearon, R. M., Oosterman, M., Cassibba, R., . . . van IJzendoorn, M. H. (2016). Narrowing the transmission gap: A synthesis of three decades of research on intergenerational transmission of attachment. *Psychological Bulletin, 142*(4), 337–366.

Waters, E., & Crowell, J. A. (1999). Atypical attachment in atypical circumstances. *Monographs of the Society for Research in Child Development, 64*(3), 213–220.

Waters, E., & Valenzuela, M. (1999). Explaining disorganized attachment: Clues from research on mild-to-moderately undernourished children in Chile. In J. Solomon & C. George (Eds.), *Attachment disorganization* (pp. 265–290). New York: Guilford Press.

Willemsen-Swinkels, S. H. N., Bakermans-Kranenburg, M. J., Buitelaar, J. K., van IJzendoorn, M. H., & van Engeland, H. (2000). Insecure and disorganized attachment in children with a pervasive developmental disorder: Relationship with social interaction and heart rate. *Journal of Child Psychology and Psychiatry and Allied Disciplines, 41*, 759–767.

Zeanah, C. H., & Gleason, M. M. (2010). *Reactive attachment disorders: A review for DSM-V.* Washington, DC: American Psychiatric Association.

CHAPTER 6

Promising Approaches to Assessing Attachment in Middle Childhood

Navigating the Options

Kathryn A. Kerns and Ashley Seibert

Research on attachment in middle childhood has accelerated rapidly in the last few years. Prior to the year 2000, there were only a few published studies in which attachment was assessed when children were ages 6–12 years. Now, however, there is a substantial amount of ongoing research and a growing published literature (see Kerns & Brumariu, 2016). In other developmental periods, the early research focused on one or two measurement techniques (e.g., the Strange Situation and the Attachment Q-set in infancy, the Adult Attachment Interview in adulthood). This has not, however, been the pattern for research in middle childhood. Although research on attachment during middle childhood was initially slowed by a lack of measures, there are currently many measures available, using a variety of measurement approaches (including behavioral observation, interviews, questionnaires, and analysis of family drawings). The main difficulty now is that no single measure has emerged as the "gold standard" for assessing attachment during this age period (Bosmans & Kerns, 2015).

There is certainly value in having multiple measures of a construct available. When researchers use only one measure, there is a concern that they are studying the measure rather than the construct (i.e., one particular way to operationalize the construct). As Ghiselli, Campbell, and Zedeck (1981) have pointed out, from a domain-sampling perspective, it is useful to have multiple measures that each tap somewhat different facets of a construct. Utilizing multiple measures also allows for a direct test of the (relative) validity of different approaches and avoids the problem of prematurely settling on a single approach, while missing the opportunity to explore alternatives that are also promising. In addition, the middle childhood period is one during which there are dramatic changes in children's social, emotional, and cognitive abilities; therefore, it would not be surprising to discover that some methods are more valid at particular ages within middle childhood.

Certain complexities do arise, however, when there are multiple measures available. The first is the burden of carefully articulating the meaning of the different measures, that is, why seemingly diverse approaches can nevertheless be said to tap the same construct. For example, what is the rationale for interpreting both behavioral responses on reunion between parent and child and analysis of themes in children's narratives as measures of attachment? This raises the question: What makes a particular measure a measure of attachment? Then there is the interpretive problem faced when different measures and measurement approaches show only low or modest associations with one another, as has occurred for measures in early childhood (e.g., Bretherton, Ridgeway, & Cassidy, 1990; van IJzendoorn, Vereijken, Bakermans-Kraneburg, & Riksen-Walraven, 2004). Finally, as will be noted in the review of available measures, there are modest validity data for most measures of attachment for 6- to 12-year-olds. This problem is partly due to the fact that investigators have adopted a variety of measures rather than focusing on extensively testing one or two.

Our goal in this chapter is to highlight the key issues in measuring attachment in children 6–12 years of age. We begin with a discussion of the nature of attachment in middle childhood, then discuss general issues in assessing attachment at this age period. We next evaluate the available measures to identify promising approaches. Finally, we conclude with an agenda for future research on the topic.

THE NATURE OF ATTACHMENT IN MIDDLE CHILDHOOD

Attachments to parents do not exist in a vacuum; it is therefore useful to place attachment within the broader developmental context. Middle childhood is a period during which children's social worlds are expanding. With the beginning of formal schooling, children are exposed to a wider and more diverse group of peers than in early childhood. There are also important changes in children's cognitive and social-cognitive abilities that affect their interpretation of their world. For example, changes in reasoning ability, improved capacity for self-reflection, and greater attention to psychological states and traits are likely to influence children's representations of attachment (Raikes & Thompson, 2005). The greater capacity for self-regulation is also likely to change both the frequency and the contexts in which children feel a need to solicit assistance from attachment figures (Marvin & Britner, 1999). The onset of puberty, with its associated changes in emotion and self-definition, is also likely to impact attachments to parents (Richardson, 2005). These changes have implications for assessment given that evaluation and interpretation of attachment behaviors and attachment representations depend in part on what is normative at a given age (e.g., would contact with an attachment figure be expected in a particular situation, and which attachment behaviors are likely to be displayed?).

There are also changes in social needs and expectations within children's social relationships. A major change in parent–child relationships within middle childhood is the gradual shift from close, moment-to-moment supervision by parents to parent and child coregulation (Maccoby, 1984). This shift may affect the attachment system by changing responsibility for regulation of contact with the attachment figure from parent to parent *and* child. For example, Waters, Kondo-Ikemura, Posada, and Richters (1991) have suggested that in middle childhood, children and parents develop a supervisory partnership in which children become increasingly responsible for regulating contact and communication with the attachment figure. This supervisory partnership is most likely to develop in the context of a secure attachment relationship (Kerns, Aspelmeier, Gentzler, & Grabill, 2001; Koehn & Kerns, 2016). Peer relationships also take on greater importance in middle childhood. Children develop the capacity and desire to form close friendships with peers (Sullivan, 1953), and also develop a concern for achieving acceptance within the broader peer group (Gottman & Mettetal, 1986). Children must also navigate the social rules regarding contacts with the other sex (Sroufe, Bennett, Englund, Urban, & Shulman, 1993). The shift toward greater interest and involvement with same-sex peers may help prepare children for the emergence of attachments to peers that is hypothesized to occur in adolescence (Allen & Land, 1999; Mayseless, 2005).

Despite all of the changes children experience, the evidence suggests that attachments to parents are still central in children's lives in middle childhood (Kerns & Brumariu, 2016). The goal of the attachment system shifts from proximity to availability of the attachment figure (Bowlby, 1987, cited in Ainsworth, 1990). There is a decline in the frequency with which children rely on attachment figures for assistance (Kerns, Tomich, & Kim, 2006; Lieberman, Doyle, & Markiewicz, 1999), but there is no decline in children's perceptions of the availability of attachment figures (Kerns et al., 2006; Lieberman, Doyle, & Markiewicz, 1999). Furthermore, although by the end of middle childhood children clearly prefer to spend time with peers when they desire companionship, they also show a clear preference for parents and other adults when attachment needs are primary (e.g., when sad or scared; Kerns et al., 2006; Kobak, Rosenthal, & Serwik, 2005; Seibert & Kerns, 2009). These findings have implications for assessment in that they suggest children form attachments to parents and not to peers in middle childhood. It is therefore not clear what measures of "peer attachment" for middle childhood are measures of (e.g., friendship or social support rather than attachment per se), but they are likely mislabeled as measures of attachment and are therefore not included in this review.

ISSUES IN ASSESSING ATTACHMENT IN MIDDLE CHILDHOOD

The alert reader has perhaps noticed that we have not yet provided an explicit definition of attachment. Instead, we have assumed an implicit and shared understanding of the construct. Unfortunately, in published papers, the failure to provide a definition of attachment is common and creates serious problems. There are important and thorny questions regarding how to define attachment, and sidestepping these questions is likely to create confusion regarding what is under study. For example, is attachment a characteristic of an individual or a relationship (Ainsworth, 1990; Cassidy, 1999; Kerns, Schlegelmilch, Morgan, & Abraham, 2005; Waters, 1981)? The question of definition cannot be avoided when designing measures, as one has to decide what a given measure is a measure of.

We define *attachment* as a close affectional bond that is not interchangeable with any other and in which the provision of security is central (Ainsworth, 1989). The attachment bond is a source of joy and security, and termination of an attachment bond leads to grief and mourning (Bowlby, 1979). In childhood, parents (or a child's parent figure) serve as primary attachment figures for children, although children may also form secondary attachments to siblings and grandparents (Ainsworth, 1989). All children are expected to form attachments as long as a parent figure is available, even if that figure provides care that is less that optimal (Bowlby, 1982).

Most research on attachment focuses on the parent–child relationship, which is assumed to be an attachment relationship (see Kerns et al., 2005, for a description of measures used to identify attachment figures). In addition, most attachment measures describe individual differences in attachment security. Children who are able to use a parent figure as a secure base from which to explore, and as a haven of safety in times of distress, are by definition securely attached (Bowlby, 1982). This secure base conceptualization of attachment is the hallmark of attachment theory (Waters & Cummings, 2000), and provides an organizing framework for assessing attachment. A child who does not form a secure attachment to a caregiver may develop a secondary insecure strategy that allows him or her to maintain the relationship with the parent; in that case, the relationship is characterized by avoidance, ambivalence, or disorganization rather than clear secure base usage (Main, 1990).

In addition to patterns of organized behavior, secure attachment at the representational level is associated with schemas and scripts of family relationships, and with the ability to openly and coherently evaluate attachment relationships (Main, Kaplan, & Cassidy, 1985; Main, 1996). Bowlby (1973) suggested that children form working models of the self and other that are mutually confirming. Sroufe and Fleeson (1986) further suggested that children develop models of the whole relationship between parent and child. Working models or representations are in turn expected to influence how children process new information (e.g., selective attention, what is remembered), and thus represent a mechanism that may contribute to continuity in attachment over time. While there are observational measures for middle childhood that involve coding secure base behavior, most available measures are designed to assess children's representations of attachment figures or family relationships.

Is attachment a characteristic of a relationship, or a characteristic of the child? Children form attachments to different relationship partners (e.g., mother and father); thus, it is possible to assess the security of a specific relationship. Across childhood and adolescence, individuals have experiences in multiple attachment relationships and by at least adolescence, children are thought to have the capacity to develop generalized representations of attachment (Allen & Land, 1999), which have been referred to as "state of mind in regard to attachment" (Main et al., 1985). We believe that the attachment construct does have dual meanings, in that it can refer to both the quality of a specific relationship and to a more general approach to or understanding of attachment relationships. An important goal for future research is understanding how these two conceptualizations of attachment are interrelated (i.e., how specific attachments influence the emergence of a state of mind in regard to attachment). To avoid interpretive difficulties, it is necessary to articulate the meaning that can be attributed to the attachment measures used in a specific study. For example, what is tested in longitudinal studies of attachment employing the Strange Situation in infancy and the Adult Attachment Interview (AAI) in adulthood is whether the security in a specific attachment relationship in infancy (usually with the mother) predicts state of mind in regard to attachment in adulthood. In middle childhood, observational measures of attachment are relationship-specific, but both relationship-specific and more general measures of attachment representations have been developed.

MEASUREMENT APPROACHES IN MIDDLE CHILDHOOD

In infancy and early childhood, the most common approach to attachment assessment is observations of secure base behavior at home or in the laboratory, whereas in adolescence and adulthood, assessments typically employ interviews or questionnaires. As shown in Table 6.1, all of these approaches have been used in middle childhood. Note that the approaches vary in terms of the type of data collected (i.e., observation of behavior, child self-reports), as well as the construct assessed (i.e., a specific relationship or a more general attachment orientation). In addition, almost all of the measures are based on the secure base construct, in that they include either observations of secure base behavior or child reports of situations in which secure base behavior is expected (e.g., story stems or autobiographical interviews, attachment questionnaires). Note, however, that the link to secure base behavior is less clear for the responses to pictured separations (which emphasize coping in the parent's absence), and interview measures include narrative coherence while

TABLE 6.1. Approaches to Assessment of Attachment in Middle Childhood

Type of data collected	Construct assessed	Relationship-specific or general?
6- to 8-year-olds		
Behavior on reunion with caregiver following long separation in lab	Secure base behavior as reflected in physical proximity, conversation, and emotional exchanges	Relationship-specific
Storytelling tasks for situations eliciting secure base behavior	Attachment representations as reflected in story themes, child–caregiver behavior depicted, and narrative coherence	Relationship-specific or general
Verbal responses to pictures of parent–child separations	Attachment representations as reflected in emotional openness and adaptive coping during separation from parents	General
9- to 12-year-olds		
Storytelling tasks for situations eliciting secure base behavior	Attachment representations as reflected in story themes, child–caregiver behavior depicted, and narrative coherence	Relationship-specific or general
Verbal responses to separation	Attachment representations as pictures of parent–child reflected in emotional openness and adaptive coping during separation from parents	General
Reports of autobiographical experiences with parents	Attachment representations as reflected in reports of actual child–caregiver interactions and narrative coherence	Relationship-specific or general
Standard structured questionnaires	Conscious representations of relationships with caregivers (feelings, secure base behavior)	Relationship-specific

discussing attachment-themed information as part of the criteria for scoring attachment security.

Laboratory-based separation–reunion measures have been employed with children 6–8 years of age. Narrative assessments have been utilized to capture representations of attachment in children 6–12 years of age, with participants asked to discuss autobiographical events or tell stories with attachment-related themes (e.g., how the secure base is involved in mitigating child distress). The narrative measures sometimes include an assessment of narrative coherence (e.g., is the story logical, believable, and internally coherent?), as well as the content of the narrative (e.g., is emotion expressed, are caregivers represented as competent and caring?). Questionnaire measures of attachment, developed for 8- to 12-year-olds, are predicated on the notion that children's perceptions of caregiver availability and secure base use can meaningfully assess one facet of the attachment construct (Kerns, Tomich, Aspelmeier, & Contreras, 2000). The limitations of self-report questionnaires are well-known (e.g., halo effects, social desirability), and there is the added concern that even a highly motivated person may have difficulty accessing his or her "true" feelings regarding attachment figures (Kerns et al., 2005). Nevertheless, it seems worthwhile to ask whether children's conscious reports of attachment can be useful, rather than to assume at the outset that their validity is zero. For that reason, questionnaire measures of attachment are included in this review. Rather than measuring attachment from only one of these perspectives, it may be more useful to develop a set of attachment-based measures of the parent–child relationship (Kerns et al., 2000). Regardless of which approach is adopted in any given study, it is critical for investigators to clearly articulate their conceptualization of attachment.

Measure validation is a complex, iterative process in which any new measure can be evaluated with reference to several criteria. While the demonstration of measure reliability is usually straightforward (e.g., test–retest reliability), demonstration of a measure's validity is not, in that typically no single test of a measure is sufficient to provide unequivocal evidence of a measure's validity, and several different types of data can be used to evaluate validity. In addition, as Patterson and Bank (1987) note, measure validation and construct validation are inextricably linked, in that tests of theory are also tests of the validity of a measure. Solomon and George (2008) specify four criteria for evaluating measures of attachment. Specifically, they argue that a measure of attachment security should be positively related to caregiver responsiveness, show consistency over time, predict important aspects of development (e.g., success on key developmental tasks), and be valid cross-culturally. Kerns, Brumariu, and Seibert (2011) have suggested three additional criteria: A new measure of attachment should be moderately related to other measures of attachment administered close in time, predict secure base behavior to the attachment figure in naturalistic contexts, and show evidence of discriminant validity (i.e., should not simply correlate with all things "good"). As readers will see, only a few types of data are currently available for most middle-childhood attachment measures.

In the review of specific measures that follows, we have divided middle childhood into the earlier (ages 6–8) and later (ages 9–12) years. This organization also highlights the fact that some measures have been used only in one age period. Whereas narrative techniques have been employed at both age periods, behavioral observation has only been extensively used with younger children, and autobiographical interviews and questionnaires have been used with older children.

ASSESSING ATTACHMENT IN 6- TO 8-YEAR-OLD CHILDREN

Three types of measures have been used to assess attachment in 6- to 8-year-old children. Behavioral observation has been adapted from infancy observational techniques (i.e., the Strange Situation), storystem narratives were adapted from procedures first used with preschoolers, and techniques that evaluate responses to pictures with attachment themes (i.e., Separation Anxiety Test [SAT]) were adapted from methods originally used with adolescents.

Behavioral Observations

Procedure

To assess attachment with behavioral observation techniques, investigators have used variations on the Main and Cassidy (1988) separation–reunion procedure, and coding is based on children's behavior during reunion with a parent following a 1-hour-long separation. Observational intervals upon reunion range from 3 to 5 minutes. In a few studies, two separations and two reunions take place. The first separation is 45 minutes long, and the second separation is 30 minutes long. The attachment classifications are based on behavior observed during both of the reunion periods (Moss, Cyr, & Dubois-Comtois, 2004; Humber & Moss, 2005; Moss & St-Laurent, 2001). During separation, the parent and the child are given attachment-related tasks to prime the attachment system. For example, parents can complete the AAI, and children can complete the SAT or family drawings. When the reunion happens, the child should be engaging in free play with the experimenter.

In the majority of studies, this classification system has been used with children between ages 5 and 7, although it has also been used with children as old as age 9 years (Graham & Easterbrooks, 2000; Moss, Bureau, Beliveau, Zdebik, & Lépine, 2009). Cassidy, Marvin, and the MacArthur Attachment Working Group, 1992) altered Main and Cassidy's separation–reunion procedure so that it would be more appropriate for preschool-age (3–5 years) children (Solomon & George, 2008). It is important for investigators to keep in mind that although the Main–Cassidy and Cassidy–Marvin procedures and coding are conceptually similar, one system may be more appropriate for children of a certain age than the other. Therefore, one should carefully consider which system to use, especially when conducting longitudinal research.

Coding

Children's responses to their parent's entrance and subsequent interactions are classified into five groups: *secure, avoidant, ambivalent, controlling,* and *unclassified.* Attachments coded as secure are characterized by confident, relaxed, and open reunion behavior. The child shows pleasure at seeing the parent, expresses interest in interacting with the parent, and seeks proximity toward the parent. The conversation is positive, and both the child and parent participate in conversation. Attachments coded as avoidant are characterized by attempts by the child to avoid interaction with the parent. The child minimizes opportunities for interaction with the parent by seeming to be busy and involved in play. The conversation is impersonal and lacks affective content. Attachments coded as ambivalent may include hostility, fear, and sadness, which are mixed with attempts to seek contact with the parent. The child's behavior may also seem to be immature or babyish. Attachments coded as controlling are characterized by behavior that shows the child has assumed control of the relationship, such as role reversal. Control may be expressed through punitive behavior (e.g., rejection, humiliation, embarrassment), or through caregiving behavior (e.g., cheering, reassuring, overly bright affect). Unclassified attachments are insecure attachment patterns that do not fit into any of the other groups. Reunion behavior is also rated on a 9-point scale of security and a 7-point scale of avoidance.

Training

Learning the coding system is a complex task that requires extensive training. It is also important to establish reliability with an expert coder. In several studies, coders were trained by members of the MacArthur Working Group on Attachment (Graham & Easterbrooks, 2000; Easterbrooks, Davidson, & Chazan, 1993). In other studies, coders were trained by recognized experts and achieved reliability with these expert coders on a separate sample of videotapes (Moss et al., 2004; Cassidy, Kirsh, Scolton, & Parke, 1996). Investigators interested in training should contact Mary Main or Erik Hesse (currently at the Department of Psychology, University of California, Berkeley) or Ellen Moss (currently at the University of Quebec at Montreal).

Observer Agreement

In most studies, interrater agreement is relatively high. Agreement for classification has been shown to range from 76% to 88% (Cassidy, 1988; Moss et al., 2004). Agreement for the rating scales is also acceptable with Easterbrooks et al. (1993) reporting agreement of 85% for both avoidance and security, and Main and Cassidy (1988) reporting correlations of .76 for avoidance and .72 for security.

TEST–RETEST RELIABILITY AND STABILITY

In their original study for the development of this attachment classification system, Main and Cassidy (1988) found that stability for reunion classification with the mother over a 1-month period was moderate (62%).

RELATIONS TO OTHER MEASURES OF ATTACHMENT

Main and Cassidy (1988) found that attachment classifications of 6-year-olds to their mothers were highly predictable from infancy attachment classifications to the mothers (84%). Predictability was not as high for attachments to the fathers (61%). Solomon and George (2008) report that Main–Cassidy classifications have been shown to be strongly related to attachment classifications based on children's responses in the Attachment Structured DollPlay Interview, as well as to classifications and security ratings based on the SAT.

VALIDATION THROUGH TESTS OF CONSTRUCT VALIDITY

The Main–Cassidy separation–reunion procedure has been validated in samples of 6- to 8-year-olds by demonstrating predictable associations between attachment classifications and mother–child interaction, children's representations of self, social competence, and academic and socioemotional adaptation (Dubois-Comtois, Cyr, & Moss, 2011; Humber & Moss, 2005; Moss & St-Laurent, 2001; Easterbrooks et al., 1993; Cassidy, 1988). This procedure has also been validated in samples of 5-year-old children (see Solomon & George, 2008, for a review).

Summary

The Main–Cassidy separation–reunion procedure has been extensively used with minor changes in procedure. As noted by Solomon and George (2008), the procedure has been shown to be reliable and valid. It appears to be the observational measure of choice for this age. Versions for older children have not yet been developed and validated.

StoryStem Narratives

Procedure

The storystem technique was originally developed for preschoolers (Bretherton et al., 1990) and has been adapted for older children. This measure is predicated on the assumption that children's storytelling about attachment-themed events can reveal their representation of attachment to caregivers. Some studies have adapted Bretherton et al.'s (1990) story set, the Attachment Story Completion Test (ASCT), for older children (e.g., Gloger-Tippelt & Kappler, 2016; Solomon, George, & De Jong, 1995; Dubois-Comtois et al., 2011; Poehlmann, 2005; Scholtens, Rydell, Bohlin, & Thorell, 2014). Other studies have used story stems from the MacArthur Story Stem Battery (MSSB; e.g., Gloger-Tippelt, Gomille, Koenig, & Vetter, 2002), which partially overlaps with the ASCT. It should be noted that the MSSB includes many stories, only a subset of which were designed to assess attachment. Other investigators have borrowed a few stories from the MSSB and combined them with their own story stems (e.g., Hodges, Steele, Hillman, & Henderson, 2003) and "Little Pig" [LP] story stems), and other studies have developed their own story stems, such as the Manchester Child Attachment Story Task (MCAST; e.g., Green, Stanley, Smith, & Goldwyn, 2000). Verschueren and Marcoen (1999) borrowed one story from the ASCT, three stories from Cassidy (1988), and included their own story. While the number and content of stories used may differ, the basic technique remains the same. The family figures used in the interview usually include a mother and/or a father, a child matched to the target child's age and sex, and an opposite-sex sibling (although Green et al. [2000] only include one child and one caregiver). The interviewer presents the child with the beginning of a story, then asks the child to "Show me and tell me what happens next," using dolls and props. Samples of attachment story themes from different story sets are presented in Table 6.2.

When using any story-stem technique, it is important first to establish rapport with the child, so he or she is relaxed and comfortable when telling his or her story. One should also use dolls that are flexible, so that the child can manipulate the dolls and make them stand while telling his or her story. One should also help the child become familiar with the dolls and props by demonstrating how to bend the dolls and letting the child help set up the props used in the story. It is also important for the interviewer to memorize the procedures and the story stems, so that he or she can pay attention to the child's story. Additionally, the interviewer should not make evaluative statements while the child is telling the story, such as, "That's great!," or other comments that may affect the child's story. If the child is having trouble telling the story, the interviewer can prompt with open-ended questions (e.g., "What happens next?") but should not push the child's story in any particular direction (e.g., "Is the mom upset?"). If there are unclear actions or events in the child's story, the interviewer should ask the child to retell and reenact the story. This should be done in a way that seems as though the interviewer did not understand, and not that the child told a bad story (e.g., "Could you remind me one more time what happened when . . . ?"). When using the story-stem technique, it is imperative that one be able to tell how the child copes with stress and how he or she portrays the attachment figure in the story. Once this is clear, the interviewer should stop prompting the child for additional story details. Stories of younger children are less detailed but are nevertheless expected to possess information regarding secure base behavior.

Coding

There has not been one definitive coding system used for the storystem technique. Dubois-Comtois et al. (2011), Scholtens et al. (2014), and Gloger-Tippelt and Kappler (2016) code for attachment classifications. Gloger-Tippelt

TABLE 6.2. Samples of Attachment Story Themes

Story set	Attachment stories
6- to 8-year-olds	
MSSB	• Child spills juice at dinner. • Child discovers the family dog is gone; dog returns. • Child is warned not to touch pot on stove; child touches pot; child gets burned. • Child tells parents he or she will climb to the top of a rock; mother warns child to be careful. • Separation of child and parental figure. • Reunion of child and parental figure.
ASCT	• Child spills juice at dinner. • Child falls off a rock and hurts knee. • Child calls for parental figure thinking he or she saw a monster. • Separation of child and parental figure. • Reunion of child and parental figure.
LP	• Child goes outside behind house; sound of crying. • Little pig gets lost; cannot see other pigs; does not know how to get back. • Children and animals feel scared when elephant stamps. • Child gets permission to ride bike with friend; mom says to be careful; child falls off bike. • Child makes a picture he or she thinks is good at school; takes picture home.
MCAST	• Child awakes at night with a nightmare. • Child is playing outside and falls over; hurts knee; pain and bleeding. • Child experiences acute abdominal pain. • Child fights with a friend at school and returns home. • Child gets lost and is alone while shopping with a parent in a large crowd. • Child completes a beautiful drawing at school; gets praise from teacher; takes it home to show to caregiver.
Cassidy (1988)	• Child gives his or her mom a present made by the child. • Child approaches mom and says, "I'm sorry mom." • Child does not like what is served for dinner. • Child has to do the one thing he or she most hates doing. • Child discovers his or her bicycle has been stolen by an unfamiliar child. • Child awakened by loud noise in the middle of the night.

Note. MSSB, MacArthur Story Stem Battery; ASCT, Attachment Story Completion Task; LP, Little Pig; MCAST, Manchester Child Attachment Story Task.

et al. (2002) used a dimensional measure of attachment security for each story (*very secure, secure, insecure, very insecure*) and a global attachment security score (*secure* or *insecure*) for the five stories. For each of the stories, Green et al. (2000) made codings on 9-point continuous scales that fall into four groups (*attachmentrelated behaviors, narrative coherence, disorganized phenomena,* and *"bizarreness" of narrative content*) and a categorical attachment assignment. Then, an overall interview classification is made according to the predominant classification across the stories. Poehlmann (2005) coded four structural codes (e.g., avoidance, coherence) and seven content codes (e.g., positive behavior of child to adult, nonpunitive discipline) for each story. Scores for each code were summed across the four stories, so that children's scores ranged from 0 (present in none of the stories) to 4 (present in all of the stories). Verschueren and Marcoen (1999) rated each story on a 5-point scale for attachment security and assigned an attachment classification (secure, insecure–avoidant, insecure–bizarre/ambivalent, and secure–insecure). Each child then received a global categorization (secure, avoidant, bizarre/ambivalent) and a global attachment security score based on the five stories.

Training

Steele, Hodges, Kaniuk, Hillman, and Henderson (2003), report that coding of children's responses is available in a manual, and a training package is available for mental health professionals. Ellen Moss offers training on the ASCT. No other studies mention their training procedure. There are many story-stem sets available to use, each with its own complexities. Therefore, it is important for one to carefully consider which system to use and make sure that training is available before choosing a particular system.

Observer Agreement

Reliability for the single stories in Gloger-Tippelt et al. (2002) ranged from kappa =.59 to .77, and the reliability of the global attachment security score was kappa = .89. Interrater reliability for Green et al. (2000) for the threeway classification was 80% (kappa = .62) and for D vs. nonD was 82% (kappa = .41). Poehlmann (2005) reported kappas ranging from .64 to .86. Verschueren and Marcoen (1999) reported a mean agreement for story classifications of 82% for mothers and 86% for fathers. The agreement for global classification was 88% (kappa = .82) for mothers and 88% (kappa = .81) for fathers. Dubois-Comtois et al. (2011) report agreement of 82% (kappa = .76) for four-way attachment classifications, and Scholtens et al. (2014) report a kappa of .69 for three-way agreement (secure, insecure–organized, disorganized). Gloger-Tipplet and Kappler (2016) report good agreement for several samples in which the German Attachment Story Completion Task was used (kappas ranged from .77 to .92).

Test–Retest Reliability and Stability

Green et al. (2000) repeated the story task after 5.5 months for 33 children. They found that 76.5% of avoidant, secure, ambivalent/resistant (ABC) cat egories and 69% of disorganized/disoriented (D) categories remained stable.

Relations with Other Attachment Measures

Gloger-Tippelt et al. (2002) reported that story completions at age 6 were significantly associated with Strange Situation classifications at 13 months. Goldwyn, Stanley, Smith, and Green (2000) reported a significant agreement between secure and insecure classification on the MCAST and the SAT, but only moderate kappa (.41). Dubois-Comtois et al. (2011) reported significant concordance between a story stem and a behavioral measure of attachment. Gloger-Tippelt and Kappler (2016) reported moderate concordance with observational and autobiographical measures of attachment.

Validation through Tests of Construct Validity

Three studies revealed that children's story-stem responses were related to maternal AAI classifications (Gloger-Tippelt et al., 2002; Goldwyn et al., 2000; Steele et al., 2003), and another study indicated that story-stem responses were related to ratings of maternal behavior (Dubois-Comtois et al., 2011). Children rated highly for disorganization were rated by teachers and parents as showing less adaptive behavior (e.g., attention or behavior problems; Goldwyn et al., 2000; Futh, O'Connor, Matias, Green, & Scott, 2008; Scholtens et al., 2014). Poehlmann (2005) found that secure relationships were more likely when children lived in a stable caregiving situation and/or when mothers were not incarcerated. Verschueren and Marcoen (1999) found that story-stem classifications of father–child attachment were related to social–emotional competence, while story-stem classifications of mother–child attachment were related to self-representations. In terms of discriminant validity, story-stem narratives are not related to temperament (Goldwyn et al., 2000), maternal education, immigrant status (Scholtens et al., 2014), or verbal skill (Gloger-Tippelt & Kappler, 2016; Poehlmann, 2005). Scholtens et al. (2014) found that disorganized children produced less coherent narratives even when the content was not attachment based.

Summary

Several studies have indicated that story-stem narratives are related to other attachment measures or to indices of social development. However, one must keep in mind that several different story-stem sets are used, each with its own coding system. Also, there are very limited validity data for each system.

Therefore, although the story-stem procedure appears to be a promising approach, one must carefully consider which system to use.

Verbal Responses to Pictures of Parent–Child Separation

Procedure

The SAT is a semiprojective technique based on responses to pictures of parent–child separation experiences. After the picture is described to the children, they are asked how the child in the picture feels, why the child feels that way, and what the child is going to do. Most studies use Klagsbrun and Bowlby's (1976) version of the SAT (Main et al., 1985; Grossmann et al., 2002). Children are shown six photographs of parent–child separation experiences, and the age and gender of the child in the picture is matched to the participant. Photographs include both mild separations (e.g., child's first day at school—at point of separation from mom; child at park with parents and told to play by him- or herself; mom putting child to bed—about to go out the door) and severe separations (e.g., parents go out for the evening—leave child at home; parents go away for the weekend—leave child with aunt and uncle; parents going away for 2 weeks—leave child at home—giving child a present). Clarke, Ungerer, Chahoud, Johnson, and Stiefel (2002) also used the Klagsbrun and Bowlby (1976) stories for children age 7 and younger, but they used photographs by Slough and Greenberg (1990). Slough and Greenberg took new photographs that preserved the same situational contexts as the original photographs, but they made a few modifications. These modifications include showing mother and father in most of the scenes; using the same setting, parents, and props for the boy and girl pictures; updating the photographs with more modern hairstyles and clothes; and showing only the children's profiles or the back of their heads to help maintain ambiguity in facial expression. Even though modifications were made to the photographs, they still portrayed the same six situational contexts listed earlier. For children ages 8 and older, Clarke et al. (2002) used a version of the SAT that was modified by Wright, Binney, and Smith (1995). The photographs still depicted mild and severe separations, but modifications were made to make the separation situations more age appropriate. For example, "The boy/girl is going away on a school trip for 2 weeks" was considered a severe separation, while "The boy's/girl's dad is going away to work" was considered a mild separation. Jacobsen, Edelstein, and Hofmann (1994) and Jacobsen and Hofmann (1997) used a picturestory sequence depicting a parent–child separation in nine separate sketches that was originally used by Chandler (1973) to measure children's perspective taking. The picture-story sequence is as follows: The child is seen standing by an adult figure (1) who is preparing to leave on an airplane (2). After waving good-bye (3) and watching the plane depart (4), the child returns home (5). A mailman delivers a package to the child (6). The child opens the package (7), finds a toy plane inside (8), and cries as the mailman looks on (9).

Coding

Although several different systems are used, most systems commonly included rating scales of coping and emotional openness or a system for classifying a broader attachment pattern. Main et al. (1985) coded for emotional openness and quality of coping. Clarke et al. (2002) rated stories using three continuous scales: attachment and selfreliance (4-point scales) and avoidance (3-point scale). Grossmann et al. (2002) based the security of children's overall response patterns on children's emotional openness, positive evaluation of the availability of supportive others, coherence of narrative, and developmentally appropriate coping behaviors. Children's overall security was rated on a 7-point scale. Easterbrooks and Abeles (2000) made ratings on 9-point scales, in which 9 indicates greater emotional security or adaptive coping. Responses were also classified into attachment categories for the entire SAT interview (secure, avoidant, ambivalent/resistant, insecure controlling). Jacobsen et al. (1994) distinguished four major attachment groups (secure, insecure–avoidant, insecure–ambivalent, and insecure–disorganized).

Training

Given the limited use of the system, consultation with an investigator who has used the system is recommended. As there is complexity in each system and clinical judgment is required, it is necessary to acquire coding manuals and training before using this technique. Easterbrooks and Abeles (2000) reported that coders trained on a sample of transcripts provided by Nancy Kaplan. In Jacobsen et al. (1994) and Jacobsen and Hofmann (1997), the main rater was trained by Nancy Kaplan. The main rater then trained two independent raters.

Observer Agreement

In Clarke et al. (2002), agreement ranged from 81 to 87% for their three continuous scales. Grossmann et al. (2002) reported a kappa of .88. Easterbrooks and Abeles (2000) reported a kappa of .86 for emotional security, .90 for coping solutions, and .92 for the attachment classifications. In Jacobsen et al. (1994), agreement for the four classification groups was 87% and 80%. Jacobsen and Hofmann (1997) reported kappas of .69 and .68 for the four attachment groups.

Test–Retest Reliability and Stability

Jacobsen and Hofmann (1997) established test–retest reliability on a subsample of children who were administered the separation story 1 year later. A significant concordance was found across 1 year for the four attachment classifications (kappa = .78).

Relations with Other Attachment Measures

Main et al. (1985) found that mother–child attachment in infancy, but not father–child attachment, was related to emotional openness and coping on the SAT. Grossmann et al. (2002) found that quality of attachment in the Strange Situation predicted children's attachment representations at age 6. Jacobsen et al. (1994) and Jacobsen and Hofmann (1997) reported significant associations between the Main and Cassidy (1988) attachment classifications and classifications of children's responses to the separation story.

Validation through Tests of Construct Validity

Clarke et al. (2002) reported that children with attention-deficit/hyperactivity disorder (ADHD) obtained lower scores on the attachment and selfreliance scales of the SAT than did control children. Easterbrooks and Abeles (2000) found that children with greater "ease of access to selfevaluations" also showed greater emotional security and quality of coping during the SAT. This finding was not due to verbal competence, since the researchers controlled for verbal skill in the analysis. Bohlin, Hagekull, and Rydell (2000) found that the attachment and avoidance scales of the SAT were associated with good social functioning, and low scores on the selfreliance scales were related to high social anxiety. Jacobsen et al. (1994) reported that children with secure attachment representations at age 7 had better cognitive functioning than children with insecure attachment representations. Jacobsen and Hofmann (1997) found that children with secure attachment representations were better in terms of attention–participation, insecurity about self, and grade point average (GPA) at school than were insecure children.

Summary

The SAT appears to be a promising method of assessing attachment for 6 to 8-year-olds. With the exception of Jacobsen et al. (1994) and Jacobsen and Hofmann (1997), most studies used the same method. There is some evidence of validity, as the SAT is related to social and cognitive adjustment, and other measures of attachment, but there is no information about the association between the SAT and maternal behavior or maternal attachment. In addition, evidence for test–retest reliability and discriminant validity are limited.

ASSESSING ATTACHMENT IN 9- TO 12-YEAR-OLD CHILDREN

Several types of measures have been used to assess attachment in 9- to 12-year-old children. Two techniques used with 6- to 8-year-olds, story-stem interviews and responses to pictures (i.e., SAT), have been modified for use with older children. An autobiographical interview initially developed for adults and used with adults and adolescents (i.e., the AAI) has also been modified for children in later middle childhood. All three of these techniques are designed to assess children's attachment representations. In addition, questionnaire measures have been developed to assess children's perceptions of attachment. Note that word prompt measures—a narrative approach that has been used with adults—have been adapted for middle childhood (e.g., Psouni & Apetroaia, 2014), but are covered in another chapter on this method (see Crowell, Chapter 9, this volume) and are not described here. Behavioral measures, in which attachment patterns are coded from parent–child interactions, have also recently been developed (Boldt, Kochanska, Grekin, & Brock, 2016; Brumariu, Giuseppone, et al., 2018). As these measures are quite new and each has only been evaluated in one study, we do not discuss them, although we do note that they show promise, in that each method was related to other measures of attachment, parenting, and child adjustment (Boldt et al., 2016; Brumariu, Giuseppone, et al., 2018).

Story-Stem Narratives

The Doll Story Completion Task (Granot & Mayseless, 2001) is a story-stem procedure in which an interviewer begins a story using dolls and props, and asks the child to complete the story. The interview procedure and the story stems were first developed for preschoolers (Bretherton et al., 1990; see ASCT story stems in Table 6.1). After a warmup story, children are presented five stories with different themes. The original story themes were later modified by David Granot and Ofra Mayseless (2001), following piloting, to make the stories more appropriate for preadolescents. For example, the story about a monster was changed to "seeing something in your room," and in another story the length of the parent–child separation was increased from 1 to 3 days. After beginning the story, the interviewer then asks the child to say and show with the dolls what happens next. The family in the story includes a mother and children matched on age and sex to the target child and his or her siblings. Kerns et al. (2011) later modified this procedure. They introduced two new story stems that were used in place of the five stories. In one story, the child is having difficulty completing a homework assignment that is due the next day. In a second story, the child is returning home after having a fight with a friend. Kerns et al. also modified the procedure by including only the target child and one parent in the story, so that stories would reflect more closely that specific relationship. See the section on story-stem narratives for 6- to 8-year-olds for additional tips on administering story stems.

Coding

Granot and Mayseless (2001) developed a coding system based in part on the coding procedures of Bretherton et al. (1990). A coder watches a videotape of an interview, and each individual story is scored as secure or insecure.

Then, after considering the entire interview, the coder rates each child on four attachment patterns—secure, avoidant, ambivalent, and disorganized—using 5-point scales. Coding criteria include expression of emotion in the story (e.g., valence and regulation), representation of caregivers (e.g., responsiveness and sensitivity of the parent), resolution of problems (e.g., was problem resolved and was there a return to normal activities?), and narrative coherence (e.g., was story logical and internally consistent?). Each participant is also assigned to a single, best-fitting classification. Kerns et al. (2011) modified the Granot and Mayseless (2001) coding criteria. The main change was that "representation of caregivers" explicitly included coordination of actions between the child and parent. A third scoring system (Kerns, Abraham, Schlegelmilch, & Morgan, 2007) is based on Waters, Rodrigues, and Ridgeway's (1998) coding of the degree to which a child's narrative reflects the secure base script. In the Kerns et al. (2011) system, interviews are first coded for markers of the secure base script, then rank ordered for similarity to a secure base prototype.

Training

Interviewers are trained on both the data collection protocol and the scoring system; training on the latter is important, so that interviewers know when to stop prompting the child for additional story details. To date, all coders using the original system (Granot & Mayseless, 2001) have established reliability with Granot and Mayseless by coding at least 20 tapes to check for reliability. The scriptedness coding system was developed and tested by one set of coders (Kerns et al., 2007).

Observer Agreement

Granot and Maysless (2001) reported high levels of agreement for their four-category attachment classification coding system, with 85% agreement for two different sets of coders (kappas = .77 and .81). Correlations for the 5-point pattern ratings were also high, ranging from .78 to .85. Kerns et al. (2007) also reported adequate agreement, reporting 68% agreement for the same four-category system (kappa = .54). Correlations for scriptedness ratings in the same study were also adequate, *r*'s = .74–.86. Using a revision of the Granot and Mayseless coding criteria, Kerns et al. (2011) rated each child using 5-point pattern ratings, and gammas were .70–.96. In Movahed-Abtahi and Kerns (2017), intraclass correlations ranged from .60 to .77.

Test–Retest Reliability and Stability

Two studies assessed test–retest reliability over a 3-month interval. Granot and Maysless (2001) reported a 94% stability rate for classifications and correlations for pattern ratings ranging from .63 to .82. Kerns et al. (2005) reported a lower but significant rate of stability in a second sample (50%), with correlations for pattern ratings ranging from .25 to .54 and correlations for scriptedness rankings ranging from .34 to .54.

Relations with Other Attachment Measures

The Doll Play Interview and the Security Scale were significantly related in three studies (Granot & Mayseless, 2001; Kerns et al., 2007; Kerns et al., 2011) but not another (Kerns et al., 2007).

Validation through Tests of Construct Validity

Attachment classifications or attachment pattern ratings derived from the interview have related in expected ways to teacher reports of school adjustment and behavior problems, peer sociometric nominations, social-information processing style, observations of mothers' parenting, and measures of emotion and internalizing symptoms (Brumariu & Kerns, 2010; Brumariu, Kerns, & Seibert, 2012; Granot & Mayseless, 2001, 2012; Kerns et al., 2007, 2011). In addition, scriptedness scores were related to children's reports of negative mood, and mother and teacher reports of emotion regulation (Kerns et al., 2007). The interview has also shown discriminant validity, in that classifications are not related to measures of language or logical thinking (Granot & Maysless, 2001) or to indices of the verbal complexity of children's narratives (Kerns et al., 2007).

Summary

Story-stem techniques can be used with 9- to 12-year-olds. The Doll Play Interview was initially developed with an Israeli sample, and in that culture, the measure has shown high test–retest reliability and evidence of convergent and discriminant validity. Results have been more modest when the interview was used in a U.S. sample, although an adaptation with different story stems that are more culturally relevant seems more promising for U.S. samples (Kerns et al., 2011; Movahed-Abtahi & Kerns, 2017). The script approach to scoring story-stem interviews is a promising alternative that is easier to use than the more complex classification system requiring substantial clinical judgment, but it requires further testing.

Verbal Responses to Pictures of Parent–Child Separation

Procedure

The SAT is a semiprojective measure in which children's responses to pictures of parent–child separations are elicited. Typically, children are shown a picture (e.g., parent leaving for 2 weeks), then are asked to say how the child is feeling, why he or she is feeling that way, and what he or she should do. The child in the picture is matched to the age and sex of the target child. Pictures of both mild separations (e.g., parents leave for the evening) and severe separations (e.g., parent is being taken to the hospital) are shown. There are two versions of the SAT for 9- to 12-year-olds. Wright et al. (1995) adapted stimuli used with 6-year-olds to make them more developmentally appropriate for older children, and Avezier, Sagi, Resnick, and Gini (2002) adapted picture stimuli that had been developed for adolescents. Although the picture sets are different, three similar pictures are common to the two sets. The pictures used by Avezier et al. depict more serious situations; two of the situations depicted in their "mild" pictures are used as "severe" pictures in the Wright et al. (1995) picture set. Children's responses have been recorded on paper (Wright et al., 1995), audiotaped (Avezier et al., 2002), or recorded with a computer-administered interview (Kerns et al., 2000). Although children usually are asked what the child in the picture would feel and do, Wright et al. (1995) administered the questions twice, first asking children what the child in the picture would feel and do (other), then asking the child him- or herself what he or she would feel and do (self).

Coding

All coding systems take into consideration children's emotional openness and coping responses. Wright et al. (1995) rated stories using three continuous scales: attachment and self-reliance (4-point scales) and avoidance (3-point scale). Aggregate scores were calculated separately for the other and self-questions. Avezier et al. (2002) used three 9-point rating scales: emotional openness, coping with separations, and narrative coherence (the latter was based on AAI criteria). Scores were highly correlated and summed to create an index of secure attachment. Kerns et al. (2000) used the same coding system as Avezier et al. (2002), although they scored for attachment classification (*secure, dismissing, preoccupied*) as well as three rating scales: Emotional Openness, Dismissing of Attachment, and Narrative Coherence. In the Kerns et al. (2000) study, the computer-administered interview was scored by a neural network whose scoring criteria were based on 200 interviews hand-scored by Gary Resnick (see Kerns et al., 2000, for details). Shmueli-Goetz, Target, Fonagy, and Datta (2008) used the same coding system by Resnick to code children as secure, ambivalent, or avoidant.

Training

Wright et al. (1995) trained on pilot subjects. In the other studies, Gary Resnick either coded the interviews or provided training on the coding.

Observer Agreement

In Wright et al. (1995), kappas for their continuous scales ranged from .58 to .84. Avezier et al. (2002) assessed agreement with intraclass correlations, which ranged from .80 to .89. Kerns et al. (2000) checked reliability of the neural network scoring by hand-scoring a subset of the cases with the coding system used by Avezier et al. (2002). Gammas for the scales ranged from .61 to .94, and kappas were .35 for three-way classifications (*secure, dismissing, preoccupied*) and .61 for two-way classifications (*secure, insecure*). Shmueli-Goetz et al. (2008) reported a kappa of .67 for three-way classifications.

Test–Retest Reliability and Stability

Wright et al. (1995) administered the SAT again after a 4-week interval to a subsample of their clinical group. None of the correlations was significant (all less that .40).

Relations with Other Attachment Measures

Avezier et al. (2002) reported a marginally significant association between mother–child attachment, assessed at age 1 in the Strange Situation, and security assessed on the SAT, but it was the opposite of prediction (early security predicted later insecurity). Kerns et al. (2000) found that attachment classifications and ratings from the SAT correlated with child reports of security and avoidant coping with mothers and fathers. Shmueli-Goetz et al. (2008) found that SAT classifications were related to attachment classifications derived from an autobiographical interview (64% agreement for 3-way classification, kappa = .36).

Validation through Tests of Construct Validity

Wright et al. (1995) found that a clinical and a control group differed on scales of attachment and avoidance, with stronger differences in the self than in the other condition. SAT scores were related to school adjustment in one study (Avezier et al., 2002) but not another (Kerns et al., 2000), and have shown some associations with measures of peer competence or friendship (Avezier et al., 2002; Contreras, Kerns, Weimer, Gentzler, & Tomich, 2000; Howes & Tonyan, 2000). One study found evidence of discriminant validity, in that SAT scores were not related to vocabulary or IQ (Avezier et al., 2002).

Summary

The review of studies presents a mixed picture. The SAT, when used with 9- to 12-year-olds, has not yet been demonstrated to have adequate test–retest reliability, and associations with other attachment measures and measures of child adjustment have been inconsistent. Thus, validity data are weaker than in studies with younger children. Wright et al. (1995) reported that children's responses to the interview were brief and could be recorded on paper. It could be that the structured nature of the interview is too constraining to allow for adequate assessment of individual differences in attachment representations in older, more verbal children. Given the availability of other measures, we recommend that investigators use a measure other than the SAT to assess attachment in 9- to 12-year-olds.

Autobiographical Narratives

Procedure

Three different autobiographical interviews, based conceptually and procedurally on the AAI, have been developed for preadolescents.[1] In all of the interviews, children are asked to describe and reflect on experiences with their caregivers, and to give specific examples, as well as more general descriptions of their relationships. The Attachment Interview for Childhood and Adolescence (AICA; Ammanti, van IJzendoorn, Speranza, & Tambelli, 2000) uses the same structure and questions as the AAI, although the language of the interview was simplified (e.g., definitions of terms were provided) and questions regarding parenting were omitted. The Child Attachment Interview (CAI; Target, Fonagy, & Shmueli-Goetz, 2003; Shmueli-Goetz et al., 2008) is based on both the Berkeley Autobiographical Interview and the AAI. It differs from the AAI in that children are asked about recent events and current relationships rather than earlier experiences. Interview questions are listed in Shmueli-Goetz et al. (2008). A third interview, the Friends and Family Interview (FFI; Steele & Steele, 2005) is somewhat similar to both of these interviews, in that children are asked about childhood relationships, and coding captures both children's experiences and discourse style (e.g., coherence). The FFI is much broader in content, including questions about family, school, and self-concept, and responses in all areas are considered in coding. Because of this breadth, the FFI may measure broader concepts than attachment per se, depending on what parts of the interview are scored.

As with any narrative procedure, it is important for the interviewer to establish rapport with the child prior to beginning a narrative interview. The interviewer should be interested and polite, and allow the child sufficient time to formulate an answer. The interviewer also should be careful not to show approval for the child's responses or make other comments that might guide the child's responses, while nevertheless steering the child back to the interview when needed. To be sure the interview can be coded later for coherence, it is very important that the interviewer follow the protocol closely, which includes prompting the child for details at appropriate times.

---

[1]Grossmann et al. (2002) reported using a fourth attachment interview with 10-year-olds. This interview is very different from the other autobiographical interviews developed, in that it asks children to report what behavioral strategies they use when feeling specific emotions (e.g., sad, angry) or when coping with challenges and disappointments. The only data reported for this measure are adequate agreement for 3-point security ratings and a significant association with mother–child attachment as assessed in the Strange Situation at age 1 (Grossmann et al., 2002). Manuscripts describing the interview in detail are written in German.

Coding

The coding systems for narrative interviews typically capture both the quality of described experiences with a parent and the coherence of the narrative. The coding system for the AICA (Ammaniti et al., 2000) closely parallels the coding system for the AAI. Trained coders rate each transcript using twelve 9-point scales. Five scales tap probable childhood experiences (e.g., parent loving, parent rejecting), and are rated separately for the mother–child and the father–child relationship. In addition, there are seven representation scales (e.g., idealization, coherence). After completing all scales, coders assign an interview one of four classifications that capture overall state of mind in regard to attachment: *dismissing, secure, preoccupied,* or *unresolved.* Coding of the CAI (Target et al., 2003; Shmueli-Goetz et al., 2008) is based on video recordings of the interview, and final classifications are based on both linguistic analysis and the child's behavior during thea interview (e.g., eye contact, signs of anxiety). The 13 language codes are rated on 9-point scales that capture both experiences (e.g., conflict resolution strategies) and representations (e.g., coherence). Although only some categories are rated separately for the mother–child and father–child relationship, an overall classification is assigned separately for mother–child and father–child attachment, using a four-category system: *secure, dismissing, preoccupied,* and *disorganized.* The coding system for the FFI has 7 scales that are rated on 4-point scales, taking into consideration responses across the entire interview (Kriss, Steele, & Steele, 2012). The scales capture coherence, secure base availability, self-esteem, peer relationships, and different defenses (e.g., idealization of parent), and children are assigned a classification (*secure–autonomous, avoidant, worried*).

Training

Learning the coding system for any of these interviews requires extensive training. The administration and scoring of these measures should not be attempted without first consulting with colleagues who are experienced in using the measures. A good understanding of attachment theory is also very helpful. Ammaniti et al. (2000) reported that coders of the AICA were all previously trained to criterion on the AAI. Target et al. (2003) reported that coders for the CAI were all familiar with current attachment assessment methodologies. Training sessions on the CAI are available (see Shmueli-Goetz et al., 2008, for information). Training procedures for the FFI are not described in Steele and Steele (2005; Kriss et al., 2012); investigators can contact Howard Steele for information.

Observer Agreement

Ammaniti et al. (2000) found good agreement for the four-category assignments coded from the AICA (82%, kappa = .64). Correlations for individual rating scales were also all acceptable, ranging from .60 to 1.00. Target et al.

(2003) also found, with the CAI, good agreement on four-way classifications with two different sets of coders (kappas for mother classifications ranged from .60 to .89, and kappas for father classifications ranged from .54 to .89). Correlations for individual ratings scales from the CAI were all acceptable (*r*'s .66–.94) with one exception (*r* = .38; see also Shmueli-Goetz et al. [2008] for data on a second sample). Borelli et al. (2010) reported a kappa of .86 for four-way classifications and a correlation of .97 for ratings of narrative coherence, and Scott, Briskman, Woolgar, Humayun, and O'Connor (2011) reported a kappa of .78 (85% agreement) for four-way classifications. Although Steele and Steele (2005) did not provide information on observer agreement for the FFI, Abrines et al. (2012) reported correlations of .67–.82 for the scales they rated from the FFI, and Psouni and Apetroaia (2014) reported a kappa of .82 (90% agreement).

Test–Retest Reliability and Stability

In a 4-year follow-up from age 10 to 14 years, Ammaniti et al. (2000) reported 71% stability (kappa = .48) for the four-category classification system of the AICA. Correlations for individual ratings were significant for four of 10 experience scales and four of six representation scales (significant *r*'s ranged from .36 to .66). The four-category classification system of the CAI (Target et al., 2003) showed high test–retest reliability over 3 months (kappas .78 for mother–child and .67 for father–child) and similarly high levels of stability over 1 year (kappas .78 for mother–child and .66 for father–child). Correlations for individual coding categories were modest, ranging from .29 to .90 (median .63) at the 3-month retest and .08 to .75 (median .40) at the 12-month retest.

Relations with Other Attachment Measures

In a longitudinal study, the Strange Situation was administered at age 1, separation–reunion and story-stem measures were administered at age 5, and the AICA was administered at age 11 (Ammaniti, Speranza, & Fedele, 2005). Three-way classification stability rates between the AICA and the earlier measures ranged from 52 to 68% but were not significant in this small sample (*n* = 21). Attachment classifications on the CAI were related to children's classifications on the SAT (64% concordance; Shmueli-Goetz et al., 2008). Steele and Steele (2005) observed infants in the Strange Situation separately with both mothers and fathers, and found that father–child attachment but not mother–child attachment predicted at age 11 children's coherence and reports of maternal secure base availability on the FFI. The FFI classifications and secure base support ratings were strongly related to secure scriptedness scores from a word prompt story task (Psouni & Apetroaia, 2014), and FFI coherence ratings are also correlated with self-reports of attachment (Kerns, Mathews, Koehn, Williams, & Siener-Ciesla, 2015; Psouni & Apetroaia, 2014).

Validation through Tests of Construct Validity

Classifications from both the CAI and AICA have been related as expected with maternal AAIs (Ammaniti et al., 2005; Target et al., 2003; Shmueli-Goetz et al., 2008). Target et al. (2003) reported that secure versus insecure classifications from the CAI were not related to Verbal IQ or child age, ethnicity, social class, or gender. Shmueli-Goetz (2008) reported that the CAI classifications were related to maternal reports of the child's personality. Scott et al. (2011) found that secure classifications from the CAI were related to parenting, and Scott et al. and Borelli et al. (2010) reported that secure classifications from the CAI were related to measures of child emotion. Borelli et al. (2016) also found that CAI ratings predicted children's internalizing symptoms. Steele and Steele (2005) found that maternal AAIs, collected prior to the child's birth, predicted 11-year-olds' narrative coherence and perceptions of their mother's secure base availability. FFI ratings of attachment security were also (negatively) related to attention problems (Abrines et al., 2012), and coherence scores were related to children's school adjustment (Kerns et al., 2015).

Summary

It appears that autobiographical interviews can be used with preadolescents. Both the AICA and CAI showed evidence of test–retest reliability. The AICA, CAI, and FFI show some associations with maternal AAIs and other measures of attachment, although other types of validity data are limited. Thus, while autobiographical interviews have been established as valid measures of attachment for adolescents, and it appears that children in middle childhood are also capable of completing autobiographical interviews adapted for younger children, there is a great need for studies that further test the validity of these interviews.

Questionnaire Assessments of Children's Perceptions of Attachment

Investigators have developed a number of different questionnaires to assess children's perceptions of attachments, but unfortunately there are serious limitations to most of them. One problem is conceptual: It is not clear that some measures assess attachment rather than related constructs. For example, some investigators have interpreted measures of social support as measures of attachment (e.g., Rubin et al., 2004), with the argument that social support measures are correlated with attachment. We find this argument unconvincing; attachment is also correlated with self-esteem, but it does not seem reasonable to conclude that self-esteem measures are therefore a good proxy for attachment. The other problem is that some measures labeled "attachment" tap parent–child relationship qualities that are only loosely related to attachment or are assessed without regard to context. For example, the Inventory of Parent and Peer Attachment (Gullone & Robinson, 2005) assesses trust, alienation, and communication. It is unclear how these properties relate to the secure base construct. For example, ambivalent attachment is not a problem of low levels of communication, but rather that communications with the attachment figure do not result in feelings of security (which might even result in high levels of communication as part of a heightening strategy). Thus, broad questionnaire measures may not be sensitive enough to context.

We only include in this review measures that tap what Bretherton (1985) has termed the *narrow* rather than the *broad* meaning of attachment; that is, the measures capture the secure base conceptualization of attachment rather than broader qualities of the parent–child relationship. Because of inherent limitations in self-report questionnaires, we also excluded questionnaire measures from this review for the following reasons: The questionnaire contained only a single item; the measure has only been validated against other self-reports obtained from the child; and/or the measure has only been used in a single study. After applying these conceptual and methodological exclusionary criteria, we identified two questionnaire measures: the Security Scale (Kerns et al., 2001) and the Avoidant and Preoccupied Coping Scales (Finnegan, Hodges, & Perry, 1996; see Brenning, Soenens, Braet, & Bosmans, 2011, for a recent adaptation of an adolescent measure to assess avoidant and anxious–ambivalent attachment).

Procedure

Both the Security Scale (Kerns et al., 2001) and the Avoidant and Preoccupied Coping Scales (also called Preoccupied and Coping Attachment Style; Yunger, Corby, & Perry, 2005) separately assess children's perceptions of the mother–child and father–child relationship. Both also use the same "Some kids . . . , Other kids . . . " format pioneered by Susan Harter (1982), in which children are presented two options for a question; they are told some kids are one way (e.g., like to tell their mom what they are thinking or feeling), while other kids are another way (e.g., don't like to tell their mom what they are thinking or feeling). The child is asked to choose which type of kid he or she is like, then to indicate whether the statement he or she chose is really true or sort of true for him or her. It is thought that asking children to identify with a group of kids, rather than having to rate the self low on an item (e.g., "share information with my mom"), may decrease socially desirable responding (Harter, 1982). The 15 items on the Security Scale assess a single, continuously scored security dimension. Lieberman et al. (1999) suggested that the scale has two distinct subscales, Availability and Dependency (termed *reliance* by Kerns et al., 2006), but Verschueren and Marcoen (2005) have questioned whether the evidence supports the distinctiveness of the two subscales. A newer version of the Security Scale, which distinguishes between secure base and safe-haven support, is not discussed here, as it has only been used in one published paper (Kerns et al., 2015). Earlier versions of the Preoccupied and Coping scales had 18 (Finnegan et al., 1996) or 15 (Hodges, Finnegan, & Perry, 1999) items per scale, although in the most recent version there are 10 item scales for each dimension (Yunger et al., 2005).

Scoring

Each item on the Security Scale is scored on a 4-point scale (see Kerns, Klepac, & Cole, 1996); rating the "Secure" option really true is scored a 4 and sort of true a 3, with the "Insecure" option sort of true scored a 2 and really true scored a 1. Item scores are averaged to calculate a total Security score. The Coping Styles Questionnaire (see Finnegan et al., 1996) uses a different scoring system in which each item is scored 0, 1, or 2. For each question, one choice is a description of either an avoidant or preoccupied coping response. If the child selects that option, s/he receives a score of 2 if it is rated really true and a score of 1 if it is rated sort of true. If the child selects the non-Avoidant or non-Preoccupied option, s/he receives a score of 0, regardless of whether the child considers the description to be really true or sort of true. Items are summed to create total scores for Preoccupied Coping and Avoidant Coping.

INTERNAL CONSISTENCY

Internal consistency is high for both instruments, with scale coefficients typically .80 or higher (see Dwyer, 2005; Kerns et al., 2005, for reviews).

TEST–RETEST RELIABILITY AND STABILITY

Test–retest reliability data are available for both instruments for children's reports of the mother–child relationship. Kerns, Klepac, and Cole (1996) reported a 2-week test–retest correlation of .75 for the Security Scale. Similarly, Finnegan et al. (1996) reported 2-week test–retest correlations of .83 for Preoccupied Coping and .76 Avoidant Coping. Two studies with the Security Scale (Kerns et al., 2000; Verschueren & Marcoen, 2005) have examined the stability of security over a 2- or 3-year interval (from age 8 to 10 or 11 years). Correlations were significant for the mother–child relationship in one study, and for the father–child relationship in both studies, although significant correlations were modest in magnitude (r's .28–.37). Hodges et al. (1999) assessed coping after 1 year in a sample that was originally assessed at ages 8–14 years of age, and found stability for both Preoccupied Coping, $r = .65$, and Avoidant Coping, $r = .53$.

RELATIONS WITH OTHER ATTACHMENT MEASURES

Kerns et al. (2000) examined associations between the Security Scale, the Preoccupied and Avoidant Coping Scales, and classifications and scale ratings from the SAT. They found some associations between the Security Scale and the SAT. In addition, children's Security Scores were inversely correlated with Avoidant Coping, but not consistently related to Preoccupied Coping.

Avoidant Coping was more strongly related to the SAT than was Preoccupied Coping. Two studies indicated that Security Scores were related in expected ways to ratings or classifications from the Doll Story Completion Task (Granot & Mayseless, 2001; Kerns et al., 2011). The Security Scale is also related to ratings of coherence from the FFI and CAI (Borelli et al., 2016; Kerns et al., 2015; Psouni & Apetroaia, 2014) and to ratings of secure base support from the FFI (Kerns et al., 2015; Psouni & Apetroaia, 2014).

VALIDATION THROUGH TESTS OF CONSTRUCT VALIDITY

The Security Scale has been significantly related to observation and questionnaire measures of parenting (Kerns et al., 2000, 2001, 2011); mothers' reports of anxious attachment (Doyle, Markiewicz, Brendgen, Lieberman, & Voss, 2000); parents' reports of the quality of the marital relationship (Harold, Shelton, Goeke-Morey, & Cummings, 2004); teacher ratings of children's school adjustment (Granot & Mayseless, 2001; Kerns et al., 2000, 2006, 2015); patterns of social-information processing (Cassidy, Ziv, Mehta, & Feeney, 2003); symptoms of anxiety and depression (Brumariu et al., 2012; Kerns et al., 2011); and observational, teacher report, peer report, and self-report measures of peer relationships (Abraham & Kerns, 2013; Contreras et al., 2000; Granot & Mayseless, 2001; Kerns et al., 1996; Lieberman et al., 1999; Verschueren & Marcoen, 2002). Although the findings are generally consistent, there is some variability (e.g., in a particular study, an effect might be found for mother–child but not father–child attachment). In addition, expected associations have been shown in samples from different countries (e.g., Belgium: Bosmans, De Raedt, & Braet, 2007; Taiwan: Chen, Lin, & Li, 2012; Israel: Bauminger & Kimhi-Kind, 2008).

Avoidant coping has been associated in predicted ways with questionnaire measures of parenting (Karavasalis, Doyle, & Markiewicz, 2003; Kerns et al., 2000; Yunger et al., 2005), peer reports of externalizing behavior (Finnegan et al., 1996), and teacher reports of school adjustment (Kerns et al., 2006). Preoccupied Coping has not related consistently to questionnaire or observational measures of parenting (Karavasalis et al., 2003; Kerns et al., 2000, 2008; Yunger et al., 2005), although it has predicted peer nominations of internalizing behavior for boys (Finnegan et al., 1996) and teacher reports of school adjustment (Kerns et al., 2006).

SUMMARY

Both the Security Scale and the Avoidant and Preoccupied Coping Scales have shown some evidence of reliability and validity, although evidence of validity is weaker for the Preoccupied Coping Scale than for the other two (see Kerns et al. [2000, 2008] for discussion of the concerns). In addition, correlations between the Avoidant Coping Scale and the Security Scale suggest the two measures may be tapping a single secure–avoidant dimension. Thus, while the Security Scale and Coping Scales were intended to complement one another, it is not clear whether the Avoidant and Preoccupied Coping Scales provide novel information beyond what is captured by the Security Scale. The Security Scale has also been validated more extensively, and a meta-analysis provides a summary of the measure's correlates (Brumariu, Madigan, et al., 2018). Validity data for the Coping Scales are not as strong, especially for the Preoccupied Coping Scale, and the Preoccupied Scale developed by Brenning et al. (2011) may hold more promise. Effect sizes with both instruments are often small in magnitude; thus, findings may not be significant in small samples. Additional research is needed to clarify how questionnaire and narrative measures of attachment overlap in preadolescence.

CONCLUSIONS

Unlike at other age periods, in middle childhood there are many approaches and measures available to assess attachment. This diversity may be necessary because of the developmental changes taking place during this time; that is, approaches that are valid for 6-year-olds may not be equally valid for 12-year-olds. For example, our review suggests that the SAT appears to work well with younger children but not with older children. In contrast, autobiographical narratives may be appropriate to use with preadolescents, but may be too cognitively demanding for younger children. Thus, in selecting measures for middle childhood, researchers need to consider which approaches are most valid for the particular age they wish to study. Longitudinal studies in middle childhood may require different measurement approaches at different ages.

There is additional complexity for assessing attachment during middle childhood, because the different measures and approaches vary substantially in terms of how they conceptualize attachment. It is important to keep in mind that when choosing a measure, one is actually choosing a particular conceptualization of one's construct. Some measures assess secure base behavior, others assess attachment representations, and still others assess child perceptions. In addition, there is also an important difference among measures in whether attachment is conceptualized as relationship specific or as an overall (general) representation of attachment relationships. Therefore, it is important for investigators to consider what it is they want to measure, to state clearly their conceptualization of the construct, and to choose a measure that can bear that interpretation.

As summarized in this chapter, investigators have now developed and begun validating several different measures. Earlier, we described seven criteria that could be used for evaluating attachment measures. As shown in Tables 6.3 and 6.4, there are currently limited validity data for most middle childhood measures. None has been validated against naturalistic observations of secure base behavior (this criterion was omitted from the table), and few measurement approaches have been evaluated against all of the other six criteria. In addition, even when validity data are available, there are often few studies for any one criterion, and evidence for validity may be mixed.

TABLE 6.3. Available Validity Data for Attachment Measures, 6- to 8-Year-Olds

Measure	Maternal responsiveness	Consistent over time	Predict development	Validate cross-culturally	Other measures of attachment	Discriminant validity
Behavioral observations						
Separation–reunion:						
Main & Cassidy (1988)	x	x	x	x	x	x
Story-stem measures						
Doll Story completion:						
Verschueren & Marcoen (1999)			x	x		
Manchester Story Task:						
Green et al. (2000)		x	x	x		
Goldwyn et al. (2000)			x		x	x
Gloger-Tippelt et al. (2002)					x	
Gloger-Tippelt & Kappler (2016)					x	x
Attachment Story completion:						
Poehlmann (2005)	x					x
Dubois-Comtois et al. (2011)	x				x	
Scholtens et al. (2014)			x			x
Verbal response to pictures of separation						
SAT:						
Jacobsen et al. (1994)			x	x	x	
Jacobsen & Hofmann (1997)		x	x	x	x	
Bohlin et al. (2000)			x			
Easterbrooks & Abeles (2000)			x			x
Grossmann et al. (2002)					x	

Note. "x" indicates the type of validity data available. It should be noted that for most of the measures, there are only one or two studies that have evaluated a particular validity criterion.

TABLE 6.4. Available Validity Data for Attachment Measures, 9- to 12-Year-Olds

Measure	Maternal responsiveness	Consistent over time	Predict development	Validate cross-culturally	Other measures of attachment	Discriminant validity
Story-stem measures						
Doll Story completion:						
Granot & Mayseless (2001)		X	X	X	X	X
Granot & Mayseless (2012)			X			
Kerns Doll Story:						
Kerns et al. (2011)	X		X		X	
Brumariu & Kerns (2010)			X			X
Brumariu et al. (2012)			X			
Verbal response to pictures of separation						
SAT:						
Wright et al. (1995)			X		X	
Avezier et al. (2002)			X	X	X	X
Autobiographical narratives						
CAI:						
Ammaniti et al. (2000)		X			X	
Shmeuli-Goetz et al. (2008)		X	X		X	X
Borelli et al. (2010)			X			
Scott et al. (2011)	X		X			
Borelli et al. (2016)			X		X	X
FFI:						
Steele & Steele (2005)					X	
Abrines et al. (2012)			X			
Psouni & Apetroaia (2014)					X	
Kerns et al. (2015)			X		X	

(continued)

TABLE 6.4. *(continued)*

Measure	Maternal responsiveness	Consistent over time	Predict development	Validate cross-culturally	Other measures of attachment	Discriminant validity
Questionnaires						
Security Scale[a]*:*						
Kerns et al. (2001)	x	x	x		x	x
Kerns et al. (2011)	x		x		x	x
Brumariu & Kerns (2010)			x			x
Granot & Mayseless (2001)			x	x	x	
De Minzi (2006)	x		x	x		
Chen (2012)			x	x		
Chen et al. (2012)	x			x		x
Scharf et al. (2016)			x	x		
Avoidance:						
Finnegan et al. (1996)	x	x	x		x	
Brenning et al. (2011)			x		x	
Preocccupied:						
Finnegan et al. (1996)		x	x			
Brenning et al. (2011)			x		x	

Note. "x" indicates the type of validity data available. It should be noted that for most of the measures, there are only one or two studies that have evaluated a particular validity criterion.

[a]The Security Scale has been used extensively and translated into several languages; only a small number of representative studies are included in this table to save space.

Behavioral observation with young children, story-stem measures, autobiographical interviews, and questionnaires for older children have been tested most extensively.

A behavioral observation procedure has been validated for 6- to 8-year-old children, but currently no observation system has been exhaustively validated for older children. Although children's displays of attachment behavior become more subtle in the middle childhood years compared to earlier (Main & Cassidy, 1988), it may nevertheless be worth exploring the measurement of secure base behavior in older children. Two different observational measures have been developed for children ages 9–12 years (Boldt et al., 2016;

Brumariu, Giuseppone, et al., 2018), both of which involve rating attachment in the context of parent–child interaction during tasks. Each has only been used in one study, and both show some promise but need more extensive validation. Representational measures are a promising approach, but no specific measure has been extensively validated yet. Especially needed are studies of representational measures that examine test–retest reliability, discriminant validity, and how the measures are related to maternal behavior. Questionnaire measures have shown some validity with older children, although these measures may be less precise and consequently may yield smaller effect sizes than other types of measures. Finally, there is a critical need for additional studies that evaluate overlap of the different measures, both within and across measurement approaches (i.e., behavioral observation, attachment representations, and questionnaires). We recommend that investigators include at least two different measures of attachment in their studies, so that overlap in assessments (and their correlates) can be evaluated directly. Finally, attachment priming has been employed with 6- to 7-year-olds as a way of manipulating secure attachment (Stupica, Brett, Woodhouse, & Cassidy, 2018), and this represents a novel way of studying attachment in middle childhood.

As we noted earlier, many of the measures of attachment for middle childhood are adaptations of measures originally developed for other age periods. Coding manuals also are often adapted from those for other ages. In testing and refining measures, we recommend that investigators not lose sight of the need to consider how attachment might operate specifically within the middle childhood period. As we noted earlier, there are many changes children experience in middle childhood that might affect the attachment system. Although there are some data on who might operate as attachment figures in middle childhood (Kerns et al., 2006; Kobak et al., 2005; Seibert & Kerns, 2009), we lack other basic descriptive information about attachment during this period. For example, if secure base behavior becomes organized as a supervisory partnership in middle childhood, what does this look like, and does it change the goal of the attachment system (e.g., does the goal change from availability of the attachment figure to mutual regulation with the attachment figure)? How might the manifestations of avoidant, ambivalent, and disorganized attachments change in the middle childhood years? To cite one example, Hans, Bernstein, and Sims (2000) have speculated that the behavior of ambivalent children in middle childhood differs from younger ages, in that older ambivalent children will, in addition to showing exaggerated emotion displays, also act in ways to create negative affect in the parent (e.g., acting passively rude) as part of their strategy to engage a parent. Careful observation of children in longitudinal studies may help illuminate how children capitalize on their more sophisticated knowledge of the social world to develop new approaches to regulating contact with the attachment figure.

Recent work in our laboratory illustrates the value of collecting normative data. When we began using doll play procedures, we used the story stems used by other investigators. We initially assumed the stories would work well for our participants. We became concerned, however, about the validity of some of the stories. For example, in the "hurt knee" stories, most American preadolescents were very nonchalant and did not express need for an attachment figure, unlike children in Israel (see Kerns et al., 2007). When we asked children about a scary figure in their room at night, many children spontaneously reported this never happened to them. This led us to wonder in what types of situations children would want contact with an attachment figure, and we interviewed 94 children between ages 7 and 12 years to find out. We asked them to tell us about a time when they were sad, and a time when they were scared (two emotions that Bowlby suggested may trigger secure base behavior). For each situation, we content-coded the answers (observer kappas for agreement were .87 and .90). For the sad question, four of seven categories were named by at least 10% of the children: performance failures (e.g., in sports or school; 22%); physical injury or illness of self or other (13%); social conflict (e.g., disagreement with a friend; 13%); and loss of a family member or pet (10%). For the scared question, four of nine categories were named by at least 10% of the children: dark or night (e.g., afraid of the dark; 19%); performance failures (e.g., sports try-out; 16%); scary media (e.g., movie; 11%); and animals/people (e.g., bullies, dogs; 10%). We suggest that investigators may want to use this information as they refine storytelling measures of attachment representations. We further recommend that investigators include some open-ended questions in all of their studies to address the need for information on how the attachment system operates in middle childhood.

Given the range of options available, which measures would we recommend? In our opinion, for the early middle childhood years (ages 6–8 years) there are three good options: the separation-reunion (behavioral) measure and the story-stem and SAT interviews (representation measures). All three of these measures have been used in multiple studies, and evidence of reliability and validity has been presented for each. We should note that there are currently many variations of story-stem techniques, so an investigator would need to choose one system. All of these techniques require careful administration and extensive training on coding procedures. An investigator would need training before using any of these techniques.

The matter is less settled for the later middle-childhood period. The most promising approaches appear to be story-stem or autobiographical interviews. The Security Scale may also be worth including in studies in which assessments of specific insecure attachment patterns are not needed, especially if a more extensive assessment of attachment is not possible. Given that all of these measures are relatively new and have not been extensively validated (the Security Scale has currently been tested the most extensively; see Brumariu, Giuseppone, et al., 2018), we recommend including two different measures of attachment in a study whenever possible.

In conclusion, while there has been substantial progress in developing measures to assess attachment in middle childhood, there is still a great deal of work to be done to more fully validate the measures. We encourage investigators to extend prior work by testing and refining measures that are already available rather than creating new measures. In doing so, it will be important to consider the implications of the developmental changes occurring in middle childhood for attachment assessment. This work will also allow the field to address questions regarding how attachment changes in middle childhood (e.g., to understand when a more general "state of mind" regarding attachment emerges), as well as facilitate longitudinal studies of attachment across childhood.

REFERENCES

Abraham, M. M., & Kerns, K. A. (2013). Positive and negative emotions and coping as mediators of the link between mother–child attachment and peer relationships. *Merrill–Palmer Quarterly, 59*, 399–425.

Abrines, N., Barcons, N., Marre, D., Brun, C., Fornieles, A., & Fumadó, V. (2012). ADHD-like symptoms and attachment in internationally adopted children. *Attachment and Human Development, 14*(4), 405–423.

Ainsworth, M. D. S. (1989). Attachments beyond infancy. *American Psychologist, 44*, 709–716.

Ainsworth, M. D. S. (1990). Epilogue: Some considerations regarding theory and assessment relevant to attachments beyond infancy. In M. T. Greenberg, D. Cicchetti, & E. M. Cummings (Eds.), *Attachment in the preschool years* (pp. 463–488). Chicago: University of Chicago Press.

Allen, J. P., & Land, D. (1999). Attachment in adolescence. In J. Cassidy & P. R. Shaver (Eds.), *Handbook of attachment: Theory, research, and clinical applications* (pp. 319–335). New York: Guilford Press.

Ammaniti, M., Speranza, A. M., & Fedele, S. (2005). Attachment in infancy and in early and late childhood: A longitudinal study. In K. A. Kerns & R. A. Richardson (Eds.), *Attachment in middle childhood* (pp. 115–136). New York: Guilford Press.

Ammaniti, M., van IJzendoorn, M. H., Speranza, A. M., & Tambelli, R. (2000). Internal working models of attachment during late childhood and early adolescence: An exploration of stability and change. *Attachment and Human Development, 2*, 328–346.

Avezier, O., Sagi, A., Resnick, G., & Gini, M. (2002). School competence in young adolescence: Links to early attachment relationships beyond concurrent self-perceived competence and representations of relationships. *International Journal of Behavioral Development, 26*, 397–409.

Bauminger, N., & Kimhi-Kind, I. (2008). Social information processing, security of attachment, and emotion regulation in children with learning disabilities. *Journal of Learning Disabilities, 41*(4), 315–332.

Bohlin, G., Hagekull, B., & Rydell, A. (2000). Attachment and social functioning: A longitudinal study from infancy to middle childhood. *Social Development, 9*, 24–39.

Boldt, L. J., Kochanska, G., Grekin, R., & Brock, R. L. (2016). Attachment in middle childhood: Predictors, correlates, and implications for adaptation. *Attachment and Human Development, 18*, 115–140.

Borelli, J. L., Crowley, M. J., David, D. H., Sbarra, D. A., Anderson, G. M., & Mayes, L. C. (2010). Attachment and emotion in school-aged children. *Emotion, 10*(4), 475–485.

Borelli, J. L., Somers, J., West, J. L., Coffey, J. K., De Los Reyes, A., & Shmueli-Goetz, Y. (2016). Associations between attachment narratives and self-report measures of attachment in middle childhood: Extending evidence for the validity of the Child Attachment Interview. *Journal of Child and Family Studies, 25,* 1235–1246.

Bosmans, G., De Raedt, R., & Braet, C. (2007). The invisible bonds: Does the secure base script of attachment influence children's attention toward their mother? *Journal of Clinical Child and Adolescent Psychology, 36,* 557–567.

Bosmans, G., & Kerns, K. A. (2015). Attachment in middle childhood: Progress and prospects. In G. Bosmans & K. A. Kerns (Eds.), *Attachment in middle childhood: Theoretical advances and new directions in an emerging field* (pp. 1–14). San Francisco: Jossey-Bass.

Bowlby, J. (1973). *Attachment and loss: Vol. 2. Separation.* New York: Basic Books.

Bowlby, J. (1979). *The making and breaking of affectional bonds.* London: Tavistock.

Bowlby, J. (1982). *Attachment and loss: Vol. 1. Attachment* (2nd ed.). New York: Basic Books. (Original work published 1969)

Brenning, K., Soenens, B., Braet, C., & Bosmans, G. (2011). An adaptation of the Experiences in Close Relationships Scale—Revised for use with children and adolescents. *Journal of Social and Personal Relationships, 28,* 1048–1072.

Bretherton, I. (1985). Attachment theory: Retrospect and prospect. In I. Bretherton & E. Waters (Eds.), Growing points of attachment theory and research. *Monographs of the Society for Research in Child Development, 50*(1/2, Serial No. 209), 3–35.

Bretherton, I., Ridgeway, D., & Cassidy, J. (1990). Assessing internal working models of the attachment relationship. In M. T. Greenberg, D. Cicchetti, & E. M. Cummings (Eds.), *Attachment in the preschool years: Theory, research, and intervention* (pp. 273–308). Chicago: University of Chicago Press.

Brumariu, L. E., Giuseppone, K., Kerns, K. A., van de Walle, M., Bureau, J., Bosmans, G., & Lyons-Ruth, K. (2018). Middle Childhood Attachment Strategies Coding System: Initial validation of a behavioral measure. *Attachment and Human Development, 20,* 491–513.

Brumariu, L. E., & Kerns, K. A. (2010). Mother–child attachment patterns and different types of anxiety symptoms: Is there specificity of relations? *Child Psychiatry and Human Development, 41,* 663–674.

Brumariu, L. E., Kerns, K. A., & Seibert, A. C. (2012). Mother–child attachment, emotion regulation, and anxiety symptoms in middle childhood. *Personal Relationships, 19,* 569–585.

Brumariu, L. E., Madigan, S., Giussepone, K. R., Movahed Abtahi, M., & Kerns, K. A. (2018). The Security Scale as a measure of attachment: Meta-analytic evidence of validity. *Attachment and Human Development, 20,* 600–625.

Cassidy, J. (1988). Child–mother attachment and the self in six-year-olds. *Child Development, 59,* 121–134.

Cassidy, J. (1999). The nature of the child's ties. In J. Cassidy & P. R. Shaver (Eds.), *Handbook of attachment: Theory, research, and clinical applications* (pp. 3–20). New York: Guilford Press.

Cassidy, J., Kirsh, S. J., Scolton, K. L., & Parke, R. D. (1996). Attachment and representations of peer relationships. *Developmental Psychology, 32,* 892–904.

Cassidy, J., Marvin, R. S., & the MacArthur Attachment Working Group. (1992). *Attachment organization in preschool children: Coding guidelines*. Unpublished manuscript, University of Virginia, Charlottesville, VA.
Cassidy, J., Ziv, Y., Mehta, T. G., & Feeney, B. C. (2003). Feedback seeking in children and adolescents: Associations with self-perceptions, attachment representations, and depression. *Child Development, 74*, 612–628.
Chandler, M. J. (1973). Egocentrism and antisocial behavior: The assessment and training of social perspective-taking skills. *Developmental Psychology, 9*, 326–332.
Chen, B. (2012). The association between self-reported mother–child attachment and social initiative and withdrawal in Chinese school-aged children. *Journal of Genetic Psychology, 173*, 279–301.
Chen, F., Lin, H., & Li, C. (2012). The role of emotion in parent–child relationships: Children's emotionality, maternal meta-emotion, and children's attachment security. *Journal of Child and Family Studies, 21*(3), 403–410.
Clarke, L., Ungerer, J., Chahoud, K., Johnson, S., & Stiefel, I. (2002). Attention deficit hyperactivity disorder is associated with attachment security. *Clinical Child Psychology and Psychiatry, 7*, 179–198.
Contreras, J. M., Kerns, K. A., Weimer, B. L., Gentzler, A. L., & Tomich, P. L. (2000). Emotion regulation as a mediator of associations between mother–child attachment and peer relationships in middle childhood. *Journal of Family Psychology, 14*, 111–124.
De Minzi, M. C. R. (2006). Loneliness and depression in middle childhood: The relation to attachment and parenting style. *Journal of Genetic Psychology, 167*, 189–210.
Doyle, A. B., Markiewicz, D., Brendgen, M., Lieberman, M., & Voss, K. (2000). Child attachment security and self-concept: Associations with mother and father attachment style and marital quality. *Merrill–Palmer Quarterly, 46*, 514–539.
Dubois-Comtois, K., Cyr, C., & Moss, E. (2011). Attachment behavior and mother–child conversations as predictors of attachment representations in middle childhood: A longitudinal study. *Attachment and Human Development, 13*, 335–357.
Dwyer, K. M. (2005). The meaning and measurement of attachment in middle and late childhood. *Human Development, 48*, 155–182.
Easterbrooks, M. A., & Abeles, R. (2000). Windows to the self in 8-year-olds: Bridges to attachment representation and behavioral adjustment. *Attachment and Human Development, 2*, 85–106.
Easterbrooks, M. A., Davidson, C. E., & Chazan, R. (1993). Psychosocial risk, attachment, and behavior problems among school-aged children. *Development and Psychopathology, 5*, 389–402.
Finnegan, R. A., Hodges, E. V. E., & Perry, D. G. (1996). Preoccupied and avoidant coping during middle childhood. *Child Development, 67*, 1318–1328.
Futh, M. A., O'Connor, T. G., Matias, C., Green, J., & Scott, S. (2008). Attachment narratives and behavioral and emotional symptoms in an ethnically diverse, at-risk sample. *Journal of the American Academy of Child and Adolescent Psychiatry, 47*, 709–718.
Ghiselli, E. E., Campbell, J. P., & Zedeck, S. (1981). *Measurement theory for the behavioral sciences*. New York: Freeman.
Gloger-Tippelt, G., Gomille, B., Koenig, L., & Vetter, J. (2002). Attachment representations in 6-year-olds: Related longitudinally to the quality of attachment

in infancy and mothers' attachment representations. *Attachment and Human Development, 4,* 318–339.

Gloger-Tippelt, G., & Kappler, G. (2016). Narratives of attachment in middle childhood: Do gender, age, and risk-status matter for quality of attachment? *Attachment and Human Development, 18,* 570–595.

Goldwyn, R., Stanley, C., Smith, V., & Green, J. (2000). The Manchester Child Attachment Story Task: Relationship with parental AAI, SAT, and child behavior. *Attachment and Human Development, 2,* 71–84.

Gottman, J., & Mettetal, G. (1986). Speculations about social and affective development: Friendship and acquaintanceship through adolescence. In J. M. Gottman & J. G. Parker (Eds.), *Conversations of friends* (pp. 192–237). New York: Cambridge University Press.

Graham, C. A., & Easterbrooks, M. A. (2000). School-aged children's vulnerability to depressive symptomatology: The role of attachment security, maternal depressive symptomatology, and economic risk. *Development and Psychopathology, 12,* 201–213.

Granot, D., & Mayseless, O. (2001). Attachment security and adjustment to school in middle childhood. *International Journal of Behavioral Development, 25,* 530–541.

Granot, D., & Mayseless, O. (2012). Representations of mother–child attachment relationships and social-information processing of peer relationships in early adolescence. *Journal of Early Adolescence, 32*(4), 537–564.

Green, J., Stanley, C., Smith, V., & Goldwyn, R. (2000). A new method of evaluating attachment representations in young school-age children: The Manchester Child Attachment Story Task. *Attachment and Human Development, 2,* 48–70.

Grossmann, K., Grossmann, K. E., Fremmer-Bombik, E., Kindler, H., Scheuerer-Englisch, H., & Zimmermann, P. (2002). The uniqueness of the child–father attachment relationship: Fathers' sensitive and challenging play as a pivotal variable in a 16-year longitudinal study. *Social Development, 11,* 307–331.

Gullone, E., & Robinson, K. (2005). The Inventory of Parent and Peer Attachment—Revised (IPPA-R) for children: A psychometric investigation. *Clinical Psychology and Psychotherapy, 12,* 67–79.

Hans, S., Bernstein, V. J., & Sims, B. E. (2000). Change and continuity in ambivalent attachment relationships from infancy through adolescence. In P. M. Crittenden & A. H. Claussen (Eds.), *The organization of attachment relationships: Maturation, culture, and context* (pp. 277–299). New York: Cambridge University Press.

Harold, G. T., Shelton, K. H., Goeke-Morey, M. C., & Cummings, E. M. (2004). Marital conflict, child emotional security about family relationships and child adjustment. *Social Development, 13,* 350–376.

Harter, S. (1982). The perceived competence scale for children. *Child Development, 53,* 87–97.

Hodges, E. V. E., Finnegan, R. A., & Perry, D. G. (1999). Skewed autonomy-relatedness in preadolescents' conceptions of their relationships with mother, father, and best friend. *Developmental Psychology, 35,* 737–748.

Hodges, J., Steele, M., Hillman, S., & Henderson, K. (2003). Mental representations and defenses in severely maltreated children. In R. N. Emde, D. P. Wolf, & D. Oppenheim (Eds.), *Revealing the inner worlds of young children* (pp. 240–267). New York: Oxford University Press.

Howes, C., & Tonyan, H. (2000). Links between adult and peer relations across four developmental periods. In K. A. Kerns, J. M. Contreras, & A. M. Neal-Barnett (Eds.), *Family and peers: Linking two social worlds* (pp. 85–113). Westport, CT: Praeger.

Humber, N., & Moss, E. (2005). The relationship of preschool and early school age attachment to mother–child interaction. *American Journal of Orthopsychiatry, 75*, 128–141.

Jacobsen, T., Edelstein, W., & Hofmann, V. (1994). A longitudinal study of the relation between representations of attachment in childhood and cognitive functioning in childhood and adolescence. *Developmental Psychology, 30*, 112–124.

Jacobsen, T., & Hofmann, V. (1997). Children's attachment representations: Longitudinal relations to school behavior and academic competency in middle childhood and adolescence. *Developmental Psychology, 33*, 703–710.

Karavasilis, L., Doyle, A. B., & Markiewicz, D. (2003). Associations between parenting style and attachment to mother in middle childhood and adolescence. *International Journal of Behavioral Development, 27*, 153–164.

Kerns, K. A., Abraham, M. M., Schlegelmilch, A., & Morgan, T. A. (2007). Mother–child attachment in later middle childhood: Assessment approaches and associations with mood and emotion regulation. *Attachment and Human Development, 9*, 33–53.

Kerns, K. A., Aspelmeier, J. E., Gentzler, A. L., & Grabill, C. M. (2001). Parent–child attachment and monitoring in middle childhood. *Journal of Family Psychology, 15*, 69–81.

Kerns, K. A., & Brumariu, L. E. (2016). Attachment in middle childhood. In J. Cassidy & P. Shaver (Eds.), *Handbook of attachment* (3rd ed., pp. 349–365). New York: Guilford Press.

Kerns, K. A., Brumariu, L. E., & Seibert, A. C. (2011). Multi-method assessment of mother–child attachment: Links to parenting and child adjustment in middle childhood. *Attachment and Human Development, 13*, 315–333.

Kerns, K. A., Klepac, L., & Cole, A. (1996). Peer relationships and preadolescents' perceptions of security in the child–mother relationship. *Developmental Psychology, 32*, 457–466.

Kerns, K. A., Mathews, B. L., Koehn, A. J., Williams, C. T., & Siener-Ciesla, S. (2015). Assessing both safe haven and secure base support in parent–child relationships. *Attachment and Human Development, 17*, 337–353.

Kerns, K. A., Schlegelmilch, A., Morgan, T. A., & Abraham, M. M. (2005). Assessing attachment in middle childhood. In K. A. Kerns & R. A. Richardson (Eds.), *Attachment in middle childhood* (pp. 46–70). New York: Guilford Press.

Kerns, K. A., Tomich, P. L., Aspelmeier, J. E., & Contreras, J. M. (2000). Attachment-based assessments of parent–child relationships in middle childhood. *Developmental Psychology, 36*, 614–626.

Kerns, K. A., Tomich, P. L., & Kim, P. (2006). Normative trends in children's perceptions of availability and utilization of attachment figures in middle childhood. *Social Development, 15*, 1–22.

Klagsbrun, M., & Bowlby, J. (1976). Response to separation from parents: A clinical test for young children. *British Journal of Projective Psychology, 21*, 7–26.

Kobak, R., Rosenthal, N., & Serwik, A. (2005). The attachment hierarchy in middle childhood: Conceptual and methodological issues. In K. A. Kerns & R. A. Richardson (Eds.), *Attachment in middle childhood* (pp. 71–88). New York: Guilford Press.

Koehn, A. J., & Kerns, K. A. (2016). The supervision partnership as a phase of attachment. *Journal of Early Adolescence, 36,* 961–988.

Kriss, A., Steele, H., & Steele, M. (2012). Measuring attachment and reflective functioning in early adolescence: An introduction to the Friends and Family Interview. *Research in Psychotherapy: Psychopathology, Process and Outcome, 15,* 87–95.

Lieberman, M., Doyle, A., & Markiewicz, D. (1999). Developmental patterns in security of attachment to mother and father in late childhood and early adolescence: Associations with peer relations. *Child Development, 70,* 202–213.

Maccoby, E. (1984). Middle childhood in the context of the family. In W. A. Collins (Ed.), *Development during middle childhood* (pp. 184–239). Washington, DC: National Academy Press.

Main, M. (1990). Cross-cultural studies of attachment organization: Recent studies, changing methodologies, and the concept of conditional strategies. *Human Development, 33,* 48–61.

Main, M. (1996). Introduction to the special section on attachment and psychopathology: 2. Overview of the field of attachment. *Journal of Consulting and Clinical Psychology, 64,* 237–243.

Main, M., & Cassidy, J. (1988). Categories of response to reunion with the parent at age 6: Predictable from infant attachment classifications and stable over a 1-month period. *Developmental Psychology, 24,* 415–426.

Main, M., Kaplan, N., & Cassidy, J. (1985). Security of infancy, childhood, and adulthood: A move to the level of representation. In I. Bretherton & E. Waters (Eds.), Growing points of attachment theory and research. *Monographs of the Society for Research in Child Development, 50*(1/2, Serial No. 209), 66–104.

Marvin, R. S., & Britner, P. A. (1999). Normative development: The ontogeny of attachment. In J. Cassidy & P. R. Shaver (Eds.), *Handbook of attachment: Theory, research, and clinical applications* (pp. 44–67). New York: Guilford Press.

Mayseless, O. (2005). Ontogeny of attachment in middle childhood: Conceptualization of normative changes. In K. A. Kerns & R. A. Richardson (Eds.), *Attachment in middle childhood* (pp. 1–23). New York: Guilford Press.

Moss, E., Bureau, J., Béliveau, M., Zdebik, M., & Lépine, S. (2009). Links between children's attachment behavior at early school-age, their attachment-related representations, and behavior problems in middle childhood. *International Journal of Behavioral Development, 33*(2), 155–166.

Moss, E., Cyr, C., & Dubois-Comtois, K. (2004). Attachment at early school age and developmental risk: Examining family contexts and behavior problems of controlling–caregiving, controlling–punitive, and behaviorally disorganized children. *Developmental Psychology, 40,* 519–532.

Moss, E., & St-Laurent, D. (2001). Attachment at school age and academic performance. *Developmental Psychology, 37,* 863–874.

Movahed-Abtahi, M., & Kerns, K. A. (2017). Attachment and emotion regulation in middle childhood: Changes in affect and vagal tone during a social stress task. *Attachment and Human Development, 19,* 221–242.

Patterson, G. R., & Bank, L. (1987). When is a nomological network a construct? In D. R. Peterson & D. B. Fisherman (Eds.), *Assessment for decision* (pp. 249–279). New Brunswick, NJ: Rutgers University Press.

Poehlmann, J. (2005). Representations of attachment relationships in children of incarcerated mothers. *Child Development, 76,* 679–696.

Psouni, E., & Apetroaia, A. (2014). Measuring scripted attachment-related knowledge in middle childhood: The Secure Base Script Test. *Attachment and Human Development, 16,* 22–41.

Raikes, H. A., & Thompson, R. A. (2005). Relationships past, present, and future: Reflections on attachment in middle childhood. In K. A. Kerns & R. A. Richardson (Eds.), *Attachment in middle childhood* (pp. 255–282). New York: Guilford Press.

Richardson, R. A. (2005). Developmental contextual considerations of parent–child attachment in the later middle childhood years. In K. A. Kerns & R. A. Richardson (Eds.), *Attachment in middle childhood* (pp. 24–45). New York: Guilford Press.

Rubin, K. H., Dwyer, K. M., Booth-LaForce, C., Kim, A. H., Burgess, K. B., & Rose-Krasnor, L. (2004). Attachment, friendship, and psychosocial functioning in early adolescence. *Journal of Early Adolescence, 24,* 326–356.

Scharf, M., Kerns, K. A., Rousseau, S., & Kivenson-Baron, I. (2016). Mother–child attachment and social anxiety: Associations with friendship skills and peer competence of Arab children. *School Psychology International, 37,* 271–288.

Scholtens, S., Rydell, A., Bohlin, G., & Thorell, L. B. (2014). ADHD symptoms and attachment representations: Considering the role of conduct problems, cognitive deficits and narrative responses in non-attachment-related story stems. *Journal of Abnormal Child Psychology, 42,* 1033–1042.

Scott, S., Briskman, J., Woolgar, M., Humayun, S., & O'Connor, T. G. (2011). Attachment in adolescence: Overlap with parenting and unique prediction of behavioural adjustment. *Journal of Child Psychiatry and Psychology, 52,* 1052–1062.

Seibert, A. C., & Kerns, K. A. (2009). Attachment figures in middle childhood. *International Journal of Behavioral Development, 33,* 347–355.

Shmueli-Goetz, Y., Target, M., Fonagy, P., & Datta, A. (2008). The Child Attachment Interview: A psychometric study of reliability and discriminant validity. *Developmental Psychology, 44,* 939–956.

Slough, N. M., & Greenberg, M. T. (1990). Five-year-olds' representations of separation from parents: Responses from the perspective of self and other. *New Directions for Child Development, 48,* 67–84.

Solomon, J., & George, C. (2008). The measurement of attachment security and related constructs in infancy and early childhood. In J. Cassidy & P. Shaver (Eds.), *Handbook of attachment* (2nd ed., pp. 383–416). New York: Guilford Press.

Solomon, J., George, C., & De Jong, A. (1995). Children classified as controlling at age six: Evidence of disorganized representational strategies and aggression at home and at school. *Development and Psychopathology,* 7(3), 447–463.

Sroufe, L. A., Bennett, C., Englund, M., Urban, J., & Shulman, S. (1993). The significance of gender boundaries in preadolescence: Contemporary correlates and antecedents of boundary violation and maintenance. *Child Development, 64,* 455–466.

Sroufe, L. A., & Fleeson, J. (1986). Attachment and the construction of relationships. In W. W. Hartup & Z. Rubin (Eds.), *Relationships and development* (pp. 57–71). Hillsdale, NJ: Erlbaum.

Steele, H., & Steele, M. (2005). The construct of coherence as an indicator of attachment security in middle childhood: The Friends and Family Interview. In K. A. Kerns & R. A. Richardson (Eds.), *Attachment in middle childhood* (pp. 137–160). New York: Guilford Press.

Steele, M., Hodges, J., Kaniuk, J., Hillman, S., & Henderson, K. (2003). Attachment representations and adoption: Associations between maternal states of mind and emotion narratives in previously maltreated children. *Journal of Child Psychotherapy, 29,* 187–205.

Stupica, B., Brett, B. E., Woodhouse, S. S., & Cassidy, J. (2019). Attachment security priming decreases children's physiological response to threat. *Child Development, 90,* 1254–1271.

Sullivan, H. S. (1953). *The interpersonal theory of psychiatry.* New York: Norton.

Target, M., Fonagy, P., & Shmueli-Goetz, Y. (2003). Attachment representations in school-age children: The development of the Child Attachment Interview (CAI). *Journal of Child Psychotherapy, 29,* 171–186.

van IJzendoorn, M. H., Vereijken, C. M. J. L., Bakermans-Kranenburg, M. J., & Riksen-Walraven, J. M. (2004). Assessing attachment security with the Attachment Q-Sort: Meta-analytic evidence for the validity of the observer AQS. *Child Development, 75,* 1188–1213.

Verschueren, K., & Marcoen, A. (1999). Representation of self and socioemotional competence in kindergartners: Differential and combined effects of attachment to mother and father. *Child Development, 70,* 183–201.

Verschueren, K., & Marcoen, A. (2002). Perceptions of self and relationship with parents in aggressive and nonaggressive rejected children. *Journal of School Psychology, 40,* 501–522.

Verschueren, K., & Marcoen, A. (2005). Perceived security of attachment to mother and father: Developmental differences and relations to self-worth and peer relationships at school. In K. A. Kerns & R. A. Richardson (Eds.), *Attachment in middle childhood* (pp. 212–230). New York: Guilford Press.

Waters, E. (1981). Traits, behavioral systems, and relationships: Three models of infant–adult attachment. In K. Immelman, G. Barlow, L. Petrinovitch, & M. Main (Eds.), *Behavioral development* (pp. 621–650). Cambridge, MA: Cambridge University Press.

Waters, E., & Cummings, E. M. (2000). A secure base from which to explore secure relationships. *Child Development, 71,* 164–172.

Waters, E., Kondo-Ikemura, K., Posada, G., & Richters, J. E. (1991). Learning to love: Mechanisms and milestones. In M. Gunnar (Ed.), *Minnesota Symposium on Child Psychology* (Vol. 24, pp. 217–255). Hillsdale, NJ: Erlbaum.

Waters, H. S., Rodrigues, L. M., & Ridgeway, D. (1998). Cognitive underpinnings of narrative attachment assessment. *Journal of Experimental Child Psychology, 71,* 211–234.

Wright, J. C., Binney, V., & Smith, P. K. (1995). Security of attachment in 8–12-year-olds: A revised version of the Separation Anxiety Test, its psychometric properties and clinical interpretation. *Journal of Child Psychology and Psychiatry, 36,* 757–774.

Yunger, J. L., Corby, B. C., & Perry, D. G. (2005). Dimensions of attachment in middle childhood. In K. A. Kerns & R. A. Richardson (Eds.), *Attachment in middle childhood* (pp. 89–114). New York: Guilford Press.

CHAPTER 7

Assessing Attachment in Adolescence

Joseph P. Allen

Adolescence is an inherently transitional period in psychosocial development, and this simple fact has profound implications for the assessment of the attachment behavioral system during this period. Any consideration of how best to assess attachment in adolescence must first begin by addressing the fundamental question raised by the myriad psychosocial transitions of this period: What becomes of the attachment system, which was once so prominent a part of the infant–caregiver relationship, as the infant grows through childhood and into adolescence and gains increasing emotional independence from his or her caregiver?

Even a passing consideration of this question and its implications makes clear that attachment in adolescence is not just be a slightly more grown-up version of what was observed during infancy, nor even of what is observed during middle childhood. In important ways, the attachment behavioral system has likely evolved into a much different entity by adolescence one that bears resemblances to and echoes of the attachment system seen in infancy and childhood, but one that is also changing in two fundamental ways, with substantial implications for the assessment of attachment during this period. First, as the adolescent seeks to gain emotional independence from parents and begins the work of forming peer bonds that will ultimately become primary, the adolescent's key attachment relationships with parents are changing dramatically in terms of their attachment functions (Rosenthal & Kobak, 2010). Second, the adolescent is simultaneously developing the capacity and increasing desire to independently and internally manage many attachment needs that formerly required interaction with an attachment figure. Both of these changes have important implications for the assessment of attachment in adolescence, and we consider each change and its implications in turn below before going on to review specific measurement approaches that have been developed to assess attachment during this period.

DEVELOPMENTAL CONSIDERATIONS IN ASSESSING ADOLESCENT ATTACHMENT

Changes in Adolescent Attachment Relationships

One of the most dramatic changes in the attachment system during adolescence is the beginning of the gradual transfer of the primary display of attachment behaviors and affect from caregivers to peers. Even quite early in adolescence, at least some teens begin identifying specific close peers to whom they turn for comfort when distressed and around whom they feel freer exploring new behaviors and environments (e.g., "I'll try out for the soccer team if Mark's trying out too"). Steadily and incrementally during this period, an adolescent's closest peer or peers are likely to begin taking on some of the functions of attachment figures (Rosenthal & Kobak, 2010). Adolescents may start to find peers at least for a time to be irreplaceable in their social world and expect a given peer to "be there" to meet future needs, even if this expectation is not entirely realistic. Adolescents may reflexively seek proximity to a given peer, and in the rare event of an unexpected death of a peer, teens may go through a period of painful mourning. These intense adolescent peer bonds, the frequent subject of popular literature and films from *The Outsiders* to *Stand by Me* (Hinton, 1967; King, 1986), no doubt capture popular interest in part precisely because they represent such a fascinating and emotion-laden shift in orientation of the attachment system from parents to peers during adolescence.

At least some close peer relationships in adolescence may, at least for a time, meet, or nearly meet, almost all of the formal criteria that have been described as characterizing an attachment relationship (see, e.g., Ainsworth, 1989; Cassidy, 1999), yet the question of whether a peer relationship in adolescence is a "real" attachment relationship misses the fundamental point. Whatever we choose to call them, many close adolescent peer relationships are, at minimum, *developing* attachment relationships, even if they have not yet reached fully mature status. Although it is true that close peer relationships in adolescence do still clearly lack the intensity and primacy of the infant–caregiver bond, it is also true that by adolescence, the adolescent–*caregiver* attachment relationship also lacks the intensity and primacy not only of the infant–caregiver bond, but even of the bonds observed in middle childhood. Rather than focusing on the precise conditions under which a given relationship in adolescence becomes an "attachment relationship," it may make more sense to recognize that some particularly intense adolescent relationships with peers are likely to increasingly take on critical attachment functions, even if such functions are manifest in less intense and durable form than is seen in earlier relationships with parents or than will be seen later in some adult pair-bonds (Allen, 2008).

One of the key features of adolescent–peer relationships that distinguish them from earlier relationships with caregivers is their increasing symmetry. Adolescents are not only beginning to get attachment needs met by close peers, but they are also beginning to *meet* the attachment needs of their peers. The caregiving system, as it begins to develop in adolescence, is clearly not isomorphic with the attachment system—a critical point to which we will return—but as it comes online, it does serve to add intensity and power to developing attachment relationships—and an element of reciprocity that will be critical in adult attachment relationships going forward. For unless an adolescent displays some capacity to provide caregiving to peers, those peers are unlikely to rely on that adolescent to meet their attachment needs or to stick around for very long to meet that adolescent's attachment needs in turn. Assessing the developing attachment functions in the increasingly complex adolescent–peer relationship provides one of the major challenges for the field going forward.

Developing Capacities for Autonomous Functioning

The gradual transfer of attachment interests from parents to peers is facilitated in part by a second major developmental change: the adolescent's increasing capacity to function with substantial emotional autonomy with respect to parents for sustained periods of time. Indeed, adolescence is unique in that it is the period of the lifespan in which the individual is most likely to actively seek *not* to depend on his or her attachment figure in times of stress (Steinberg, 1990). This stance is not completely without developmental precedent; exploration has always been the complement to the securely functioning attachment system, and toddlers also display well-documented pushes for autonomy. What is striking in adolescence, however, and what is relatively unprecedented to this point in the lifespan, is the extent to which the adolescent will at times feel enough distress and anxiety to strongly activate his or her attachment system, then *consciously choose* to avoid seeking help from a primary attachment figure in handling this distress.

The adolescent struggle for autonomy thus becomes an omnipresent background against which attachment processes play out, and this will have important implications for assessment of attachment processes during this period, as we consider below. The adolescent's rapidly developing competence is decreasing his or her need for dependence on parental attachment figures, and the strong need to explore and master new environments is promoting healthy growth in the exploratory system. Given these changes, the adolescent seeks to develop a new balance between attachment behaviors and the adolescent's exploratory needs (Allen, Porter, McFarland, McElhaney, & Marsh, 2007). Because the attachment system is homeostatic, balancing safety and exploration, it makes sense that as increasing maturity increases safety and self-sufficiency, the balance of exploration and overt attachment behaviors would shift in favor of exploration.

When the parent–adolescent relationship is functioning well, it becomes increasingly goal-corrected (Kobak & Duemmler, 1994) in a way that facilitates this shift. As the adolescent gains communication and perspective-taking skills, it becomes possible for both parent and teen to modify (or correct) their attachment-related behavior as needed to best meet the teen's evolving attachment needs, while balancing other needs as well. However, whereas the goal-corrected partnership in infancy and childhood might be described as reflecting a *coordinated* effort between parent and child, in adolescence, it seems more appropriate to consider this as a *negotiated* effort (Allen, 2008), and this negotiation will also become an important part of efforts to assess attachment in adolescence. Yet, for all these changes, the parental relationship still remains primary in attachment terms: Adolescents will still typically turn first and foremost to parents under conditions of extreme stress (Kobak, Rosenthal, Zajac, & Madsen, 2007). Thus, even as the attachment system of the adolescent is in the midst of fundamental changes in orientation and level of activation, the parent still remains a primary attachment figure for the vast majority of teens.

One of the factors that facilitates both increased reliance on (sometimes unreliable) peers for meeting attachment needs, as well as efforts to decrease reliance on parents for meeting those same needs, is the remarkable growth in the adolescent's capacity for self-regulation and self-soothing. This growing capacity changes the operation of the attachment behavioral system in fundamental ways. These changes are ultimately qualitative and not just quantitative; they stem from the changing nature of situations likely to activate the attachment behavioral system beginning in adolescence, and they fundamentally impact a number of approaches to assessing attachment during this period. Unlike at earlier points in development, for example, adolescents only rarely experience fundamental physical safety threats that send them seeking their attachment figures. Furthermore, the extreme distress and emotional disorganization that infants routinely experience is rare for most teens.

These changes likely have important implications for the ways in which the attachment behavioral system is activated and can be observed. We now know, for example, that there is a broad array of neural, physiological, and psychological systems underlying attachment behavior (Coan, 2010). The functions of these systems range from the primitive activation of the "fight-or-flight" response to more complex regulation of centers related to felt emotional security (Coan, Schaefer, & Davidson, 2006; Cummings & Davies, 1996; Hofer, 2006; Taylor et al., 2000). As the adolescent gets more adept at judging (and avoiding) fundamental physical and emotional threats and stressors, the degree to which these various systems are activated in attachment-relevant environments is likely to shift. Primitive "fight-or-flight" responses are likely to come online less often, whereas higher-order processes may increasingly operate in regulating attachment behavior.

Indeed, even the role of the attachment system in the survival of the organism changes during this period. Unlike infancy, during which severe attachment disorders are associated with an immediate threat to survival (and likely posed an even greater threat in evolutionary time), in adulthood, recent national surveys indicate that 1 adult in 4 reports having *no one* with whom to discuss important issues in their lives (McPherson, Smith-Lovin, & Brashears, 2006). The evolving attachment system will clearly maintain an important role as the adolescent matures, but not one that is necessarily critical to survival except in extremely rare instances. Conversely, while the immediate safety/survival functions of the attachment system in adolescence are decreasing in importance, the importance of the attachment system for basic emotional and even physical regulation clearly does not disappear. Witness, for example, the remarkable finding that in adulthood, social isolation and a corresponding lack of available attachment figures has been identified as creating a great a long-term risk for mortality as cigarette smoking (Holt-Lunstad, Smith, & Layton, 2010). The point of this discussion is simply that the attachment system is evolving on social, cognitive, and even neural levels, from being fundamental to human survival to ultimately serving as an optional (though important) aspect of adult human functioning. Unvarnished attachment behavior may be less easily seen, even as the attachment system retains long-term importance in terms of adolescent and adult functioning.

As the adolescent increases in cognitive sophistication over the course of development, one result is a growing capacity to *internalize* key functions of the attachment behavioral system. This growing capacity creates a heretofore unheard of degree of independence from attachment figures. Adolescents can function for increasingly long stretches, for example, without *any* substantial contact with their attachment figures (e.g., for weeks at a time at summer camps). They can do so in part precisely because they have internalized important functions of past attachment relationships, which will be critical to assess in order to understand the role of attachment in adolescence. This internalization may happen via a developed capacity to imagine (and be soothed by imagining) what an attachment figure might say or do in a given stressful situation, or simply by having learned to self-soothe over time given the scaffolding provided by attachment figures. In at least this one important respect, the attachment system is becoming subsumed as just one component of a broader emotion regulation system (Allen & Manning, 2007). Turning to attachment figures for comfort and security becomes just *one* option for maintaining equilibrium and capacity for exploration in the face of stressful experiences, but many other options are coming online.

An additional important feature of the internalization of the attachment system in adolescence is the capacity to represent past attachment experiences in complex, integrative ways. While evidence suggests that even significantly younger children may operate on internalized "scripts" reflecting past attachment experiences and guiding future behaviors (Waters & Waters, 2006), by adolescence, the development of formal operational thinking capacity allows the individual to metacognitively evaluate and assess these scripts in terms of their accuracy and utility—at least under some conditions.

Implications of Developmental Changes in Adolescence

The two major developmental changes of adolescence most relevant to attachment—an increasing orientation toward peers and away from parents, and an increasing capacity and interest in establishing autonomy with respect to attachment figures and attachment needs—each have major implications for the assessment of attachment during this period. Increasingly, we can and must, for example, consider not only observations of ongoing dyadic relationships but also the internalized representations of those relationships. Peer relationships are also going to become increasingly important to assess, not simply as correlates of attachment status, but as attachment contexts themselves. And parental relationships are going to change in nature, with attachment behaviors being less frequent, less visible, and therefore less easily observed, even as they no doubt remain of great importance.

In addition, the functioning of the attachment system is now going to become increasingly closely linked to broader emotion regulation capacities. When the emotion regulation system is functioning optimally, and is relatively untaxed, the attachment system may seldom be activated, and therefore difficult to observe. Conversely, for individuals in which emotion regulation remains an ongoing struggle, the attachment system may be frequently activated, the adolescent difficult to soothe, and the risk for insecurity greater, just as it is with temperamentally difficult infants.

Together, the complexities created by these developmental changes pose a unique set of challenges to the assessment of attachment during adolescence. As we now turn to looking at how we currently assess attachment in adolescence, these complexities should offer a continuous cautionary note: No single measure of attachment processes in adolescence, no matter how successful or useful, is likely to capture all of these important complexities. As adolescents have grown in sophistication, so too have attachment dynamics, and increasingly we are going to need a very substantial array of measurement tools to begin to capture this complexity. Let's now turn to look at some of the available tools.

MEASUREMENT APPROACHES FOR ASSESSING ADOLESCENT ATTACHMENT

Interview-Based Assessments

In terms of the sheer volume and quality of findings generated for the field, by far, the most productive approach to assessing attachment phenomena in adolescence has been the downward extension of the Adult Attachment Interview (AAI; George, Kaplan, & Main, 1996; Main, Goldwyn, & Hesse, 2002).

The AAI is a semistructured interview that examines individuals' descriptions of their childhood relationships with parents. The adolescent version is a slight modification of the adult version, with changes only to make the questions more natural and easily understood for an adolescent population (Ward & Carlson, 1995). It should be noted, however, that while adolescents may readily understand the questions in the AAI, adolescents are often quite reticent about engaging in in-depth, personal conversations about emotionally evocative material. Unless interviewers make significant efforts to establish adequate rapport with teens, the teens' willingness to engage in the work of the interview and the likelihood of obtaining a valid interview from which to code all are suspect. Thus, the "warm-up" part of the interview, though relatively unstructured (for both adolescents and adults) becomes particularly crucial when interviewing adolescents.

The AAI can be coded to yield classifications (autonomous, dismissing, preoccupied, unresolved/disoriented) that parallel infant classifications from the Strange Situation (secure, avoidant, ambivalent/resistant, and disorganized) (Main et al., 2002). This interview can also be coded using a Q-sort methodology that yields continuous scores for security versus insecurity, hyperactivation versus deactivation of attachment, preoccupation, and dismissal of attachment experiences (Kobak, Cole, Ferenz-Gillies, Fleming, & Gamble, 1993). These continuous scores have been found to bear a high degree of concordance with the classification-based coding system (Allen & Hauser, 1996).

Security/autonomy in the AAI is manifested in coherent and believable accounts of past relationship experiences, *regardless of whether those experiences were positive or negative*. Secure individuals are able to provide a balanced perspective on their relationships, while also expressing a high degree of valuing of attachment relationships, as well as insight into the ways in which these relationships have affected them (Main et al., 2002). Other facets of the interview matter are also considered closely, including whether the individual values versus devalues attachment relationships, though these other facets are often secondary to overall coherence in both coding systems. For example, an idealizing individual can appear to value attachment relationships, yet still be coded as nonautonomous (the AAI analogue of insecurity).

The AAI has yielded a wealth of findings linking security/autonomy in the interview to social functioning. Most striking have been findings linking classifications derived from the AAI to the Strange Situation behavior of one's offspring, with concordance rates as high as 70–80% (van IJzendoorn, 1995). These predictions have been obtained with both adolescent and adult mothers, and can be found even when maternal AAIs are obtained prior to the birth of the child in question. This degree of continuity across individuals, across time, and across vastly different assessment methods (observation of infant behavior with his or her mother vs. coding of a transcribed interview) is among the most remarkable such continuities obtained in the social sciences.

More importantly for the purposes of this chapter, the AAI has also displayed relations to a wide array of indices of psychosocial functioning in adolescence, including parent–teen interaction qualities (Allen et al., 2003, 2007, Kobak et al., 1993; Roisman, Madsen, Hennighausen, Sroufe, & Collins, 2001); ability to manage close friendships, romantic relationships, and broader peer interactions (Allen, Moore, Kuperminc, & Bell, 1998; Allen et al., 2007; Dykas, Woodhouse, Ehrlich, & Cassidy, 2012; Furman, Simon, Shaffer, & Bouchey, 2002; Larose & Bernier, 2001; Lieberman, Doyle, & Markiewicz, 1999; Sroufe, Egeland, Carlson, & Collins, 2005; Weimer, Kerns, & Oldenberg, 2004; Zimmermann, 2004); capacity to manage emotion regulation challenges without developing internalizing symptoms (Adam, Sheldon-Keller, & West, 1996; Bernier, Larose, & Whipple, 2005; Cole-Detke & Kobak, 1996; Kobak, Sudler, & Gamble, 1991; Larose & Bernier, 2001; Rosenstein & Horowitz, 1996; Zimmermann, Maier, Winter, & Grossmann, 2001); adjustment difficulties at school (Scott, Briskman, Woolgar, Humayun, & O'Connor, 2011); and avoidance of externalizing behavior patterns, particularly those reflecting a lack of social skills (Allen et al., 2002). (For an in-depth description of the role of the AAI in explaining key aspects of adolescent development and functioning, see Allen, 2008). The AAI also displays very high levels of test–retest stability over the course of adolescence (Allen, McElhaney, Kuperminc, & Jodl, 2004; Ammaniti, van IJzendoorn, Speranza, & Tambelli, 2000; Zimmermann & Becker-Stoll, 2002).

One area in which relations to the AAI have been more equivocal is assessments of continuity from infant attachment security to security/autonomy as assessed via the AAI in adolescence. This continuity appears modestly robust when environments are generally stable and benign but can disappear entirely in more fluid environments (although assessment of intervening environmental factors can account for some apparent discontinuities) (Hamilton, 2000; Waters, Hamilton, & Weinfield, 2000; Weinfield, Sroufe, & Egeland, 2000; Weinfield, Whaley, & Egeland, 2004). Within adolescence, security/autonomy assessed via the AAI displays only very modest correlations with maternal security assessed contemporaneously with this same measure (Allen et al., 2004), although modest concordances have been observed between adolescent and parental states of mind scales on the AAI (Scharf, Mayseless, & Kivenson-Baron, 2012). This is quite different from the consistently high parent–offspring concordances observed in infancy, however.

In several important respects, the AAI can be distinguished from most all other existing approaches to assessing the attachment system. First, and most importantly, the AAI does not assess attachment relationships, past or present. This is crucial, not as a criticism of the AAI, but because it suggests that regardless of the value of the AAI, there remains a giant gap in our knowledge about attachment in adolescence if we rely solely on this measure. Rather, the AAI assesses an internalized state of mind, and it does so in a way that relies on the adolescent's newly developing perspective-taking ability that allows him or her to reflect on and consider attachment experiences with increasing objectivity.

Second, the AAI does not primarily assess the content of an individual's working model of attachment relationships. While the processes of speaking coherently about attachment experiences may indeed result from qualities of the individual's internal working models, assessment of coherence in speaking about such models is far different from direct judgments about the content of those models, or about the expectations built into them. This focus of the AAI on the process by which attachment is described, but not on the specific content of internal working models of attachment relationships, while clearly of great value, nonetheless also leaves a gap in our knowledge, which researchers are just beginning to fill.

Third, the AAI is distinguished by its capacity to identify unresolved states of mind regarding attachment (analogous to infant insecure–disorganized states). Such states in adolescence have been reliably linked to past experiences of trauma and childhood sexual abuse, as would be predicted by theory, as well as to dissociative thought problems in adolescence (Bailey, Moran, & Pederson, 2007; Madigan, Vaillancourt, McKibbon, & Benoit, 2012).

It is also noteworthy that the AAI and its coding system were developed not by establishing its relation to other markers of adult attachment, but rather as a *predictor* of the attachment of an adult's infant offspring. At first reading, this might seem to be a distinction without an important difference. The critical point, though, is that a parent interview that predicts infant security is most logically and properly construed as more a measure of the parent's *caregiving* system than of the parent's attachment system. The AAI "works" as a predictor of infant attachment security, because it predicts with remarkable accuracy something about the quality of the parenting behavior that will be provided to that infant.

Undoubtedly, the caregiving system and the attachment system are related, but the two are not identical. Past attachment experiences (and current attachment relationships and thinking about attachment) are likely to influence the caregiving system, but so are other factors. The single parent who is not in an attachment relationship and not seeking one, perhaps due to a belief that such relationships are unlikely to work out well in adulthood, can nevertheless still provide a secure base to his or her infant. Expectations about one's own attachment needs either in the past as a child or currently as an adult bear only an indirect relationship to one's capacity to meet an infant's needs.

Indeed, close examination even suggests the AAI may actually be capturing a broader quality of the capacity to regulate strong affect (aroused in describing attachment experiences). From this perspective, the AAI may be less directly a measure of attachment processes, yet also more broadly applicable to an array of aspects of human psychosocial functioning. Indeed, a close examination of what is coded in the AAI indicates that it is the capacity to flexibly and coherently discuss emotionally charged experiences that is seen as most indicative of a state of autonomy with respect to attachment.

To be even more precise and to take full advantage of Mary Main's care in labeling classifications from the AAI, "autonomy" with respect to attachment, as Main labels the analogue to infant security, is explicitly not the same as security *within* attachment relationships. Indeed, the development of a degree of autonomy with respect to attachment is precisely what many adolescents seek. This developing autonomy may also be what leaves adolescents able to function without their attachment figure for long periods of time, and what leaves some particularly impressive single parents able to raise secure infants even though they may lack attachment figures in their own lives.

Conversely, it should also be noted that coherence in the AAI is not assessed in abstract, decontextualized terms, but rather is assessed primarily in terms of discourse regarding attachment figures and close relationships. Whether this means, however, that coherence in the AAI solely reflects an attachment process versus a broader emotion regulation capacity that is well-captured when discussing attachment relationships remains an open question. Indeed, the breadth of the correlates of the AAI, together with its somewhat ambiguous relationship to infant attachment assessments, only adds force to this question.

None of this is in any way to denigrate the AAI and the remarkable advances it represents, but simply to suggest that in assessing attachment in adolescence, the AAI at most gets at one aspect of attachment processes. We still have more work to do and as primary and productive a role as the AAI has taken to date, researchers would be foolish simply to rely on it going forward as capturing all relevant attachment phenomena during adolescence. Hence, while the AAI remains the "gold standard" for assessing attachment processes in adolescence, other measures increasingly merit consideration in addressing aspects of attachment not as well-assessed with the AAI.

Although far less widely used, a second, interview-based approach has been developed and applied in research with individuals in late childhood and early adolescence (up through age 12). The Child Attachment Interview (Shmueli-Goetz, Target, Fonagy, & Datta, 2008) is explicitly informed by the AAI but utilizes a more structured question format designed to be more accessible to individuals in late childhood and early adolescence. The measure has demonstrated strong psychometric properties and been found to yield classifications for children and early adolescents with significant relations to maternal AAI classifications (Shmueli-Goetz, et al., 2008). It may be most apt for younger adolescents or those for whom the AAI is for some reason not readily applicable.

Secure Base Scripts and Projective Assessments

Beyond the AAI, several other approaches exist to get at the internalized thought processes related to attachment that are held by adolescents. One promising approach is based on the key tenet of attachment theory that as a result of attachment experiences, all individuals form and then utilize a series of scripts reflecting their experiences with secure base behaviors, and that these scripts then guide future actions in attachment-relevant contexts (Waters & Waters, 2006).

To assess these scripts, Harriet Waters developed a projective approach using a prompt-word outline method (Waters, 1981; Waters & Hou, 1987). This approach involves providing a participant with a story title and 12–14 prompt words that loosely suggest a prototypical story line. Participants are then asked to formulate a story that uses each of these words. This story is then coded in terms of the presence and completeness of an underlying script or schema reflecting a secure base that emerges from this prompt. Given that one of the central tenets of lifespan attachment theory is that individuals form internal working models of themselves in attachment relationships, which then influence future behavior in such relationships, this approach has the advantage of assessing the expectations implicit in such models, in a way that nonetheless minimizes demand characteristics of the measure.

In research using this approach thus far, qualities of narratives around secure base scripts for mothers (though not for fathers) have been found to predict qualities of scripts regarding other adolescent relationships, suggesting these scripts are indeed tapping into generalized models of secure base interactions (Dykas, Woodhouse, Cassidy, & Waters, 2006; Steiner, Rafferty, & Waters, 2008). Further, these qualities of maternal scripts have also been found linked to AAI coherence of mind scores, to avoidance and anxiety scores from the Experiences in Close Relationship Inventory, and to prior observations of mother–child attachment in the first 3 years of life (Dykas et al., 2006; Steele et al., 2014). Similarly, this measure, when employed with adults, has also been found to have concordances with the Strange Situation behavior of an adult's infant offspring of similar magnitude to that found via the AAI (Tini, Corcoran, Rodrigues-Doolabh, & Waters, 2003).

This measure has the potential advantage that it may well be more engaging for adolescents than the AAI, which requires extended, focused thought about attachment behaviors with one's parents—a topic that many adolescents find developmentally challenging given the normative push to establish autonomy with respect to parents as attachment figures during this period. Furthermore, given that the coding for this measure relies far less on subtle linguistic cues and extended transcripts than does the AAI, it also appears far easier to apply to reticent and nonverbose adolescents.

Along somewhat similar lines, the Adult Attachment Projective Picture System (AAP; George, West, & Pettem, 1997; George & West, 2012) presents individuals with pictures depicting attachment-related stimuli and asks them to create narratives describing these pictures. The measure yields the same three primary classifications plus the Unresolved classification, as does the AAI. It has recently been used with adolescents and has been found to be linked to prior security as assessed in the Strange Situation in infancy and early childhood (Aikins, Howes, & Hamilton, 2009). Research with adults has also established the AAP test–retest reliability, interrater reliability, and concordance with the AAI for the four major attachment groups (George & West, 2012).

Relationship-Based Approaches

Moving away from approaches assessing implicit aspects of models of attachment relationships, the Relationship Questionnaire developed by Bartholomew and Horowitz (1991) directly assesses an individual's internalized representations of relationships via self-reports about consciously recollected experiences in close relationships. In contrast to both the AAI and the prompt-word approach, this approach explicitly focuses on assessing conscious aspects of internal working models, including attitudes, feelings, and behaviors with regard to specific relationships. Most studies to date, primarily focusing on adults, have yielded only low to null relations between this measure and the AAI (Bernier, Larose, & Boivin, 2007; Crowell, Fraley, & Shaver, 1999; De Haas, Bakermans-Kranenburg, & van IJzendoorn, 1994; Mayseless & Sagi, 1994; Mayseless & Scharf, 2007; Shaver, Belsky, & Brennan, 2000). However, the research that has examined both attachment states of mind (as assessed by the AAI) and attachment styles (as assessed by the Relationship Questionnaire) have indicated that both measures contribute significant, if independent, variance to explaining important outcomes (Mayseless & Scharf, 2007). Furthermore, although this measure taps overt, conscious thinking about attachment, it has been extensively related to subliminal, nonconscious beliefs and associations with regard to attachments in late adolescent (e.g., college-student) populations (Shaver & Mikulincer, 2002a, 2002b).

The Experiences in Close Relationships Scale (Brennan, Clark, & Shaver, 1998) takes a similar approach to that of the Relationship Questionnaire in assessing consciously reported approaches to attachment relationships. This 36-item scale taps secure versus insecure dimensions of attachment styles, yielding subscales for both attachment-related avoidance and anxiety. Though originally developed for adults, this measure has now been used with adolescents and linked to both depressive symptoms (Lee & Hankin, 2009), and the degree of synchrony versus discrepancy in parent and teen, and peer and teen reports, regarding parent behavior (Ehrlich, Cassidy, Lejuez, & Daughters, 2013).

The Behavioral Systems Questionnaire (Furman & Wehner, 1999) takes a similar approach geared specifically toward adolescents and assessing relational styles with parents from an attachment perspective. Resulting scales have been linked to high levels of maternal monitoring and support and lower levels of negative interactions, as well as to indirect effects on changes in substance use over time (Branstetter, Furman, & Cottrell, 2009).

Perhaps the measure with the longest history of targeting the assessment of the parent–teen attachment relationship is Armsden and Greenberg's (1987) Inventory of Parent and Peer Attachment (IPPA). This self-report measure asks teens to report on the teen–parent relationship in terms of the qualities of communication, trust, and alienation (reverse-scored) in the relationship. Although the IPPA has good psychometric properties and has been widely validated as a measure of parent–adolescent relationship quality, the individual items in this questionnaire are not particularly focused on attachment processes (e.g., secure base behaviors, caregiving under stress), nor does the instrument purport to in any way tap unconscious aspects of adolescents' internal working models of parents. Rather, the IPPA provides a general assessment of the current quality of the parent–adolescent relationship. Its empirical overlap with other more widely validated measures of attachment organization (e.g., the AAI) is very low (Crowell, Treboux, & Waters, 1993; Zimmermann, 2004). Although this measure appears to provide a useful general assessment of an overall parent–adolescent relationship, it does not appear particularly sensitive to the attachment processes within this relationship.

Assessing the Changing Target of Attachment Behaviors

As noted earlier, one of the defining features of attachment in adolescence is the beginning of a long-term transition toward using peers (or a particular peer) as primary attachment figures. Tracking this transition during adolescence appears likely to be a central task in identifying and understanding attachment processes during this period. Clearly, peer relationships in adolescence will only rarely meet the full criteria outlined in defining the presence of an attachment relationship (e.g., proximity seeking under stress, freer exploration in the presence of the figure; irreplaceability of the figure; mourning the loss of the figure; and expectations of an enduring relationship) (Ainsworth, 1989; Cassidy, 1999). At the same time, as noted earlier, peers are gradually taking on these functions, and there is simply no reason to assume that attachment is a dichotomous, all-or-nothing phenomenon, particularly in adolescence and young adulthood.

Several measures of attachment hierarchies have been designed to identify those persons who adolescents and young adults utilize to fulfill three main functions of attachment relationships: proximity seeking, safe haven, and secure base functions (Ainsworth, 1989; Hazan, Hutt, Sturgeon, & Bricket, 1991). Hazan and colleagues initially developed the WHOTO Interview, which consists of three questions asked with respect to each of these three attachment functions. For proximity seeking, participants are asked, "Who is the person you don't like to be away from?" Similarly, respondents are asked, "Who is the person you most want to be with when you are feeling upset or down?" (safe haven) and "Who is the person you feel you can always count on?" (secure base). For each question, participants are asked either to choose one person from a set list (e.g., mother, father, best friend, girlfriend/boyfriend, self, other) or to rate any number of persons for each one. There have been several revisions of the original WHOTO measure, rewording and adding questions and response choices, including versions by Fraley and Davis (1997) and Trinke and Bartholomew (1997) (Attachment Network Questionnaire) and Rosenthal and Kobak (2007) (Important People Interview).

To date, these measures have primarily been used to assess developmental changes in attachment relationships over time more than to capture functional correlates of individual differences in such relationships.

Observational Approaches

Last, we turn to what is in some ways the least developed aspect of assessment of adolescent attachment relationships—direct observations of adolescents interacting with their attachment figures. That this area is among the least developed is ironic given that the true secure base of attachment research for years, the base from which the field itself sprung up, was a solid underpinning in observational research.

One of the more widely reported observational approaches for assessing aspects of the parent–adolescent attachment relationship builds both on Main's view of the importance of autonomy in the context of valuing of relationships (Main et al., 2002), and on the fundamental role of exploration from a secure base in attachment processes (Bowlby, 1988; Crowell & Waters, 2005; Waters, Crowell, Elliott, Corcoran, & Treboux, 2002). Allen, Hauser, Bell, and O'Connor (1994) have developed an observational approach that assesses the adolescent's ability to establish cognitive and emotional autonomy in discussing a disagreement with a parent, while also maintaining the relationship in the midst of that discussion. This task—in which the adolescent seeks to explore the world of intellectual independence from a parent while maintaining a relationship with the parent—has been described as an analogue to the infant's task of exploring the physical world from the secure base of the parental relationship (Allen et al., 2003).

Thus far, this measure, and in particular the scales within it that focus on relationship maintenance in the face of disagreement, have been linked to adolescents' attachment security as assessed via the AAI in several studies (Allen & Hauser, 1996; Allen et al., 2003, 2007). Perhaps more significantly, this adolescent-era measure has also been found to display continuity with Strange Situation attachment assessments in infancy even when the AAI did not capture such continuity in adolescence (Zimmermann et al., 2000; Zimmermann, Fremmer-Bombik, Spangler, & Grossmann, 1995). This suggests a potentially ongoing role for this and similar approaches to relationship assessment in efforts to understand attachment processes in adolescence.

Within peer observational studies, supportive behaviors and, in particular, a teen's willingness to make a bid for emotional support from a close friend, have been related to attachment security as assessed via the AAI (Allen et al., 2007). Although this research, which focused on friendships of 13- to 15-year-olds, stops well short of establishing that these peer relationships are attachment relationships, it does suggest that qualities of attachment processes, and at least the early signs of seeking out peers as a secure base, may indeed be appearing and displaying continuity with other aspects of a teen's internal working models of attachment relationships.

FUTURE DIRECTIONS

Although this review considers a number of quite promising measures of attachment processes, models, and relationships in adolescence, striking gaps in our measurement (and theory) toolbox also exist. While those interested in assessing attachment in adolescence have many promising tools at their disposal, as the summary in Table 7.1 indicates, perhaps the greatest single danger for the future development of the field would be for researchers to assume that because we now have some well-tried measures that are linked to attachment processes and have strong external correlates, there is little need for further measure and theory development. The former assumption may be increasingly true, but it in no way does it support the latter conclusion.

Some of the most important outstanding questions that challenge both measurement of adolescent attachment processes (and the theory supporting this measurement) surround the normative development of attachment in adolescence. For example, in spite of the progress acknowledged earlier, we are only beginning to develop ways to assess the process by which the parent–adolescent attachment relationship changes in terms of its attachment functions as development progresses. Questions abound in this regard. How and when does the process develop by which the individual learns to pull back from seeking parents out when attachment needs arise? How do we distinguish this normative move toward independence from forced precocity among adolescents who have poor relationships with their parents?

Similarly, as peers take on an increasing role in adolescents' lives—moving toward someday serving as primary attachment figures for adults—the development of attachment processes within these peer relationships is just beginning to be explored. Important questions for future development efforts to address include the following: At what ages and in what domains (e.g., relationships with other peers) are adolescents most likely to start turning to peers as *primary* sources of support and comfort when attachment needs arise? How is this process different for adolescents with more versus less secure models of attachment relationships? And in what ways do peer attachment relationships share qualities with parental relationships, and in what ways are they fundamentally different?

Important questions also remain about the assessment of individual differences in attachment relationships in adolescence. Most noteworthy is the fact, illustrated in Table 7.2, that the field does not yet have a solid grip on how to assess qualities of security and insecurity within specific dyadic attachment relationships during this period, particularly as these relate to qualities of broader working models of attachment. As efforts are made to develop such tools, generalizations from infancy are likely to carry us only so far, particularly given the far greater complexity of attachment relationships in adolescence. At a minimum, attachment relationships in adolescence involve far more, and more strongly competing, behavioral systems than are present in infancy. In relationships with parents, for example, power and control

TABLE 7.1. Overview of Adolescent-Era Measures of Attachment Processes

Measure	Measurement approach	Specificity to adolescence	Overall target of assessment	Related to which other assessments?
Adult Attachment Interview (AAI; George et al., 1996; Main et al., 2002)	Coded interview (questions about episodic and semantic memories of attachment experiences)	Slight adaptation of adult version	Internal working models (coherence, autonomy, and valuing of attachment in descriptions of)	Strange Situation (SS) behavior of future offspring; SS in infancy (inconsistent relations); secure base scripts; psychosocial functioning; Relationship Questionnaire (low)
Secure base scripts (Waters & Waters, 2006)	Projective (provides story title and word prompts)	Versions specific to adolescence	Internal working models (expectations of secure base)	AAI; SS; Relationship Questionnaire
Relationship Questionnaire (Bartholomew & Horowitz, 1991)	Self-report (explicit conscious evaluation of recollected experiences in close relationships)	Usable for both adults and adolescents	Generalized relationship behavior (security, anxiety, avoidance)	Low to AAI; unconscious measures; nonconscious beliefs and associations regarding attachment; functional outcomes
Inventory of Parent and Peer Attachment (Armsden & Greenberg, 1987)	Self-report (explicit, conscious evaluation of ongoing quality of current relationship with parents and peers)	Designed for adolescents	Specific relationships (trust, communication, and alienation)	Very low to AAI; functioning

WHOTO (Hazan et al., 1991) and subsequent revisions	Self-report (explicit, conscious evaluation of attachment functions of various relationships)	Designed for adolescents	Specific relationships (hierarchy of relationships for three main attachment functions)	Theoretically predicted changes with age
Autonomy and Relatedness Coding System (Allen et al., 1994)	Observational (coded behaviors during observed disagreements)	Designed for adolescents	Specific relationships (autonomy and relatedness in disagreements)	Linked to AAI and functioning; predicted by SS
Adult Attachment Projective (George et al., 1997; George & West, 2012)	Projective (provides line drawings used as story prompts)	Usable for adults and adolescents	Internal working models (expectations of secure base)	Predicted by SS
Child Attachment Interview (Shmueli-Goetz et al., 2008)	Coded interview (questions about episodic and semantic memories of attachment experiences)	Late childhood and early adolescence	Internal working models (similar to AAI)	Concurrent maternal AAIs
Experience in Close Relationships Scale (Brennan et al., 1998)	Self-report (explicit conscious evaluation of attachment style in close relationships)	Usable for both adults and adolescents	Generalized relationship behavior (security, anxiety, avoidance)	Low to AAI; synchrony in reporting between teens and parents or peers; depressive symptoms
Behavioral Systems Questionnaire (Furman & Wehner, 1999)	Self-report (explicit conscious evaluation of attachment style with parents)	Designed for adolescents	Generalized relationship behavior (security, anxiety, avoidance)	Reported parent–child interactive behavior; functional outcomes

TABLE 7.2. Interrelations among Measures of Attachment Processes in Adolescence and Related Measures

Measure	AAI	Secure base scripts	Relationship Questionnaire	Infant Strange Situation	Offspring Strange Situation	IPPA	A & R Coding System	Psychosocial functioning
Adult Attachment Interview (George et al., 1996; Main et al., 2002)	—	**	+	+	**	+	**	**
Secure base scripts (Waters & Waters, 2006)	**	—	**	**	**	??	??	**
Relationship Questionnaire (Bartholomew & Horowitz, 1991)	+	**	—	??	??	??	??	**
Inventory of Parent and Peer Attachment (Armsden & Greenberg, 1987)	+	??	??	??	??	—	??	**
Autonomy and Relatedness Coding System (Allen et al., 1994)	**	??	??	**	??	**	—	**
Adult Attachment Projective (George et al., 1997; George & West, 2012)	**[a]	??	??	**	??	??	??	**
Child Attachment Interview (Shmueli-Goetz et al., 2008)	**[a]	??	??	??	??	??	??	**
Experience in Close Relationships Scale (Brennan et al., 1998)	+	??	**	??	??	??	??	**
Behavioral Systems Questionnaire (Furman & Wehner, 1999)	??	??	**	??	??	??	??	**

Note. ** = clear, substantial relationship; + = weak/inconsistent relationship; ?? = no relationship found to date.

[a]Links to AAI classifications were found for adults; not examined yet for adolescents.

negotiations are ongoing and often primary, and are likely to fundamentally alter the nature of attachment relationships. Most teens know, for example, that crying on a parent's shoulder tends to undermine their ability to establish autonomy vis a vis that parent.

With regard to peer relationships, attachment researchers studying adolescents are viewing a world, unlike infancy and childhood, in which two parties are both vying to get their attachment (and other) needs met within the same relationship. Adolescents are seeking to become both care receivers and caregivers in such relationships, and are doing so with other adolescents, each having his or her own independent attachment histories, expectations, and states of mind regarding attachment. Clearly the range of permutations of types of attachment relationships that can exist under these conditions is likely to be far greater than those found in infancy.

Capturing this complexity is likely to require not only the development of new assessment tools but also recognition that a three- or four-category system may in important ways be insufficient for classifying such relationships. In spite of the promise suggested in the review of measurement approaches in this chapter, the field is nevertheless still ripe for future advances in measurement.

Observational measures to date, for example, have largely been based on laboratory paradigms that only loosely mirror the adolescent's social world. Although adolescence creates difficulties in assessing attachment processes, it also opens up new windows into these processes. Social networking sites, for example, Facebook, routinely capture real-time, unfiltered, and highly salient interactions of adolescents with their peers. Promising work is now under way to capture meaningful aspects of the interactions on these sites, which, with proper consent, offer an unparalleled view into the social and emotional lives of teens (Mikami, Szwedo, Allen, Evans, & Hare, 2010; Szwedo, Mikami, & Allen, 2011).

Similarly, assessments of the changing nature and hierarchy of attachment processes in adolescence (e.g., the WHOTO), while simple, effective, and easy to administer and score, nevertheless provide only the most cursory understanding of how adolescent attachment hierarchies are changing. Future work could enhance our understanding of these changes via both in-depth interview and questionnaire measures.

Finally, as we seek to dramatically enhance our understanding of attachment *relationships* in adolescence, great promise lies in the direction of obtaining reports from *both* participants in those relationships. Many of the limitations of self-report assessments can be addressed by the use of other reports, whether the other be a parent, a close peer, or a romantic partner. Furthermore, most of the measurement approaches described in this chapter for assessing attachment relationships could be readily adapted to reports *about* a teen, not just *by* a teen.

In summary, while the field has clearly made great progress over the past decade, much work remains to be done. Our theoretical understanding of the normative social-developmental changes of adolescence suggest numerous ways in which attachment processes are likely to change (yet remain of critical importance) over the course of adolescence. In order to further develop our understanding of attachment processes in adolescence, we need to continue to work to develop multiple measurement approaches that can begin to capture the complexities involved as the attachment system is itself developing to keep pace with the adolescent's increasingly sophisticated social and emotional world.

REFERENCES

Adam, K. S., Sheldon-Keller, A. E., & West, M. (1996). Attachment organization and history of suicidal behavior in clinical adolescents. *Journal of Consulting and Clinical Psychology, 64,* 264–272.

Aikins, J. W., Howes, C., & Hamilton, C. (2009). Attachment stability and the emergence of unresolved representations during adolescence. *Attachment and Human Development, 11*(5), 491–512.

Ainsworth, M. D. S. (1989). Attachments beyond infancy. *American Psychologist, 44,* 709–716.

Allen, J. P. (2008). The attachment system in adolescence. In J. Cassidy & P. R. Shaver (Eds.), *Handbook of attachment: Theory, research and clinical applications* (2nd ed., pp. 419–435). New York: Guilford Press.

Allen, J. P., & Hauser, S. T. (1996). Autonomy and relatedness in adolescent–family interactions as predictors of young adults' states of mind regarding attachment. *Development and Psychopathology, 8*(4), 793–809.

Allen, J. P., Hauser, S. T., Bell, K. L., & O'Connor, T. G. (1994). Longitudinal assessment of autonomy and relatedness in adolescent–family interactions as predictors of adolescent ego development and self-esteem. *Child Development, 65*(1), 179–194.

Allen, J. P., & Manning, N. (2007). From safety to affect regulation: Attachment from the vantage point of adolescence. *New Directions in Child and Adolescent Development, 117,* 23–39.

Allen, J. P., Marsh, P., McFarland, C., McElhaney, K. B., Land, D. J., Jodl, K. M., & Peck, S. (2002). Attachment and autonomy as predictors of the development of social skills and delinquency during midadolescence. *Journal of Consulting and Clinical Psychology, 70*(1), 56–66.

Allen, J. P., McElhaney, K. B., Kuperminc, G. P., & Jodl, K. M. (2004). Stability and change in attachment security across adolescence. *Child Development, 75,* 1792–1805.

Allen, J. P., McElhaney, K. B., Land, D. J., Kuperminc, G. P., Moore, C. M., O'Beirne-Kelley, H., & Liebman, S. M. (2003). A secure base in adolescence: Markers of attachment security in the mother–adolescent relationship. *Child Development, 74,* 292–307.

Allen, J. P., Moore, C., Kuperminc, G., & Bell, K. (1998). Attachment and adolescent psychosocial functioning. *Child Development, 69*(5), 1406–1419.

Allen, J. P., Porter, M. R., McFarland, F. C., McElhaney, K. B., & Marsh, P. A. (2007). The relation of attachment security to adolescents' paternal and peer relationships, depression, and externalizing behavior. *Child Development, 78,* 1222–1239.

Ammaniti, M., van IJzendoorn, M. H., Speranza, A. M., & Tambelli, R. (2000). Internal working models of attachment during late childhood and early adolescence: An exploration of stability and change. *Attachment and Human Development, 2*(3), 328–346.

Armsden, G. C., & Greenberg, M. T. (1987). The Inventory of Parent and Peer Attachment: Individual differences and their relationship to psychological well-being in adolescence. *Journal of Youth and Adolescence, 16*(5), 427–454.

Bailey, H. N., Moran, G., & Pederson, D. R. (2007). Childhood maltreatment, complex trauma symptoms, and unresolved attachment in an at-risk sample of adolescent mothers. *Attachment and Human Development, 9*(2), 139–161.

Bartholomew, K., & Horowitz, L. M. (1991). Attachment styles among young adults: A test of a four-category model. *Journal of Personality and Social Psychology, 61,* 226–244.

Bernier, A., Larose, S., & Boivin, M. (2007). Individual differences in adult attachment: Disentangling two assessment traditions. *European Journal of Developmental Psychology, 4*(2), 220–238.

Bernier, A., Larose, S., & Whipple, N. (2005). Leaving home for college: A potentially stressful event for adolescents with preoccupied attachment patterns. *Attachment and Human Development, 7*(2), 171–185.

Bowlby, J. (1988). *A secure base: Parent–child attachment and healthy human development.* New York: Basic Books.

Branstetter, S. A., Furman, W., & Cottrell, L. (2009). The influence of representations of attachment, maternal–adolescent relationship quality, and maternal monitoring on adolescent substance use: A 2-year longitudinal examination. *Child Development, 80*(5), 1448–1462.

Brennan, K. A., Clark, C. L., & Shaver, P. R. (1998). Self-report measurement of adult attachment: An integrative overview. In J. A. Simpson & W. S. Rholes (Eds.), *Attachment theory and close relationships* (pp. 46–76). New York: Guilford Press.

Cassidy, J. (1999). The nature of the child's ties. In J. Cassidy & P. R. Shaver (Eds.), *Handbook of attachment: Theory, research, and clinical applications* (pp. 3–20). New York: Guilford Press.

Coan, J. A. (2010). Adult attachment and the brain. *Journal of Social and Personal Relationships, 27*(2), 210–217.

Coan, J. A., Schaefer, H. S., & Davidson, R. J. (2006). Lending a hand: Social regulation of the neural response to threat. *Psychological Science, 17,* 1032–1039.

Cole-Detke, H., & Kobak, R. (1996). Attachment processes in eating disorder and depression. *Journal of Consulting and Clinical Psychology, 64*(2), 282–290.

Crowell, J. A., Fraley, R. C., & Shaver, P. R. (1999). Measurement of individual differences in adolescent and adult attachment. In J. Cassidy & P. R. Shaver (Eds.), *Handbook of attachment: Theory, research, and clinical applications* (pp. 434–465). New York: Guilford Press.

Crowell, J. A., Treboux, D., & Waters, E. (1993, April). *Alternatives to the Adult Attachment Interview: Self-reports of attachment style and relationships with mothers and partners.* Paper presented at the biennial meetings of the Society for Research in Child Development, New Orleans, LA.

Crowell, J., & Waters, E. (2005). Attachment representations, secure-base behavior, and the evolution of adult relationships: The Stony Brook Adult Relationship Project. In K. E. Grossmann, K. Grossmann, & E. Waters (Eds.), *Attachment from infancy to adulthood: The major longitudinal studies* (pp. 223–244). New York: Guilford Press.

Cummings, E. M., & Davies, P. (1996). Emotional security as a regulatory process in normal development and the development of psychopathology. *Development and Psychopathology, 8*(1), 123–139.

De Haas, M. A., Bakermans-Kranenburg, M. J., & van IJzendoorn, M. H. (1994). The Adult Attachment Interview and questionnaires for attachment style, temperament, and memories of parental behavior. *Journal of Genetic Psychology, 155*(4), 471–486.

Dykas, M. J., Woodhouse, S. S., Cassidy, J., & Waters, H. S. (2006). Narrative assessment of attachment representations: Links between secure base scripts and adolescent attachment. *Attachment and Human Development, 8*(3), 221–240.

Dykas, M. J., Woodhouse, S. S., Ehrlich, K. B., & Cassidy, J. (2012). Attachment-related differences in perceptions of an initial peer interaction emerge over time: Evidence of reconstructive memory processes in adolescents. *Developmental Psychology, 48*(5), 1381–1389.

Ehrlich, K. B., Cassidy, J., Lejuez, C. W., & Daughters, S. B. (2014). Discrepancies about adolescent relationships as a function of informant attachment and depressive symptoms. *Journal of Research on Adolescence, 24,* 654–666.

Fraley, R. C., & Davis, K. E. (1997). Attachment formation and transfer in young adults' close friendships and romantic relationships. *Personal Relationships, 4,* 131–144.

Furman, W., Simon, V. A., Shaffer, L., & Bouchey, H. A. (2002). Adolescents' working models and styles for relationships with parents, friends, and romantic partners. *Child Development, 73*(1), 241–255.

Furman, W., & Wehner, E. A. (1999). *The Behavioral Systems Questionnaire—Revised.* Unpublished measure, University of Denver, Denver, CO.

George, C., Kaplan, N., & Main, M. (1996). *Adult Attachment Interview* (3rd ed.). Unpublished manuscript, Department of Psychology, University of California at Berkeley, Berkeley, CA.

George, C., & West, M. L. (2012). *The Adult Attachment Projective Picture System: Attachment theory and assessment in adults.* New York: Guilford Press.

George, C., West, M., & Pettem, O. (1997). *The Adult Attachment Projective.* Unpublished protocol and classification manual, Mills College, Oakland, CA.

Hamilton, C. E. (2000). Continuity and discontinuity of attachment from infancy through adolescence. *Child Development, 71,* 690–694.

Hazan, C., Hutt, M. J., Sturgeon, J., & Bricket, T. (1991, April). *The process of relinquishing parents as attachment figures.* Paper presented at the biennial meetings of the Society for Research in Child Development, Seattle, WA.

Hinton, S. E. (1967). *The outsiders.* New York: Viking Press.

Hofer, M. (2006). Psychobiological roots of early attachment. *Current Directions in Psychological Science, 15*(2), 84–88.

Holt-Lunstad, J., Smith, T. B., & Layton, J. B. (2010). Social relationships and mortality risk: A meta-analysis. *PLOS Medicine, 7*(7), 1–20.

King, S. (Writer) & Reiner, R. (Director). (1986). *Stand by me.* New York: Columbia Pictures.

Kobak, R. R., Cole, H., Ferenz-Gillies, R., Fleming, W., & Gamble, W. (1993).

Attachment and emotion regulation during mother–teen problem-solving: A control theory analysis. *Child Development, 64*, 231–245.

Kobak, R. R., & Duemmler, S. (1994). Attachment and conversation: Toward a discourse analysis of adolescent and adult security. In K. Bartholomew & D. Perlman (Eds.), *Attachment processes in adulthood: Advances in personal relationships* (Vol. 5, pp. 121–149). London: Jessica Kingsley.

Kobak, R., Rosenthal, N. L., Zajac, K., & Madsen, S. D. (2007). Adolescent attachment hierarchies and the search for an adult pair-bond. In M. Scharf & O. Mayseless (Eds.), *New directions for child and adolescent development. Attachment in adolescence: Reflections and new angles* (pp. 57–72). San Francisco: Jossey-Bass.

Kobak, R. R., Sudler, N., & Gamble, W. (1991). Attachment and depressive symptoms during adolescence: A developmental pathways analysis. *Development and Psychopathology, 3*(4), 461–474.

Larose, S., & Bernier, A. (2001). Social support processes: Mediators of attachment state of mind and adjustment in late adolescence. *Attachment and Human Development, 3*(1), 96–120.

Lee, A., & Hankin, B. L. (2009). Insecure attachment, dysfunctional attitudes, and low self-esteem predicting prospective symptoms of depression and anxiety during adolescence. *Journal of Clinical Child and Adolescent Psychology, 38*(2), 219–231.

Lieberman, M., Doyle, A.-B., & Markiewicz, D. (1999). Developmental patterns in security of attachment to mother and father in late childhood and early adolescence: Associations with peer relations. *Child Development, 70*(1), 202–213.

Madigan, S., Vaillancourt, K., McKibbon, A., & Benoit, D. (2012). The reporting of maltreatment experiences during the Adult Attachment Interview in a sample of pregnant adolescents. *Attachment and Human Development, 14*(2), 119–143.

Main, M., Goldwyn, R., & Hesse, E. (2002). *Adult Attachment Scoring and Classification Systems, Version 7.1.* Unpublished manuscript, University of California at Berkeley, Berkeley, CA.

Mayseless, O., & Sagi, A. (1994). *The association between the Adult Attachment Interview and attachment patterns in romantic relationships.* Paper presented at the 7th International Conference on Personal Relationships, Groningen, the Netherlands.

Mayseless, O., & Scharf, M. (2007). Adolescents' attachment representations and their capacity for intimacy in close relationships. *Journal of Research on Adolescence, 17*(1), 23–50.

McPherson, M., Smith-Lovin, L., & Brashears, M. E. (2006). Social isolation in America: Changes in core discussion networks over two decades. *American Sociological Review, 71*, 353–375.

Mikami, A. Y., Szwedo, D. E., Allen, J. P., Evans, M. A., & Hare, A. L. (2010). Adolescent peer relationships and behavior problems predict young adults' communication on social networking websites. *Developmental Psychology, 46*, 46–56.

Roisman, G. I., Madsen, S. D., Hennighausen, K. H., Sroufe, L. A., & Collins, W. A. (2001). The coherence of dyadic behavior across parent–child and romantic relationships as mediated by the internalized representation of experience. *Attachment and Human Development, 3*(2), 156–172.

Rosenstein, D. S., & Horowitz, H. A. (1996). Adolescent attachment and psychopathology. *Journal of Consulting and Clinical Psychology, 64*(2), 244–253.

Rosenthal, N., & Kobak, R. R. (2007). *Assessment of adolescent attachment hierarchies: Individual differences and developmental change.* Newark: University of Delaware Press.

Rosenthal, N. L., & Kobak, R. (2010). Assessing adolescents' attachment hierarchies: Differences across developmental periods and associations with individual adaptation. *Journal of Research on Adolescence, 20*(3), 678–706.

Scharf, M., Mayseless, O., & Kivenson-Baron, I. (2012). Intergenerational concordance in Adult Attachment Interviews with mothers, fathers and adolescent sons and subsequent adjustment of sons to military service. *Attachment and Human Development, 14*(4), 367–390.

Scott, S., Briskman, J., Woolgar, M., Humayun, S., & O'Connor, T. G. (2011). Attachment in adolescence: overlap with parenting and unique prediction of behavioural adjustment. *Journal of Child Psychology and Psychiatry, 52*(10), 1052–1062.

Shaver, P. R., Belsky, J., & Brennan, K. A. (2000). The Adult Attachment Interview and self-reports of romantic attachment: Associations across domains and methods. *Personal Relationships, 7*(1), 25–43.

Shaver, P. R., & Mikulincer, M. (2002a). Attachment-related psychodynamics. *Attachment and Human Development, 4*(2), 133–161.

Shaver, P. R., & Mikulincer, M. (2002b). Dialogue on adult attachment: Diversity and integration. *Attachment and Human Development, 4*(2), 243–257.

Shmueli-Goetz, Y., Target, M., Fonagy, P., & Datta, A. (2008). The Child Attachment Interview: A psychometric study of reliability and discriminant validity. *Developmental Psychology, 44*(4), 939–956.

Sroufe, L. A., Egeland, B., Carlson, E. A., & Collins, W. A. (2005). *The development of the person: The Minnesota Study of Risk and Adaptation from Birth to Adulthood.* New York: Guilford Press.

Steele, R. D., Waters, T. E. A., Bost, K. K., Vaughn, B. E., Truitt, W., Waters, H. S., . . . Roissman, G. I. (2014). Caregiving antecedents of secure base script knowledge: A comparative analysis of young adult attachment representations. *Developmental Psychology, 50,* 2526–2538.

Steinberg, L. D. (1990). Interdependence in the family: Autonomy, conflict and harmony in the parent–adolescent relationship. In S. S. Feldman & G. R. Elliott (Eds.), *At the threshold: The developing adolescent* (pp. 255–276). Cambridge, MA: Harvard University Press.

Steiner, M. A., Rafferty, M. M., & Waters, H. S. (2008). *Development of secure base script knowledge in adolescence.* Unpublished manuscript.

Szwedo, D. E., Mikami, A. Y., & Allen, J. P. (2011). Qualities of peer relations on Facebook and MySpace: Predictions from negative mother–teen interactions. *Journal of Research on Adolescence, 21*(3), 595–607.

Taylor, S. E., Klein, L. C., Lewis, B. P., Gruenewald, T. L., Gurung, R. A. R., & Updegraff, J. A. (2000). Biobehavioral responses to stress in females: Tend-and-befriend, not fight-or-flight. *Psychological Review, 107*(3), 411–429.

Tini, M., Corcoran, D., Rodrigues-Doolabh, L., & Waters, E. (2003, April). *Maternal attachment scripts and infant secure base behavior.* Paper presented at the poster symposium presented at the biennial meetings of the Society for Research in Child Development, Tampa, FL.

Trinke, S. J., & Bartholomew, K. (1997). Hierarchies of attachment relationships in young adulthood. *Journal of Social and Personal Relationships, 14*(5), 603–625.

van IJzendoorn, M. H. (1995). Adult attachment representations, parental responsiveness, and infant attachment: A meta-analysis on the predictive validity of the Adult Attachment Interview. *Psychological Bulletin, 117*(3), 387–403.

Ward, M. J., & Carlson, E. A. (1995). Associations among adult attachment representations, maternal sensitivity, and infant–mother attachment in a sample of adolescent mothers. *Child Development, 66,* 69–79.

Waters, E., Crowell, J., Elliott, M., Corcoran, D., & Treboux, D. (2002). Bowlby's secure base theory and the social/personality psychology of attachment styles: Work(s) in progress. *Attachment and Human Development, 4*(2), 230–242.

Waters, E., Hamilton, C. E., & Weinfield, N. S. (2000). The stability of attachment security from infancy to adolescence and early adulthood: General introduction. *Child Development, 71*(3), 678–683.

Waters, H. S. (1981). Organizational strategies in memory for prose: A developmental analysis. *Journal of Experimental Child Psychology, 32*(2), 223–246.

Waters, H. S., & Hou, F. T. (1987). Children's production and recall of narrative passages. *Journal of Experimental Child Psychology, 44*(3), 348–363.

Waters, H., & Waters, E. (2006). The attachment working models concept: Among other things, we build script-like representations of secure base experiences. *Attachment and Human Development, 8*(3), 185–197.

Weimer, B. L., Kerns, K. A., & Oldenberg, C. M. (2004). Adolescents' interactions with a best friend: Associations with attachment style. *Journal of Experimental Child Psychology, 88*(1), 102–120.

Weinfield, N. S., Sroufe, L. A., & Egeland, B. (2000). Attachment from infancy to early adulthood in a high-risk sample: Continuity, discontinuity, and their correlates. *Child Development, 71,* 695–702.

Weinfield, N. S., Whaley, G. J. L., & Egeland, B. (2004). Continuity, discontinuity, and coherence in attachment from infancy to late adolescence: Sequelae of organization and disorganization. *Attachment and Human Development, 6*(1), 73–97.

Zimmermann, P. (2004). Attachment representations and characteristics of friendship relations during adolescence. *Journal of Experimental Child Psychology, 88*(1), 83–101.

Zimmermann, P., & Becker-Stoll, F. (2002). Stability of attachment representations during adolescence: The influence of ego-identity status. *Journal of Adolescence, 25*(1), 107–124.

Zimmermann, P., Becker-Stoll, F., Grossmann, K., Grossmann, K. E., Scheuerer-Englisch, H., & Wartner, U. (2000). Longitudinal attachment development from infancy through adolescence. *Psychologie in Erziehung und Unterricht, 47,* 99–117.

Zimmermann, P., Fremmer-Bombik, E., Spangler, G., & Grossmann, K. E. (1995, March–April). *Attachment in adolescence: A longitudinal perspective.* Paper presented at the meeting of the Society for Research in Child Development, Indianapolis, IN.

Zimmermann, P., Maier, M. A., Winter, M., & Grossmann, K. E. (2001). Attachment and adolescents' emotion regulation during a joint problem-solving task with a friend. *International Journal of Behavioral Development, 25*(4), 331–343.

CHAPTER 8

Measuring Attachment Representations as Secure Base Script Knowledge

The Prompt-Word Outline Method in Adulthood, Adolescence, and Middle Childhood

Harriet Salatas Waters and Theodore E. A. Waters

John Bowlby recast Freud's image of a clingy, dependent infant, focused on drive reduction, and replaced it with a view of infants as much more competent, inherently motivated to exploration and mastery, and skilled at using one or a few primary attachment figures as a secure base from which to explore (Bowlby, 1969/1982). He also borrowed from cognitive psychology the notion that experience can be represented as a "working model" and argued that beyond infancy, attachment relationships are guided by mental representations. Such models could then influence memory, expectations, and response availability in subsequent social interactions.

The term *working model* referred to a cognitive representation of the environment and the self, emphasizing the dynamic aspects of a model versus a more static type of representation. But providing the details of such a model was beyond the cognitive psychology of Bowlby's day. Instead, Bowlby relied on Craik's (1943) formulation of a mental model that was at best an informal sketch of how information about the world can be used to interpret experience and make predictions in the future.

More recent advances in cognitive psychology, however, are better suited to address this challenge. There are numerous and varied modes of representation—images, lists of expectations, propositions, schemas, scripts, and so forth. Furthermore, we know quite a bit about how each one works. They differ in being episodic or semantic; implicit or explicit; available to awareness or not; parallel and effortless, or serial, slow, and effortful. Each one has distinctive effects on accessing relevant information in real-time social interactions and problem solving, memory, content elaboration, preparation and smoothness of behavior, and so forth (Epstein, 1994; Paivio, 2006; Kihlstrom, 1987; Schank, 1982, 1999).

The choice is not between one mode of representation or another. It is not as if attachment working models are comprised of scripts *OR* images *OR* lists of expectations. Multiple modes of representation are likely in play in guiding social behavior. The key is to be explicit in referring to them, and to stick to their known operating characteristics. Students of attachment representation should study the relevance of each of these in turn. As we establish the relevance of a specific mode of representation to attachment behavior, we immediately know a great deal about what roles it can and cannot play. In doing so, we iterate our way to a more detailed and specific accounting of attachment working models.

WHAT IS ATTACHMENT REPRESENTATION THE REPRESENTATION OF?

The question "What is attachment representation the representation of?" gained prominence after the introduction of the Adult Attachment Interview (AAI; Main, Kaplan, & Cassidy, 1985). The AAI prompted additional measures of adult attachment representations (e.g., projective methods; George & West, 2004) and various adaptations for children that try to obtain a sample of narrative from which loose inferences can be made about an underlying attachment representation (Oppenheim & Waters, 1995). For all of these measures, the focus has been on the coherence of a product rather than the structure or content of the underlying representation implied by the narrative. In fact, none specifically addresses what it is in early experience that is represented.

No doubt, lots of things capture secure base experience: images of specific caregiver-related experiences; somatic and affective memories of comfort and distress; narrative representations of specific interactions; and, in many instances, dynamically important meanings associated with them. We can add expectations cued by specific (and to some degree generalized) contexts, words, and behaviors, built up from relationship-specific experiences with one's own caregiver(s) and generalized to caregiver–offspring relationships more broadly. The full suite of representation structures, however, is beyond the scope of this chapter. Instead we focus on script-like representations of secure base experience (i.e., a secure base script).

Script-Like Representations of Recurring Events

Scripts were introduced by Schank and Abelson (1977) as generalized representations of familiar events with a clear temporal–causal structure organized around a goal. Scripts enable a person to fill in all kinds of details once the circumstance is identified as an exemplar of the scripted event. Not only can the person fill in the details, he or she can anticipate likely action sequences and how the actors in the script are likely to behave. With increasing experience, scripts become more elaborate with optional as well as obligatory actions. They also acquire more of a hierarchical structure, with subgoals embedded in the script (Abelson, 1981). Oftentimes, researchers refer to "going to a restaurant" as a prototypic script. The restaurant script includes entering, ordering, eating, and exiting scenes, each of which has its own script. Within the restaurant script there are variations marked, depending on type of restaurant (e.g., fast-food establishments vs. fine dining).

Bower, Black, and Turner (1979) explored the effects of scripts on human memory. They reported that there is broad consensus across individuals, for example, about what typically happens when a person goes to a restaurant, indicating that general scripts about everyday, routine activities do have some psychological validity. Bower et al. took their investigation one step further, demonstrating that people falsely recall script-consistent information that was not presented in a story containing a familiar script, and that they reorder information to conform more closely to a particular script. Smith and Graesser (1981) added to the memory findings by reporting that more typical, scripted information is recalled better, particularly over time.

Although some of the memory findings suggest that script memory is more dynamic and flexible than Schank and Abelson's original description suggested (Schank, 1982, 1999), the basic script framework has proven very useful, particularly for understanding children's event representations (Nelson, 1986, 1996). Research on early script development has shown that children do organize everyday activities in script-like representations (e.g., eating lunch at day care, birthday parties, getting dressed), and that the scripts become more elaborate with age and with increasing experience with the events in question (Nelson & Gruendel, 1986; Fivush & Slackman, 1986). In addition, the social context in which scripts develop is influenced by how mothers talk about the events as they occur, in the natural back-and-forth between mother and child (Nelson, 1986). Studies of autobiographical memory highlight individual differences in how mothers talk with their children about real-world events (Reese, Haden, & Fivush, 1993), and more recent discussions of children's representations of the experienced world have introduced concepts such as "collaborative construction" (Nelson, 1996). In summary, scripts serve as appropriate descriptions of how individuals represent familiar, regular occurrences, and are also evident at a very early age, making them a good candidate mechanism for how early attachment experiences are represented and carried forward across development.

The Definition of a Secure Base Script

Inge Bretherton (1991) first suggested that attachment scripts might be the building blocks of attachment representations. But the AAI and other adult assessments were too broad-based and complex in their scoring to be associated with a specific representational framework. Children-based assessments that followed (e.g., the Attachment Story Completion Task; Bretherton, Ridgeway, & Cassidy, 1990) relied on global ratings of security as well, obscuring which features of the protocols were key to understanding the structure of the underlying attachment representations.

In response to these limitations, Waters, Rodrigues, and Ridgeway (1998) offered a definition of a secure base script that could advance the investigation of the cognitive structure of "attachment working models." Following Ainsworth's work on infant–mother interaction (Ainsworth, Blehar, Waters, & Wall, 1978/2015), and secure base behavior (Ainsworth et al., 1978/2015; E. Waters, 1995), the key components of the secure base script were defined as (1) a child (or infant) and mother (or two adult attachment partners) are constructively engaged, (2) a challenge/obstacle is encountered that disrupts activity and/or leads to a level of distress, (3) the child (or one adult) signals for assistance, (4) the other dyad member recognizes the signal and responds in a manner consistent with the message, (5) the assistance is accepted, (6) the assistance is effective in resolving the challenge, (7) comforting/affect-regulating behavior occurs as well, and (8) the attached individual/dyad resume activity or initiate new activity (see Figure 8.1). The difficulty and/or distress can be dealt with in a variety of manners, either by removing the difficulty, removing the individual, providing the individual with an explanation of the situation that neutralizes the difficulty, or some combination of these. Furthermore, the script broadly encompasses a range of circumstances from ordinary to more emergency-type situations.

ASSESSING AN ADULT'S KNOWLEDGE OF THE SECURE BASE SCRIPT

Support for a secure base script was first found in the H. S. Waters et al. (1998) reanalysis of a developmental study of young children's attachment narratives. Attachment-related story completions of 24 children at age 37

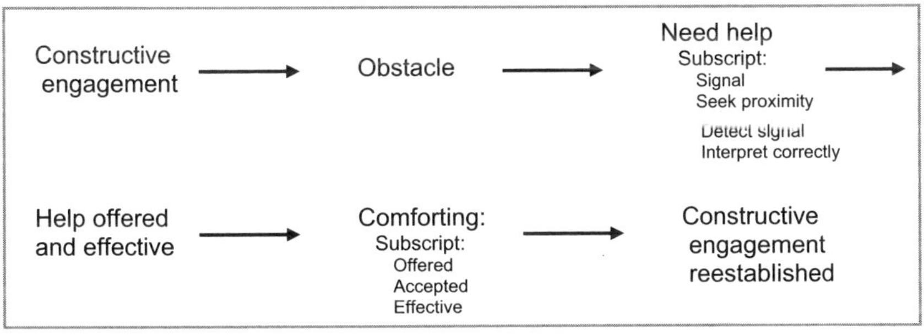

FIGURE 8.1. Content of a generalized (dyadic) secure base script.

months, and then again at 54 months, from the Bretherton et al. (1990) study were examined using a more formal cognitive analysis. The story completions were scored for the scriptedness of the story ending (i.e., whether a prototypic secure ending was used). Results indicated that children whose story completions conformed to a secure base script also had higher security scores on the Attachment Q-set based on observational data of mother–child interactions. Furthermore, children who produced more scripted story completions at 37 months did so as well when they were much older (at 54 months), showing stability in their script scores.

The promising results from H. S. Waters et al. (1998) led to the extension of the secure base script coding methodology and the development of the Attachment Script Assessment (ASA) for adult individuals. If young children who are only just beginning to represent their secure base experiences could express a secure base script in their stories, then there clearly was both a rationale and the promise of success in developing a script assessment that could be used with adults. Adapting existing narrative production techniques to prompt attachment-related narratives in adults was the next step. The prompt-word outline methodology developed by Harriet Waters in a series of developmental studies examining narrative production seemed most appropriate, since it had been used with both children and young adults (H. S. Waters & Hou, 1987; H. S. Waters, Hou, & Lee, 1993). Sets of prompt words are generated that outline a possible story line for the topic (e.g., a story about Susie having a birthday party). These words are grouped together on a page in several columns, so that if the individual follows along with the groups of words, he or she will be able to produce a coherent story. The advantages of this method include (1) everyone produces some minimal amount of story content with a beginning, middle, and end; (2) although the topic is identified and prompt words guide story production, there is enough flexibility in how the story is elaborated that a wide range of narratives is produced; and (3) the method can be adapted to elicit underlying scripts for all kinds of attachment relationships across age and across cultures.

Designing the ASA

In the current adaptation of this procedure, numerous story lines were selected based on attachment-related and nonattachment scenarios. Preliminary prompt-word outlines were then constructed to frame these situations. In all of attachment-related outlines, the general secure base script described earlier was used in the selection of appropriate word prompts. Embedded in each story line, there is some distress or situation(s) that can be addressed by providing secure base support by one of the characters (mother or spouse). Four attachment narrative topics (Baby's Morning, The Doctor's Office, Jane and Bob's Camping Trip, Sue's Accident) and two neutral narrative topics (Trip to Park, An Afternoon Shopping) were settled upon. Table 8.1 presents the final versions of the six prompt-word outlines.

TABLE 8.1. Attachment Script Assessment: Prompt-Word Outlines

A. Baby's Morning (mother–child attachment story)		
mother	hug	teddy bear
baby	smile	lost
play	story	found
blanket	pretend	nap
B. The Doctor's Office (mother–child attachment story)		
Tommy	hurry	mother
bike	doctor	toy
hurt	cry	stop
mother	shot	hold
C. Trip to Park (neutral story; child)		
Susie	swings	tired
bike	sandbox	bench
park	game	comics
friend	run	coke
D. Jane and Bob's Camping Trip (adult–partner attachment story)		
Jane	tent	campfire
Bob	wind	shadow
bags	collapse	sounds
hurry	upset	hug
E. Sue's Accident (adult–partner attachment story)		
Sue	wait	home
road	Mike	dinner
accident	tears	bed
hospital	doctor	hug
F. An Afternoon Shopping (neutral story; adult)		
Emily	browse	hungry
car	buy	food
mall	money	talk
friend	gift	home

Note. The same prompt-word outlines are used for both males and females, except for a modified version of one of the neutral stories: Afternoon Shopping becomes a trip to Home Depot rather than a trip to the mall.

The four attachment narrative topics differed on two dimensions. The first was age. Since security classifications have been shown to influence both child and adult relationships, story lines that covered both types of relationships were included. Two of the prompt-word outlines involve a child as the central character, thus exploring parent–child relations (Baby's Morning, The Doctor's Office). The second set of attachment prompt-word outlines center around adult-type situations and relations (Jane and Bob's Camping Trip, Sue's Accident). Each of the two neutral narrative topics was also either a story line that included child characters (Trip to Park) or adult characters (An Afternoon Shopping). Neutral outlines were included as a control and to provide greater variation in story lines. They evoke little to no emotional response, and do not include characters that share an attachment relationship.

The attachment narrative topics also varied in the degree of distress, in order to cover a broad range of secure base behavior. The first level of stress was introduced using scenarios depicting serious situations where someone was injured (The Doctor's Office, Sue's Accident). These outlines suggested emotionally stressful content, which should elicit secure base responses. The second level represented scenarios that were less emotionally stressful (Baby's Morning, Jane and Bob's Camping Trip), but still required some secure base interaction.

The prompt-word outlines for these story lines were constructed following the formula developed by Waters (H. S. Waters & Hou, 1987; H. S. Waters et al., 1993). Columns of words (three or four usually) are presented on a page from left to right. Each column of words can be used to discuss some activity of the main characters. Nonetheless, the interpretations can vary according to the participant. For example, "mother, baby, play, blanket" in the "Baby's Morning" story could prompt a narrative about a mother and her baby playing on a blanket, or about a baby playing and the mother covering him or her with a blanket, or a number of various other possibilities. Thus, the use of prompt-word outlines provides some guidance of content generation but still allows for distinctive story content across individuals.

Additionally, the prompt words were structured in such a way that the first column of words suggests an introduction to the story line, while the second column describes the main event/activity of the story; finally, the third column concludes the story. For example, in "The Doctor's Office" outline, the first set of words introduces the idea of Tommy out riding his bike and getting hurt. The second set of words cuts to the heart of the story, in that Tommy is taken to the doctor to have his injuries attended to. Finally, the last set of words provides a conclusion to the story, in which Tommy and his mom leave the doctor's office, ending the episode. Once again, all of the attachment-related story lines contain an underlying secure base script. Thus, those individuals who have an available secure script are likely to use that script in elaborating the story line, providing an opportunity to score their narratives on scriptedness. At the same time, the prompt words allow those who do not have a secure base script to produce a coherent story, albeit one that does not reflect the secure base script.

The preliminary outlines were revised through several iterations, until they were able to reliably prompt coherent narratives and the generated narratives varied in their secure base content. With repeated presentations to new participants, modifications continued on the outlines, until the prompt-word outlines were refined to the point that they appeared to successfully tap into a secure base script. It is particularly important to test prompt-word outlines in target populations, since it is difficult to fully anticipate how subjects will interpret the word prompts. There is always the possibility that they have a different take from the researchers developing the prompt-word outlines. Along the same lines, when researchers move to a new population, piloting of the prompt-word outlines is in order.

Administering the ASA

Each prompt-word outline consists of a story title and 12–14 prompt words, printed in three columns on a single sheet of paper (approximately 18-point type; 3–4 words per column). At the beginning of the session, each participant is told that he or she will be asked to produce six different narratives based on prompt-word outlines. They are told that three of the stories deal with children and another three deal with adult-type relationships (or vice versa). Participants are then presented with the first prompt-word outline. They are asked to use the columns of words to frame their story, going from left to right. Although they are asked to use the prompt-word outline as a guide, elaborations are welcomed, and participants are free to use the words in any way they like, and may change the order around if they wish. There is no demand that every word be used, although omissions are rare and are not critical (and not part of the scoring). Participants are told to tell their story, putting in as much information and as many details as they can, in order to tell the best possible story. In terms of length, they are asked to produce a narrative that would approximate a page in length, if written.

For each prompt-word outline, participants are given up to 2 minutes to review the words and formulate a story line. When they are ready, a digital recorder is turned on, and their generated stories are recorded. The prompt-word outline sheet remains in front of them as they go from column to column, generating their story. The same procedure is followed for the remaining five prompt-word outlines. Individual sessions range from 20 to 30 minutes.

In order to obtain spontaneous content and organization, the passages are always recorded rather than written. This is an important aspect of the procedure, because when writing, we have time; indeed, we are taught to edit our thoughts to a greater extent than possible or necessary when speaking. Oral production taps into the underlying scripts that guide production without encumbering participants with the need for online editing.

Finally, there are a number of caveats about the successful administration of the script assessment. The stories need to be in the third person, and participants are stopped if they begin in the first person, reflecting an autobiographical narrative. Our goal is to tap generalized relationship expectations, not to sample a *specific* autobiographical event from a person's life involving, for example, a car accident. The characters in the adult stories are always introduced as husband and wife, or as close partners (whatever works for a particular culture/sample). Stories about brother/sister, or characters who are just friends should be avoided, because these are not typically attachment figures. As a precaution, this point about the adult characters is reiterated for each of the adult attachment narratives.

Scoring the ASA

The secure base script scoring is focused on the person's knowledge and access to a script-like representation of the secure base cycle (represented in Figure 8.1). It is not a general assessment of the person's psychological attachment status of "secure" or "insecure." We broadly define the prototypic secure script as one in which the secure base (mom/partner) helps the individual (character in story) deal with some distress or obstacle and helps to get the attached individual back to meaningful engagement with the environment.

To score attachment narratives on the full range of secure base scriptedness, a 7-point scale was created (see Table 8.2). The highest ranked stories are those with extensive elaboration of the secure base script and a strong interpersonal framework (scale scores 7–6). Moving down the scale, stories have less and less explicit details related to the secure base script but still follow the basic structure of the script (scale scores 5–4). Narratives presenting a more "matter-of-fact," event-focused presentation, without explicit secure base content, receive a score of 3. The lowest scoring stories (scale points 2 and 1) are often disjointed (i.e., do not have a clear script-based temporal causal structure) and/or contain unusual atypical content. *Atypical content* refers to elements of the narrative that are either inconsistent with, or directly contradict, the secure base script. Emotional content may be present (e.g., Jane was upset); with no follow-up or reaction from the secure base character. The lowest scoring stories might even eliminate the partner in the secure base pairing (child or adult partner) as an active participant in the story or redirect the story to some other aspect of the situation, and away from the relationship content (e.g., a "Doctor's Office" story that focuses on the paperwork at the hospital).

Secure Base Script Content

For all of the attachment story lines, how the secure base script is instantiated is context specific for the particular scenario reflected in the prompt-word outline. Keeping that in mind, narratives organized around a secure base script have a number of features:

TABLE 8.2. Scriptedness Scoring System

Score	Description
7	These are the very best examples of secure base content in the narrative. There is a rich interplay between the two principal characters. There is a great deal of attention to the psychological state of the other, and the "secure base" is very responsive to that psychological state. Important to the secure base script is the resolution of the problem/distress with a return to normalcy.
6	These narratives fall short of the richness of secure base content that is evidenced in stories ranked "7." Nonetheless, these stories to contain a reasonable amount of secure base content.
5	These narratives have a medium amount of secure base content but not as much elaboration as those that are ranked "7" or "6."
4	These narratives have some secure base content, but not very much. Thus, they are weak on secure base content, but there is no unusual or atypical content contained in the story either.
3	These narratives seem mostly event-related stories, in which what is happening is presented, with very little commentary on the give-and-take between the characters, or on the psychological content of the story.
2	These are event-related as well, but so brief as to seem disjointed. Also included in this category are narratives that contain some unusual or atypical content that is inconsistent with a secure base script. The intrusion of this content, however, is not as consistent or pervasive as the narratives that are scored "1."
1	These narratives are theme-based variations that come across as quite peculiar interpretations of the implied story line. Not only is the secure base script not recognized, but a quite different script is in its place. The narratives can be quite detailed, with generated content consistent with the peculiar interpretation of the story line. These are not that common. Narratives that have significant unusual or atypical content but fall short of a complete theme-based variation also receive a "1."

1. The secure base helping to select and implement strategies for getting things back to normal and defusing the emotional distress, when that is possible, or avoiding distress altogether by facilitating transitions to other activities (for a baby or child) and providing explanatory frameworks to help understand the situation (for young child). For example:

- "Well, let's think really hard. If I were a teddy bear where would I be?" (memory retrieval strategy used by Mom to help child find lost Teddy Bear)
- "Mom gently laid the baby in the crib and told her that it was time for a nap, and that she would see her in just a little while when she woke up.

And Mom kissed the baby on the cheek and quietly walked out the room and said, 'Good night, baby.' " (transition to nap time)

- "Tommy started to cry again, but the mother was able to hold him, and he stopped crying. The doctor needed also to stitch up his chin, so Tommy started to cry again. And his mother said, 'Doctor can you just stop for one minute? Let me hold him and I'll be able to calm him down.' " (strategy for defusing emotional distress)
- (Doctor says) "We'll have to give you a stitch. But only a few stitches. But everything will be OK. And his mother reassured him. 'It might hurt for a minute Tommy, but it's going to be OK.' Tommy was still very upset, held his mother's hand real tight, with his mom standing right next to him." (mother provides comfort, both in the way of explanation and physical closeness)
- "And now Jane is like, 'Bob, come on. It's time for the hotel, we gotta get out of here.' And he explains to her, 'You know, we can reset this up (tent). If you really want to go to a hotel, we can, but we really wanted to get away from just all the people and the commotion, and the confusion.' And she says, 'Well, all right. If you really feel we can recover this and make it OK.' " (secure base offers strategy to make everything work out)
- "When Mike arrived, Sue had tears in her eyes, because she was very shaken by the accident. The doctor said, 'There's nothing to be worried about. Everything will be OK. Sue will just need to have some rest and relaxation for the next few days.' So Mike went over to his wife, gave her a really big hug, and said, 'Why don't we go home honey?' " (secure base comforts Sue, recognizing she needs the comforting, and then initiates the next step to getting things back to normal, going home)

2. The secure base reconfiguring the person's representation to focus on more positive aspects, thereby diffusing the negative emotion. This often involves pointing out the "bright" side of a situation (e.g., "We'll certainly talk about this trip for years to come"; this feature would not be relevant for Baby's Morning). For example:

- "Tommy was proud of himself and his mother said, 'Tommy, you did a wonderful job. You did real good, Mom was very proud. You didn't cry too much, and see, now your leg is gonna heal up real nice and be all better.' " (mother focuses on positive outcome, leg looks better, as well as how good Tommy was)
- "After they got the tent set up (after it had collapsed), they worked together to get it set up, and Jane was really enjoying herself. She told Bob that it was more that they were together than where they actually took their vacation." (Jane focuses on positive aspect of experience, in part because she knows that Bob is concerned about how things went badly early on)

- "And the wind started to howl like those coyotes and those wolves, and the tent started flapping around. It flapped so hard that it collapsed right on top of Jane and Bob. And Jane was so upset that their anniversary trip was ruined. But Bob looked at her, gave her a big hug and said, 'Don't worry honey, this will be an anniversary to remember.'" (Bob recasts experience into positive terms)
- "Sue and Mike looked at the unprepared dinner on the counter and it reminded them how precious life is, and that things can take a turn immediately, without warning. With this on their mind, they went to bed early and thought of how fortunate they were that everything turned out OK. They fell asleep, and because they realized their lives were so full, they never even thought about dinner." (accident experience is recast in relationship terms)
- "And on the way home, Sue remembered that all the food for dinner was in her car that was towed away to the repair shop. Seeing as they had nothing in the house to eat, they both made a big bag of popcorn, and they had a can of Kool-Aid that was left over in the refrigerator. Afterwards they went to bed and Sue said, 'I'm so sorry. I planned this really big dinner for you.' And Mike just gave her a really big hug and said, 'The best kind of gift I have is you, home safe with me.'" (dinner disaster is recast in positive relationship terms)

3. An interpersonal focus, that is, a sensitivity to and awareness of the other person's psychological/emotional state. The content of secure base narratives focuses on the interaction between the two individuals rather than simply describing the sequence of events in the story. The secure base responds to requests, cues from child/partner, modifying his or her own behavior as a consequence. There is give-and-take, with each partner making his or her own unique contribution to the situation, activity, but working together "as a team." There is also emotional give-and-take, with an expressed emotion in one leading to an emotional response in the other. For example:

- "Baby wanted to play hide and go seek, so mother went and got a blanket from the baby's room." (responding to request)
- "And the mom would just smile at her, and the baby would coo and laugh at the mom. She liked to laugh at the faces mom made." (emotional give-and-take)
- "And pretend that the teddy bear is hiding. The baby is looking for the teddy bear, and it pops out from behind mom. And the baby is very happy because he's found the teddy bear. They play for a little bit longer. The baby seems to be getting tired and mom puts the baby down for a nap." (awareness of baby's psychological state)
- "So, Tommy was such a big boy, though, that he made his mother proud, and said, 'OK, I'll be really good, Mom. I promise.' And his mother

was so happy with him that she said, 'OK, we'll go to the toy shop and we'll be able to pick up a toy that you might like as a reward for being so good.' " (emotional give-and-take)

- "And, of course, now (after telling scary campfire stories), every little twig that is out there starts to drive her crazy, cause, of course, now, it's this monster or that monster coming through. He reassures her that it's a fox or whatever, although in his mind, he's thinking, well it could be a bear, but you don't tell her that." (sensitivity to other's psychological state)
- "The sounds of the cricket and the wind in the leaves were all very romantic, and Jane agreed that this was the perfect vacation. Bob thanked Jane for agreeing to come, and Jane thanked Bob for showing her that camping could be a good vacation as long as they were together. The night ended with a big hug and they went into their tent." (emotional give-and-take, a team)
- "Sue was a little groggy right now, and still very upset and shaken from the accident. As soon as she saw Mike, she went into tears. 'Oh, I can't believe I did this. This is so bad. I feel terrible. I didn't realize how tired I was [in this story, Sue nodded at the wheel].' Mike said, 'We're just lucky that you're OK, and that the gentleman in the truck is fine.' " (emotional give-and-take, Sue breaks down, now that her secure base is here, and Mike reassures her that everyone is fine)

Event-Focused Narratives

Narratives outside the 7–4 secure base script range of the scale, range from nonscript, event-focused narratives to those that may be brief/disjointed or contain atypical, unusual content. An event-focused narrative that follows the events implied by the prompt-word outline, presenting a coherent accounting of the particular scenario, will receive a 3. These stories often have an "and then, and then" flavor, in which the events are enumerated with little emotional give-and-take or interactive engagement between the characters. They may track the prompt words and thus include emotion words such as *smile, hug, cry, upset,* and so forth, but do not have the more dynamic back-and-forth that characterizes secure base script content. The words are used, but the narrative content falls short of clear evidence of the interpersonal sensitivity to the other person's (child/partner) psychological state or signals for help that indicate secure base script knowledge. For example:

- "Mother and the baby wake up and they decided they're gonna spend the morning playing. They have breakfast together, and then they play peekaboo with a blanket, and the baby laughs and smiles. And then the mom plays a game with the baby, and hugs her. And they read a story together." (an "and then, and then" narrative format)

- "They rushed him to the doctor. He was crying and his leg had been badly hurt, and when the doctor saw it, they told him that he needed a shot. They told her that she had to hold him down. He was still crying. They gave him a shot so that he wouldn't get an infection and he stopped crying and he felt a little better." (no explicit interaction between mother and child as the events unfold, even though child is upset)

- "Jane and Bob tried and tried to get the tent up, but every time, it kept collapsing. Bob thought this was incredibly funny, and Jane was very, very upset. Eventually, they got the tent standing; they laid out their sleeping bags and started their camp fire. The rain had stopped and they made a beautiful fire. They took out their hot dogs and marshmallows and roasted away." (listing of events, no explicit interactions, even though both Bob and Jane express emotional reactions to the tent collapsing)

- "She had to wait a few minutes for the emergency room doctor to see her and to call her husband Mike. He finally got to the hospital in tears after an hour and a half. Finally, the doctor came and saw her and said, 'We think we need to give you some X-rays to make sure you'll be OK.' That's what they did. The X-rays showed that nothing was broken and she just had some bad bruises but that she could probably go home and wouldn't have to stay there overnight. Mike and Sue went home." (listing of events, very matter of fact, no explicit interactions between Sue and Mike)

Atypical, Unusual, Nonscript Content

As noted earlier, narratives outside of the secure base script range will nonetheless reflect the prompt-word outlines as the producer elaborates a particular story line. Since the prompt-word outlines serve as a guide, there is a wide range of possible elaborations on the story. Within that narrative diversity there can be noteworthy unusual, atypical interactions between the characters that are inconsistent with a secure base script, or significant redirection of the story line. Such narratives fall into the 2–1 range of the scriptedness scale. Given the range of possible ways in which unusual, atypical content can be introduced, we present just a sampling from low-scoring stories.

- "And the child cannot find the teddy bear and she is upset and she takes a nap, and when she wakes up she finds the teddy bear next to her." (although the child is upset, Mom is nowhere to be found, and the resolution also does not explicitly involve Mom)

- "The baby started crying a lot, like she was hungry or wanted to be held, so the mother had gone up to the baby and picked up the baby and gave her a nice hug, but the baby was still crying. . . . So she took the teddy bear and laid the teddy bear next to the baby and she was saying hello to the baby with the teddy bear, and that didn't do the trick. So she picked up the baby again and gave the baby a nice big hug, and the baby still was crying and wouldn't do anything." (Mom seems to be having repeated difficulty in calming down the baby, not the usual secure base "mom" character)

- "His mother had hurried on over to him to see what was wrong. She saw all the blood. She got so nervous, she picked him up and threw him in the car, and they ran to the doctor's office." (Mom's reaction is unusual, focus is on mom being nervous, does not address any upset Tommy might feel)

- "He [the doctor] said, 'All right, let me get the nurse and we'll give you a tetanus shot.' So he starts to cry. Mom's upset because he's all bloody and a mess. She says, 'All right, if you handle it like a big boy, I promise I'll take you to the toy store.' He says, 'Well, would you buy me the toy that I've been wanting?' She said, 'Well, depending on how you are at the doctor's office, sure.' " (interaction between Mom and Tommy is unusual, it is more of a negotiation about getting a toy, no effort to comfort Tommy, who is upset about the tetanus shot)

- "By the time he got home, he was late and Jane was hurrying him to put the bags into the truck and off they went. . . . They put the tent up in a hurry. Since they didn't secure all of the poles, when the wind came, the whole tent collapsed and Jane was very upset because there was no reason that Bob should have been late to begin with. After they finished putting the tent back up, they built a campfire." (unusual content in that Jane maintains her anger/annoyance at Bob's lateness, Bob doesn't deal with Jane being upset)

- "Sue was calling the hospital, because she was going into labor, and the doctor told her that she'd have to wait until he finished with dinner. Well, Sue got a little pissed off, because Mike wasn't home from getting ice cream. . . . She was upset, she started crying, tears came down flowing off her face, she ended up screaming and crying on her bed, waiting for her husband Mike. Finally, a phone call came. 'Your husband was in an accident.' That's all Sue needed to hear, being 9 months pregnant, going into labor. She said, 'There's been an accident, well, we're going to have another accident; the baby's on the way if somebody doesn't get here and get me to a hospital.' " (story redirected to Sue's pregnancy, Sue is annoyed/angry at Mike throughout the story)

Strategies for Script Scoring

Overall, scoring secure base script knowledge is very much a process of pattern matching. Assuming access to a secure script and the events implied by the particular prompt-word outline, we can describe how the secure base script is instantiated for each of the attachment scenarios. Once this is accomplished, we can ask whether a particular narrative matches a prototypic story that might be generated with reference to the secure base script. Higher script scores reflect a better match. In fact, it is not a matter of what percentage of the script elements the person uses. It is more a matter of how certain the rater can be that the person is using the script. The metaphor we often use during training sessions is that of trying to discern the outline of a sea serpent in a body of water. You don't have to see every element—you may see a part here and a part there. Where a story falls in the 7–4 script range is determined by how much of the script is elaborated in the story and therefore how confident the scorer is that the person used a secure base script to guide its production. In terms of our metaphor, we might ask how much of the monster is visible above the water.

In approaching secure base script scoring, it is worth noting that scripts are learned as a whole (Schank & Abelson, 1977; Bower et al., 1979; Mandler, 1984). For example, the restaurant script elements are not learned separately. If someone is handing you a menu, you can be certain that the next step will be an opportunity to read the menu and the waiter/waitress will return to take your order. The remaining elements of the script will follow in the expected order. In the same vein, the basic elements of the secure base script (constructive engagement, problem/distress, rescue, resolution) are part of a whole. As such, our script scoring, and the 7-point scriptedness scale, is focused on the narrative as a whole. After scorers identify content that signal secure base script knowledge and/or possible atypical content inconsistent with a secure base script, the scorer gives each narrative an overall 7–1 score.

Complete sample narratives, along with their script scores, are presented in Appendix 8.1. Several Baby's Morning narratives are included from one that is well-scripted to one that is event-focused, with no secure base content, to one that has unusual content. For the other three attachment-relevant scenarios, only well-scripted narratives are presented. In examining the sample Baby's Morning narratives, it is important to note that those passages not organized along lines of a secure base script are nonetheless well-formed narratives. The key to receiving a high script score is not the production of a well-organized narrative but producing one that is guided by, and that elaborates on, a secure base script. Scorers rely on evidence of the prototypical pattern of secure base support in the narrative, one of signaling and response, resolution of the problem, and reengagement with the environment.

Methodological Advantages of the ASA

In contrast to other measures of attachment representations, it is worth noting that the ASA is more easily administered and scored than many of these measures (e.g., the AAI, the Adult Attachment Projective). Even difficult attachment narratives require only minutes of rereading and parsing before being scored. Furthermore, the ASA prompt-word format offers some important methodological advantages:

1. It is possible to construct distinct but parallel prompt-word sets that would allow multiple independent assessments. This in turn would allow

researchers to increase reliability by aggregating scriptedness scores across several parallel prompt-word sets. The availability of multiple prompt-word sets would also make it easier to ensure that results are not specific to a particular set of materials. Finally, it would make it possible to avoid contamination by using different test materials in repeated-measures designs.

2. A recurring problem in AAI-type assessments is the inability to disentangle contributions and expectations of the mother versus the father. This problem is easily resolved using separate prompt-word sets that refer to "me and my mother" or "me and my father." It would also be easy to develop secure base prompt-word sets involving nonparental attachment figures such as teachers, mentors, or therapists.

3. Prompt-word sets can also be constructed specific to parent–child versus adult–adult relationships. This would be helpful in research on the hypothesis that experience in parent–child relationships establishes a prototype that influences secure base relationships in adulthood. The prompt-word methodology could also be adapted for assessments of relationship specific versus generalized relationship representations (first person—"me and my child" or "me and my spouse" vs. third person—"a mother and child" or "a husband and wife" prompt sets). Such distinctions cannot be disentangled in the AAI or its counterpart for adult close relationships (Current Relationship Interview [CRI]; Owens et al., 1995).

4. Finally, prompt-word sets and the scriptedness scoring procedures are easily adapted for use in different family and cultural contexts.

VALIDATION STUDIES OF THE ASA

The hypothesis that attachment representations include script-like representations of early secure base experience was the starting point on validation. A series of studies examined (1) the structure of such representations, and then links between (2) secure base script knowledge and AAI coherence, (3) relations between maternal script knowledge and Strange Situation classifications, AQS security scores, (4) the presence of script-like secure base representations in a variety of cultures, and (5) mother–child co-construction interactions that support script construction. We can also report on a number of extensions of the prompt-word outline method to examine the development and integration of attachment representations in adolescence and late middle childhood, and on the other side of the developmental time line, adult–child/aging parent script representations. Some progress has also been made on current relationships and student/mentor script representations.

One of the advantages of the prompt-word method is that it has allowed questions about the structure and organization of attachment representations to be pursued. Our first question concerned the generality versus specificity of secure base representations. Is there a single broadly generalized secure base script, or are parent–child and adult-type relationships represented differently? H. S. Waters and Rodrigues-Doolabh (2001) explored this in a community sample of adults by looking at the correlations among script scores from mother–child and adult–adult prompt-word sets, and nonsecure base materials (see Table 8.3). The results from this analysis indicated that secure base script scores from mother–child prompt-word sets were highly correlated (r = .80–.90), as were scores from adult–adult prompt-word sets. In addition, correlations across the two kinds of prompt-word sets (r's > .60) indicated that a common secure base script is relevant to both types of relationship. This is an important result consistent with the hypothesis that infant–mother and adult–adult relationships are similar in kind. Finally, neither mother–child nor adult–adult scores were significantly correlated with the scriptedness of non-secure base passages (e.g., script for going to the mall), indicating that the prompt-word method is not simply assessing a general narrative production skill or cognitive ability.

In a recent study, T. Waters, Fraley, et al. (2015) examined the latent structure of secure base script knowledge, taking advantage of two large samples, one of 714 adults and another of 674 adolescents, from subsequent research using the ASA with adults and an ASA adaptation for adolescents. The findings support the conclusions of the original validation study. Factor analyses indicated that secure base script knowledge is generalized across relationships, mother–child and adult close relationships for adult subjects, and mother–child and father–child relationships for adolescents. Thus, at least by late adolescence, secure base script knowledge is generalized and brought to bear across a variety of attachment relationships.

TABLE 8.3. Testing the Generalized Secure Base-Script Hypothesis: Convergent–Discriminant Validity

	Scriptedness	
	Pilot sample (N = 16)	Replication (N = 40)
Convergent validity		
Within mother–child stories	r = .89***	r = .83***
Within adult–adult stories	r = .78***	r = .60**
Across mother–child and adult–adult stories	r = .83***	r = .74***
Discriminant validity (general script knowledge)		
Mother–child vs. non-Attachment stories	r = –.15, ns	r = –.03, ns
Adult–adult vs. non-Attachment stories	r = –.16, ns	r = .05, ns

*p < .05; **p < .01; ***p < .001.

Next, in order to establish the relevance of script-like attachment representations to current attachment theory, H. S. Waters and Rodrigues-Doolabh (2001) looked at links between secure base script knowledge and AAI coherence (see Table 8.4). The results indicated that script knowledge was highly correlated with AAI coherence (r = .50–.60) in their community sample. Moreover, the correlations were comparable with mother–child and adult–adult prompt-word sets. In addition to demonstrating the relevance of script knowledge to current attachment theory, this is very useful information about the secure base relevance of the AAI. Indeed, correlations with secure base script knowledge seem a useful and easily implemented check on both the breadth and secure base relevance of AAI interviews across age and in different samples and cultures. In more recent research with adolescents, Steele et al. (2014) reproduced the strong link between secure base script knowledge and the AAI in a sample of late adolescents. Even more relevant to this issue, is the development of the AAI Secure Base Script Scale (AAI_{SBS}; see T. Waters & Facompré, Chapter 10, this volume). Using the AAI_{SBS} scale, T. Waters, Ruiz, and Roisman (2017) demonstrated that secure base script content in AAIs was correlated with AAI coherence scores, and showed stability of the relation between AAI_{SBS} scores and AAI coherence in late adolescence and again in early adulthood.

Once research established the link between the ASA and AAI coherence, further validation of the ASA was pursued by checking whether the ASA and the AAI have important correlates in common. Two measures can be substantially correlated, yet share few, if any, of the same correlates. With this in mind, Tini, Cochran, Rodrigues-Doolabh, and Waters (2003) examined links between maternal secure base script knowledge and infant Strange Situation

TABLE 8.4. Relations among AAI Coherence, Scriptedness, and IQ Scores

	AAI coherence	
	Pilot sample (N = 16)	**Replication (N = 40)**
Mother–child stories Scriptedness	r = .65**	r = .52***
Adult–adult stories Scriptedness	r = .57*	r = .51***
Combined—all stories Scriptedness	r = .64**	r = .55***
IQ (Henmon–Nelson Tests)	r = –.09, ns	r = –.13, ns

Note. Correlations between script scores and IQ scores were also nonsignificant; r = .16 for the pilot sample, r = .23 for the replication sample.
*p < .05; **p < .01; ***p < .001.

classifications. Scores from several mother–child and adult–adult passages were averaged to yield a single reliable estimate of maternal script knowledge. When these were dichotomized—script scores >4 (at least some evidence of secure base scriptedness) versus <4 (no evidence of secure base script use)—concordance with secure–insecure Strange Situation classification (74%) was comparable to that summarized in van IJzendoorn's (1995) meta-analysis of AAI–Strange Situation concordance. More recent studies using the AQS add to the list of shared correlates by linking maternal script scores to children's AQS security scores as well (Bost et al., 2006; Monteiro, Verissimo, Vaughn, Santos, & Bost, 2008; Vaughn et al., 2007; Verissimo & Salvaterra, 2006; Wong et al., 2011). Monterio et al. (2008) also reported parallel parental script–child attachment results with fathers, extending use of the ASA to both parents. Demonstrating that script knowledge and AAI coherence are not only correlated but also share theoretically significant correlates provides important evidence of the relevance of secure base script knowledge to current attachment theory and research. It also strengthens the claim that script-like representations of the secure base phenomenon are an important component of what are generically referred to as attachment representations or working models.

In addition, we cannot take for granted that adults in other cultures organize or represent their close relationships along the same lines as adults in Western cultures. Rodrigues-Doolabh, Wais, Zevallos, and Rodrigues (2001) and Rodrigues-Doolabh, Zevallos, Turan, and Green (2003) asked adult women from a wide range of cultures to produce stories from the ASA secure base prompt-word outlines. The cultures included Switzerland, Romania, Colombia, Zimbabwe, Turkey, and United Arab Emirates. Prompt-word sets were adapted in several cases to be appropriate to the respective cultures (e.g., because camping is not a usual male–female activity for young adults in the United Arab Emirates, this prompt-word set was replaced with "The Lost Purse"). Results indicated that within each of these cultures, script knowledge scores were comparable to those in U.S. samples (see Table 8.5). In addition, the correlations among and between scores based on mother–child and adult–adult prompt-word sets were similar to those in U.S. samples.

Although a wider range of cultures should be sampled, these results suggest that script-like representation of secure base experiences is not unique to adults living in middle class, Western, industrial societies. As attachment theory predicts, secure base use and support are important themes across a wide range of cultures. Subsequent studies using translated ASA versions have reported significant relations between AAI coherence, script scores, and mother sensitivity in an Italian sample (Coppola, Vaughn, Cassibba, & Constantini, 2006), and maternal script scores and child AQS security scores in Colombian and Portuguese samples (Monteiro et al., 2008; Vaughn et al., 2007; Verissimo & Salvaterra, 2006; Wong et al., 2011).

Finally, it is important to recognize that organized mental representations are not simply the passive memory residue of experience. Active construction

TABLE 8.5. Cross-Cultural Generality of Secure Base Script Representations

	US	Switzerland	Romania	Colombia	Zimbabwe	Turkey	UAE
Mean script score (max = 7)							
Mother–child	3.95	4.12	3.67	3.91	3.72	3.97	3.98
SD	1.71	1.36	1.18	1.12	1.48	1.26	1.23
Adult–adult	3.96	4.14	3.75	3.72	3.44	3.88	3.57
SD	1.56	1.26	.97	1.20	1.15	1.31	1.22
Correlations between . . .							
Mother–child stories	.83	.68	.49	.65	.64	.51	.50
Adult–adult stories	.60	.65	.41	.46	.74	.67	.73
Across story types	.74	.78	.63	.68	.77	.58	.72

Note. N = 40 participants for US sample, 24 participants for cross-cultural samples. All correlations are significant at the .05 level or greater.

and elaboration are also important. Accordingly, H. S. Waters, Steiner, Zaman, Apetroaia, and Crowell (2018) examined links between maternal secure base script knowledge and co-construction of secure base themes during both storytelling and open discussions of affect-laden vignettes. In the storytelling task, mothers were asked to help their preschool children tell attachment-relevant stories suggested by a series of picture prompts. In the other task, mothers were asked to discuss hypothetical situations, some of which contained positive emotional content, some that contained negative content (e.g., "How would you feel if mommy didn't let you sleep in the bed with her?" vs. "Mommy watches you at the beach"). All mothers were tested in advance on the AAI and on secure base script knowledge (ASA). The mother–child interactions were video-recorded, transcribed, then scored on the quality of the co-construction partnership, the mother's skill in prompting elaboration, and helping build an explanatory framework. Results indicated that both AAI coherence and secure base script knowledge were significantly related to the mothers' communication effectiveness, quality of the co-construction partnership, and mothers' ability to encourage content elaboration.

Additional studies have also shown links between maternal script knowledge and mother–child narrative styles in memory talk (Bost et al., 2006) and with children's attachment story completions (Apetroaia & Waters, 2018; Wong et al., 2011). All of these studies highlight how mother–child communication can build understanding and representation of secure base support and how maternal attachment script representations may contribute to cross-generation consistency in attachment security through mothers' co-construction skills. They also suggest that new research investigating the mechanisms underlying cross-generation transmission of attachment by describing mothers' attachment representations more specifically in terms of secure base script knowledge is needed. As noted by Posada and Waters (2018), the patterning of children's secure base behavior when interacting with their mother is also related to the structure of children's knowledge of secure base relationships (i.e., secure base script knowledge). These studies do not imply that script knowledge, in both parent and child, is the only factor in mother–child secure base interactions. A wide range of cognitive, defensive, and experience-specific factors are likely to contribute as well. However, it will be easier to appreciate these when the effects of script knowledge can be measured and controlled.

EXTENDING SCRIPT ASSESSMENTS TO DIVERSE RELATIONSHIPS

The original ASA contains secure base prompt-word sets that elicit narratives about mother–child or adult–adult interactions and was designed for use with adults. Since then, researchers have extended the range of prompt-word sets to include a number of other relationships following the ASA prompt-word formula. First efforts involved the development of adolescent "me and mom" and "me and dad" script assessments (see Appendix 8.2 for the adolescent ASA). The adolescent prompt-word outlines were first tested with eighth- and 11th-grade students to establish that narratives from these outlines could be scored on scriptedness (Steiner, Arjomand, & Waters, 2003). Dykas, Woodhouse, Cassidy, and Waters (2006) then administered the adolescent script assessment to a new sample of 11th graders and validated the adolescent script assessment against adolescent AAI coherence scores. Results indicated that adolescents have a general secure base script for mother and father, that these scripts are related, and that both are linked to attachment security as measured by the AAI. Steele et al. (2014) subsequently administered the adolescent script assessment to a sample of 673 18-year-olds from the National Institute of Child Health and Human Development (NICHD) Study of Early Child Care and Youth Development. They reported significant relations between ASA script scores and adolescent AAI coherence and security classifications, mother–child attachment in the first 3 years of life and with observations of maternal and paternal sensitivity from childhood to adolescence. Vaughn et al. (2016) continued the analysis of the NICHD study data, reporting that multiple domains of parental secure base support during childhood also contributed to adolescent attachment script representations.

T. Waters, Bosmans, Vandevivere, Dujardin, and Waters (2015) continued the push to earlier ages by developing a middle-childhood script assessment appropriate for later childhood, 10 to 12 years of age (see Appendix

8.2 for the Middle Childhood ASA). They reported three critical pieces of evidence in support of secure base script representations in middle childhood. Script scores across attachment narratives showed high consistency in two different Western cultures, the United States and Belgium, and demonstrated that the script assessment successfully tapped into a stable underlying script. In addition, they reported evidence of intergenerational transmission of secure base script knowledge, with mothers' script scores related to their children's and, finally, evidence of relations to symptoms of psychopathology (Child Behavior Checklist). Parallel efforts by Psouni and Apetroaia (2014) showed significant relations between their Secure Base Script Test and other middle childhood attachment measures, the Kerns Security Scale (e.g., Kerns, Klepac, & Cole, 1996), and the Friends and Family Interview (Kriss, Steele, & Steele, 2013). Overall, these studies indicate that secure base script knowledge is an important component of attachment representations in middle childhood.

There also has been a push to extend attachment script assessments toward older adults as they encounter different attachment challenges. Chen, Waters, Hartman, Zimmerman, and Miklowitz (2013) adapted the ASA prompt-word outline method to develop an adult–child/aging parent script assessment (e.g., parent falls during a visit) that they then used with a sample of adult children caring for an elderly parent with some signs of dementia. The quality of adult child–elderly parent interactions was assessed using the Level of Expressed Emotions Scale (Cole & Kazarian, 1988), along with self-report measures of the extent to which caregivers experienced caregiving as difficult or demanding. Caregivers' secure base script knowledge significantly predicted lower levels of negative expressed emotion. Furthermore, this effect was moderated by the extent to which the participants experienced caring for their elderly parents as difficult, with adult child–elderly parent secure base script representations playing a greater role when the caregiving situation is perceived as difficult.

Additional extensions include Wais's (2003) development of a current relationship script assessment for use in husband–wife-type relationships relying on a range of scenarios in which one or the other partner could provide support (e.g., a difficult job decision, partner falls ill). Two of the four prompt-word outlines involve the husband as a potential caregiver, and there are two in which the wife is the potential caregiver; all are framed within a current relationship and are produced in the first person, "Me and my spouse." Once developed and piloted, the current relationship script assessment was administered to 48 women who had been part of original validation sample of the ASA, women for whom there were also script scores from the ASA, coherence scores from the AAI, and coherence scores from the Current Relationship Interview (parallel format to the AAI; Owens et al., 1995). The relationship script scores were correlated with both attachment measures (AAI, ASA) and relationship-specific measures (CRI, secure base behavior in videotaped interactions).

Finally, Zevallos, Waters, and Waters (2009) investigated whether secure base script representations lead to positive expectations and goals concerning mentor–student relationships. Freshmen university students were administered both the original ASA and a new mentor–student script assessment that captured secure base use of mentors. Additional measures included questions about student expectations of college mentor–student opportunities and their previous mentoring experiences in high school. Overall, the results indicated that freshmen with higher script scores on the ASA were more likely to be open to close mentoring relationships with other adults (other than parent) and experience these relationships in a positive light. Furthermore, they cast the hypothetical scenarios presented in the mentor–student script assessment (e.g., Choosing a Major) within secure base terms, even though they have not yet dealt with these situations in their short university experience to date.

CONCLUSION

Modern attachment theory has maintained its prominence in the field of developmental psychology for over 50 years, due in part to John Bowlby's reconceptualization of the infant–mother tie as a secure base relationship (Bowlby, 1958, 1969/1982) and the lasting value of Mary Ainsworth's (1967; Ainsworth et al., 1978/2015) early studies of infant attachment. Continued advances in attachment theory have been heralded by progress in behavioral assessment beyond infancy (e.g., Greenberg, Cicchetti, & Cummings, 1990) and the move to representation in the 1980s (Main, Kaplan, & Cassidy, 1985). Its coherence across these advances in theory and a rich expansion of empirical findings can be credited to the central "secure base construct" that integrates insights about affect, cognition, and behavior in close relationships across age (E. Waters & Cummings, 2000). Keeping that in mind, H. S. Waters et al. (1998) proposed that an individual's history of secure base support is represented in memory as a "secure base script" characterizing the dynamic interplay between caregiver and child in moments of distress and exploration of the environment within a temporal–causal framework. This chapter documents 20 years of investigation on secure base script representations from early childhood (toddlerhood) to adulthood, providing a range of validation data, including both behavioral and cognitive–representational empirical support.

Key validation findings for the ASA include (1) significant relations to AAI coherence for both adolescent and adult individuals, (2) positive relations between maternal script knowledge and child attachment security, (3) links between maternal script knowledge and co-construction skills of secure base themes during children's storytelling and open discussions of affect-laden vignettes, (4) evidence of secure base script knowledge across cultures and links to the AAI, as well as associations with child security, (5) evidence of origins of adolescent and adult script knowledge in early caregiving experiences, (6) evidence of secure base script knowledge from story-stem completions from 3- to 4½-year-olds to middle childhood and adolescent age ranges and into adulthood, even extending to middle-aged individuals.

In light of results obtained in these studies, and a number of methodological advantages, including ease of scoring of attachment narratives from toddlerhood to adulthood, future research on the emergence and developmental progression of secure base script representations is possible. In part, this is due to the very nature of script-like representations. Because the organization of scripts originates in and is influenced by experience, and in turn influences behavior, researchers have an opportunity to track the interplay between experience and representation across the developmental time frame, checking the impact that maternal sensitivity, maternal co-construction skills, and other factors have on both secure base behavior and secure base representations across age (see Posada & Waters, 2018). The adaptability of the secure base script scoring and the application of the prompt-word method to different ages and relationship contexts encourages longitudinal designs that can bridge important developmental periods. That same adaptability gives attachment researchers a valuable tool for clarifying and helping resolve issues surrounding attachment representations and the Internal Working Model concept (H. S. Waters, Waters, & Waters, 2021).

Secure base script representations also direct researchers' attention to the type of mother–child verbal–cognitive engagement that can encourage the construction of attachment script representations (e.g., maternal use of open-ended questions), helping build a causal–explanatory framework about children's experience, intentions, feelings (H. S. Waters, Corcoran, & Waters, 2018). As sensitive parenting shifts from physical behavior to include more verbal exchanges with age, narrative-based script assessments can gauge the impact of these changes on children's attachment script representations and serve as an important developmental tool to evaluate the role that individual differences in parental communication styles play. Some recent attachment intervention approaches have in fact incorporated elaborative and emotion-rich reminiscing as part of parenting training, all of which is consistent with an overall attachment script framework (Valentino, 2017), specifically that parental script knowledge guides effective communication about attachment-relevant and emotion-laden experiences.

Furthermore, reported links between maternal script knowledge and both children's secure base use and secure base script representations (Apetroaia & Waters, 2018; Vaughn et al., 2007; Wong et al., 2011) open the door for examining how secure base script knowledge might influence a mother's view of mother–child interactions and what constitutes effective secure base support. Because script representations structure knowledge about events, influence memory, and impact expectations about what is to happen (Nelson, 1986), it is likely that they influence what a mother perceives in a particular situation and, consequently, her behavior. In a recent study, Waters, Corcoran, et al. (2018) demonstrated that mothers with a broader understanding of the secure base script were better able to describe contingent secure base support during a typical mother–child play day at a park. They also had a clearer "eye" for observing differences between more and less skillful mother–child interactions during joint storytelling. These findings are consistent with the hypothesis that secure base scripts frame an individual's perceptions and expectations of how mother–child interactions proceed in a range of contexts.

In conclusion, multiple secure base script assessments spanning different ages offer opportunities for a wide range of developmental investigations that enable researchers to track developmental and individual changes in attachment script representations (e.g., Bosmans, van de Walle, Heylen, De Winter, & Bijttebier, 2017) and explore the predictive power of secure base script representations in terms of later developmental outcomes (e.g., Ruiz, Waters, & Yates, 2020). Not only can researchers explore important behavioral, affective, and cognitive correlates of secure base script knowledge at different ages, but they also can advance our understanding of how scripted attachment representations may change and evolve over time. T. Waters et al. (2019) recently reported a taxometric analysis of middle childhood secure base script knowledge revealing a categorical latent structure, in contrast to comparable analyses with adolescent and adult script knowledge that suggested continuous latent structure (T. Waters, Fraley, et al., 2015). This intriguing finding suggests a shift from categorical to dimensional latent structure from middle childhood to adulthood. Future research should explore how script knowledge is organized, generalized, and elaborated with age—questions that have been mostly unexamined to date (but see T. Waters, 2021).

REFERENCES

Abelson, R. P. (1981). Psychological status of the script concept. *American Psychologist, 36,* 715–729.

Ainsworth, M. D. S. (1967). *Infancy in Uganda: Infant care and the growth of love.* Baltimore: Johns Hopkins University Press.

Ainsworth, M. D. S., Blehar, M. C., Waters, E., & Wall, S. (2015). *Patterns of attachment: A psychological study of the Strange Situation.* New York: Taylor & Francis (Psychology Press). (Original work published 1978)

Apetroaia, A., & Waters, H. S. (2018). Intergenerational transmission of secure base script knowledge: The role of maternal co-construction skills. In G. Posada & H. S. Waters (Eds.), The mother–child attachment partnership in early childhood: Secure base behavioral and representational processes. *Monographs of the Society for Research in Child Development, 83*(4), 91–105.

Bosmans, G., van de Walle, M., Heylen, J., De Winter, S., & Bijttebier, P. (2017, April). *The development of the secure base script from middle childhood to early adolescence: A two-year longitudinal study.* Paper presented at the biennial meeting of the Society for Research in Child Development, Austin, TX.

Bost, K. K., Shin, N., McBride, B. A., Brown, G. L., Vaughn, B. E., Coppola, G., . . . Korth, B. (2006). Maternal secure base scripts, children's attachment security, and mother–child narrative styles. *Attachment and Human Development, 8,* 241–260.

Bower, G. H., Black, J. B., & Turner, T. J. (1979). Scripts in memory for text. *Cognitive Psychology, 11,* 177–220.

Bowlby, J. (1958). The nature of the child's tie to its mother. *International Journal of Psychoanalysis, 39,* 350–373.

Bowlby, J. (1982). *Attachment and loss: Vol. 1. Attachment.* New York: Basic Books. (Original work published 1969)

Bretherton, I. (1991). New wine in old bottles. In M. Gunnar & L. A. Sroufe (Eds.), *Minnesota Symposia on Child Psychology: Vol. 23. Concepts of self* (pp. 1–34). Hillsdale, NJ: Erlbaum.

Bretherton, I., Ridgeway, D., & Cassidy, J. (1990). Assessing internal working models of the attachment relationship: An attachment story completion task for 3-year-olds. In M. Greenberg, D. Cicchetti, & E. M. Cummings (Eds.), *Attachment in the pre-school years: Theory, research and intervention* (pp. 273–308). Chicago: University of Chicago Press.

Chen, C. K., Waters, H. S., Hartman, M., Zimmerman, S., & Miklowitz, D. J. (2013). The relationship between secure base script knowledge and expressed emotion among adult children caring for parents with dementia. *Attachment and Human Development, 15,* 332–348.

Cole, J. D., & Kazarian, S. S. (1988). The Level of Expressed Emotion Scale: A new measure of expressed emotion. *Journal of Clinical Psychology, 44,* 392–397.

Coppola, G., Vaughn, B. E., Cassibba, R., & Costantini, A. (2006). The attachment script representation procedure in an Italian sample: Associations with Adult Attachment Interview scales and with maternal sensitivity. *Attachment and Human Development, 8,* 209–219.

Craik, K. (1943). *The nature of explanation.* Cambridge, UK: Cambridge University Press.

Dykas, M. J., Woodhouse, S. S., Cassidy, J., & Waters, H. S. (2006). Narrative assessment of attachment representations: Links between secure base scripts and adolescent attachment. *Attachment and Human Development, 8,* 221–240.

Epstein, S. (1994). An integration of the cognitive and psychodynamic unconscious. *American Psychologist, 49,* 709–724.

Fivush, R., & Slackman, E. (1986). The acquisition and development of scripts. In K. Nelson (Ed.), *Event knowledge: Structure and function in development* (pp. 71–96). Hillsdale, NJ: Erlbaum.

George, C., & West, M. (2004). The Adult Attachment Projective: Measuring individual differences in attachment security using projective methodology. In M. Hersen (Series Ed.) & M. Hilsenroth & D. Segal (Vol. Eds.), *Comprehensive handbook of psychological assessment: Vol. 2. Personality assessment* (pp. 431–447). Hoboken, NJ: Wiley.

Greenberg, M., Cicchetti, D., & Cummings, M. (Eds.). (1990). *Attachment in the preschool years: Theory, research, and intervention.* Chicago: University of Chicago Press.

Kerns, K. A., Klepac, L., & Cole, A. (1996). Peer relationships and preadolescents' perceptions of security in the child–mother relationship. *Developmental Psychology, 32,* 457–466.

Kihlstrom, J. F. (1987). The cognitive unconscious. *Science, 237*(4821), 1445–1452.

Kriss, A., Steele, H., & Steele, M. (2013). Measuring attachment and reflective functioning in early adolescence: An introduction to the friends and family interview. *Research in Psychotherapy: Psychopathology, Process and Outcome, 15,* 87–95.

Main, M., Kaplan, N., & Cassidy, J. (1985). Security in infancy, childhood and adulthood: A move to the level of representation. In I. Bretherton & E. Waters (Eds.), Growing points of attachment theory and research. *Monographs of the Society for Research in Child Development, 50*(1–2), 66–104.

Mandler, J. M. (1984). *Stories, scripts, and scenes: Aspects of schema theory.* Hillsdale, NJ: Erlbaum.

Monteiro, L., Veríssimo, M., Vaughn, B. E., Santos, A. J., & Bost, K. K. (2008). Secure base representations for both fathers and mothers predict children's secure base behavior in a sample of Portuguese families. *Attachment and Human Development, 10,* 189–206.

Nelson, K. (1986). *Event knowledge: Structure and function in development.* Mahwah, NJ: Erlbaum.

Nelson, K. (1996). *Language in cognitive development: The emergence of the mediated mind.* Cambridge, UK: Cambridge University Press.

Nelson, K., & Gruendel, J. (1986). Children's scripts. In K. Nelson (Ed.), *Event knowledge: Structure and function in development* (pp. 21–46). Hillsdale, NJ: Erlbaum.

Oppenheim, D., & Waters, H. S. (1995). Narrative processes and attachment representations: Issues of development and assessment. In E. Waters, B. Vaughn, G. Posada, & K. Kondo-Ikemura (Eds.), Caregiving, cultural, and cognitive perspectives on secure-base behavior and working models: New growing points of attachment theory and research. *Monographs of the Society for Research in Child Development, 60*(2–3), 197–215.

Owens, G., Crowell, J. A., Pan, H. S., Treboux, D., O'Connor, E., & Waters, E. (1995). The prototype hypothesis and the origins of attachment working models: Parent–child relationships and adult–adult romantic relationships. In E. Waters, B. Vaughn, G. Posada, & K. Kondo-Ikemura (Eds.), Culture, caregiving, and cognition: Perspectives on secure base phenomena and attachment working models. *Monographs of the Society for Research in Child Development, 60*(2–3), 216–233.

Paivio, A. (2006). *Mind and its evolution: A dual coding theoretical approach.* Mahwah, NJ: Erlbaum.

Posada, G., & Waters, H. S. (Eds.). (2018). The mother–child attachment partnership in early childhood: Secure base behavioral and representational processes. *Monographs of the Society for Research in Child Development, 83*(4).

Psouni, E., & Apetroaia, A. (2014). Measuring scripted attachment-related knowledge in middle childhood: The Secure Base Script Test. *Attachment and Human Development, 16,* 22–41.

Reese, E., Haden, C., & Fivush, R. (1993). Mother–child conversations about the past: Relationships of style and memory over time. *Cognitive Development, 8,* 403–430.

Rodrigues-Doolabh, L., Wais, D., Zevallos, A., & Rodrigues, R. (2001). *Attachment scripts across cultures.* Paper presented at the meeting of the Society for Research in Child Development. Retrieved from *www.psychology.sunysb.edu/attachment/srcd2001/crossculture/lr-srcd2110.pdf.*

Rodrigues-Doohlab, L., Zevallos, A., Turan, B., & Green, J. (2003). *Attachment scripts across cultures.* Paper presented at the meeting of the Society for Research in Child Development. Retrieved from *www.psychology.sunysb.edu/attachment/srcd2003/posters/srcd2003_rodrigues.pdf.*

Ruiz, S., Waters, T. E. A., & Yates, T. M. (2020). Secure base script knowledge as a mediator between early life stress and later child behavior problems. *Attachment and Human Development, 22*(6), 627–642.

Schank, R. (1982). *Dynamic memory: A theory of reminding and learning in computers and people.* London: Cambridge University Press.

Schank, R. (1999). *Dynamic memory revisited.* Cambridge, UK: Cambridge University Press.

Schank, R., & Abelson, R. (1977). *Scripts, plans, goals, and understanding.* New York: Wiley.

Smith, D. A., & Graesser, A. C. (1981). Memory for actions in scripted activities as a function of typicality, retention interval, and retrieval task. *Memory and Cognition, 9,* 550–559.

Steele, R. D., Waters, T. E. A., Bost, K. K., Vaughn, B. E., Truitt, W., Waters, H. S., . . . Roisman, G. I. (2014). Caregiving antecedents of secure base script knowledge in the NICHD Study of Early Child Care and Youth Development (SECCYD). *Developmental Psychology, 50,* 2526–2538.

Steiner, M., Arjomand, M., & Waters, H. S. (2003). *Adolescent representations of close relationships: Organized around a secure base script?* Paper presented at the meeting of the Society for Research in Child Development. Retrieved from *www.psychology.sunysb.edu/attachment/srcd2003/srcd2003.htm.*

Tini, M., Cochran, D., Rodrigues-Doolabh, L., & Waters, E. (2003). *Maternal attachment scripts and infant security.* Paper presented at the meeting of the Society for Research in Child Development. Retrieved from *www.psychology.sunysb.edu/attachment/srcd2003/srcd2003.htm.*

Valentino, K. (2017). Relational interventions for maltreated children. *Child Development, 88,* 359–367.

van IJzendoorn, M. H. (1995). Adult attachment representations, parental responsiveness, and infant attachment: A meta-analysis on the predictive validity of the Adult Attachment Interview. *Psychological Bulletin, 117,* 387–403.

Vaughn, B. E., Coppola, G., Veríssimo, M., Monteiro, L., Santos, A. J., Posada, G., . . . Korth, B. (2007). The quality of maternal secure base scripts predicts children's secure base behavior at home in three socio-cultural groups. *International Journal of Behavioral Development, 31,* 65–76.

Vaughn, B. E., Waters, T. E. A., Steele, R. D., Roisman, G. I., Bost, K. K., Truitt, W., . . . Booth-LaForce, C. (2016). Multiple domains of parental secure base support during childhood and adolescence: Contributions to adolescents' representations of attachment as a secure base script. *Attachment and Human Development, 18,* 317–336.

Veríssimo, M., & Salvaterra, F. (2006). Maternal secure-base scripts and children's attachment security in an adopted sample. *Attachment and Human Development, 8,* 261–273.

Wais, D. (2003). *Script assessment of partner-specific attachment representations.* Unpublished doctoral dissertation, State University of New York at Stony Brook, Stony Brook, NY.

Waters, E. (1995). The Attachment Q-Set (Version 3). In E. Waters, B. Vaughn, G. Posada, & K. Kondo-Ikemura (Eds.), Caregiving, cultural, and cognitive perspectives on secure-base behavior and working models: New growing points of attachment theory and research. *Monographs of the Society for Research in Child Development, 60*(2–3), 234–246.

Waters, E., & Cummings, M. C. (2000). A secure base from which to explore close relationships. *Child Development, 71,* 164–172.

Waters, H. S., Corcoran, D. M., & Waters, T. E. A. (2018). Maternal secure base script knowledge and judgements of mother–child interactions. In G. Posada & H. S. Waters (Eds.), The mother–child attachment partnership in early childhood: Secure base behavioral and representational processes. *Monographs of the Society for Research in Child Development, 83*(4), 106–120.

Waters, H. S., & Hou, F. (1987). Children's production and recall of narrative passages. *Journal of Experimental Child Psychology, 44*, 348–363.

Waters, H. S., Hou, F., & Lee, Y. (1993). Organization and elaboration in children's repeated production of prose. *Journal of Experimental Child Psychology, 55*, 31–55.

Waters, H. S., Rodrigues, L. M., & Ridgeway, D. (1998). Cognitive underpinnings of narrative attachment assessment. *Journal of Experimental Child Psychology, 71*, 211–234.

Waters, H. S., & Rodrigues-Doolabh, L. (2001). *Are attachment scripts the building blocks of attachment representations?* Paper presented at the meeting of the Society for Research in Child Development. Retrieved from *www.psychology.sunysb.edu/attachment/srcd2001/srcd2001.htm.*

Waters, H. S., Steiner, M. A., Zaman, W., Apetroaia, A., & Crowell, J. A. (2018). Co-construction of attachment representations and affect-regulating cognitions: The role of maternal attachment security. In G. Posada & H. S. Waters (Eds.), The mother–child attachment partnership in early childhood: Secure base behavioral and representational processes. *Monographs of the Society for Research in Child Development*, *83*(4), 60–73.

Waters, H. S., Waters, T. E. A., & Waters, E. (2021). From internal working models to script-like attachment representations. In R. A. Thompson, J. A. Simpson, & L. J. Berlin (Eds.), *Attachment: The fundamental questions*. New York: Guilford Press.

Waters, T. E. A. (2021). Representational measures of attachment: A secure base script perspective. In R. A. Thompson, J. A. Simpson, & L. J. Berlin (Eds.), *Attachment: The fundamental questions*. New York: Guilford Press.

Waters, T. E. A., Bosmans, G., Vandevivere, E., Dujardin, A, & Waters, H. S. (2015). Secure base representations in middle childhood across two Western cultures: Associations with parental attachment representations and maternal reports of behavior problems. *Developmental Psychology, 51*, 1013–1025.

Waters, T. E. A., Facompré, C. R., Dujardin, A., van de Walle, M., Verhees, M., Bodner, N., . . . Bosmans, G. (2019). Taxometric analysis of secure base script knowledge in middle childhood reveals categorical latent structure. *Child Development, 90*, 694–707.

Waters, T. E. A., Fraley, R. C., Groh, A. M., Steele, R. D., Vaughn, B. E., Bost, K. K., . . . Roisman, G. I. (2015). The latent structure of secure base script knowledge. *Developmental Psychology, 51*, 823–830.

Waters, T. E. A., Ruiz, S. K., & Roisman, G. I. (2017). Origins of secure base script knowledge and the developmental construction of attachment representations. *Child Development, 88*(1), 198–209.

Wong, M., Bost, K. K., Shin, N., Verissomo, M., Maia, J., Monteiro, L, . . . Vaughn, B. E. (2011). Preschool children's mental representations of attachment: Anteced ents in their secure base behaviors and maternal attachment scripts. *Attachment and Human Development, 13*, 489–502.

Zevallos, A., Waters, H. S., & Waters, E. (2009, April). *The building blocks of positive mentor–student expectations: Contributions from attachment and mentoring experiences*. Poster presented at the meeting of the Society for Research in Child Development, Denver, CO.

APPENDIX 8.1. Sample Attachment Narratives: Attachment Script Assessment for Adults

1. Baby's Morning: Secure Base Script

Every morning, Mother went in to see baby as she lay in the crib. She was such a good baby. She would play and she would gurgle, and she would play with her little mobile up above her head. And every morning that mother went in to baby, she found that baby kicked the blanket. So Mother would pick the baby up and she would give her a big, big hug and a nice smile, and lots of little kisses all over her face. Then they would go downstairs and they would have breakfast. Baby didn't like oatmeal too much. So Mother would make up a story and pretend that there was a little teddy bear that would come to visit. And the teddy bear would come and baby would eat her oatmeal. But one day, they lost her little teddy bear. Mom had always made the story about the teddy bear, because baby loved her little teddy bear and would call her "teddy, teddy." And teddy bear was lost. Mother and baby looked all over for the bear, but they couldn't find it. They had looked high; they had looked low. So Mother brought baby up to bed, up to her little crib and there, underneath the crib, they found the teddy. Now baby was able to go to sleep. And every time baby went to sleep with the teddy, she had a wonderful sound little nap.

2. Baby's Morning: No Secure Base Script, Matter-of-Fact Presentation of Events

It's 6 o'clock in the morning and the baby's morning begins. A loud cry from the crib awakens mother to a smiling happy baby, that wants to be fed, changed, and played with. Mom picks up the baby, tucked in the blanket, with a hug and a smile and takes care of the baby's needs. After an early breakfast, Mom puts the baby in a playpen, while she begins her day. After she gets herself together, her and baby play a pretend game with the teddy bear. The teddy bear is good company for the baby, because the baby is just learning to talk and the teddy bear is a good listener. The teddy bear is also a good teething ring, since the baby is beginning to teethe. After a little more play and another quick snack, the baby is put down for a nap.

3. Baby's Morning: No Secure Base Script, Atypical Content, Mom Is Nervous, Teddy Not Found in Time for Nap

A new mother woke up one of the first mornings she was alone with her baby to play. She took out the pink blanket, spread it on the floor, gave her newborn baby and big hug, a smile, and put her on the blanket. The mother was very nervous, as this was the first time she was alone with her new baby. She sat on the blanket and played with her, and started to tell her a pretend story of the three little bears. It was the only story she knew. As she was telling the story, she took out one of her new baby's teddy bears to play with it, to make her story seem more real, but the doorbell rang, and she got up to answer the door and when she came back, the teddy bear was lost. Now her new baby had fallen asleep and taken a nap. The mother panicked because she couldn't find the new teddy bear. She looked everywhere—under the couch, behind the door, and in the couch. Then she found it, under her new born baby while she was taking a nap.

4. The Doctor's Office: Secure Base Script

It was bright and sunny day. Tommy decided to go outside to ride his bicycle. He put on his helmet, he got on his bike, and started to ride up and down the block. His mother told him to be careful not to ride too fast so he doesn't get hurt. Tommy was riding up and down the block for a while without any problem, and then he decided to be a little more adventurous and wound up hitting a curb and falling over. Tommy realized he was very hurt and started to cry. When his mother heard him crying, she hurried out the door and picked him up. She realized that he had been hurt pretty bad and she should take him to the doctor. In the car on the way to the doctor, Tommy asked his mother if he needed to get a shot. And Tommy's mother said, "Well, it would depend on how hurt you are." So on the way to the doctor they stopped at a store and bought Tommy a toy, just in case he needed a shot, so he wouldn't cry. When they got to the doctor's office, the doctor decided that Tommy would need a shot, so his mother held him very close and told Tommy not to worry, that the shot would only hurt for a minute, and as soon as it was over they would stop for ice cream on the way home.

5. Jane and Bob's Camping Trip: Secure Base Script

Jane and Bob were all excited cause for their first-year anniversary they were going on a camping trip to the Adirondacks. And Jane and Bob had woken up early and decided they were gonna pack up the car and head up to the north country. Jane, unfortunately, had quite a few bags to pack in the car. And Bob kept saying hurry up because traffic was starting to build on the roadway. When they got to the campsite, they set up the tent, and they went for a long walk in the woods to enjoy the out of doors. When they came back, they made a campfire, and sat near the campfire. And there were many sounds that were going on at the campfire, in the hillside; sounds like coyotes, and wolves, all sorts of things. And Jane was very upset, because there were shadows that were playing on the side of the tent. But that's OK because Bob said, "There's nothing out there to be afraid of." They decided they were gonna go to bed. So they go to bed. And a big storm had come in to the area, and they didn't realize that a big storm was coming. And the wind started to howl like those coyotes and those wolves, and the tent started flapping around. It flapped so hard that it collapsed right on top of Jane and Bob. And Jane was so upset that their anniversary trip was ruined. But Bob looked at her, gave her a big hug and said, "Don't worry, honey, this will be an anniversary to remember."

6. The Accident: Secure Base Script

Sue was racing home from work with groceries in the car because she was ready to make dinner. She wanted to have a special dinner for Mike because he had just gotten a big promotion at work. Well, the weather had turned ugly, and it started to rain. While Sue was driving on the road she had an accident. Luckily it wasn't serious, but just to be on the safe side, the policeman said that "I would recommend you going to the hospital to just check out those bruises." So Sue went to the hospital. She got checked out by the doctor. She waited in the waiting room for Mike to get there. When Mike arrived, Sue had tears in her eyes, because she was very shaken by the accident. The doctor said, "There's nothing to be worried about. Everything will be OK. Sue will just need to have some rest and relaxation for the next few days." So Mike went over to his wife, gave her a really big hug, and said, "Why don't we go home, honey?" And on the way home, Sue remembered that all the food for dinner was in her car that was towed away to the repair shop. Seeing as they had nothing in the house to eat, they both made a big bag of popcorn, and they had a can of Kool-Aid that was left over in the refrigerator. Afterwards they went to bed, and Sue said, "I'm so sorry. I planned this really big dinner for you." And Mike just gave her a really big hug, and said, "The best kind of gift I have is you, home safe with me."

APPENDIX 8.2. Adolescent and Middle Childhood ASA Prompt-Word Outlines

I. ADOLESCENT ATTACHMENT SCRIPT ASSESSMENT (UPDATED 2014)

"Me and Mom" Prompt-Word Outlines

A1. Acne

Sunday	Mom	laugh
mirror	talk	bathroom
acne	herself	experiment
embarrassed	acne	make-up

A2. Haircut (Male Version of the Acne Story)

weekend	Mom	clippers
barber	talk	experiment
bad haircut	we laugh	fix
embarrassed	bathroom	hug

B. The Party

Friday night	sulk	movie
party	couch	popcorn
uninvited	Mom	smile
miserable	talk	bed

"Me and Dad" Prompt-Word Outlines

C. Tennis Match (Sport Can Be Changed)

championship	opponent	losing
nervous	discuss	look
Dad	strategy	Dad
ask	game begins	thumbs-up

D. Studying for an Exam

studying	Dad	tutor
exam	newspaper	discuss
difficult	look up	smile
worried	help	sleep

II. MIDDLE CHILDHOOD ATTACHMENT SCRIPT ASSESSMENT (T. WATERS, BOSMANS, ET AL., 2015)

"Me and Mom" Prompt-Word Outlines

A. Scary Dog in the Yard

outside	sniff	mom	dog gone
play	bark	broom	go inside
big dog	I cry	chase	play

B. At the Beach

Mom and I	climb	mom	bandage
picnic	rocks	hurry	hug
beach	I'm cut	doctor	home

C. Soccer Game

morning	play	I miss	Mom
big game	tired	lose	talk
nervous	easy shot	upset	practice

CHAPTER 9

The Adult Attachment Interview

A Guide for New Researchers and Research Consumers

Judith A. Crowell

The Adult Attachment Interview (AAI) was developed "to assess the security of the adult's overall working model of attachment, that is, the security of the self in relation to attachment in its generality rather than in relation to any particular present or past relationship" (Main, Kaplan, & Cassidy, 1985, p. 78). More recent formulations describe the AAI as assessing an individual's "state of mind" with respect to attachment (Steele & Steele, 2008; Main, Hesse, & Goldwyn, 2008). Analyses of large numbers of AAIs suggest that discourse in the AAI is distributed along two dimensions (Crowell, Fraley, & Roisman, 2016): (1) the degree to which adults freely evaluate their childhood experiences or are dismissing of them, and (2) variation in preoccupation (see Crowell, 2021).

The AAI's history, conceptual underpinnings, and validity are well described in several lengthy articles (Main, 2000; Hesse, 2008) and in the *Handbook of Attachment, Third Edition* (Cassidy & Shaver, 2016). A chapter by Main et al. (2008) in the important book *Clinical Applications of the Adult Attachment Interview* (Steele & Steele, 2008), is especially rich with examples from AAI transcripts and discusses in detail the role of language analysis in AAI scoring and classification decisions.

These sources reflect the advantaged perspective of the AAI's authors and their sense of the strategies and difficulties in bringing such a complex measure into general use. This chapter, too, focuses on the interview, its structure, and scoring principles. However, the perspective is my own—informed by having attended the very first AAI training seminar in 1985 and another 7 years further into the AAI's development, having taught AAI administration and scoring to several cohorts of researchers in our Stony Brook attachment research group, and having used the AAI extensively in research on marriage and early adult development. My perspective is also informed by 25 years of clinical experience in child and family psychiatry. While existing descriptions and discussions of the AAI remain as useful as ever, there is clearly room in the AAI literature for additional perspectives.

ADULT ATTACHMENT: THEORETICAL ISSUES

Drawing on ideas from cognitive psychology, in particular, the work of Craik (1943) and Piaget (1952), Bowlby (1969/1982, 1973) hypothesized that individuals develop an "internal working model" (IWM) of the world. Bowlby's conceptualization of the IWM included complementary models of the self and others, the acceptability of the self and the availability/responsiveness of the attachment figures (Bowlby, 1973). Such models would operate automatically, without the need for conscious appraisal, guiding behavior in relationships with parents and influencing expectations, strategies, and behavior in later relationships (Bretherton, 1985).

Revision of Representations

Bowlby assumed that attachment representations would tend to be relatively stable because of (1) the tendency to assimilate experience to existing schemas; (2) the substantial base of experience underpinning IWMs; and (3) the stabilizing influence of relationship partners, their thoughts, reactions, and behaviors, and their interpretations of the individual and the relationship (Bretherton & Munholland, 1999). Nonetheless, he used the term *working* models to indicate that they remain open to revision in light of significant attachment-related experiences. In childhood, this would ordinarily mean change in the quality of the attachment relationship (Bowlby, 1973).

Developmental advances in cognitive sophistication can lead to remapping and elaboration of early relationship experiences. In addition, beginning in adolescence and early adulthood, experience in committed relationships can be a catalyst to change by illustrating (or requiring) new ways of working in relationships. Such change often enriches a person's understanding and attachment-related competence (Bowlby, 1973; Crowell, Treboux, & Waters, 2002; Oppenheim & Waters, 1995; Owens et al., 1995; Treboux, Crowell, & Waters, 2004).

Defensive Processes

Despite this openness to change and the fact that attachment representations tend toward greater coherence over time, Bowlby (1979, 1980) recognized that defensive processes can limit the prospects for change. Individuals can selectively exclude available information to consider more salient and/or less distressing experiences, both in the external world and internally. Thus, Bowlby argued that chronic distressing, anxiety-provoking experiences in a close relationship can divert attention and distort perception in ways that limit the "updating" of IWMs and render the attachment system less effective. The alerting and activation of the attachment system, and the ensuing thoughts, feelings, and behaviors, would be limiting or misregulated. In Bowlby's experience, young children seemed especially vulnerable to the effects of defensive exclusion, perhaps because of their limited cognitive abilities and the fact that so many of the obstacles they encounter are experienced as attachment related or dealt with through attachment behavior.

Over time, defensive exclusion can cause attachment representations to become unintegrated or incoherent—the same individual hosting a conscious and acceptable IWM based on distorted or selected information, and a relatively inaccessible model based on actual but unacceptable or unassimilable experiences (Bowlby, 1973, 1979; Main, 1991, 2000). These models would not be coordinated and, indeed, would be separately recollected (Bretherton, 1990; Bretherton & Munholland, 1999; Schank, 1982; Schank & Abelson, 1977).

The IWM concept has taken attachment theory considerably beyond early behavioral control system models and opened the door to a rich lifespan perspective on the attachment behavior system. Without this, it would be difficult to understand developmental changes in the expression of attachment and its enduring influence in and across relationships and as a system that regulates affect and cognition, as well as behavior. Bowlby would have valued, and current attachment theorists need to master, advances in cognitive psychology relevant to how early experiences are represented in the mind. Although such work did not play a major role in the development of the AAI, it is likely the key to understand links between attachment-related experiences and autobiographical narratives such as the AAI.

USING NARRATIVES TO ASSESS ATTACHMENT REPRESENTATIONS

In infancy, overt behavior is a reliable sign of activation in the attachment system. Not so in adults, whose attachment system is less closely linked to overt behavior. This necessitates alternative assessment strategies.

The use of narrative to assess attachment is based on the idea that "mental processes vary as distinctively as do behavioral processes" (Main et al., 1985, p. 78), and that language is the better indicator for adult assessment. Moreover, it is theoretically grounded, Bowlby's ideas about IMWs having played an important role in the design of the interview questions and the scoring system (Main et al., 1985). Key attachment theory postulates that influenced the development of the AAI system include the following:

1. Infants develop models that guide behavior in attachment relationships in the first year of life that are elaborated over time (Fonagy, Gergely, Jurist, & Target, 2002; Main et al., 1985).

2. Working models are based on repeated attachment-relevant experiences in the infant's daily life with the caregiver. The repetitive and consistent nature of the experiences are encoded as in memory as "generalized event representations" (Main et al., 1985, p. 76), as is any kind of experience that is repeatedly experienced (e.g., bedtime rituals, mealtime routines). As such, it has been hypothesized that part of the underlying structure of the attachment working model is script-like in nature (Bretherton, 1985, 1990; Main et al., 1985; Waters & Rodrigues-Doolabh, 2001).

3. IWMs operate at least partially outside of conscious awareness. The highly repetitive and frequent nature of attachment-related experiences in infancy and the associated script-like aspect of the representations means that they are "overlearned" and operate automatically. They are not so much "unconscious" processes, but rather processes that typically are not purposefully considered. Furthermore, to the extent that they are script-like, their conscious explication requires a real base of experience and knowledge that may be lacking in certain forms of insecure attachment.

4. The IWM provides guidelines for behavior, attention, and the affective appraisal of experience. It is a behavioral guide: If *x* event occurs, then a series of predictable steps should follow from it. The activation of attachment behavior is triggered by an emotional alerting or arousal, and in infancy many internal and external events or stimuli result in the expression of attachment behavior. With age, competence, experience, and input from the attachment figure(s), appraisal elements become more differentiated.

5. Autobiographical memories and personal narrative are powerful organizers of experience over time and with respect to causation. Thus, IWMs are not considered simply templates or scripts, behavioral guides, and/or emotional appraisal systems, but are processes that serve to "obtain or to limit access to information" (Main et al., 1985, p. 77; Main, 1991, 2000). Experience itself is attended to, understood, interpreted, and given meaning through the representational frame.

6. Formal operational thought allows the individual to observe and assess a given relationship system; hence, the model of the relationship can be altered without an actual change in the relationship. Such processes are associated with self-reflection and the understanding of other people's mind states as distinct from one's own (Fonagy et al., 2002). With respect to the AAI, this process is understood as the means by which adults who had "insecure" attachment experiences in childhood, but who are believable, balanced, and coherent regarding attachment in interview, are classified as secure.

7. The scoring system strongly reflects Bowlby's ideas about secondary strategies, defensive processes, and incompatible models.

THE AAI

The AAI consists of 20 autobiographical questions presented in a strategic order (see Table 9.1). The questions focus on the parent–child relationship under age 14 under the assumption that (1) younger children experience a greater frequency and intensity of attachment experiences that underpin the IWM, and (2) the parent–adolescent relationship has greater variability, and potentially more conflict, thus making identification of attachment patterns more challenging. Some of the questions have follow-up components, and

TABLE 9.1. Topics Discussed in the Adult Attachment Interview
Introduction
1. Family Background
Activating the Attachment System
2. Childhood Relationship with Parents 3. Adjectives for Childhood Relationship with Mother 4. Adjectives for Childhood Relationship with Father 5. Closer Parent?
Memory of Attachment Experiences
6. Reactions to Being Upset, Ill, and Injured 7. Experiences of Separation from Parents 8. Feelings of Being Rejected by Parents 9. Experiences of Being Threatened by Parents
Assessment of Experiences and Their Impact
10. Impact of Early Experience on Adult Personality 11. Understanding of Parents' Behavior
Other Key Experiences
12. Other Significant Adults 13. Losses of Important People 14. Traumatic Experiences—Abuse
Relationships over Time
15. Changes over Time in Relationship with Parents 16. Current Relationship with Parents
Being a Parent and What It Means (if applicable)
17. Relationship with Own Children 18. Three Wishes for Own Children 19. Important Lessons Learned from Parents 20. Important Lessons to Be Learned by Own Children

interviewers are trained to prompt strategically for important scoring-related information.

The first question (Q1) focuses on family background, where the individual grew up, the composition of the family, the occupations of the parents, and access to and relationships with extended family and other close individuals. This familiar material provides important context for later questions. It also provides a baseline against which to compare language use when discussing more attachment-relevant or difficult material. (See the "Coherence of Mind" and "Special Note on Clinical Samples" sections below.)

The interviewer then asks (Q2) the adult for his or her overview of the relationship with parents in childhood and for five adjectives describing his or her relationships with the mother (Q3), the father (Q4), and/or other primary attachment figures in childhood. These questions are intended to "surprise the unconscious," in the sense that they are unusual, provocative, and unexpected challenges to the attachment system. This provides useful clues as to the individual's comfort with attachment-related topics. It is also a first step toward activating the person's primary attachment strategy. The interviewee is then asked to illustrate each adjective by recalling a relevant childhood experience or interaction. The relationship between the generic (semantic) memories reflected in the adjectives and the specific (episodic) memories provided as illustrations reveals a great deal about the coherence and integration of underlying attachment representations. In addition to the logical coherence of the interviewee's answers, their comfort, flexibility, and consistency in moving back and forth between overarching assessments (adjectives) and specific events can be an important factor in determining their ultimate classification. Wrapping up this section, the interviewer asks about which parent the individual felt closer to in childhood (Q5) and why he or she felt that way.

The interviewer then inquires about childhood experiences with parents in which the attachment system is activated (upset,[1] injury, illness [Q6], and separations from parents [Q7], whether they had ever felt rejected [Q8] or threatened by their parents [Q9] in childhood). As in the Strange Situation's repeated separations, cycling through one source of distress and then another escalates the degree of attachment-related challenge, seeking further to activate the interviewee's primary attachment strategy. As in the adjective questions, coders examine comfort, consistency, and believability across the several responses for clues about the coherence and integration of the underlying attachment representation. And analogous again to the Strange Situation, how the upsetting events are resolved, and the manner, clarity, and completeness

[1]Following as it does questions about interviewees' early relationships with their parents, interviewees may respond to this question as if it asks about having been upset by the parents. They may say they went to their rooms or wanted to be alone. This interpretation and the seemingly avoidant response are understandable. However, parents as a source of upset is not what is intended by the question, and interviewers and scorers should be aware of this "bug" in what is otherwise a very elegantly formulated interview.

with which the resolutions are described, tell a great deal about the person's access to organized attachment responses.

The interview then moves from interviewees discussing specific attachment-related events to questions about the meanings they attach to them. Interviewees are asked (Q10) how experiences with their parents in childhood have influenced the development of their adult personality, and if applicable, their behavior as parents. They are also asked (Q11) about their views on why their parents acted as they did. They are asked about other adults who may have been important in their lives, especially adults who may have had a caregiving role (Q12).

The adults are next asked whether they have experienced the loss of important figures in their lives (Q13) and about experiences that they consider to have been abusive (Q14). If an interviewee reports such experiences, the responses are used to assess whether the individual is disorganized and unresolved about the experiences. The analogy here is to the disorganized and fearful behavior sometimes observed in the Strange Situation.

Questions to interviewees about changes in the relationship with the parents in adolescence (Q15) and about their current relationship to their parents (Q16) challenge interviewees to examine the consistency and/or evolution of their experiences and personal narrative. There is an underlying assumption in the scoring that the parent–child relationship develops and changes as children grow, and also that individuals may see events differently as adults than they did as children. Thus, this section may elicit metacognitive monitoring by the adult (see below).

The interview ends (Q17–Q20) with questions about hopes for the individuals' children, what they feel is the most important thing learned from their childhood experiences with their parents, and what they hope their own child(ren) will learn from them. These questions again call on the adults to distill and summarize ideas that they have presented across the interview, and again offer the coder the opportunity to examine the degree to which there is integration/coordination of ideas regarding attachment. They also restore the individual to the present and allow for a smooth exit to the interview.[2]

Interviewing

The AAI covers deeply personal topics that most adults do not discuss casually. Thus, the interviewer is more than someone who asks a list of questions. The act of explaining significant childhood experiences *to another person* is key to eliciting the characteristic discourse patterns on which scoring and classification are based. There is an *Interviewer's Guide* to the AAI, that

[2]Although the AAI has been used for over 20 years (over 10,000 interviews reported in the literature), there is no recorded instance of ill effects from participating in the interview, although participants may certainly become distressed in responding to some of the questions. The interview is routinely approved without revision by university institutional review boards.

in addition to presenting the items, explains the intent of each question and how the interviewer should respond in various situations (George, Kaplan, & Main, 1985). Training typically requires several practice interviews, which are audiotaped and discussed with a trainer.

The challenge for the interviewer is to present the questions clearly and patiently, to understand what kind of information scorers require, and to allow interviewees to respond in their own style. Probing for content and asking follow-up questions that can assist scorers is an acquired skill. Probing cannot be allowed to shape the interviewee's narrative. Nor can the interviewer allow him- or herself to become distracted or caught up in the interviewee's narrative. Yet it is critical that interviewees feel they are revealing their story to an interested listener, and that the interviewer listen and maintain a sense of the situation and what is being said. If the questions are too rote, interviewees understandably become annoyed, the interview takes on a stilted quality, and the depth and scorability of the interview is diminished.

For some interviewers (and some interviewees), the concentrated, almost relentless format of the interview at times, especially in the section covering loss, presents particular difficulties. It is common to hear accounts of loss, abuse, rejection, anger, sadness, and fear. Interviewees are usually very, almost surprisingly, cooperative, but occasionally one will react with hostility to the questions. Whatever the situation, the interviewer must proceed without overreacting or cutting off the flow of the interview because of his or her own discomfort. Nonetheless, many participants appreciate the opportunity to share their past experiences. Indeed, in some cases, these experiences may be more difficult for the interviewer to hear than for the participant to share. For this reason, it is often useful, although not a requirement, for interviewers to have some clinical background or be trained as an AAI coder. It is also helpful to have an interview trainer randomly check audiotapes and to be available to interviewers who have questions or have been distressed by a particular interview experience.

The most effective interview strikes a delicate balance between inquiring and letting people tell their own story as they understand it, motivated by an interested and nonjudgmental listener. Table 9.2 summarizes important skills for maximizing the quality of AAI interviews.

Transcription

The AAI cannot be scored from a video or audio record, or from the interviewer's recall (were he or she a trained coder). Scoring requires a verbatim transcript that can be carefully examined for expressed and for unintended qualities of discourse and signs of incoherence and inconsistency. It is also very helpful to include both page numbers and line numbers for easy reference during and after scoring. Because the scoring system leans heavily on cognitive and linguistic criteria, typists should not insert information about the individual's emotional expression during the interview. To ensure accurate

TABLE 9.2. Conducting the Interview: Some Do's and Don'ts

It is important to . . .

- Listen with interest
- Pay attention to what the interviewee is telling you
- Ask all the questions
- Probe only as much as indicated in the interviewing manual
- Acknowledge when the interviewee has already partly or mostly answered a question earlier in the interview, and ask if he or she wants to add anything to what he or she has already said
- Listen to your interviews
- Tell a senior person if you have found an interview upsetting

It is important* not *to . . .

- Go off topic
- Avoid questions that make you uncomfortable
- Get so focused on the next question that you forget to listen and respond to what the interviewee says
- Respond negatively to interviewee challenges (e.g., "What do you mean?"; "What a stupid question!"), but answer questions as best you can
- "Help" the interviewee with your own interpretation

transcription, it is important to have someone (preferably the interviewer and preferably promptly) check the initial transcription against the audiotape. Scoring is then undertaken using the corrected transcript.

Technically, scoring and classification comprise an assessment of the *transcript,* a particular narrative on a particular topic at a particular time, not of the individual (Main & Goldwyn, 1998; Main et al., 1985). Accordingly, accurate scoring depends on accurate transcription—including a verbatim record of language, phrasing, identification of "ums" and "ers," and an indication (with ellipses) of the duration of pauses. Unfortunately, typists have a tendency to automatically "correct" language to make more sense, or they simply hear what would be more expectable. This can create significant problems for coders, who are alert to inconsistencies and hoping to take advantage of convergent evidence from different parts of the interview.

CODING THE AAI

Rationale Underlying AAI Scoring

The original AAI scoring system (Main & Goldwyn, 1998) was developed by examining interviews of 44 parents whose infants' Strange Situation (SS) classifications were known (Hesse, 1999; Main & Goldwyn, 1998). Mary

Main and Ruth Goldwyn identified qualities of content and discourse that distinguished parents of children with differing SS classifications. Thus, the scoring system was expressly developed to capture features of the attachment system also tapped by the SS. It is important to note that the coding of the AAI was not solely "pattern-focused," but that it identified the ability of the individual to use the attachment figure as a secure base. In addition, the scoring very much follows on Bowlby's hypotheses regarding IWMs, including close attention to defensive cognitive processes. The system has been refined and expanded over the past 20 years, but it continues to have this focus.

The transcript of the AAI is a sample of verbal behavior from which we infer something about the adequacy and effectiveness of the underlying attachment representation. A coherent, clear, well-supported narrative is considered a reflection of an adaptive, flexible, comprehensive IWM. A disorganized, limited, unsupported, stereotypical, illogical, and/or contradictory narrative reflects an inflexible, narrow, uninformed and/or distorted model of attachment.

Scoring involves a series of assessments about the coherence and quality of the narrative based on the coder's judgments about the (1) likely nature of interviewees' early experience, and (2) their state of mind or subjective stance about their experiences. Coherence is judged with respect to Grice's maxims of quality, quantity, relevance, and manner (Main, Goldwyn, & Hesse, 2003). A number of scales are used to characterize the nature of likely experience, as well as states of mind. These ratings ensure close reading of the transcript. Although scoring pays considerable attention to detail, the ultimate strategy is to focus on coherence and consistency across the whole transcript and on the convergence of evidence rather than single oddities. Thus, consistency of scale scores in the two broad domains, as well as with overarching prototypical descriptions, aims the coder toward a classification. Identification of patterns or classification of the AAI is useful in helping the coder and the researcher in understanding the coherence and meaning of the transcript, but it is not theoretically necessary (Waters & Beauchaine, 2003). Secure versus insecure qualities can be dimensionalized.

Training

Learning to code the AAI requires significant commitment, as it is difficult, complex, and expensive in terms of both time and money. The training occurs at a 2-week-long intensive institute or "boot camp" conducted by Mary Main and Erik Hesse or one of a handful of qualified trainers. Prior to the training, the prospective coder is expected to interview at least one person and to be interviewed with the AAI. Training involves group sessions in the mornings and afternoons, with scoring homework in the evenings. To be an official AAI coder, the trainee must demonstrate high coding agreement with the trainers on several sets of transcripts following the training institute. The AAI is also expensive because of the labor-intensive interviewing, transcription, and scoring, including demonstration of agreement in each sample (optimally, there are two trained coders in a research laboratory, or one or two such coders are paid by the research team).

The Scoring System

Scoring is based on (1) the coder's assessment of the individual's childhood experiences with parents and (2) the language used in the interview. It is also based on the individual's (3) ability to give an integrated, believable account of experiences and their meaning, both within and across sections of the interview, in particular, autobiographical continuity and the degree of overlap between the semantic and episodic memories provided. Coding draws on scores assigned on two sets of scales, the Experience and the State of Mind scales, described below. After scale scores are assigned, the coder examines correspondence among the scales, the interview as a whole, and prototypic descriptions of the major classifications. It is through these processes that a final classification is obtained.

All of the scales use 9 points. A score of 1 indicates the characteristic is not present, and a score between 5 and 9 indicates a significant level for each characteristic. There are some interviews that do not provide the coder with enough information to assign a score for certain scales. In these instances, the coder has two choices: (1) A tentative score may be given, in parentheses, as a "best guess," indicating that the characteristic being scored is present at least at that level, but may possibly be higher; or (2) a score of can't rate (CR) can be given. This rating can be given for experience scales when the coder finds the transcript so lacking in content regarding the domain in question that he or she is unable to render a score. This rating is not helpful in identifying type of insecurity, but it is frequently a sign of a notably incoherent, and therefore insecure, transcript.

The Experience Scales

These scales describe parental behavior and are rated separately for the mother and father. If the interviewee identifies a parenting role for other caregivers, those individuals are scored as well. The scales are used to rate the degree to which parents demonstrated loving, supportive behavior, demanded premature independence in the child (rejection), engaged in involving, role-reversing behavior, and pressed the child to achieve and/or neglected the child. Scale scores are based on direct and indirect evidence provided in the interview for these parental behaviors, *not on the opinion expressed by the interviewee.* The ratings of these behaviors by the coder are compared with the assessment provided by the interviewee, and thus contribute to identifying particular discourse styles, strategies, and defensive processes employed by the individual.

The ratings of experience are inferred, being based on retrospective accounts and taking into account discourse style. As such, the interview cannot be used as a proxy for childhood attachment status or a source of accurate biographical information.

Loving Behavior is scored from descriptions of supportive, caring behavior directed to the individual in childhood, and take into account the various ways in which a parent can be scored as "unloving," that is, rejecting, neglecting, and so forth. As a parent can be unloving in ways other than those described by the specific experience rating scales (e.g., being abusive), the Loving scale incorporates this information as well. The emphasis is on loving behavior from an attachment perspective; thus, descriptions of affection, caring, concern, physical and emotional comforting, and support of the child's development as an individual are sought. Memories of the parents being available and responsive when the child was distressed, ill, or injured are especially important. Positive parental behaviors such as material generosity (e.g., buying gifts, sending the child to expensive summer camps), joking with the child, going on vacations together, and transporting them to activities, carry little weight in the scoring of loving behavior, as they are not considered secure base behaviors. Indeed, if they are the *only* positive parental behaviors described, this inclines the coder to consider whether idealization (see the section on the State of Mind scale) is being used as a strategy. A high score on the Loving scale is strongly associated with a secure and coherence stance in the interview.

Scoring of *Rejecting Behavior* is based on parental behaviors of avoiding or turning away the child's attachment needs or approaches. It does not imply abusive behavior or dislike; rather, it refers to minimizing the child's needs and sometimes distance and coldness. The descriptions may give direct evidence of such experiences ("We weren't one of those huggy families") or the behavior may be inferred indirectly through the lack of evidence for availability, responsiveness, and support. The experiences coded on this scale are often associated with an avoidant, dismissing stance in the interview, characterized by idealization and lack of recall, or even derogation.

The *Involving, Role-Reversing, Preoccupying Behavior* scale captures the degree to which a parent seems to have needed the child, or was confused and/or incompetent enough to have trouble caring for the child. At the mid- to high range of the behavior, the descriptions indicate the parent used guilt to engage the child, had a true need of the child's care and attention, and/or used other forms of role reversal, such as spousification. Descriptions of involving behaviors by the parent are often associated with a discourse style that is actively angry or passive and confused.

The *Neglecting Behavior* scale addresses the extent to which the parent ignored the child or was unable/unwilling to care for his or her needs. To be scored as neglecting, the parent must have had the opportunity to be responsive and engaged but chose to be involved with other activities, such as sleeping, watching television, or frequent evenings out, and so forth.

The last inferred Experience scale is the *Pressure to Achieve* scale, which assesses the degree to which the parent pushed the child to be successful in academic or other domains, or to take an adult role in the family. Of particular importance in rating this behavior is the question of whether the relationship seems to be based around the child's achievement and the extent to which the child's well-being may be ignored at the expense of parental drive. This scale, like the Neglecting Behavior scale, is not closely connected to a particular defensive strategy or classification.

The State of Mind Scales

The State of Mind scales assess current discourse style and particular forms of incoherence that indicate strategic adaptations or defensive processes. These include idealization, insistence on lack of recall, active anger, derogation, fear of loss, and passivity of speech. Several of these strategies directly parallel the behavioral strategies observed in the SS. For example, idealization is comparable to the infant avoidance, as the interviewee presents a positive overview of the parent while apparently ignoring or dismissing the significance of the parent's actual behavior or its emotional impart. Active anger expressed toward the parent in the AAI is comparable to an infant's angry resistant behavior in the SS, and passive speech to the passive behavior of the helplessly passive (C2) infant.

IDEALIZATION

This scale assesses the difference between the individual's positive presentation of the parent or attachment-relevant events and the actual evidence that is provided for such an overview. Thus, the highly idealizing transcript presents an "image" of a normal or even wonderful parent, with little supporting evidence or even reports that outright contradict such a description. In some cases, in the midrange of idealization, the discrepancy between the overview and the reported experience is not extreme, and the individual may have some evidence for positive parental behavior and/or may acknowledge some negative behavior on the part of the parent. In this instance, the individual makes statements about negative experiences being "normal" or that the behavior of the parent or the impact of the experience is not important or meaningful. Idealization is often accompanied by minimal descriptions of events, and tends to violate Grice's maxims of quantity and quality in particular. Idealization is scored with respect to each parent.

Idealization can be seen in the following examples: The individual uses the highly positive adjectives (e.g., *loving, caring, supportive, honest*) to describe the relationship with his father. When asked for a specific memory that would capture the loving and caring aspects of the relationship, the answers fail to support the positive adjective:

ADULT: Well, he was just there all the time, day in and day out, not matter which way you cut it. Always around. . . . No matter which way you cut it, he was just there, just a regular dad.

INTERVIEWER: What about caring?

ADULT: Just the same, always there. He was really caring. I remember one time my friend was over and he lied and told my dad that I had cheated on Monopoly when I really hadn't. My dad got really mad and sent my friend home and made me go to bed without dinner. He was a typical dad. . . . Just cared so much about what was best for me and that I would do the right thing.

Idealization is often associated with statements that negative experiences are deserved and ultimately beneficial:

ADULT: One time my dad was angry at me and he took out a belt and started hitting me. He must have hit me 20 times on my back and I couldn't walk or sleep for a few days.

INTERVIEWER: Why was he angry?

ADULT: I don't know, I'm sure I deserved it, probably did some stupid thing.

INTERVIEWER: (*Subsequently asks about the effects of such childhood experiences.*)

ADULT: They made me strong and independent. They made me a better person. My parents spoiled me rotten.

INSISTENCE ON INABILITY TO RECALL

This discourse pattern is often associated with idealization. For this scale, the coder rates the frequency the individual states that he or she cannot remember, insistence that he or she cannot remember, and his or her use of this kind of statement to stop further questioning. An example of lack of recall is seen when the interviewer queries.

INTERVIEWER: You mentioned that your relationship with your father was "loving." Can you think of a specific memory or incident from childhood to illustrate how your relationship with him was "loving"?

ADULT: I can't remember.

INTERVIEWER: Take your time.

ADULT: It was all the time, just always happening. Nothing comes to mind.

DEROGATION OF ATTACHMENT

This scale assesses the cold, sharp, and contemptuous dismissal of attachment figures and/or attachment experiences, either directly experienced or witnessed. Derogation is expressed in brief statements about people or events being "foolish, laughable, or not worth the time" (Main, Goldwyn, & Hesse, 2003, p. 82). In its mild form, derogation is often humorous, but in its more intense forms, the individual's statements have a nasty, biting, sarcastic tone. Derogation is scored with respect to each parent, and with respect to attachment overall. An example of derogation can be seen in this brief response to an interviewer asking,

> INTERVIEWER: Did the loss of your mother have an impact on your adult personality?
>
> ADULT: My mother? That witch? Meant nothing to me.

FEAR OF LOSS OF THE CHILD THROUGH DEATH

This scale describes a discourse pattern discovered to be associated with infant avoidance in the course of developing the coding system. It can only be scored from the individual's discussion of his or her own child. The scale is used to rate the expressed fear that the child may die. If this concern is not expressed, a score is not given. However, in the event the individual expresses this anxiety, a low score is given if the individual can clearly connect this fear to current or previous experience, such as having a very ill child or a close connection to a child that did die. The highest scores are given when there is no obvious link to previous experience and the individual indicates that the fear is impacting his or her parenting behavior:

> ADULT: I never let her ride in a car with anyone else, because I am sure she will die in an accident and I won't be there.

INVOLVING AND PREOCCUPYING ANGER

Discourse of this type parallels the angry, resistant behavior observed in anxious–resistant (C1) infants in the SS. The anger in the interview is active and intense in its expression, with little to no self-monitoring, and as such, differs from cold, controlled derogation or *intentional* and clear descriptions of having been or being angry. In addition to violating Grice's maxims of relevance and manner, the individual often says too much, thus violating the maxim of quantity. Main, Goldwyn, and Hesse (2003, pp. 95–100) identify nine ways in which involving anger is manifested, including run-on sentences and paragraphs that identify an attachment figure's faults or offenses, quotations without preface such that the individual appears to be lost in a conversation or argument with the parent, exaggerative language, and attempts to engage the interviewer into agreeing with his or her viewpoint and to elicit common ground with the interviewer. As with idealization and derogation, involving anger is scored with respect to each parent.

An example of involving anger that includes exaggeration, run-on statements, and quotations without preface follows:

INTERVIEWER: Can you think of a specific memory that would illustrate your choice of the word *controlling* to describe the relationship with your mother?

ADULT: I can only think of about a million. . . . She was always nagging, nagging at me, beating on me, telling me what she wanted. Blah, blah, blah, blah, blah, do this, do that, clean the dishes, put the kids to bed, take out the garbage, cook the dinner. She never let up; she was always, always nagging at me. Stop yelling at me—can't you take care of your own kids? Can't you let me be? What do you want from me?

PASSIVITY OF DISCOURSE

This discourse pattern parallels the passive, helpless behavior that characterizes the C2 anxious–resistant infant in the SS. There are a number of ways in which passivity can be expressed in the interview, but all indicate a helpless, confused, vague, even lost, position with respect to attachment and attachment figures. Unlike the apparently deliberate minimal response that may characterize a dismissing state of mind, the limited discourse of passivity appears unintentional. The tone is often overtly positive, yet it has an ominous underlying quality. The interview is examined for seven forms of passivity that include the use of nonsense words or vague expressions ("kind of a thing") to fill in for "real" ideas, wandering into irrelevant topics or difficulty expressing meaning, the use of childish language, failing to complete sentences/thoughts, and/or slips into confusion between the self and the parent. Transcripts that are given high ratings on passivity are very difficult to follow, and it can be very challenging, if not impossible, to deduce the experiences of the individual from the content of the transcript. An example of passive speech that includes a positive but ominous tone, childish speech, nonsense words and unfinished sentences, can be seen in the response to the following query:

INTERVIEWER: I'd like you to give me a general description of your childhood relationship with your parents.

ADULT: Oh, it was lovely. So happy, so pretty, with flowers and oh. . . . stuff like that . . . all around . . . sometimes we sang. . . . da da da da da da. She was so. . . . I didn't mean to. . . . and mommy told me I was the goodest girl, and. . . . That.

METACOGNITIVE MONITORING

This scale assesses monitoring and awareness discourse typically manifested in three ways. There may be a recognition of "appearance–reality distinction," expressed awareness of "representational diversity," and/or identification of "representational change." This scale is intended to be associated with security, but it is still a "work in progress."

Appearance–reality distinction is the idea that things are not always as they appear to be. In expressing this form of awareness, an individual might comment that although his or her parent's behavior on a particular occasion might have appeared harsh or unloving, it is difficult to understand what forces may have motivated or even compelled such behavior at the time it was happening. Representational diversity is the idea that the same event or experience may be seen, experienced, or understood differently by different people, an idea closely related to mentalization (Fonagy et al., 2002). Representational change is the idea that present understanding of experience may be quite different from the individual's past views. An individual might comment that with greater experience he or she has achieved a more in-depth and complex understanding of past events. This increased awareness does not diminish the importance or validity of the childhood perspective.

UNRESOLVED OR DISORGANIZED STATES OF MIND

Two scales are used to identity unresolved or disorganized states of mind that are associated with the traumatic attachment experiences of loss and abuse. In each case, the individual must identify that he or she has had the experience before a score can be given on the scale. The *Unresolved State of Mind with Respect to Loss* scale captures discourse regarding the death(s) of close others that is disorganized and disoriented, and the *Unresolved State of Mind with Respect to Abuse* scale captures similar discourse regarding experiences of abuse and abusers. Even when the events described are in the past, the disorganization can give the impression that the event was recent. Indeed, recent traumatic events should be coded with caution, as some disorganization is normal in such situations. There are several ways in which disorganized and disoriented language is manifested, but they all show "lapses in the monitoring of reasoning or discourse" (Main, Goldwyn, & Hesse, 2003, p. 131).

Lapses in reasoning regarding death include indications of the belief that the deceased is not really dead or that simple, unrelated acts may have caused the death. A lapse in reasoning regarding abuse can include denial of the abuse (after stating it happened) and/or feelings that it was deserved. Such lapses also include psychologically confused statements that suggest impossible mental actions used to cope with the trauma.

Lapses in monitoring of discourse include confusion about when the event occurred, where it occurred, or confusion between self and the deceased or abuser. They may also include sudden changes in topic or, in the case of loss, the use of flowery, poetic language in describing the events surrounding the loss or the deceased individual. Extreme behavioral reactions in response to loss are also considered in the scoring, especially suicidal reactions or serious decline in functioning. Such lapses in reasoning and monitoring can be seen in the following excerpts:

INTERVIEWER: Have your feelings about your grandmother's death changed over time [occurred 6 years ago]?

ADULT: Well, I'm still upset about it; I can't get over the fact that she is dead.

INTERVIEWER: Were you able to attend the funeral?

ADULT: She didn't want one. She had her body cremated and she wants a spring service around her tombstone . . . in the spring.

INTERVIEWER: Did this loss have any effect on your adult personality?

ADULT: Yes, 'cause now I am really, really depressed and—constantly think about what I could do to see my grandma again and be with my grandma.

COHERENCE

The secure versus insecure dimension assessed with the AAI maps most directly onto attachment theory (Ainsworth, Blehar, Waters, & Wall, 1978/2015; Bowlby, 1969/1982). The *Coherence of Transcript* score is the strongest correlate of adult attachment security and the strongest predictor of the individual's infant's attachment security. It is often used in data analysis as a proxy for security.

First, high coherence means that scores on the previously discussed scales that indicate defensive or confused discourse, such as idealization, derogation, passivity, involving anger, and unresolved discourse, are low. The Coherence of Transcript score includes the assessments of these qualities of discourse. Thus, by definition, an individual cannot be highly coherent if he or she employs one or more forms of specific rated incoherence (e.g., idealization, active anger) as described earlier.

Second, a highly coherent narrative demonstrates consistency, clarity, and collaboration with the interview process. This concept of coherence is based on Grice's maxims regarding discourse (Main, 2000). The maxims are quality, quantity, relevance, and manner.

1. Quality reflects the believability of the discourse; that it is without contradictions or illogical conclusions.
2. Quantity reflects the amount of information given, that there is enough, but not too much, given to understand the narrative.
3. Relevance indicates that the individual answers the questions that are asked of him or her.
4. Manner is the use of orderly, clear, free-flowing language rather than jargon, canned speech, or nonsense words.

Coherence is illustrated in the following interview excerpt, in the consistency between the adjective and the ready access to memories of availability and support, and in the clear, direct, and cooperative response to the question.

Note that the concept of coherence is not synonymous with sophisticated or highly articulate language. Coherence discourse often anticipates later AAI questions, as in this case when the adult spontaneously brings up an example of being upset.

> INTERVIEWER: Can you think of a specific memory or incident to illustrate why you chose loving to describe your childhood relationship with your mother?
>
> ADULT: Oh, wow! There are so many things! She read to me every night and tucked me in. She always took really good care of me when I was sick. . . . Let me think of a specific incident. . . . One time I came home from school and I was so upset, I was crying. I must have been about 9 years old. She hugged me and sat down with me on the couch, got me tissues, and just got the whole story out of me. (*Tells of getting in trouble with teacher unfairly.*) I felt so much better after I'd told her and she believed me, and she said she would call my teacher and let her know what had really happened.

COHERENCE OF MIND

The Coherence of Mind scale often corresponds to the Coherence of Transcript score, and in such cases does not add to the overall scoring. However, it can be very useful in particular situations to integrate specific phenomena into the classification procedure. First, it allows the rater to code unusual beliefs that contradict or challenge basic tenets of attachment theory but are not internally inconsistent within the interview. Most commonly the Coherence of Mind scale is useful in understanding and coding individuals who may have acquired unusual beliefs (e.g., belief in ghosts, possession, omens) in the context of traumatic experiences, such as loss or abuse. In such cases, it is associated with Unresolved status. In such situations, the Coherence of Mind score can be significantly lower than the Coherence of Transcript score.

The scale also allows the coder to compensate for a discourse presentation or problem that is not related to attachment. In this case, the Coherence of Mind score may be higher than the Coherence of Transcript score. Indeed, particular care must be taken in scoring transcripts of individuals who are not native English speakers, or those who manifest a pervasive dysfluency that may be related to a speech and language disorder rather than reflecting a defensive process. Discourse difficulties that are unrelated to attachment will present themselves throughout the transcript, regardless of the topic being discussed, whereas attachment-related incoherence emerges most strongly in aspects of the interview that most strongly challenge the attachment system, such as the parental adjective section and the upset, illness questions. Similarly, unresolved discourse patterns are most obvious in the discussion of loss and abuse, and tend to be absent from discussions of other topics.

SPECIAL NOTE ON CLINICAL SAMPLES

Clinical samples can be especially challenging to the coder, as mental illnesses often broadly impact on discourse style (e.g., depression, attention-deficit/hyperactivity disorder [ADHD], or psychosis) in ways that are not specifically related to attachment. These disorders can reduce coherence overall, especially by impacting on the maxims of quantity (e.g., depression), manner (e.g., psychosis), and relevance (e.g., ADHD). The Coherence of Mind scale provides the opportunity to carefully consider this possibility. While, clearly, it makes sense that clinical samples do have a higher proportion of transcripts classified as insecure, failure to consider the impact of mental illness and language disabilities on discourse patterns will lead to "false positives," that is, artificially elevate the percentage of insecure transcripts.

AAI Classifications

After scale scores are obtained, the coder proceeds to assigning a major classification to the transcript, usually secure, dismissing, or preoccupied. In some specific circumstances, the classification of "can't classify" (CC) is assigned rather than one of the three major classifications. The determination of whether the transcript should be additionally classified as unresolved is also made. The relations among scale scores, classifications, and subclassifications are presented in Figure 9.1.

There are abbreviations for the classifications: The major infant classification designations are A (avoidant), B (secure), and C (resistant), and the major adult classifications are Ds (dismissing), E (enmeshed or preoccupied), and F (autonomous/secure). The infant "disorganized" classification is associated with the unresolved (U) classification in an adult.

A WORD ABOUT LABELS

The scale scores and classifications have labels that describe processes within the context of the attachment system. All too often, these labels have been confused or linked with broad personality traits; security equated with trait-like sociability, affection, honesty; dismissing "translated" to mean hostile, unfriendly, and antisocial; and preoccupation confused with overt anxiety and neediness. None of these interpretations is intended by the AAI classifications. Problems also arise from the fact that labels derived from the AAI classification system have been adopted as titles for widely used self-report measures. It cannot be overemphasized that these measures are rarely correlated more than .30, and never strongly enough to suggest that they measure the same constructs or that the measures are interchangeable. Moreover, they have very different patterns of correlates (e.g., Simpson, Rholes, Orina, & Grich, 2002; Waters, Crowell, Elliot, Corcoran, & Treboux, 2002). Thus, the measures should not be viewed as interchangeable in research or in literature reviews.

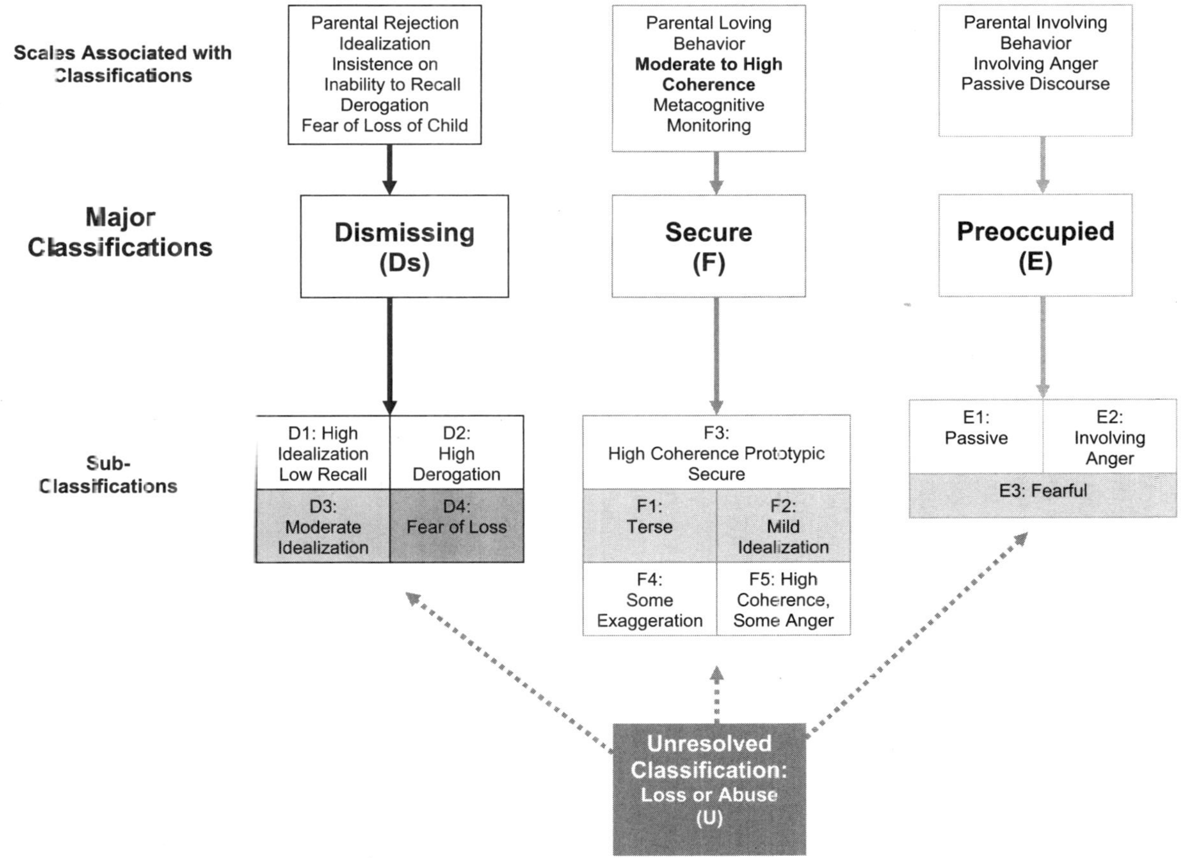

FIGURE 9.1. Schematic representation of the AAI classification system showing scales that are most related to major classifications, subclassifications, and similarities among subclassifications.

THE SECURE/AUTONOMOUS[3] CLASSIFICATION

Individuals classified as secure (F) present a balanced, flexible view of early relationships, value attachment relationships, and view attachment-related experiences as influential in their development. In parallel to the direct approach of the infant, the secure adult's approach to the interview is one of comfort and engagement with the topic. They are generally open, direct, and cooperative, regardless of how difficult the material is to discuss. If they decline to discuss a topic because they consider it too personal or emotionally painful, they are cooperative and straightforward about it. Their balanced view of experience is often apparent in an empathic discussion of the imperfections of the self and parents, presented with warmth, humor, lack of blame, and/or other attempts to understand behavior (evidence of mentalization). Individuals assigned to this classification are able to identify both positive and negative effects of experience on their development, and do not identify with or support negative parental behavior. Even if they do not engage in metacognitive monitoring, their self-awareness shows in their efforts to be clear and understood by their listener.

The "secure" transcript contains coherent, believable reports of parental behavior; simply put, the adult's summarizing descriptions (semantic memories) of the parenting he or she received matches the specific (episodic) memories given of parental behavior. The responses not only meet Grice's criteria of quality and quantity, but the discourse also fits the criteria for manner and relevance; thus, it is fresh and to the point. Scores on the Coherence scale are midrange (5) to high (9). Because security is inferred from coherence, *any kind of childhood experience* may be associated with being classified as secure, although, in most cases, there are clear and specific examples of loving behavior by the parents.

As shown in Figure 9.1, the scales typically associated with security are moderate to high coherence, moderate to high parental loving behavior, and metacognition. There are five subclassifications of the secure classification that are comparable to the four subclassifications of infant attachment in the SS. Thus, they range from those that have a more dismissing stance, with some tendency toward idealization, less access to memory, or derogation (F1 and F2 are comparable to B1 and B2) to those that are more preoccupied (F4, which corresponds to the B4 infant category, and F5). The prototypic secure classification is the F3 category. The F3, and interestingly, the F5 classifications correspond to the B3 infant classification in studies of the AAI and SS (Hesse, 1999).

[3]The term *autonomous* initially was intended to reflect flexibility of attention in attachment-relevant situations and the free-flowing ability to consider and discuss attachment experiences. Unfortunately, it carries an unintended, and potentially confusing, association with the idea of being independent. The term *autonomous* has largely fallen into disuse, and the classification is most often referred to simply as *secure*.

EARNED SECURITY

The term *earned security* has been used in adult attachment research to refer to those individuals who report parental behavior that is coded as unloving, yet have coherent transcripts and state of mind. Their attachment behavior with close others resembles that of "naturally" secure individuals, that is, those people whose parents are scored as loving and are high in coherence (Cohn, Cowan, Cowan, & Pearson, 1992; Cohn, Silver, Cowan, Cowan, & Pearson, 1992).

Subsequent to the identification of this pattern of scales scores, retrospective research suggested that this presentation is associated with depressive symptoms (Pearson, Cohn, Cowan, & Cowan, 1994). Indeed, in longitudinal research, Roisman, Padrón, Sroufe, and Egeland (2002) found that parent–child observations of children subsequently classified as "earned" secure in adulthood revealed their parents actually were behaviorally supportive and responsive, but that these adults had significant depressive symptoms in the intervening years. These findings clearly illustrate that the interviews do not represent actual experience but are reflections of current state of mind.

INSECURE CLASSIFICATIONS

In and of themselves, the insecure classifications are not pathological. They represent normal variations in attachment patterns in the general population. They are not traits or temperament patterns (see section "A Word about Labels"), and do not "explain" all behavioral responses; they should not be used to predict behavioral responses outside of the domain of attachment. For example, using the AAI to predict food choices or investment behavior is a costly way to study a domain that would be difficult to integrate into attachment theory were someone to report significant correlations. There is considerable evidence, however, that AAI insecurity is a risk factor for problems in relationships and relationship behavior, impaired adaptation to stress, and some forms of psychopathology (e.g., Allen et al., 2003; Cohn, Cowan, et al., 1992; Cohn, Silver, et al., 1992; Collins & Feeney, 2000; Collins & Read, 1990; Crowell, O'Connor, Wollmers, Sprafkin, & Rao, 1991; Crowell & Feldman, 1988; Crowell, Treboux, Gao, et al., 2002; Dykas, 2003; Fonagy, Steele, & Steele, 1991; Furman, Simon, Shaffer, & Bouchey, 2002; Goldberg, Gotowiec, & Simmons, 1995; Greenberg, 1999; Guttmann-Steinmetz, Cuva, Brockmeyer, & Crowell, 2005; Hesse, 1999; Kobak, Cole, Ferenz-Gillies, Fleming, & Gamble, 1993; Lyons-Ruth & Jacobvitz, 1999; Main et al., 1985; Paley et al., 2005; Posada, Waters, Crowell, & Lay, 1995; Roisman, Madsen, Hennighausen, Sroufe, & Collins, 2001; Simpson et al., 2002; Treboux et al., 2004; van IJzendoorn, 1995; Wampler, Shi, Nelson, & Kimball, 2003).

Insecure classifications are associated with incoherent accounts, which means that interviewees' broad assessments of experience are not matched by their actual descriptions of parental behavior (reflecting the maxim of poor quality in Grice's terms), and are consistent with Bowlby's hypotheses regarding defensive processes. Little evidence is provided for the parent serving as a secure base, and discourse, whether dismissing or preoccupied, mirrors the lack of exploration, inflexibility, and anxieties of insecure infants. The adult classifications reflect the secondary strategies used to manage the anxiety of having a parent who was significantly limited in his or her role as a secure base. Coherence scores fall below 5.

THE DISMISSING CLASSIFICATION

Adults classified as insecure-dismissing (Ds) seem uncomfortable with the topic of the interview, deny the impact of early attachment relationships on their personality development, have difficulty recalling specific events, and often idealize their experiences. The transcript has a distant, limited quality, often violating Grice's maxim of quantity. Three of the coded forms of incoherence capture the most prominent features of the dismissing category: idealization, dismissing derogation, and insistence on lack of recall. In addition, Fear of Loss of the Child is a scale associated with the Ds classification.

The classification is associated with descriptions of rejection in the coder's opinion (pushing the child away in attachment-activating situations) in the context of the adult giving an overarching assessment of having normal or typically loving parents. Other features of the category include an emphasis on strength and independence; little to no description of need, sadness, or distress; and sometimes an emphasis on fun and material aspects of the relationship. There is a minimization of negative experiences, if they are acknowledged at all, and a positive frame is put on negative parental behaviors as being normal or even beneficial.

There are four subclassifications (see Figure 9.1). Two are empirically associated with the more avoidant forms of infant behavior (A1) (Hesse, 1999): The Ds1 subclassification is characterized by marked idealization and minimal description, and the Ds2 subclassification is characterized by derogatory statements regarding attachment or attachment figures. The two other subclassifications are associated with less avoidant infant behavior (A2) in the SS. The transcript of the Ds3 subclassification typically contains some descriptions of negative experiences but with restriction of negative feeling associated with those experiences. Thus, the feelings reported are much more likely to be annoyance rather than sadness. There is minimal valuing of attachment. The Ds4 subclassification reflects fear of loss of the child and was derived from its association with the A2 classification in the SS, not because it has a specific comparable infant behavioral component. It is rare and is given with a best fitting alternative classification.

THE PREOCCUPIED CLASSIFICATION

Adults classified as insecure-preoccupied (E) may display angry preoccupation regarding attachment figures; they may display confusion or oscillation about past experiences, or in rare instances, they may appear overwhelmed and preoccupied by frightening experiences that are not clearly described in the transcript. Descriptions of relationships with parents are typically marked by active anger or passivity, and these scale scores are specifically tied to the preoccupied classification.

The preoccupied classification is associated with reports in the coder's opinion of nonloving, involving, even role-reversing parenting in which the child needed to be alert to parental needs in preference to his or her own. The individual is not balanced in his or her descriptions and may cast blame on him- or herself or others for various events either overtly or implicitly. The past and present may be mixed or blurred in discourse. Another common characteristic of these transcripts is the use of formulaic responses (violations of Grice's maxim of manner) that include jargon or "psychobabble," such that the interviewee seems to be very "familiar" with the topic and implies that the interviewer is as well (e.g., "I'm the adult child of an alcoholic, and well, you know what that means"). In this case, the individual uses a "canned" phrase instead a direct statement, such as "My mother was an alcoholic," and attempts to engage the interviewer in the illusion of having made an insightful remark.

There are three subclassifications (see Figure 9.1): The E1 subclassification is associated with marked passivity of discourse that parallels the passive behavior of the C2 infant classification. The E2 subclassification is associated with active anger, jargon, and definitive, but often oscillating, statements regarding the motives and thoughts of others, and it parallels the angry, resistant behavior associated with the C1 classification in infancy. The E3 classification is characterized by fear and/or traumatic loss of memory and is essentially a clinical classification.

CAN'T CLASSIFY

In some instances, most commonly in high-risk samples, the transcript review yields a mixed pattern of scale scores. For example, the individual may highly idealize the mother and use angry speech with respect to the father. This combination of scores suggests a lack of integration in strategy that does not allow the coder to settle on a predominant secondary stance of preoccupied or dismissing. In such cases, a classification of can't classify (CC) is given, in association with the best fitting major classifications. Such interviews are often markedly incoherent and thus are considered to reflect a high degree of insecurity. The CC category is specifically defined, and is not given for borderline secure–insecure transcripts or for a poorly conducted or transcribed interview. There are other specific discourse patterns in high-risk samples that are currently being researched (Lyons-Ruth, Yellin, Melnick, & Atwood, 2005).

THE UNRESOLVED CLASSIFICATION

Individuals may be classified as unresolved in addition to one of the three major classifications or a CC designation. Unresolved adults report attachment-related traumas of loss and/or abuse, and there is confusion and disorganization in the discussion of those topics.

In the traditional scoring system, the unresolved classification has been considered an insecure classification, and is assigned when one or both of the Unresolved scale scores are greater than 5. This approach may oversimplify the meaning of the unresolved category. AAI coding considers the designation of unresolved for loss and unresolved for trauma/abuse as equivalent; individuals may receive the classification for either reason and are typically grouped together for data-analytic purposes. However, empirical findings and the abuse/posttraumatic stress disorder (PTSD) literature increasingly do not support this approach, as there is evidence from both the attachment literature and the trauma literature that abusive experiences and traumatic loss differentially impact the individual (e.g., Breslau, Chilcoat, Kessler, & Davis, 1999; Crowell, Treboux, & Waters, 2002; Kilpatrick et al., 2003; Kitamura, Sakamoto, Yasumiya, Sumiyama, & Fujihara, 2000; Leon, Jacobvitz, & Hazen, 2004; Lyons-Ruth & Jacobvitz, 1999; Lyons-Ruth, Yellin, Melnick, & Atwood, 2003; Lyons-Ruth et al., 2005; van der Kolk, 1988).

Assigning a Classification

Determination of classifications is based on the patterns of scale scores and on the transcripts' best fit to the description of a specific category. The coder examines the transcript carefully and closely, marking discourse strategies and impressions of the child's experiences, as well as the fit to the classification overviews. Attention is paid to the skill of the interviewer; for example, the interviewee should not be penalized for relevantly answering a poorly worded or off-topic question. Scoring should, in effect, summarize the interview and transcript.

Classification is done with what is referred to as a "top-down, bottom-up" approach to scoring. The "top-down" approach involves the coder's overall gestalt of the interview, that is, its correspondence to a "prototypic" description of the classification. For example, a lively, balanced transcript should yield a secure classification; an abrupt, "shut down" transcript is typically dismissing; and a long, jargony, oscillating, angry interview is typically preoccupied. "Bottom-up" scoring involves examination of the scale scores and how they "add up" to a particular classification; for example, high scores on the Loving and Coherence scales should yield a secure classification. High scores on the Rejecting, Idealization, and Lack of Recall scales should yield a dismissing classification, and high scores for the Role-Reversing scales and Active and Involving Anger should yield a preoccupied classification.

The gestalt of the interview and summation of the scale scores should lead to the same classification, and if they do not, reevaluation of the transcript is imperative. Similarly, high scores on incompatible scales (e.g., high Loving and high Rejecting scores for the mother, in combination with a high passivity score (not associated with either a loving or rejecting experience), should lead to careful reevaluation of the transcript before a classification can be assigned. In the event that there is a true discrepancy between apparent experience and State of Mind scores, *state of mind always has priority in determining classification*. In addition, state of mind manifested in the descriptions of childhood experiences takes precedence over state of mind about current relationship experiences.

POSSIBLE SCORING CONFUSION AMONG MAJOR CLASSIFICATIONS

There are several ways in which the transcripts can appear similar that can lead to classification errors. Confusion between dismissing and passive preoccupied transcripts can occur, because both may have minimal content, dismissing ones because of the use of avoidant strategies and preoccupied transcripts because of confused, limited, passive discourse. Similarly, both active anger and derogation present strongly negative views of parents that may lead to confusion between preoccupied and dismissing classifications.

Preoccupied and secure transcripts can also be mistaken for one another. Both may contain statements indicating valuing of attachment, and preoccupied discourse can appear "open" because of the sharing of intimate or highly personal details, or willingness to take blame or express apparent forgiveness toward parents. Indeed, parents of preoccupied individuals probably had variable, inconsistent behavior that may have ranged between loving and very unloving (Ainsworth et al., 1978/2015), and a parallel fluctuation in discourse style can be seen in the preoccupied transcript.

Dismissing and secure transcripts can also be mistaken for one another, and the line between the dismissing and the secure classification can be a fine one. Some secure transcripts can be quite terse, lacking in the detail that is helpful to the coder. Some of the more coherent dismissing transcripts can show consistency between general descriptions and specific events—they differ from secure transcripts mainly in moderate idealization: Negative feelings in response to negative experience are more likely to be expressed as annoyance or irritability rather than sadness. The impact of attachment experiences on personal development is largely dismissed (e.g., "It was no big deal").

DESCRIPTIVE STUDIES OF THE AAI

Distribution of Classifications

The distribution of AAI classifications in nonclinical samples of women, men, and adolescents is as follows: secure, 58%; dismissing, 24%; preoccupied, 18% (Bakermans-Kranenburg & van IJzendoorn, 1993; van IJzendoorn & Bakermans-Kranenburg, 1996). About 19% of individuals also receive an unresolved classification. Within normative samples, about 11% of individuals classified as secure, 26% of the dismissing group, and 40% of the preoccupied group are also classified as unresolved; and of those classified as unresolved, 38% have a major classification of secure, 24% are dismissing, and 38% are preoccupied. There are no gender differences in distribution of classifications when the original scoring system is used (van IJzendoorn & Bakermans-Kranenburg, 1996), but with the Q-sort method of scoring (see below), men may be more likely to be classified dismissing (Borman, Allen, Carter, Cole, & Hauser, 1998).

The base rate of insecurity in clinical and at-risk samples is much higher: secure 8%, dismissing, 26%, preoccupied, 25%, and unresolved 40% (van IJzendoorn & Bakermans-Kranenburg, 1996). The CC category is also much more common in such samples, and is often combined with either the preoccupied or unresolved categories in data analyses.

Stability and Validity

Stability of the major attachment classifications is high, as reported in a number of studies using the original AAI scoring system; there is 78–90% consistency across periods ranging from 2 weeks to 6 years for the three major classification groups. For example, 86% of individuals over a 21-month transition to marriage received the same classification (secure vs. insecure) at each assessment, kappa = .73, p = .01, 96% for the secure classification, 75% for the insecure combined (predominantly due to high stability of the dismissing classification). Over 4.5 years in the same sample, the stability was 83%, kappa = .59, p = .01 (Crowell, Treboux, & Waters, 2002; Crowell & Waters, 2005).

Similarly, the overall stability of classifications within adulthood of a clinical/high-risk sample of adults who had been psychiatrically hospitalized in adolescence was 84%, kappa = .51, p = .01, over up to 13 years (Crowell & Hauser, 2008). However, within this high-risk sample, attachment insecurity was found to be much more stable (95%) than the secure classification (33%). Within the insecure classifications, stability was low, 54% of those classified as dismissing were consistent across the 13 years, only 25% of those classified as preoccupied, and no participant with a CC designation received that classification more than once (n = 8).

Stability for the unresolved classification is consistently lower than that of the major classifications (van IJzendoorn & Bakermans-Kranenburg, 1996). For example, across the transition to marriage, stability for being classified as unresolved or not unresolved was 81% overall (kappa = .41, p < .001) (Crowell, Treboux, & Waters, 2002). However, for those who were scored as unresolved before marriage, only 46% maintained their unresolved classification, whereas 91% of individuals who were not unresolved before marriage were classified as not unresolved 21 months later. In contrast, in the high-risk sample noted earlier (Crowell & Hauser, 2008), neither the unresolved nor the not unresolved classification was stable over time, 54% overall, nonsignificant (*ns*), suggesting that within a high-risk group there is much variability in discourse related to traumatic events, possibly because the frequency of such events is relatively high in such a sample.

Validity

The AAI has been validated against a number of attachment assessments. Most importantly, it is consistently correlated with attachment behavior and interactions, indirectly through its connection to the SS and directly with observations of adults' attachment behavior with their partners and their children (e.g., Cohn, Cowan, et al., 1992; Cohn, Silver, et al., 1992; Crowell & Feldman, 1988; Crowell, Treboux, Gao, et al., 2002; Lyons-Ruth et al., 2005; Paley et al., 2005; Posada et al., 1995; Simpson et al., 2002; Wampler et al., 2003).

The AAI has been used in studies of adolescent behavioral interactions as well (e.g., Allen et al., 2003; Dykas, 2003; Kobak et al., 1993). The measure is not as well validated in younger populations as it is in adults. For example, many studies indicate that the proportion of individuals classified as insecure is higher in adolescence than in childhood and adulthood, and this is likely a normative developmental phenomenon (e.g., Ammaniti, van IJzendoorn, Speranza, & Tambelli, 2000; Crowell, Treboux, Gao, et al., 2002). We know little about these processes, as studies tracking the evolution of individuals' interviews over time are uncommon, (e.g., Ammaniti et al., 2000; Crowell, Treboux, & Waters, 2002; Crowell & Hauser, 2008). The meaning of dismissing or preoccupied qualities in an adolescent's transcript remains open, and the factors associated with "adolescent limited" insecurity are not known.

AAI training institutes and research have been conducted in a number of different countries (The Netherlands: Bakermans-Kranenburg & van IJzendoorn, 1993; Schuengel, Bakermans-Kranenburg, & van IJzendoorn, 1999; Germany: Grossmann & Grossmann, 2003; Israel: Sagi et al., 1994; Sagi-Schwartz, Koren-Karie, & Joels, 2003; Norway: Ivarsson, 2008; Sweden: Almqvist & Broberg, 2003; Italy: Ammaniti & Speranza, 1995; Ammaniti et al., 2000). The results of these studies are generally consistent with studies using the AAI in the United States and the United Kingdom. However, the training of the coders, the translation, and use of the scoring system for transcripts of non-English speakers has not been the subject of research or even much discussion (Crowell & Treboux, 1995).

Discriminant Validity

These important studies followed quite closely upon the development, teaching, and dissemination of the AAI. Security assessed with the AAI is not associated with memory, social desirability, or discourse style on an unrelated topic (Bakermans-Kranenburg & van IJzendoorn, 1993; Crowell et al., 1996; Sagi et al., 1994). There is a low but significant correlation with questionnaire-based IQ scores (e.g., Crowell et al., 1996), that is associated with participants classified as preoccupied achieving lower IQ scores.

Sensitivity and Change

Recent research with both normative and clinical samples has addressed whether the AAI is sensitive enough to predict change and development in individual functioning. Two studies have found an association between day-to-day social functioning and AAI security in a high-functioning group of mothers of preschoolers (Crowell et al., 1996) and a relatively low-functioning, high-risk sample (Crowell & Hauser, 2008). These differences between secure and insecure classifications were not related to outlying individuals. Thus, it appears that the AAI is sensitive enough to detect individual differences even within a narrow range, that is, among healthy people and within a high-risk group.

AAI coherence scores have also been shown to predict who is going to change. The same study of high-risk participants noted earlier (Crowell & Hauser, 2008) found that the less coherent/secure participants were, the more likely their day-to-day functioning was to decline over a 5-year interval between ages 34 and 39 years, and, of course, the opposite. *None* of the other domains assessed, including self-reported psychiatric symptoms, drug and alcohol use, and relationship quality, were significantly associated with functional outcomes. This supports the idea that AAI coherence and its representational underpinnings are built over time and are based on many experiences. As such, they appear to be stably predictive and unlikely to vary with contextual circumstances or smaller-scale life events, as are domains such as drug use or symptom expression.

What kinds of experiences do lead to change in AAI coherence and classifications? This remains an open question. The most notable period of change identified to date is in early adult life. Many longitudinal studies find that samples of late adolescents/young adults have a higher proportion of insecure participants than samples of older adults (e.g., Creasey, 2002; Treboux et al., 2004; van IJzendoorn & Bakermans-Kranenburg, 1996), indicating a trend toward greater security/coherence in this developmental period. One study examined factors associated with change across a 21-month transition to marriage (Crowell, Treboux, & Waters, 2002). About 12% of the young adults originally classified as insecure were subsequently classified as secure. Exposure to new ideas and new relationships, as well as physical and psychological distance from parents, were associated with this change. High relationship satisfaction and coherence in talking about the relationship with the partner were also associated with change, although partners' attachment security was not. The study concluded that life events, even important ones such as the transition to marriage, were themselves not the impetus for change. Rather, new experiences, especially in the attachment domain, and perceptions of those experiences, were factors associated with increased security/coherence.

Data Analysis

The choice of data-analytic strategy should be guided by the research questions, of course. Comparisons of secure versus insecure classifications are common (two groups), as are those that compare secure, dismissing, and preoccupied classifications (three groups). In these comparisons, diverse strategies have been used to handle the unresolved classifications that (1) exclude individuals classified as unresolved, (2) include them as insecure, or (3) use only the major classification to designate group placement (see below). Data analysis rarely utilizes the fine distinctions among subclassifications, largely because of sample-size issues and the challenges of obtaining coder agreement for subclassifications.

Discriminant function analysis using over 500 transcripts scored in several laboratories has enabled AAI security to be represented as a continuous variable (Fyffe, 1997). The coder rating of "coherence of transcript" correlates $r = .96$ with the security function, indicating that the secure–insecure judgment made by coders is virtually identical with the "coherence" judgment.

Regarding data analysis with the unresolved classification, there are several important considerations. It has been relatively common for studies to use four group analyses (secure, dismissing, preoccupied, and unresolved). However, there is growing evidence that the unresolved classification should not be considered equivalent to the three major classifications (Creasey, 2002; Crowell & Hauser, 2008; Crowell, Treboux, & Waters, 2002; Ward, Lee, & Polan, 2006). Unresolved-secure individuals are generally similar to those classified as secure, although with some vulnerabilities (e.g., Creasey, 2002; Posada et al., 1995; Ward et al., 2006). In contrast, the pairing of the unresolved classification with an insecure classification is likely to be associated with impaired attachment behavior and with psychopathology. For these reasons, many investigators are electing to use three (secure, dismissing, preoccupied) by two (not unresolved, unresolved) analyses of variance. Planned comparisons may also be used, comparing secure with all insecure, then unresolved with other insecure, and dismissing versus preoccupied.

Sample size is an important consideration when planning a study with the AAI. In the general population, the secure–insecure distribution is close to 50/50%, but it is not unusual for high-risk samples to have a 20/80% distribution or to be even more skewed toward insecurity. There are also cultural variations in AAI distributions. An adequate sample size is in the range of 30 individuals in each group (e.g., secure, dismissing, and preoccupied) to examine differences among groups. Although a continuous variable, coherence, can be used in analyses to achieve greater power, again, it is clear that studies using the AAI are expensive and require considerable other resources as well.

Alternative Forms of Scoring

Q-Sort Scoring System

The Adult Attachment Q-Sort was derived from the original scoring system (Kobak, 1993; Kobak et al., 1993). Its underlying structure parallels that of the Main and Goldwyn (1998) system, but it emphasizes the relation between affect regulation and attachment representations by examining the use of secure versus insecure emotional strategies and minimizing (deactivating) versus maximizing (hyperactivating) emotional strategies. An individual's transcript is rated by two or more coders using 100 Q-sort items and instructions that impose a forced-normal distribution along a 9-point continuum (Kobak et al., 1993). The interview is scored with a forced distribution of descriptors and yields scores for two dimensions: security–anxiety and deactivation–hyperactivation.

Security is defined as coherence and cooperation within the interview, and usually, although not necessarily, memories of supportive attachment figures in the coder's opinion. Deactivation corresponds to dismissing strategies, whereas hyperactivation refers to the excessive detail and active anger seen in the transcripts of many preoccupied subjects. These two strategies, deactivating and hyperactivating, lie at opposite ends of a single dimension, and this dimension is assumed to be orthogonal to the secure–anxious or secure–insecure dimension. The individual's sorts on each dimension can then be correlated with expert-based prototypic sorts for the dimensions. The scores can be used to classify the adult into the categories of the Main and Goldwyn (1998) system. About 80% of individuals receive the same classification with the Q-sort as is obtained with the original system (r =.65), with more overlap on the deactivation–hyperactivation dimension than on the secure–insecure dimension (Kobak et al., 1993).

Expanding the Unresolved Mental States

Karlen Lyons-Ruth and colleagues (2005) have developed additional scales for coding the AAI that are potentially very useful in clinical samples, and for work with parents and infants. Their scales address specifically hostile and helpless states of mind that may be evidenced in AAI transcripts. These scales appear to correspond more directly to infant disorganization in the SS and to problematic parental behavior in parent–child interactions than do the original AAI coding scales.

THE AAI IN MARRIAGE: THE CURRENT RELATIONSHIP INTERVIEW

As a complement to the AAI, several research groups have developed narrative assessments of a specific representation of adult attachment relationships (Cowan & Cowan, 2009; Crowell & Owens, 1996; Dickstein, Seifer, & Albus, 2009). One of these, the Current Relationship Interview (CRI; Crowell & Owens, 1996), has been used to explore development and possible change of representational patterns in the context of an adult attachment relationship. As described earlier, the AAI was intended to assess the generalized representation of attachment or state of mind of an adult, as it develops from relationships with childhood attachment figures. The situation of engaging a "new" attachment figure (i.e., a partner) presents the individual with the challenge of fitting the partner's and the self's own behavior to the generalized representation. Furthermore, given the reciprocal nature of adult attachment, this integration must include the roles of both the attachment figure and the attached (i.e., "support provider" and the "support seeker"). Attachment experiences, both observed and directly experienced, with romantic partners in general, and with the partner in particular, appear to lead to the development of this relatively specific representation or state of mind about adult attachment, at least early in adult attachment relationships (Owens et al., 1995). As with the generalized attachment representation, the adult partnership representation is hypothesized to be organized around the secure base phenomenon but with specific reference to the partner. It seems likely that such representations are informed by (1) the actual attachment experiences and explicit discussion with the partner, (2) the understanding of attachment in a general or fundamental way, and (3) how well the experiences fit within that generalized frame or foundation.

The interview intentionally parallels the AAI in format and inquires about attachment experiences in adult partnerships, especially focusing on the current relationship. As with the AAI, the individual is repeatedly given the opportunity to convey the secure base script, but in this case with respect to the reciprocal seeking and provision of secure base support by the self and the partner in a variety of situations. The CRI differs from the AAI in its emphasis on the present rather than recall of the past, and there is greater emphasis on the reported behaviors of the self than on those of the partner.

The scoring system parallels the AAI scoring system in the use of rating scales that characterize the individual's behavior, the partner's behavior, and the individual's discourse style. The measure yields classifications similar to those of the AAI that reflect state of mind with respect to attachment in the adult relationship: Secure$_{\text{CRI}}$, Insecure-Dismissing$_{\text{CRI}}$, and Insecure-Preoccupied$_{\text{CRI}}$. Classifications reflect the behavior and thoughts of the participant with respect to adult attachment. Security or Coherence reflects participants' ability to present an integrated, believable account of their own and their partners' attachment-related behaviors and their meaning. Thus, it is not synonymous with relationship satisfaction or having a supportive partner. The Coherence scale is highly correlated with a continuous Security score derived from discriminant function analysis (Crowell & Waters, 1997).

The Insecure-Dismissing$_{\text{CRI}}$ classification is characterized by idealization or normalization in the descriptions of behavior of the self and/or experiences with the partner/relationship, a strong emphasis on independence in the relationship, on fun, material possessions, and acquisitions, with avoidance of providing support to the partner and/or of approaching the partner for help. The Insecure-Preoccupied$_{\text{CRI}}$ classification is characterized by descriptions of ineffective support seeking from and support provision to the partner (e.g., anger, whining, nagging, helplessness, feeling high anxiety when the partner expresses distress), and active anger or confusion and passivity of thought about the relationship.

Before marriage, 18 months of marriage, and 6 years of marriage, the distribution of the classifications was $\text{Secure}_{\text{CRI}}$, 46% (*n* = 144), 46% (*n* = 83), and 47% (*n* = 108), respectively; $\text{Insecure-Dismissing}_{\text{CRI}}$ 37% (*n* = 116), 39% (*n* = 70), 41% (*n* = 94), respectively; and $\text{Insecure-Preoccupied}_{\text{CRI}}$, 17% (*n* = 54), 15% (*n* = 26), 12% (*n* = 28), respectively (Treboux et al., 2004).

The correspondence between AAI and CRI security just prior to marriage (*r* = .51) suggests that the generalized and specific representations are significantly related but are not equivalent (Crowell, Treboux, Gao, et al., 2002; Owens et al., 1995). As noted earlier, there is evidence that high coherence of the CRI, as well as positive perceptions of the relationship before marriage, are associated with change from generalized insecurity (AAI) to security (Crowell, Treboux, & Waters, 2002). It also appears that concordance versus discordance of security of AAI and CRI has important implications for marital outcome and functioning, especially in situations where there are high numbers of stressful events (Treboux et al., 2004). This is to say, there is evidence that the fit between cognitions about attachment in general and about attachment in the current adult relationship may be as or more relevant to marital processes than the quality of either set of cognitions alone (Dickstein et al., 2009; Treboux et al., 2004).

CONCLUSION

The AAI and the adult attachment self-report assessments that followed shortly thereafter (Bartholomew & Horowitz, 1991; Hazan & Shaver, 1987) all emphasized identification of adult attachment patterns that corresponded to the attachment patterns observed in the SS. Following from this, the study of adult attachment has focused heavily on individual differences in the organization of attachment behavior and in expectations regarding attachment relationships rather than on the normative, developmental aspects of attachment beyond childhood. Indeed, although it is fundamentally a developmentally based assessment, the AAI is not easy to use in the study of development because of the challenges associated with its administration and scoring—challenges that are even more daunting when the AAI is administered more than once.

The challenges associated with the AAI are many: It has not been published. Considerable training is required to administer the interview, and extensive and expensive training is essential to learning to score it. It is expensive to use, as it requires hours of skillful interviewing and transcriptions, as well as trained coders. Logistics aside, the AAI is a complex assessment with many components that are difficult to quantify. It is hard to say what is being measured with the AAI; there is no clear and direct link between an AAI classification and a well-defined "representation of attachment." Indeed, it seems that the "shape" of a representation or IWM must emerge from the shadows cast by the measures that attempt to assess it. These issues all present considerable obstacles to the researcher who would like to use the AAI.

That said, there is no measure of adult attachment that is as well-researched and validated regarding core aspects of attachment theory or that presents such a rich database about an individual's autobiographical recollections of attachment experiences and behaviors. The AAI and its scoring system are firmly grounded in attachment theory. More than any other measure of attachment, it addresses each of the legs of the attachment control system, behavior, cognition, and emotional appraisal and regulation (Crowell, 2009). In all these ways, the AAI is more than a tool to identify attachment patterns and their correlates; it can be extremely valuable in the study of the attachment system across the lifespan, as a number of longitudinal studies have shown (e.g., Allen, Hauser, & Borman-Spurrell, 1996; Crowell & Hauser, 2008; Crowell, Treboux, & Waters, 2002; Fonagy, Steele, & Steele, 1991; Kaplan, 2003; Main et al., 1985; Roisman et al., 2002; Treboux et al., 2004; Waters, Merrick, Treboux, Crowell, & Albersheim, 2000). Expensive and difficult to use, the AAI is nonetheless, if not the "gold standard" in adult attachment research, certainly worth its weight in gold.

REFERENCES

Ainsworth, M. D. S., Blehar, M., Waters, E., & Wall, S. (2015). *Patterns of attachment: A psychological study of the Strange Situation*. New York: Taylor & Francis (Psychology Press). (Original work published 1978)

Allen, J., Hauser, S., & Borman-Spurrell, E. (1996). Attachment theory as a framework for understanding sequelae of severe adolescent psychopathology: An 11-year follow-up study. *Journal of Consulting and Clinical Psychology, 64*(2), 254–263.

Allen, J. P., McElhaney, K. B., Land, D. J., Kuperminc, G., Moore, C., O'Beirne-Kelly, H., & Kilmer, S. L. (2003). A secure base in adolescence: Markers of attachment security in the mother–adolescent relationship. *Child Development, 74*, 292–307.

Almqvist, K., & Broberg, A. (2003). Young children traumatized by organized violence together with their mothers: The critical effects of damaged internal representations. *Attachment and Human Development, 5*, 367–380.

Ammaniti, M., & Speranza, A. M. (1995). Maternal representations and disorganized patterns of attachment in children. *Giornale di Neuropsichiatria dell'Età Evolutiva, 15*, 27–34.

Ammaniti, M., van IJzendoorn, M., Speranza, A. M., & Tambelli, R. (2000). Internal working models of attachment during late childhood and early adolescence: An exploration of stability and change. *Attachment and Human Development, 2*, 328–346.

Bakermans-Kranenburg, M., & van IJzendoorn, M. (1993). A psychometric study of the Adult Attachment Interview: Reliability and discriminant validity. *Developmental Psychology, 29*(5), 870–879.

Bartholomew, K., & Horowitz, L. M. (1991). Attachment styles among young adults: A test of a four-category model. *Journal of Personality and Social Psychology, 61,* 226–244.

Borman, E., Allen, J., Carter, A., Cole, H., & Hauser, S. (1998). *Assessing adult attachment: A comparison of interview-based and self-report methods.* Unpublished manuscript, Harvard University, Cambridge, MA.

Bowlby, J. (1973). *Separation: Vol. 2. Anxiety and anger.* New York: Basic Books.

Bowlby, J. (1979). *The making and breaking of affectional bonds.* London: Tavistock.

Bowlby, J. (1980). *Attachment and loss: Vol. 3. Loss, sadness, and depression.* New York: Basic Books.

Bowlby, J. (1982). *Attachment and loss: Vol. 1. Attachment.* New York: Basic Books. (Original work published 1969)

Breslau, N., Chilcoat, H. D., Kessler, R. C., & Davis, G. C. (1999). Previous exposure to trauma and PTSD effects of subsequent trauma: Results from the Detroit Area Survey of Trauma. *American Journal of Psychiatry, 156,* 902–907.

Bretherton, I. (1985). Attachment theory: Retrospect and prospect. In I. Bretherton & E. Waters (Eds.), Growing points of attachment theory and research. *Monographs of the Society for Research in Child Development, 50*(1–2, Serial No. 209), 3–35.

Bretherton, I. (1990). Open communication and internal working models: Their role in the development of attachment relationships. In R. A. Thompson (Ed.), *Nebraska Symposium on Motivation* (Vol. 36, pp. 59–113). Lincoln: University of Nebraska Press.

Bretherton, I., & Munholland, K. A. (1999). Internal working models in attachment relationships: A construct revisited. In J. Cassidy & P. R. Shaver (Eds.), *Handbook of attachment: Theory, research, and clinical applications* (pp. 89–111). New York: Guilford Press.

Cassidy, J., & Shaver, P. R. (Eds.). (2016). *Handbook of attachment, third edition: Theory, research, and clinical applications.* New York: Guilford Press.

Cohn, D., Cowan, P. A., Cowan, C. P., & Pearson, J. (1992). Mothers' and fathers' working models of childhood attachment relationships, parenting styles, and child behavior. *Development and Psychopathology, 4,* 417–431.

Cohn, D., Silver, D., Cowan, P., Cowan, C., & Pearson, J. (1992). Working models of childhood attachment and couples' relationships. *Journal of Family Issues, 13*(4), 432–449.

Collins, N., & Feeney, B. C. (2000). A safe haven: An attachment theory perspective on support seeking and caregiving in intimate relationships. *Journal of Personality and Social Psychology, 78,* 1053–1073.

Collins, N. L., & Read, S. J. (1990). Adult attachment, working models, and relationship quality in dating couples. *Journal of Personality and Social Psychology, 58*(4), 644–663.

Cowan, C., & Cowan, P. (2009). A family system view of adult attachment and couple attachment in predicting children's adaptation to school. *Attachment and Human Development, 11,* 29–46.

Craik, K. (1943). *The nature of explanation.* Cambridge, UK: Cambridge University Press.

Creasey, G. (2002). Psychological distress in college-aged women: Links with unresolved/preoccupied attachment status and the mediating role of negative mood regulation expectancies. *Attachment and Human Development, 4*(3), 261–277.

Crowell, J. (2009). A life-span perspective: Elements of continuity and discontinuity in the attachment system. In L. Carli, D. Cavanna, & G. C. Zavattini (Eds.), *Psicologia delle relaizioni di coppia* (p. 2). Chicago: il Mulino.

Crowell, J. A. (2021). Measuring the security of attachment in adults. In R. A. Thompson, J. Simpson, & L. Berlin (Eds.), *Attachment: The fundamental questions.* New York: Guilford Press.

Crowell, J. A., & Feldman, S. S. (1988). Mothers' internal models of relationships and children's behavioral and developmental status: A study of mother–child interaction. *Child Development, 59,* 1273–1285.

Crowell, J. A., Fraley, R. C., & Roisman, G. I. (2016). Measurement of individual differences in adult attachment. In J. Cassidy & P. R. Shaver (Eds.), *Handbook of attachment: Theory, research, and clinical applications* (3rd ed., pp. 598–635). New York: Guilford Press.

Crowell, J., & Hauser, S. (2008). AAIs in a high-risk sample: Stability and relation to functioning from adolescence to 39 years. In H. Steele & M. Steele (Eds.), *Clinical applications of the Adult Attachment Interview* (pp. 341–370). New York: Guilford Press.

Crowell, J., O'Connor, E., Wollmers, G., Sprafkin, J., & Rao, U. (1991). Mothers' conceptualizations of parent–child relationships: Relation to mother–child interaction and child behavior problems. *Development and Psychopathology, 3,* 431–444.

Crowell, J. A., & Owens, G. (1996). *Current Relationship Interview and Scoring System.* Unpublished manuscript, State University of New York at Stony Brook, Stony Brook, NY.

Crowell, J. A., & Treboux, D. (1995). A review of adult attachment measures: Implications for theory and research. *Social Development, 4*(3), 294–327.

Crowell, J. A., Treboux, D., Gao, Y., Fyffe, C., Pan, H., & Waters, E. (2002). Assessing secure base behavior in adulthood: Development of a measure, links to adult attachment representations, and relations to couples' communication and reports of relationships. *Developmental Psychology, 38*(5), 679–693.

Crowell, J. A., Treboux, D., & Waters, E. (2002). Stability of attachment representations: The transition to marriage. *Developmental Psychology, 38,* 467–479.

Crowell, J. A., & Waters, E. (1997, April). *The secure base phenomenon in adult attachment relationships: Exploration of the core of the attachment system.* Poster presented at the biennial meeting of the Society for Research in Child Development, Washington, DC.

Crowell, J. A., & Waters, E. (2005). Attachment representations, secure-base behavior, and the evolution of adult relationships. In K. E. Grossmann, K. Grossmann, & E. Waters (Eds.), *Attachment from infancy to adulthood: The major longitudinal studies* (pp. 223–244). New York: Guilford Press.

Crowell, J. A., Waters, E., Treboux, D., O'Connor, E. O., Colon-Downs, C., Feider, O., . . . Posada, G. (1996). Discriminant validity of the Adult Attachment Interview. *Child Development, 67*(5), 2584–2599.

Dickstein, S., Seifer, R., & Albus, K. E. (2009). Attachment patterns across multiple family relationships in adulthood: Associations with child outcomes. *Attachment and Human Development, 11,* 5–27.

Dykas, M. J. (2003). *Adolescent secure base use and parental secure base support: Relations with adolescent attachment security.* Unpublished master's thesis, University of Maryland, College Park, MD.

Fonagy, P., Gergely, G., Jurist, E., & Target, M. (2002). *Affect regulation, mentalization, and the development of the self.* New York: Other Press.

Fonagy, P., Steele, H., & Steele, M. (1991). Maternal representations of attachment during pregnancy predict the organization of infant–mother attachment at one year of age. *Child Development, 62,* 891–905.

Fonagy, P., Steele, M., Steele, H., Moran, G., & Higgitt, A. (1991). The capacity for understanding mental states: The reflective self in parent and child and its significance for security of attachment. *Infant Mental Health Journal, 12,* 201–218.

Furman, W., Simon, V. A., Shaffer, L., & Bouchey, H. A. (2002). Adolescents' working models and styles for relationships with parents, friends, and romantic partners. *Child Development, 73,* 241–255.

Fyffe, C. (1997). *Empirical classification of adult attachment status: Predicting group membership.* Poster presented at the biennial meeting of the Society for Research in Child Development.

George, C., Kaplan, N., & Main, M. (1985). *The Adult Attachment Interview.* Unpublished manuscript, University of California at Berkeley, Berkeley, CA.

Goldberg, S., Gotowiec, A., & Simmons, R. J. (1995). Infant–mother attachment and behavior problems in healthy and clinically ill preschoolers. *Development and Psychopathology, 7,* 267–282.

Greenberg, M. T. (1999). Attachment and psychopathology in childhood. In J. Cassidy & P. R. Shaver (Eds.), *Handbook of attachment: Theory, research and clinical applications* (pp. 469–496). New York: Guilford Press.

Grossmann, K. E., & Grossmann, K. (2003, July). *Attachment, exploration and psychological security across 22 years: From mothers' and fathers' sensitivity and support to later attachment and partnership representations.* Paper presented at the conference Attachment from Infancy and Childhood to Adulthood (ATICA), Regensberg, Germany.

Guttmann-Steinmetz, S., Cuva, S., Brockmeyer, S., & Crowell, J. (2005, April). *Associations between the secure base scripts of children and their mothers: Are they mediated by their interactions (and/or influenced by children's symptoms)?* Presented at the biennial meeting of the Society for Research in Child Development, Atlanta, GA.

Hazan, C., & Shaver, P. (1987). Romantic love conceptualized as an attachment process. *Journal of Personality and Social Psychology, 52*(3), 511–524.

Heider, F. (1958). *The psychology of interpersonal relations.* New York: Wiley.

Hesse, E. (1999). The Adult Attachment Interview: Historical and current perspective. In J. Cassidy & P. R. Shaver (Eds.), *Handbook of attachment: Theory, research, and clinical applications* (pp. 395–433). New York: Guilford Press.

Hesse, E. (2008). The Adult Attachment Interview: Protocol, method of analysis, and empirical studies. In J. Cassidy & P. R. Shaver (Eds.), *Handbook of attachment: Theory, research, and clinical applications* (2nd ed., pp. 552–598). New York: Guilford Press.

Ivarsson, T. (2008). Obsessive–compulsive disorder in adolescence: An AAI perspective. In H. Steele & M. Steele (Eds.), *Clinical applications of the Adult Attachment Interview* (pp. 213–235). New York: Guilford Press.

Johnson-Laird, P. N. (1983). *Mental models.* Cambridge, MA: Harvard University Press.

Kaplan, N. (2003). *Attachment from infancy to young adulthood in the Bay Area*

Longitudinal Study: Predictions from early and middle childhood. Paper presented at a meeting of the Society for Research in Child Development, Tampa, FL.

Kilpatrick, D. G., Ruggiero, K. J., Acierno, R., Saunders, B. E., Resnick, H. S., & Best, C. L. (2003). Violence and risk of PTSD, major depression, substance abuse/dependence, and comorbidity: Results from the National Survey of Adolescents. *Journal of Consulting and Clinical Psychology, 71,* 692–700.

Kitamura, T., Sakamoto, S., Yasumiya, R., Sumiyama, T., & Fujihara, S. (2000). Child abuse, other early experiences and depression: II. Single episode and recurrent/chronic subtypes of depression and their link to early experiences. *Archives of Women's Mental Health, 3,* 53–58.

Kobak, R. R. (1993). *The attachment Q-sort.* Unpublished manuscript, University of Delaware, Newark, DE.

Kobak, R. R., Cole, H. E., Ferenz-Gillies, R., Fleming, W. S., & Gamble, W. (1993). Attachment and emotion regulation during mother–teen problem solving: A control theory analysis. *Child Development, 64,* 231–245.

Leon, K., Jacobvitz, D., & Hazen, N. L. (2004). Maternal resolution of loss and abuse: Associations with adjustment to the transition to parenthood. *Infant Mental Health Journal, 25,* 130–148.

Lyons-Ruth, K., & Jacobvitz, D. (1999). Attachment disorganization: Unresolved loss, relational violence, and lapses in behavioral and attentional strategies. In J. Cassidy & P. Shaver (Eds.), *Handbook of attachment: Theory, research, and clinical applications* (pp. 520–554). New York: Guilford Press.

Lyons-Ruth, K., Yellin, C., Melnick, S., & Atwood, G. (2003). Childhood experiences of trauma and loss have different relations to maternal unresolved and hostile–helpless states of mind on the AAI. *Attachment and Human Development, 5,* 409–414.

Lyons-Ruth, K., Yellin, C., Melnick, S., & Atwood, G. (2005). Expanding the concept of unresolved mental states: Hostile/helpless states of mind on the Adult Attachment Interview are associated with disrupted mother–infant communication and infant disorganization. *Development and Psychopathology, 17*(1), 1–23.

Main, M. (1991). Metacognitive knowledge, metacognitive monitoring, and singular (coherent) versus multiple (incoherent) models of attachment: Findings and directions for future research. In C. M. Parkes, J. Stevenson-Hinde, & P. Marris (Eds.), *Attachment across the life cycle* (pp. 127–159). London: Routledge.

Main, M. (2000). The organized categories of infant, child, and adult attachment: Flexible vs. inflexible attention under attachment-related stress. *Journal of the American Psychoanalytic Association, 48*(4), 1055–1096; discussion 1175–1087.

Main, M., & Goldwyn, R. (1998). *Adult Attachment Rating and Classification Systems, Version 7.0.* Unpublished manuscript, University of California at Berkeley, Berkeley, CA.

Main, M., Goldwyn, R., & Hesse, E. (2003). *Adult Attachment Rating and Classification Systems, Version 7.2.* Unpublished manuscript, University of California at Berkeley, Berkeley, CA.

Main, M., Hesse, E., & Goldwyn, R. (2008). Studying differences in language usage in recounting attachment history: An introduction to the AAI. In H. Steele & M. Steele (Eds.), *Clinical applications of the Adult Attachment Interview* (pp. 31–68). New York: Guilford Press.

Main, M., Kaplan, N., & Cassidy, J. (1985). Security of infancy, childhood, and adulthood: A move to the level of representation. In I. Bretherton & E. Waters (Eds.), Growing points of attachment theory and research. *Monographs for the Society for Research in Child Development, 50*(1–2, Serial No. 209), 66–106.

Oppenheim, D., & Waters, H. (1995). Narrative processes and attachment representations: Issues of development and assessment. In E. Waters, B. Vaughn, G. Posada, & K. Kondo-Ikemura (Eds.), Caregiving, cultural, and cognitive perspectives on secure-base behavior and working models: New growing points of attachment theory and research. *Monographs of the Society for Research in Child Development, 60*(2–3), 197–215.

Owens, G., Crowell, J., Pan, H., Treboux, D., O'Connor, E., & Waters, E. (1995). The prototype hypothesis and the origins of attachment working models: Adult relationships with parents and romantic partners. In E. Waters, B. Vaughn, G. Posada, & K. Kondo-Ikemura (Eds.), Caregiving, cultural, and cognitive perspectives on secure-base behavior and working models: New growing points of attachment theory and research. *Monographs of the Society for Research in Child Development, 60*(2–3), 216–233.

Paley, B., Cox, M. J., Kanoy, K. W., Harter, K. S., Burchinal, M., & Margand, N. A. (2005). Adult attachment and marital interaction as predictors of whole family interactions during the transition to parenthood. *Journal of Family Psychology, 19*(3), 420–429.

Pearson, J., Cohn, D., Cowan, P., & Cowan, C. P. (1994). Earned- and continuous-security in adult attachment: Relation to depressive symptomatology and parenting style. *Development and Psychopathology, 6,* 359–373.

Piaget, J. (1952). *The origins of intelligence in children.* New York: International Universities Press.

Posada, G., Waters, E., Crowell, J. A., & Lay, K. L. (1995). Is it easier to use a secure mother as a secure base?: Attachment Q-sort correlates of the Adult Attachment Interview. In E. Waters, B. Vaughn, G. Posada, & K. Kondo-Ikemura (Eds.), Caregiving, cultural, and cognitive perspectives on secure-base behavior and working models: New growing points of attachment theory and research. *Monographs of the Society for Research in Child Development, 60*(2–3), 133–145.

Roisman, G. I., Madsen, S. D., Hennighausen, K., Sroufe, L. A., & Collins, W. A. (2001). The coherence of dyadic behavior across parent–child and romantic relationships as mediated by the internalized representation of experience. *Attachment and Human Development, 3,* 156–172.

Roisman, G. I., Padrón, E., Sroufe, L. A., & Egeland, B. (2002). Earned-secure attachment status in retrospect and prospect. *Child Development, 73,* 1204–1219.

Sagi, A., van IJzendoorn, M., Scharf, M., Korne-Karje, N., Joels, T., & Mayseless, O. (1994). Stability and discriminant validity of the Adult Attachment Interview. *Developmental Psychology, 30*(5), 771–777.

Sagi-Schwartz, A., Koren-Karie, N., & Joels, T. (2003). Failed mourning in the Adult Attachment Interview: The case of Holocaust child survivors. *Attachment and Human Development, 5*(4), 398–408; discussion 409–314.

Schank, R. C. (1982). *Dynamic memory: A theory of reminding and learning in computers and people.* Cambridge, UK: Cambridge University Press.

Schank, R. C., & Abelson, R. P. (1977). *Scripts, plans, goals and understanding.* Hillsdale, NJ: Erlbaum.

Schuengel, C., Bakermans-Kranenburg, M., & van IJzendoorn, M. (1999). Attachment and loss: Frightening maternal behavior linking unresolved loss and disorganized infant attachment. *Journal of Consulting and Clinical Psychology, 67,* 54–63.

Simpson, J., Rholes, W. S., Orina, M. M., & Grich, J. (2002). Working models of attachment, support giving, and support seeking in a stressful situation. *Personality and Social Psychology Bulletin, 28,* 598–608.

Steele, H., & Steele, M. (2008). Ten clinical uses of the Adult Attachment Interview. In H. Steele & M. Steele (Eds.), *Clinical applications of the Adult Attachment Interview* (pp. 3–30). New York: Guilford Press.

Treboux, D., Crowell, J. A., & Waters, E. (2004). When "new" meets "old": Configurations of adult attachment representations and their implications for marital functioning. *Developmental Psychology, 40*(2), 295–314.

van der Kolk, B. (1988). The trauma spectrum: The interaction of biological and social events in the genesis of the trauma response. *Journal of Traumatic Stress, 1,* 273–290.

van IJzendoorn, M. (1995). Adult attachment representations, parental responsiveness, and infant attachment: A meta-analysis on the predictive validity of the Adult Attachment Interview. *Psychological Bulletin, 117,* 387–403.

van IJzendoorn, M., & Bakermans-Kranenburg, M. (1996). Attachment representations in mothers, fathers, adolescents, and clinical groups: A meta-analytic search for normative data. *Journal of Consulting and Clinical Psychology, 64*(1), 8–21.

Wampler, K. S., Shi, L., Nelson, B. S., & Kimball, T. G. (2003). The Adult Attachment Interview and observed couple interaction: Implications for an intergenerational perspective on couple therapy. *Family Process, 42*(4), 497–515.

Ward, M. J., Lee, S. S., & Polan, H. J. (2006). Attachment and psychopathology in a community sample. *Attachment and Human Development, 8,* 327–340.

Waters, E., & Beauchaine, T. (2003). Are there really patterns of attachment?: Theoretical and empirical perspectives. *Developmental Psychology, 39,* 417–432.

Waters, E., Crowell, J., Elliot, M., Corcoran, D., & Treboux, D. (2002). Bowlby's secure base theory and the social/personality psychology of attachment styles: Work(s) in progress. *Attachment and Human Development, 4,* 230–242.

Waters, E., Merrick, S., Treboux, D., Crowell, J., & Albersheim, L. (2000). Attachment security in infancy and early adulthood: A twenty-year longitudinal study. *Child Development, 71,* 684–689.

Waters, H., & Rodrigues-Doolabh, L. (2001, April). *Are attachment scripts the building blocks of attachment representations?: Narrative assessment of representations and the AAI.* Paper presented at the biennial meeting of the Society for Research in Child Development, Minneapolis, MN.

CHAPTER 10

Measuring Secure Base Script Knowledge in the Adult Attachment Interview

Theodore E. A. Waters and Christopher R. Facompré

The secure base concept—that the primary caregiver acts as both the child's haven of safety and as a secure base from which to explore—is central to the logic of attachment theory (Ainsworth, 1967, 1972; Ainsworth, Blehar, Waters, & Wall, 1978/2015; Bowlby, 1969/1982; Feeney, 2004; Sroufe & Waters, 1977; E. Waters & Cummings, 2003). It is surprising, therefore, that the term *secure base* is nowhere mentioned in the scoring manual for the Adult Attachment Interview (AAI; Main, Goldwyn, & Hesse, 2003–2008). This reflects the fact that, unlike attachment research in infancy, which emphasizes secure base behavior (Ainsworth et al., 1978/2015), attachment research in adulthood privileges narrative discourse (e.g., Main, Kaplan, & Cassidy, 1985).

It is understandable that attachment researchers interested in adolescence and adulthood have placed such importance on narrative discourse. Indeed, the parallels between discourse patterns in the AAI and Ainsworth's patterns of infant attachment are striking. In addition, they have a wide range of theoretical and clinically significant correlates (Sroufe, Egeland, Carlson, & Collins, 2009).

Coherent narrative, however, does little in the way of explaining how skillful and consistent secure base use and support manifests. Individuals may recall early caregiving experiences free from defensive strategies associated with dismissing or preoccupied attachment, but secure base behavior is far more than the absence of defense. It also relies on detailed knowledge of how and when to seek support, what to expect when that support is offered, and how to recognize signals and provide effective support for others. From this perspective, attachment representations reflect an understanding (or lack thereof) of secure base use and support acquired from lived experiences with primary caregivers. This knowledge is then carried forward and brought to bear in novel developmental contexts (e.g., romantic partnership). These same secure base representations are elicited during the AAI, thereby providing a parsimonious explanation for how narratives of early experience relate to adaptive relationship functioning. Although it could be argued that the secure base concept is implicitly represented in traditional AAI scoring, the fact remains that coders primarily focus on Grice's (1975) conversational maxims. This represents an opportunity to expand current views on the AAI by *explicitly* including the secure base concept.

Guided by recent work on script-like attachment representations (H. Waters & Waters, 2006), we present in this chapter a novel coding system focused on assessing secure base content in the AAI. We provide a descriptive account of how secure base script knowledge manifests in the AAI and a method for quantifying it. In addition, we discuss validation efforts and preliminary results using the coding system. Finally, we present a framework for understanding how the secure base script might explain the coherence of narrative discourse during the AAI.

THE SECURE BASE SCRIPT

As defined by Schank and Abelson (1977; see also Nelson, 1986), a *script* is a schematic representation of the temporal–causal structure of a frequently experienced class of events, such as going to a restaurant or visiting a doctor's office. Accessing or activating such representations generates expectations that shape social perception and help organize behavior. A great deal of cognitive psychology research has investigated the structure of script-like representations (Abelson, 1981) and demonstrated that they have significant effects on attention (e.g., Fiske & Taylor, 1991), memory (e.g., Bower, Black, & Turner, 1979; Graesser, Gordon, & Sawyer, 1979), and behavior (e.g., Bargh, 1996; Langer, 1992).

Drawing on Schank and Abelson's (1977) work on the script-like temporal–causal structure of everyday events, Bretherton (e.g., 1987) suggested that the script concept might be useful for understanding attachment representations. Subsequently, Waters and Waters (2006) defined a secure base script in which (1) the individual is meaningfully engaged in exploration/interaction, (2) the engagement is disrupted; (3) distressed, the individual signals distress and seeks support from the primary attachment figure; (4) the attachment figure offers support; (5) the support is accepted; (6) the support effectively solves the problem; (7) the comforting is effective, and (8) the individual reengages in meaningful activity in the environment. Importantly, this definition highlights Ainsworth's concept of the attachment–exploration balance, rather than the separation–reunion sequence familiar from the Strange Situation Procedure (SSP; Ainsworth et al., 1978/2015).

Attachment theory and research have long been plagued by the tendency to view attachment as synonymous with "love" or social relationships in general (e.g., including peer relationships and many facets of diverse adult–adult relationships). Bowlby's attachment theory, however, is not a theory of relationships in general. Instead, it focuses specifically on a few special relationships characterized by secure base use, persistence, separation protest, and grief and mourning in response to loss (Petters, Waters, & Schönbrodt, 2010). Viewing adult attachment representations in terms of a script focuses attention on the secure base aspect of attachment relationships. In addition, by focusing attention on representations of early secure base experience, the secure base script concept suggests a bridge between early experience and adult attachment representations (T. Waters, Brockmeyer, & Crowell, 2013).

SECURE BASE CONTENT IN THE AAI

Mary Ainsworth stated that the goal of her *Infancy in Uganda* project was not to prove the validity of Bowlby's secure base concept but to see whether it was an apt description of infants' actual interactions with the primary caregiver (Ainsworth & Marvin, 1995). We have approached the issue of secure base script content in the AAI in much the same way. To date, over 10,000 AAIs have been analyzed in published attachment research (Bakermans-Kranenburg & van IJzendoorn, 2009). Yet, because secure base content is not a designated scoring criterion for any of the AAI scales or classifications (Main et al., 2003–2008), little attention has been explicitly paid to such content.

There are certainly ample opportunities for interviewees to introduce secure base content into their AAI narratives. Such content is often found when describing relationship experiences in response to the Relationship Adjectives, Closest Parent questions, and in the questions about distress, rejection, and trauma. When we examined 15 AAI transcripts (16,955 lines of narrative response) from the Stony Brook Longitudinal Attachment Study (Crowell & Waters, 2005), 2,745 lines (16.2%) contained direct or indirect references to secure base use or support. Interestingly, 59% of the secure base script-related material was found in just three questions: Q3 and Q4 ("Choose five adjectives or words that reflect your relationship with your mother/father"), and Q6 ("When you were upset as a child, what would you usually do?"). The distribution of secure base content across all interview questions is summarized in Table 10.1.

We identified a wealth of relevant content when viewing AAI transcripts from a secure base script perspective. Secure base content fell into two basic categories: secure base expectations (SBEs) and secure base scenes (SB scenes).

SBEs are general comments that reflect an interviewee's use of the secure base script. They either summarize or refer to identifiable elements of the secure base script. SBEs commonly refer to expectations of availability, responsiveness, or support for exploration (e.g., "Mom always wanted me to try new things, she always supported what I wanted to do"). Although SBEs sometimes occur in detailed recounting of a particular event, they more often occur as simple assertions or generalizations about early experiences. In contrast, SB scenes retell specific experiences in which the secure base is needed and responds in a way that is either consistent or inconsistent with the secure base script.

TABLE 10.1. Distribution of Secure Base-Related Content across AAI Questions

Content	% of total
1. Family background	6%
2. Early relationship	6%
3. Adjectives (mother)	21%
4. Adjectives (father)	17%
5. Closest parent	2%
6. Upset	19%
7. Separation	6%
8. Rejection	6%
9. Threatening/discipline	4%
10. Effect of childhood experience	3%
11. Why parents behaved as they did	1%
12. Other significant adults	2%
13. Loss	4%
14. Change relationship to parents	1%
15. Current relationship with parents	1%
16. Three wishes	0%
17. Lessons learned	0%
18. Hopes for children	0%
	100%

Note. $n = 15$.

Secure Base Expectations

Secure base-related expectations are often the most obvious indication that a person is conceptualizing his or her relationship with their caregivers in terms of an underlying secure base script. Table 10.2 lists a range of positive SBEs that commonly appear in AAI transcripts. The categorization of such content provides an organizing framework for interpreting and scoring SBEs. Importantly, for an utterance to qualify as an SBE, the interviewee must express a distinct expectation (i.e., not merely emotional states) that bears directly on secure base support. Thus, when searching for SBEs, emphasis is placed on content that points to script-like representations of early secure base experience, not on the loving quality or warmth of the relationship.

Whereas positive SBEs advance secure base interactions by focusing attention, cueing goals, and recruiting/organizing behaviors, expectations that are incompatible with the secure base script (i.e., negative SBEs) explicitly or implicitly contradict one or more features central to the secure base script. Such expectations block, derail, or otherwise undermine secure base use and support; for example, "I never knew what she was going to do" (i.e., not predictable) or, "She was as frightened as I was" (i.e., not stronger and wiser).

As in any AAI scoring scale, individual utterances are difficult to evaluate in isolation and should not be used as a basis for important decisions. Coders, when possible, should assign scores based on converging evidence from multiple indicators rather than a single SBE. Below are brief definitions of the SBE categories we have identified, accompanied by a brief note on their relevance to the secure base concept. Additionally, we provide several positive and negative examples reflecting each type.

TABLE 10.2. Secure Base Expectations in the AAI

- Open communication
- Stronger and wiser
- Always there for me
- Available
- Responsive
- Motivated
- Fond of child
- Supports exploration
- Predictable
- Effective comforting
- Proximity seeking

Open Communication

Open Communication is the expectation that one's needs/bids for support will be recognized and resolved by the secure base figure and that seeking support is a welcomed behavior. Positive examples of open communication typically describe the caregiver as approachable and reflect a degree of comfortability and confidence when requesting support.

> INTERVIEWEE: If I ever had any problems I could always talk to [my mother] . . . any problem, I could always ask her for something I needed and I would feel better.

In contrast, negative examples of open communication describe a strong belief that one should not share personal problems with caregivers, based on their unwillingness to take the time to listen or the feeling that bids for support will be met with hostility. The following example illustrates this point, depicting the parent as unwilling to listen and unable to "[make] everything alright."

> INTERVIEWEE: Ummm, well [my father] always had a kind of frame of mind where you were supposed to be tough about things and um, he wasn't real good at listening and making everything alright. So . . . I don't think my sister and I ever really went to him with, you know, I'm feeling bad or I need to tell you about this.

Stronger and Wiser

Stronger and Wiser is the expectation is that the secure base has the necessary knowledge, skill, or ability to resolve challenges and distress, and provide support. This is an important basis for establishing confidence when exploring away from the attachment figure or exploring new domains. Expectations of stronger and wiser should therefore be connected to well-founded feelings of trust (i.e., they should not include unfounded idealizations).

> INTERVIEWEE: I feel like if [my mother] thinks that this is what I should do, then she probably knows best, you know? And basically, one of the big reasons that I remember wanting to start school early was that I wanted to be with my one particular friend, but I also think I trusted her enough that, if she was going [to suggest this], it would be OK. She tested me and thought that it would be OK.

In contrast, negative examples cast considerable doubt on the caregiver's competency to resolve conflict in most situations. Assertions to this effect often describe the caregiver as irrational or unable to control/structure the environment for the child.

INTERVIEWEE: [Child gets injured on bicycle.] My next-door neighbor came over and he took care of me and patched me up 'cause my mother wasn't good with things like that. . . . She just can't handle it, especially to see one of us in pain. It just totally destroys her.

In the positive example, not only does the interviewee believe that the caregiver knows best, he or she also connects this with a concrete example of how this belief impacted behavior. Idealizing statements do not usually provide this kind of rationale. In contrast, the negative example portrays the mother as fragile and "[not] good with things like that."

Always There for Me

Always There for Me is the expectation that the caregiver is always available and vigilant, prepared to respond when secure base support is needed. A word search returned the expression "always there" in nearly 50% of the AAI transcripts used to develop the secure base coding system. In most instances, it was just an easy figure of speech that could mistakenly be taken as evidence of secure base script knowledge. It is critical, therefore, that the expectation "always there for me" appear in an attachment context (i.e., when the individual needs help or support), as in the following example.

INTERVIEWEE: As I look back, I think [my father] has always been there when I . . . kind of when I step off, or get off track a little; he's always been there just to nudge me back on and just kind of tell me what's on his mind and it's usually right so . . .

INTERVIEWER: Letting you know that he is paying attention to what's going on with you?

INTERVIEWEE: Yup, and letting me know that he's always there, and he's kind of watching out and if I kinda fall off a little bit he's always there to kind of push me back on.

Importantly, statements to the effect of "always there for me" should not be confused with mere presence in the home (e.g., "My mom was a stay-at-home mom, so she was always around"). Such examples frequently appear in the transcripts of individuals whose idea of supportive parenting largely includes instrumental care. It is worth noting here that these instances are not *necessarily* treated as negative examples of the "always there for me" expectation given their indirect relation to beliefs about availability and vigilance in an attachment sense.

INTERVIEWEE: [My father] wasn't always there to support me. Any number of reasons. [. . .] Even when I tried killing myself at 14, it kinda dawned on me that night, that my father . . . I didn't expect my father to show up at the hospital when they were giving me the charcoal and stuff like that. I didn't expect him to be at the hospital. My mother had called him and he was . . . I was so surprised when he showed up that I asked him what he was doing there. [. . .] He was just . . . soccer games he missed, dance recitals he missed for no real reason. He was just . . . a lot of times for all those specific childhood events he was never there for.

In this example, there is an evident need for secure base support following an attempted suicide. It is rather telling that the interviewee is "surprised" when his or her father shows up at the hospital. If the interviewee held the SBE of "always there for me," the father's arrival would have been anticipated, not surprising. The statement "he wasn't always there to support me" is even further substantiated when the interviewee provides countless additional examples of events the father missed, absences that he had "no real reason for."

Available

Available is the expectation that there is an "open door" to the secure base; in other words, the belief that the child can always go to the caregiver for support and comfort. In contrast to "always there for me," these examples are more specific to the caregiver's literal availability or accessibility (i.e., on a day-to-day, moment-to-moment basis) than to the caregiver's motivation to provide support. In this sense, it is more focused than "always there for me." This distinction is included to ensure that both senses of caregiver support are identified as SBEs. In practice, these SBEs often co-occur.

INTERVIEWEE: [My mother] was always interested in what we had to say. She was always, you know, loving in that respect . . . she was always around when we needed her to be there. She would always sit there to listen to anything we had to say. She was always, you know, always open, like the door was always open there, she was always very receptive to our feelings. [. . .] If we needed her she was always there and it's like . . . she always said the door was always open, anything we had to talk to her about.

Negative examples focus on physical absence and dismissal of the child's support-seeking behavior. As a result, alternative (and less effective) strategies for regulating emotion and distress are often adopted (e.g., taking care of oneself). In the example below, the interviewee emphasizes the caregiver's emotional distance by what is viewed as outright rejection of support seeking and prioritizing work over being physically available.

INTERVIEWEE: I would always, like, call [my mother]. And she kind of—every time would say, like you have to stop calling me, like I'm at work, leave me alone. And so I guess in that way, I felt kind of distant 'cause she wasn't really, like, there. Um, she worked a lot so [it was] like distant and she would never come—she would never come home and deal with the issue, and I felt kind of, not neglected, but the situation was neglected.

Responsive

Responsive is the expectation is that signals for support will be recognized by the attachment figure and promptly addressed through instrumental and emotional support. It is often seen as a "caregiver's intuition" or a dedicated caregiver who always "saves the day."

> INTERVIEWEE: [My mother] just loves me to death . . . would do anything for me. If I would cry, she'd wipe the tear . . . if I was sad, she'd make me laugh . . . if I was bored, she'd do something with me . . . play a game with me . . . or take me somewhere . . . she was just the best.

In this example, the interviewee expects the mother to respond across a wide range of attachment-relevant contexts, both with respect to physical and emotional pain, as well as when the child feels the need to explore the environment. Alternatively, negative examples of "responsive" describe caregivers who offer little in the way of instrumental and/or emotional support during times of need. When the child's needs are signaled to the caregiver in these instances, action is either not taken or delayed in favor of the parent's needs.

> INTERVIEWEE: [What would you do when you were upset?] Probably cry and then go to my dad 'cause he was the only one around and then he'd probably just complain and tell me to leave him alone. That's usually what happened.

Although the interviewee regularly sought support from their father, the negative expectation is implied in the undermining qualification "[because] he was the only one around." This is then made explicit when the interviewee adds " . . . and then he would probably just complain and tell me to leave him alone."

Motivated

Motivated is the expectation that the caregiver consistently extends extra effort to support the child's goals and ambitions. Interviewees with the motivated SBE describe their caregivers as regularly going above and beyond what is ordinarily required to support the child's exploration.

> INTERVIEWEE: [My father] would do anything for us. He's sacrificed a lot for us, always puts his kids first, like the type who would give you anything before he went out and did something for himself. Although I'm beginning to think that's just the way men are.

In this example, the interviewee expects that their father will be motivated to place her needs ahead of his own. Interestingly, the interviewee has generalized that expectation to all men. Certainly, all men are not like this, but perhaps the interviewee seeks partners who resemble the qualities of a good secure base. This illustrates how script-like representations might explain continuity across different types of relationships. In contrast to the previous excerpt, negative examples typically reflect an interviewee's view of being unimportant or a low priority.

> INTERVIEWEE: [My father] would never put any effort into anything [with us]. It was always kind of like the last action [or his last thought], like "well I did something, [interviewee's name]," you know . . . so he wouldn't feel so guilty.

In this example, the child is markedly low on the father's priority list. Furthermore, the father's efforts toward the relationship are discussed in terms of the bare minimum, focusing to a great extent on alleviating his own negative affect (i.e., feelings of guilt) as opposed to supporting the child.

Fond of the Child

Fond of the Child is when the caregiver displays genuine enjoyment in the role as a parent, which translates to the child feeling loved and cared for. These expectations should be rooted in concrete experience and go beyond simply saying, "I know my mother loved me."

> INTERVIEWEE: [My mother] used to pick me up and swing me around all the time. And she liked to show me off to her friends. She was always there. Very sympathetic, always interested. It was made out of caring, I guess.

This example would receive credit, because the expectation is grounded in specific recurring interactions, such as "[My mother] used to pick me up" and "show me off to her friends." Importantly, the interviewee infers that the mother's behavior was "made out of caring." This connects the mother's actions to a positive motivation and argues against a self-serving motive.

Negative examples include harsh parenting, such as caregivers withholding love or expressing outright rejection. Interactions such as those described below, often lead to feelings of inadequacy and worthlessness, and are therefore incompatible with the secure base script.

> INTERVIEWEE: Um, [my father] never could say "I love you." He um, he could never show emotion. If I would ask him to show his feelings, he would just shut down. He wasn't able to. He would never make me feel like I was important. He would just make me feel that everything, or everyone else, came before I did. I would leave [his house] crying because I was "needing" to be told certain things that he never would say . . . so I left there feeling inadequate, I mean that was just an everyday occurrence with him. Every time I left, I was looking for what I needed to hear and it never came.

Supports Exploration

Supports Exploration is the expectation that the caregiver places high priority on the child's exploration and development. This is often illustrated in examples describing caregivers as supporting or actively encouraging goal-oriented activities and interests.

> INTERVIEWEE: [My father] always encouraged us to do whatever we wanted to do. When I was about nine, I decided that I wanted to play little league baseball with all guys, and there were no other girls. And um . . . most fathers were like, I would never let my daughter do that, and he was like "if that's what you want to do, that's fine, you know, we'll get 'ya out there and, you know, see how you do." And he went to all my games and he would stand right behind the plate, and the whole time I was at bat he would be talking to me, telling me "OK, you know, this looks good . . . step in and swing." I mean he was really very encouraging.

Supporting exploration involves more than simply allowing the child to pursue certain activities; it also requires cooperative engagement and enrichment. This is evident in the previous example. In addition to allowing his daughter to play on the boys' team, the father actively contributes to her success ("if that's what you want to do, that's fine . . . we'll get 'ya out there . . ." and also "he would stand right behind the plate and the whole time I was at bat he would be talking to me"). In this way, the secure base helps the child to live a bigger life than she could have otherwise.

In contrast, negative examples depict caregivers as dismissive of the child's interests and goals. In some cases, these can include accounts of caregivers actively preventing the child's exploration and the pursuit of new experiences, as in the following example.

> INTERVIEWEE: I was around like 10, I just really wanted to start getting involved in things at school, like extracurricular things. And um, [my father] just didn't want me to do it and I would sit there and argue with him and try to explain to him why I wanted to do it, and it would be like talking to a wall. [. . .] he would be like, "Well, you know, your grades aren't that great" and stuff like that. Or he'd just be like, "Well, I never did them so I don't think you should do them." And . . . it made it really hard for me, because those were things that I started wanting to get into and he just didn't feel that it was necessary for me to do it.

Predictable

Predictable is the expectation that the attachment figure is consistent in providing secure base support. This is often described as the belief that the child can predict how the caregiver will respond to requests for support.

> INTERVIEWEE: Our relationship was good, it was comfortable . . . it was safe . . . it was secure. Um, there were no surprises, you know, I knew

what they expected from me and it was consistent. You know, they were really loving. It was . . . it was healthy.

This example highlights how the parents' predictable behavior and rules/ expectations led the interviewee to feel safe and secure. Importantly, the predictability must be framed in an attachment context. Merely eating the same breakfast every morning, while predictable, is not relevant to secure base script knowledge.

Interviewees who lack access to the secure base script may say nothing at all about predictability or they may discuss feeling less than comfortable using their caregivers as a secure base. More explicit descriptions include erratic and irrational caregiving behaviors. In such cases, interviewees often describe having to "walk on eggshells" during their childhood in the hopes of avoiding conflicts with caregivers.

INTERVIEWEE: Well back then, we didn't know what was going on, you know? One minute [my father] was nice, the next minute he wasn't . . . and you know, you didn't know what his mood was gonna be when he walked in the front door and everybody was you know . . . edgy . . . what kind of mood was he gonna be in?

In the negative example, the father's unpredictable nature leads to feelings of uneasiness in the home. Such insecurities are likely to negatively impact the child's own attachment needs given that attention is focused on the caregiver as opposed to exploration.

Effective Comforting

Effective Comforting is the belief that caregiver's support and comfort during times of distress are helpful or linked to feeling better and reengaging in constructive activities. This is often described in terms of caregivers knowing what to do to make the child feel better and get back on track.

INTERVIEWEE: But basically [my parents would] figure out what was wrong and they'd just talk to me about it, and it wasn't, they never really did the thing that would in a sense rile me up more, and get me more upset, they would always calm me down and try to get what was really going on out, so they could you know help me look forward or . . .

Here, the expectation that caregivers will provide effective comfort is presented from two angles: first in saying that the parents never caused more distress when seeking support ("they never really did the thing that would rile me up more"), and second by stating that they "would always calm me down." In stating that the goal was to help them look forward, it is clear that the interviewee is conceptualizing the caregivers' efforts to comfort in terms of the secure base script.

Negative examples indicate that efforts to provide support typically fail in resolving the distress. The expectation that their caregiver is likely incapable of effectively resolving distress usually signals to the child that support should generally not be sought out. As shown in the following example, it is not uncommon for such individuals to describe having to turn to alternative strategies for regulating emotion and distress (e.g., needing to care for themselves).

> INTERVIEWEE: [My mother] was always the uh alarmist, so when it came to that, she was just like callin' my father. [. . .] I can remember another time like I sliced my finger open with a knife and the same thing, I tried to hide it from her because she'd get me more scared 'cause she was upset . . . like any kinda blood or anything she'd pass out.

Proximity Seeking

Proximity Seeking is the expectation that the primary response to distress is to seek out an attachment figure. In higher scoring transcripts, this SBE most frequently appears in Q6 of the AAI ("What would you do when you were upset?) and reflects a causal connection between distress and seeking support.

The interviewee in the example below articulates a general assumption that when upset or having some difficulty, the first response was most likely to seek out his or her secure base.

> INTERVIEWEE: If ever anything came up, I probably went to my mother with it. I mean even if I like had a fight with somebody at school, I would probably come home and tell my mother.
>
> INTERVIEWER: When you were upset as a child, what would you do? Now this would not be upset with your parents, this would be upset generally.
>
> INTERVIEWEE: Upset over something. Um, again, like let's say something happened at school, I think the chances are I would have been coming home to my mother. So, she'd probably be the one I would be running to if something happened.

Alternatively, in the presence of clear distress, negative examples reference failures to seek secure base support, explicit avoidance of attachment figures, or decisions to opt for self-care in lieu of caregivers' assistance.

> INTERVIEWER: Alright, so when you were upset as a child what would you do?
>
> INTERVIEWEE: I would, I wouldn't go to anyone, that's for sure, I probably just cried in my room or just sit in my room or just talk to my friends, but I would never go to my parents.

Instrumental Support

When evaluating secure base content in the AAI, it is important to distinguish between attachment-related expectations and more general expectations about the parent–child relationship (i.e., those not specific to secure base behavior). The latter often deal with resource-related aspects of parental support such as the provision of food, clothing, and shelter. For our purposes, we classify such statements as examples of "Instrumental support." Although important aspects of child care, these expectations do not necessarily point to secure base script knowledge. For example, many insecurely attached adults in the United States grow up in secure environments with adequate clothing and shelter. Similarly, material poverty per se does not preclude a child from learning the secure base script so long as consistent sensitive and supportive care is provided from a secure base figure. The following illustrates examples of instrumental support that would not, in their own right, suggest access to or use of the secure base script.

> INTERVIEWEE: Secure . . . I guess . . . I mean I know that I was distant from [my father] and all, but I know that we always had a roof over our head and that I always had a family, and I know that Dad would never leave my mother, so I knew that I was secure in that aspect.

> INTERVIEWEE: [in reference to the relationship] It felt secure . . . I didn't feel like, you know, I might have to sleep out in the street the next day.

Researchers should be cautious not to infer secure base script knowledge from singular adjectives or statements that lack information to support or confirm the interviewee's intended meaning. In the previous (second) example, the interviewee describes the relationship as "secure." Yet without additional qualifying information, we cannot assume that his or her security is thought of in the same way as an individual who conceptualizes security in terms of the secure base script. This is made clear when the interviewee states, "I didn't feel like, you know, I might have to sleep out in the street the next day." Likewise, researchers should be careful not to overlook other, perhaps less obvious descriptors of secure base script knowledge (e.g., "funny"). Only through additional detail can the interviewer discern whether the adjective or description is organized around the secure base script. This highlights the importance of asking good follow-up questions in the AAI, especially when initial interviewee responses are vague or unclear.

Secure Base Scenes and Scene Fragments

The AAI often elicits accounts of *specific* attachment-related events from childhood. Unlike the basic assertions and generalizations linked to SBEs, these passages reflect fully formed event representations. Specific event descriptions of secure base interactions, termed secure base scenes (SB Scenes), are valuable indicators when determining whether an individual has organized his or her experiences around the secure base script.

SB Scenes can touch on a range of event characteristics, including antecedents, interactions, and consequences that involve the use of a secure base.

SB Scenes can be recounted in considerable detail, or they can be so brief that they contain only fragments of a significant event. Fully developed scenes carry the most secure base script content/structure and serve as the strongest evidence that the interviewee has encoded early experiences in terms of the secure base script. In contrast to SBEs, most AAIs include only a few (if any) such well-developed passages.

Somewhat more common than complete scenes are SB Scene Fragments. Fragmented scenes include some, though not all, of the elements of the secure base script. Consequently, inferences about the interviewee's use of a secure base script are supported to a lesser extent than fully elaborated passages. SB Scenes and scene fragments can be specific, generic, or event focused. Specific scenes describe secure base-relevant one-time events (e.g., "One time I got a D in eighth grade math and my mom . . . "). Generic scenes do not refer to a specific event, but rather reflect a more general secure base-relevant context (e.g., "Whenever I got bad grades, my parents . . . "). Finally, event-focused scenes are specific event narratives that describe instrumental care and/or caregiver interactions that neither fully reflect nor contradict the secure base script. For example, "I got a D in math once. After that, my mom started reminding me to do my homework." These episodes are generally ignored in scoring secure base script content unless the interviewee indicates that the caregiver's response was in some way at odds with what he or she needed/expected or made the situation worse.

Secure Base Scenes

Each of the following SB Scenes clearly articulates a specific event from the interviewee's childhood, with varying degrees of elaboration and detail. The degree of elaboration around SB Scenes can vary widely within and across AAI transcripts. Despite differences in length and elaboration, each of the following scenes contain four basic or fundamental elements of the secure base script, specifically (1) proximity seeking/signaling for support, (2) instrumental response from caregiver, (3) emotional support from caregiver, and (4) clear resolution of the distress. These elements manifest in the example below.

INTERVIEWEE: I had an incident that uh, one of the uh, the uh . . . neighborhood boys uh wanted to play doctor with me. And uh it was uh, you know, I knew it was wrong as soon as it had happened and it was difficult for me to tell [my mother], I guess I was about seven. And I knew, I didn't tell her, didn't tell her, and then finally it just built up in me and I decided I had to tell her and I knew that she would do the right thing.

INTERVIEWER: And how did she react?

INTERVIEWEE: Uh she was um . . . she just took it in stride like she, she told me that, you know, I was right in coming to her and um she wasn't angry with me. I guess she was angry with the neighbor, the neighbor of the boy, and she spoke to his mother. But um . . . after it was over, I felt much better and um . . . I just felt like I could trust her with this terrible burden that I had on me before I told her.

Despite the delay in seeking support, the child ultimately brings the situation to the mother's attention. Indeed, children are often afraid that they may get in trouble for bad behavior. The motivation to finally seek support, however, overrides this anxiety. This is confirmed by the statement "I knew that she would do the right thing."

In the example below, the provision of secure base support is elaborated to a lesser extent than in the previous SB Scene. Nevertheless, the key elements are implied.

INTERVIEWER: What would you do when you were upset?

INTERVIEWEE: I'd probably go to my mom.

INTERVIEWER: What would she do?

INTERVIEWEE: [She'd comfort me], one time I had um a fist fight when I was younger with one of my best friends. And I don't particularly remember what it was over, but I remember being very, very upset. And . . . you know, of course, I went to my mother, and my mother wanted to call her mother and, you know and . . . work the whole thing out and, and she did, she called up and, you know, we had all gotten together. But um . . . you know, I felt . . . she, she wasn't angry at me that I had this fight, she, you know, felt for me, she really, you know, went outta her way to make, you know, make everything OK.

Here we find several clear indications that (1) a signal for support is made and recognized by the secure base, (2) instrumental support is provided when the mother calls the parents of the other child involved in the conflict, and (3) an effective resolution is achieved given the statement "she went out of her way to make everything OK." Element 3 (emotional support) should be inferred from the statement, "[when] I had this fight, she, you know, felt for me." Whereas inferred empathy reflects the support component for this scene, hugging or showering the child with warmth may fill this role in other examples.

A third example illustrates that the key elements of a secure base script can be present even in the absence of elaboration.

INTERVIEWEE: Uh, I got bit by a dog and uh, you know, but I ran home and uh [my mother] . . . she took, you know, she came right for me, I was crying, she hugged me, she got ice, she cleaned it, she explained to me we had to go to the doctor. And she, just uh, very calm about the whole thing and uh, you know, she made me feel safe.

Although script-like representations serve as a foundation for elaboration, lack of elaboration per se is not necessarily a negative indication. This is especially true when an interviewer has not been providing appropriate probes or follow-up questions. Requests for specific examples are essential in determining whether a generalization is well founded or evasive. Taken together, this highlights the importance of rigorous interviewer training and ongoing review of transcripts as they are completed.

Secure Base Fragment

The SB Scenes found in the previous section illustrate variation in the length and elaboration of autobiographical narratives. In addition to narrating complete scenes, interviewees often recall specific secure base-related events that contain some, but not all, of the four secure base script elements. In the absence of elaboration, but some elements can be inferred, the passage is considered a SB Fragment.

> INTERVIEWEE: [Not picked first during dance tryout] There was a time that . . . um I wasn't put in the front line for the show and uh I talked to [my mother] about it and 'cause I was sad, I wanted to be in the front line and she explained to me that everyone can't be and, you know, you're a good dancer and that's why you're in that class. And she tried to find ways to build me up even though I wasn't picked as one of the best at the time.

> INTERVIEWEE: I had sprained my ankle, I was playing with my cousin and I was crying, and my father came out and just swooped me up and brought me into the house. You know, he was just always there for things like that, you know, he wouldn't let us get hurt and would come to our rescue.

> INTERVIEWEE: My dog died, and I remember finding out she died and going to my mom. And my mom just, you know, just holding you and kinda listening to you and just patting me and saying, you know, "We're so sorry," you know?

> INTERVIEWEE: I remember going to perform a piano piece and sing a song in sixth grade [for a recital]. And I was very nervous 'bout doing it and [my father] just kept telling me that I can do it, not to worry about it and I could definitely do it, you like to do it, and just enjoy myself.

In each example, the narrative describes specific events and contains clear articulations of *some, but not all,* scene elements. The first three contain clear examples of proximity seeking/signaling for support, followed by a sensitive response. Although proximity seeking is not explicitly stated in the fourth example, this can be inferred given the secure base figure's apparent presence during the critical moment of need. Notably, none of the examples contains a clear indication that the support provided (instrumental or emotional) effectively resolved the distress. The presence of one or more SB Scene elements nonetheless points to the secure base relevance in each example.

Although the secure base relevance of scene fragments is evident from one or a few script elements, we cannot be confident from a single example that the interviewee has constructed a *complete* script-like representation of his or her early secure base experiences. However, in the course of responding to one or several AAI questions, an interviewee might provide multiple attachment-related event narratives that are more or less developed. As in most assessments, the best evidence is a convergence of multiple indicators—fully developed scenes, multiple scene fragments, and/or multiple SBEs.

Generic Scene

Similar to SB Scenes and SB Fragments, Generic Scenes incorporate the same four elements. Yet, rather than referring to a specific one-time event, these narratives refer to a "class" of events framed as temporal–causal generalizations about secure base experiences. Abstracting commonalities from experience is efficient in terms of storage and retrieval and, in many contexts, is more useful than retaining the particulars of any specific experience itself. Indeed, it is often more valuable to know *how* secure base interactions are likely to unfold than to recall one (or every) specific instance from past experience. Therefore, even though Generic Scenes are often lacking in detail, they are considered strong evidence that the interviewee knows the secure base script.

> INTERVIEWER: What would your parents do when you were upset?
>
> INTERVIEWEE: They would figure out what was wrong and they'd just talk to me about it, they never really did the thing that would in a sense rile me up more, and get me more upset, they would always calm me down and try to get what was really going on out, so they could you know help me look forward.

> INTERVIEWEE: [in response to the adjective *caring*] Caring? Um, I guess caring I think of. . . . like whenever I was little and got hurt? I can remember one time falling off my bike, really hurting my knee. . . . coming and crying and. . . . [my mother] could always comfort me and take care of me, make it better.

Generic Scenes can also be organized around negative SBEs, as in the following examples:

> INTERVIEWER: What would your parents do when you were upset?
>
> INTERVIEWEE: I . . . well, I would go to my mother . . . and ask her for advice and she would say something like um . . . you know, "Oh you think you have problems now? Wait till you get older" . . . you know, she wouldn't help me with solving them . . .

> INTERVIEWER: You said sometimes your mom would do things that upset you.
>
> INTERVIEWEE: Yeah, I just remember her yelling a lot and hitting me.

INTERVIEWER: What would you typically do during those times?

INTERVIEWEE: Um, I would curl up in a ball and just cry and just like, "I'm sorry, I'm sorry, I'm sorry, I'm sorry" and, and then eventually she'd calm down. I'd like clean myself up and then I'd go lie in bed.

In the AAI, Generic Scenes can provide concise, relevant replies to many questions. Notably, however, Main et al. (2003–2008) highlight instances in which AAI interviewees say they cannot recall examples of early interactions with an attachment figure. Instead, those who seemingly struggle with these questions often provide vague (and unfounded) generalizations, faltering when asked to provide illustrative examples. Such "lack of recall" is traditionally interpreted in terms of conflict or defensive processes, or incompatible mental models of caregivers, and points toward insecure or unresolved attachment classifications (e.g., Main, 1991; Main et al., 2003–2008).

For the current coding scheme, lack of detail is not necessarily viewed as negative, nor is it critical to resolve such issues to decide whether an interviewee is working from a secure base script. From a script perspective, difficulty in retrieving a specific event or detail can be interpreted in two ways: as a matter of the interviewee having schematized/scripted the experiences, or as a vague attempt to articulate secure base experience in the absence of having truly had it. If a Generic Scene contains key secure base script elements, then we can infer an underlying script-like representation, even if the interviewee cannot provide specific examples. If not, then the issue is decided on the basis of SB Scenes, SB Fragments, and SBEs in the rest of the transcript. Each of these can be evaluated in its own right.

That said, confidence that a narrative is guided by an underlying secure base script is greater if the script elements are unambiguous. Seemingly positive statements, such as "My mother could always . . . make it better," may or may not reflect secure base script knowledge, depending on what the interviewee means by "make it better." This kind of ambiguity can be observed in both Generic Scenes and SB Fragments, and thus are given equal weight in the coding system.

Scenes That Do Not Indicate Secure Base Script Knowledge

The preceding sections have focused primarily on secure base-related scenes that suggest an underlying script. However, not every scene that describes interactions with a caregiver is secure base-related or indicative of the secure base script. This is illustrated by event memories in which secure base resolutions are absent, or a sequence of acts is strung together without any apparent secure base content. When specific event narratives provided by the interviewee directly violate the elements or structure of the secure base script, these are assigned the lowest scores on the coding scale.

Secure Base Misses

Occasionally, a scene will at first seem to unfold along the lines of the secure base script (e.g., situation calls for secure base use), only to bring the expectant reader up short, without any kind of secure base-related ending. These passages are termed secure base misses (SB Miss). Akin to prototypical SB Scenes, some distress or challenge in the environment elicits a bid for help. However, in the case of a SB Miss, the narrative ends abruptly or trails off, without any concrete description of comfort or resolution of the distress. In such instances, the caregiver misses the opportunity to provide support.

> INTERVIEWEE: One day, when I was home, it must have been just [my mother] and I were there and I was in my room and um, I was kinda down 'cause there wasn't anyone to play with and um, I told her that and she, you know, said that there's a lot of things to do and just kind of, you know, said a few things and left me alone, but, which was OK, but it didn't make me feel a lot better.

> INTERVIEWEE: Um, oh um one time I was getting a fever, and then I was like freezing cold, and I was sitting in the living room but my dad—I told him that like I was getting a fever, and he wouldn't believe me and then, I did end up getting a fever um so I just went to bed and I was like freezing still, but my dad wouldn't believe me. So, I just took the medicine and went to sleep.

Coders are not necessarily looking for negative experiences with caregivers per se. Rather, the focus is primarily placed on how those experiences are organized, interpreted, and linked to more general expectations. What is critical is not the valence of the event, but how the interviewee frames the experience in terms of secure base needs.

Secure Base Failures

In contrast to SB Misses, a secure base failure (SB Fail) arises when a secure base-related scene concludes with caregiver behavior that is irrelevant or counterproductive to a secure base resolution. Memories of childhood experiences discussed in the AAI are sometimes frightening, harsh, or even abusive. If, instead of responding effectively, or missing the opportunity to provide secure base support, the caregiver's response makes the distress *worse*, the scene is coded as an SB Fail. Whereas SB Misses are characterized by a *lack of response*, SB Fails are characterized by a *counterproductive response*.

In the examples below, the caregiver exacerbates negative affect and does not get the child meaningfully reengaged in the environment. As a result, each of these examples is considered an SB Fail.

INTERVIEWEE: . . . had banged myself up pretty well.

INTERVIEWER: Oh dear, and then what happened?

INTERVIEWEE: Um, [my parents] just came rushing out and they just saw that I was bumped and bruised up and scrapped up but nothing serious. But I think it scared my mom bad enough that she got really mad. I think, they get, I don't know if it scared her or what, but she, I remember she got really mad about it. [. . .] I just remember her yelling and [. . .] throwing fits about riding the bike and not being in, and not watching where I was going and things like that.

INTERVIEWER: [Child becomes upset during a visit to a playground and decides to sit down and pout instead of playing.] Do you remember how your parent reacted? What the response was?

INTERVIEWEE: [. . .] pretty much ignored me. I was just left alone to pout and, now that I think about it, might have even kind of made fun of me. Um, which really kind of make me feel bad, like more upset than I was, because I was upset about something small probably, but I was still upset, and then getting ignored and teased a little just—it made me feel like whatever I was feeling was less important, I guess.

Alternative Schemas

The secure base script evolves from experiencing countless sensitive responsive and co-constructive caregiver interactions over a considerable period of time. If an individual's early relationships with caregivers are unresponsive, intrusive, unpredictable, or predictably difficult, they are likely to abstract the common themes in terms of very different schemas. In our review of several hundred AAI transcripts, we encountered recollections organized around conflictual or unsatisfying alternatives to secure base organization. These seemed to reflect alternative ways of understanding relationships. Moreover, their organization often seemed more thematic than script-like.

Unlike SB Scenes, which are formulated in a series of temporally related events, alternative schemas are often painted in broader strokes in the way interviewees interpret the AAI questions and form themes that recur throughout the transcript. Accordingly, we describe each alternative schema with a title, as if they are maxims or worldviews rather than scripts (see Appendix 10.1). Yet, like the secure base script, they can serve as a basis for expectations. These alternative expectations serve in place of the secure base script. Thus, transcripts organized around alternative schemas rank at the bottom of the scale for scoring secure base script knowledge and receive the lowest possible score (Table 10.3).

At present, it is not clear how many more alternative schemas might be identified in larger and more diverse samples. Nor is it clear whether some alternative schemas are used more frequently than others, or whether enough examples would suggest a taxonomy of alternative schemas. These alternatives to the secure base script are likely to arise more often in clinically and

TABLE 10.3. Scale for Scoring Secure Base Script Knowledge from the Adult Attachment Interview (AAI_{sbs})

9.	Two or more positive scenes that have clear secure base script organization and multiple positive secure base expectations. Positive scene fragments or generic scenes may also be present.
8.	One positive scene that has clear secure base structure plus one or more additional positive scene fragments or generic scenes. Multiple clear positive secure base-related expectations.
7.	One positive secure base scene and several positive secure base expectations.
6.	Several positive scenes fragments or generic scenes accompanied by multiple positive secure base expectations.
5.	One positive secure base scene fragment or generic scene. No clear positive secure base scenes, but multiple examples of positive secure base expectations.
4.	Transcript contains no positive scenes, fragments, or generic scenes. Instead, coder observes several positive secure base expectations. Some negative SBEs may be present, but the majority are positive, and the transcript generally suggests expectations consistent with the secure base script.
3.	Transcript contains no positive scenes, fragments, or generic scenes. Instead, the transcript contains largely negative SBEs or is event/instrumental care focused. There may be some positive SBEs, but the majority are negative.
2.	One or more clear examples of secure base misses or failures paired with multiple negative SBEs. Little or no evidence of an alternative schema present.
1.	Relationship viewed through the lens of an alternative schema that contradicts or is inconsistent with the secure base script.

historically underserved populations. Developmentalists and clinicians will wonder, as well, whether the presence of consolidated alternative schemas represents a greater challenge to attachment-based interventions than the mere absence or incomplete formulation of a secure base script. Alternative schemes clearly deserve attention in both clinical and cross-cultural contexts, and in different childrearing configurations.

SCORING SECURE BASE SCRIPT KNOWLEDGE FROM ATTACHMENT NARRATIVES: THE AAI SECURE BASE SCRIPT SCALE

After identifying and describing secure base script content in the AAI, attention naturally turns toward quantifying this content in a meaningful way. For this, we developed the AAI Secure Base Script scale (AAI_{sbs}). The scale for scoring secure base script content in the AAI focuses on (1) explicit and implied SBEs, and (2) secure base script elements in specific attachment-related events. Unlike traditional AAI scales and overall Coherence scoring, secure base script scoring does not focus on positive or negative affect or narrative coherence per se. Nor does secure base script scoring focus on sentence structure or idiosyncrasies of expression. This is not to say that these cannot convey important information, only that script theory directs attention elsewhere.

Like the scoring of passages based on prompt-word outlines (H. Waters & Waters, 2006), an AAI_{sbs} score is akin to a confidence rating. As a transcript is read, secure base content is noted and viewed as accumulating evidence that the interviewee is using a secure base script as a retrieval cue and tool to organize recall. The highest scores are reserved for transcripts that provide clear SB Scenes, Generic Scenes, or SB Fragments. The scale clearly indicates what score should be assigned, based on the frequency with which these types of content appear in AAI transcripts. Most importantly, coders must correctly identify and distinguish between varying types of secure base content, as this weighs heavily in coding decisions.

Scores in the middle of the AAI_{sbs} scale are assigned when transcripts do not have any content that could be coded as a SB Scene (or an SB Miss/SB Fail). In such cases, the coder is required to distinguish between scores based on SBEs alone. When a transcript seems to evidence a great number of positive SBEs, a score of 4 is usually given. Transcripts that largely reflect negative or neutral SBEs are usually assigned a score of 3. As can often be the case, SBEs may differ across caregivers. In these situations, the coder places greater weight on the SBEs for the *primary* caregiver (i.e., the person with the most investment in the child) to resolve this discrepancy, the logic being that the secure base script is acquired through repeated interactions, so whoever the interviewee had more interactions with is likely the better indicator of secure base script knowledge.

The lowest AAI_{sbs} scores are assigned to transcripts that consist mostly of negative SBEs and contain SB Misses and/or SB Fails. Some interviewees may also employ alternative schemas that are inconsistent or that contradict the secure base script. To receive the absolute lowest score, an AAI_{sbs} score of 1, the interviewee must employ an alternative schema across several questions, with minimal, or not, positive secure base content.

Validation

Several lines of evidence point to the validity and utility of the AAI_{sbs}. In terms of convergent validity, combined data ($N = 134$) from studies by Crowell and Waters (2005) and Dagan, Asok, Steele, Steele, and Bernard (2018) revealed that AAI_{sbs} scores were highly correlated with secure base script knowledge assessed using the H. Waters and Waters (2006) prompt-word based Attachment Script Assessment ($r = .50$, $p < .001$; Waters et al., in press). AAI_{sbs} scores from the Stony Brook Longitudinal Attachment Study (T. Waters et al., 2013) were also highly correlated with AAI coherence scores (AAI_{COH};

$r = .64$, $p < .001$). Moreover, AAI_{sbs} was significantly correlated with AAI_{COH} even in the Minnesota Longitudinal Study of Risk and Adaptation (MLSRA; T. Waters, Ruiz, & Roisman, 2017), a high-risk longitudinal sample, ($r = .23$, $p = < .01$ and $r = .29$, $p < .01$ at ages 19 and 26 years, respectively). AAI_{sbs} was also significantly stable across the 7-year interval in the MLSRA ($r = .55$, $p < .001$). In the same dataset, T. Waters et al. (2017) examined the developmental origins of secure base script knowledge using the AAI_{sbs} scale. A composite of maternal sensitivity across the childhood period significantly predicted secure base script knowledge at ages 19 and 26 years (r's = .33 and .37, p's < .001, respectively). This suggests that secure base script knowledge, as reflected in the AAI, is learned in the context of sensitive parental care. Notably, both stability and maternal sensitivity correlations were stronger for the AAI_{sbs} than for parallel analyses employing the AAI_{COH}.

In addition, the AAI_{sbs} has proven useful in accounting for adult romantic functioning. T. Waters et al. (2013), for example, found significant links between adults' secure base script knowledge and both caregiving and care-seeking behaviors in the context of romantic relationships. Furthermore, T. Waters, Raby, Ruiz, Martin, and Roisman (2018) found that AAI_{sbs} scores were significantly correlated with self-reported romantic relationship satisfaction, observed romantic relationship quality, and interview-assessed romantic relationship effectiveness. AAI_{sbs} has also been associated with parent–child relationship quality. Specifically, T. Waters et al. found significant correlations of AAI_{sbs} with supportive parenting and offspring SSPs (Ainsworth et al., 1978/2015). Taken together, this evidence suggests that the AAI_{sbs} system captures secure base script knowledge and produces theory-consistent results in terms of developmental antecedents and predictive significance. Furthermore, the AAI_{sbs} provides a much-needed additional assessment of secure base script knowledge and opens the door for the inclusion of multiple measures of secure base script knowledge within studies. It also affords opportunities for scoring secure base script knowledge from existing AAI's and for economizing by administering brief versions of the AAI for research that only requires secure base script scores.

Are There Insecure Attachment Scripts?

The most commonly asked question during AAI_{sbs} training workshops is whether there are also scripts corresponding to avoidant and resistant attachment styles. Thus far, we have not identified or observed avoidant or resistant attachement scripts. Rather, we have found a tremendous variety of alternative schemas. In the absence of consistent supportive care, individuals are more idiosyncratic than typological in how they deal with stress and secure base needs.

The kinds of behaviors associated with the categories of insecurity often manifest during times of stress or conflict that do not resolve quickly or with any direct cause such as contact with the secure base. It is the *consistent* resolution of stress or conflict provided by the secure base that allows for the formation of a temporally and causally linked script to emerge. Our coding suggests that insecurely attached individuals still form generalized expectations or schemas associated with relationships. However, because they lack a consistent and predictable social environment, they fail to abstract a secure base script.

In many ways, the identification of alternative schemas is more informative than avoidant or resistant scripts would have been. Simply saying a child is avoidant tells us little about what specific parenting behaviors led that child to lose trust in the caregiver. Alternative schemas paint a clearer picture of the kinds of experiences children are exposed to in lieu of supportive secure base experience. We hope attention to an individual's unique profile of alternative schemas will not only provide a detailed, descriptive clinical account of his or her attachment history but also inform intervention efforts.

SCRIPT KNOWLEDGE AND NARRATIVE COHERENCE

Research examining the development of infants and children's ability to construct representations of experiences/events suggests that even before the second year of life, infants can encode simple sequences of events and recall those sequences over long delays of up to a year (Bauer, 2006). Each time an infant experiences distress, signals for support, and receives that support, he or she is likely constructing an event representation of this sequence (i.e., episodic memory). As children's language abilities develop and improve, they begin to represent and recall events using rudimentary narratives (e.g., Nelson, 1986; Nelson & Fivush, 2004; Fivush & Waters, 2019). These rudimentary event representations/narratives are often generalized and follow a temporal–causal structure, much like a cognitive script (e.g., Fivush & Slackman, 1986). Young children readily abstract scripts from commonly occurring events and even begin this process after their first encounter with an event category (Fivush & Slackman, 1986). As children develop a sense of self, their event representations take a qualitative turn and shift from being script-like to being autobiographical (i.e., "this event happened to *me*"). By late adolescence, individuals begin integrating individual autobiographical memories into a larger narrative (i.e., life story) of who they are and how they came to be that way (e.g., Habermas & Reese, 2015; McAdams, 2001). The coherence of this narrative is a critical marker of healthy psychological development and adjustment (e.g., Baerger & McAdams, 1999; T. Waters & Fivush, 2015). This research regarding the development of event representations suggests that the secure base script precedes the development of the ability to construct discrete autobiographical memories/narratives or the kinds of overarching coherent and integrative autobiographical representations tapped by the AAI.

In addition to clarifying the emergence and developmental sequence of attachment-related event representations, it is also important to ask *how* the secure base script influences the construction of a coherent attachment narrative. The answer may lie in the reconstructive nature of autobiographical memory (e.g., Bartlett, 1932; Conway, 2005; Neisser, 1967). Generations of memory literature illustrate the prominent role of schemas/scripts in organizing and reconstructing autobiographical narrative (Markman, 1999). This literature highlights a wide range of mechanisms through which a secure base script could shape the content and organization of adult attachment narratives. Relevant here would be the influence of secure base script knowledge on conformity to Grice's (1975) maxims (quality, quantity, relation, and manner of conversational implicature).

Quality

Grice's first maxim, *Quality*, is simple. Be truthful; have evidence for what you say. Of course, AAI coders cannot be sure that an interviewee's statements are historically accurate. Instead, they judge whether the interviewee believes them to be so from the consistency with which similar/related information is asserted across questions or examples.

For those individuals who view relationships in terms of the secure base script, attachment-relevant caregiving experiences will have been encoded and stored in a script-like structure, making it is less likely that reproduced event memories would resemble structural or factual contradictions in the AAI. In addition, the secure base script is a stable form of representation. Its use in recollecting the past provides an underlying consistency to narrative accounts in the AAI. This is not only because each reconstruction is essentially using the same temporal–causal blueprint, but also because each memory that is selected may be using the same retrieval cue, resulting in consistency across recollections during the interview.

Quantity

Grice's second maxim, *Quantity,* is to be concise; provide what is needed and nothing more. This is a hallmark of narrative coherence in the AAI. This maxim is maintained when the interviewer is neither struggling to elicit complete responses nor overwhelmed with details. Conceptualizing and relating an experience as a secure base interaction provides a template that maps memories onto a well-defined narrative structure with a clear beginning, middle, and end. This helps an interviewee locate material in memory and distinguish between what is essential and what, though accessible, is not.

Individuals who lack secure base script knowledge have less ready access to attachment-relevant examples and complete recollections of early experiences with primary caregivers. Without effective retrieval cues, they easily fall into the pattern of "I don't know," or "I don't remember," often associated with the Dismissing classification in traditional AAI coding. Alternatively, a lack of secure base script knowledge may also yield narratives that are far longer than they are informative. Without a clear sense for the boundaries of a responsive and cooperative reply, interviewees may struggle to find a conclusion to the autobiographical narrative they are providing. This is often associated with Preoccupied transcripts.

Relation

Grice's *Relation* maxim highlights the importance of staying on topic throughout a conversation. In the AAI, this entails (1) understanding the interviewer's intentions in asking about early family relationships and (2) providing consistently relevant information.

Viewing early family interactions through the lens of the secure base script provides a consistent interpretation of the interviewer's questions and goals. Family interactions are about secure base use and support; the interviewer is asking about family interactions; the questions should be answered in terms of secure base use and support. Without access to a secure base script, one might not abstract a common theme from the interview and stray off topic or fail to interpret follow-up questions as being related to the core attachment themes in the interview.

In addition to understanding the nature of the interviewer's questions, individuals who have focused on secure base use and support in their early experiences will have encoded a rich store of interrelated episodes from which they can draw, using the secure base script as a retrieval cue. This lends coherence to the interviewee's narrative across the full range of AAI questions.

Manner

Grice's final maxim, *Manner,* instructs the speaker to be clear, avoid ambiguity, and provide an orderly presentation. Clarity and order are manifest within and across AAI questions. Individuals who score high on AAI coherence are easy to follow. The what, when, and where of their narrative is clearly marked. Violations of manner arise when the interviewee is unclear or inconsistent in referring to events, time frames, or speakers. These are often expressed in run-on sentences that are difficult to follow or in sentence fillers such as "blah blah blah" in place of meaningful content. Odd causal explanations and unfinished thoughts are also violations of Manner.

Access to a script-like representation of secure base interactions facilitates retrieving early experiences in full and retelling them in an orderly manner from beginning to end. Moreover, because script-like representations encode the causal, as well as the temporal structure of experiences, they focus attention on relevant, believable explanations. This avoids the struggling and grasping for straws that underlie vague and irrelevant explanations characteristic of incoherent AAI narratives.

In brief, script-like representations are well positioned to influence the coherence of AAI narratives. Yet they do so in broad strokes. They operate primarily through effects on attention, memory access/retrieval, and narrative organization. Thus, while scripts influence the overall coherence of attachment narratives, they do not account for all the nuances Main et al. (2003–2008) highlight in traditional AAI scoring. Many of the specific narrative elements they cite as violating Grice's maxims (e.g., specific lapses into jargon, slips of the tongue, use of filler phrases such as "you know" or "I mean," and run-on sentences) are too fine-grained to be explained in terms of script theory (or, for that matter, attachment theory). Clearly, a wide range of processes, from the purely linguistic to arousal and emotion-related (and perhaps even psychodynamic) are also involved in constructing the final form of an individual's AAI narrative. Thus, the significance of script theory lies not in explaining the AAI in detail but in clarifying how early secure base experiences are related to adult attachment representations, and why the link is to coherence rather than some other facet of autobiographical memory or narrative style.

CONCLUSION

The secure base phenomenon is the key descriptive insight underlying Bowlby–Ainsworth's attachment theory (Holmes, 1993; E. Waters, Bretherton, & Vaughn, 2015; E. Waters & Cummings, 2000). Yet reference to the secure base concept has been largely missing in traditional AAI coding scales. Instead, attention to narrative discourse and coherence of mind predominately reflects current thinking on the manifestation of attachment-related representations in adulthood (Main et al., 2003–2008). This does little, however, in explaining how secure base expectations in infancy and childhood give rise to attachment-related representations in adulthood.

The cognitive and developmental properties of the secure base script, and cognitive scripts in general, provide a well-formulated blueprint for understanding how individuals construct attachment representations. In this chapter, we have proposed that indications of secure base script knowledge appear frequently in the AAI and have put forward a method for quantifying such content (i.e., in the form of secure base-related expectations and scenes). Furthermore, we have argued from a script perspective that access to a secure base script would facilitate conformity to Grice's maxims and thus contribute to the coherence of adult attachment narratives. This is supported by recent empirical research in which T. Waters et al. (2017) demonstrated that the link between maternal sensitivity experienced during childhood and AAI coherence in adulthood is mediated by secure base script knowledge.

Script theory goes a considerable way toward explaining *what exactly* the development of attachment representations is the development *of*. It also helps in clarifying questions about developmental change and focusing the scope of attachment research by proposing a sequence whereby early experience leads to secure base script knowledge and the construction of a coherent autobiographical representation of attachment experiences. In addition, script theory addresses the important question, "Why is early attachment security related to later narrative coherence?"

As with many of the chapters in this volume, our work on secure base script knowledge in the AAI and the development of the AAI_{sbs} scale illustrates the way in which a measurement program can advance pressing theoretical issues in attachment theory. The ability to assess secure base script knowledge and coherence in the same interview can only contribute to the continuing good health and productivity of research in the AAI tradition. Thus, this volume should serve as a useful tool toward integrating current methods in attachment assessment for clinicians and researchers alike.

REFERENCES

Abelson, R. P. (1981). Psychological status of the script concept. *American Psychologist, 36*(7), 715–729.

Ainsworth, M. D. S. (1967). *Infancy in Uganda: Infant care and the growth of love.* Baltimore: Johns Hopkins University Press.

Ainsworth, M. D. S. (1972). Attachment and dependency: A comparison. In J. L. Gewirtz (Ed.), *Attachment and dependency* (pp. 97–137). Washington, DC: Winston.

Ainsworth, M. D. S., Blehar, M. C., Waters, E., & Wall, S. (2015). *Patterns of attachment: A psychological study of the Strange Situation.* New York: Taylor & Francis (Psychology Press). (Original work published 1978)

Ainsworth, M. D. S., & Marvin, R. S. (1995). On the shaping of attachment theory and research: An interview with Mary D. S. Ainsworth (Fall 1994). *Monographs of the Society for Research in Child Development, 60*(2–3), 3–21.

Baerger, D. R., & McAdams, D. P. (1999). Life story coherence and its relation to psychological well-being. *Narrative Inquiry, 9*(1), 69–96.

Bakermans-Kranenburg, M. J., & van IJzendoorn, M. H. (2009). The first 10,000 Adult Attachment Interviews: Distributions of adult attachment representations in clinical and non-clinical groups. *Attachment and Human Development, 11*(3), 223–263.

Bargh, J. A. (1996). Automaticity in social psychology. In E. T. Higgins & A. W. Kruglanski (Eds.), *Social psychology: Handbook of basic principles* (pp. 169–183). New York: Guilford Press.

Bartlett, F. C. (1932). *Remembering: A study in experimental and social psychology.* New York: Cambridge University Press.

Bauer, P. J. (2006). Constructing a past in infancy: A neuro-developmental account. *Trends in Cognitive Sciences, 10*(4), 175–181.

Bower, G. H., Black, J. B., & Turner, T. J. (1979). Scripts in memory for text. *Cognitive Psychology, 11*(2), 177–220.

Bowlby, J. (1982). *Attachment and loss: Vol. 1. Attachment* (2nd ed.). New York: Basic Books. (Original work published 1969)

Bretherton, I. (1987). New perspectives on attachment relations: Security, communication, and internal working models. In J. Osofsky (Ed.), *Handbook of infant development* (2nd ed., pp. 1061–1100). Oxford, UK: Wiley.

Conway, M. A. (2005). Memory and the self. *Journal of Memory and Language, 53*(4), 594–628.

Crowell, J., & Waters, E. (2005). Attachment representations, secure base behavior, and the evolution of adult relationships: The Stony Brook Adult Relationship Project. In K. E. Grossmann, K. Grossmann, & T. E. A. Waters (Eds.), *Attachment from infancy to maturity: The major longitudinal studies* (pp. 245–304). New York: Guilford Press.

Dagan, O., Asok, A., Steele, H., Steele, M., & Bernard, K. (2018). Attachment security moderates the link between adverse childhood experiences and cellular aging. *Development and Psychopathology, 30*(4), 1211–1223.

Feeney, B. C. (2004). A secure base: Responsive support of goal strivings and exploration in adult intimate relationships. *Journal of Personality and Social Psychology, 87*(5), 631–648.

Fiske, S., & Taylor, S. (1991). *Social cognition.* New York: McGraw-Hill.

Fivush, R., & Slackman, E. (1986). The acquisition and development of scripts. In K. Nelson (Ed.), *Event knowledge: Structure and function in development* (pp. 71–96). Hillsdale, NJ: Erlbaum.

Fivush, R., & Waters, T. E. A. (2019). Development and organization of autobiographical memory form and function. In J. Mace (Ed.), *The organization and structure of autobiograpghical memory* (pp. 52–71). Oxford, UK: Oxford University Press.

Graesser, A. C., Gordon, S. E., & Sawyer, J. D. (1979). Recognition memory for typical and atypical actions in scripted activities: Tests of a script pointer + tag hypothesis. *Journal of Verbal Learning and Verbal Behavior, 18*(3), 319–332.

Grice, H. P. (1975). Logic and conversation. In P. Cole & J. L. Morgan (Ed.), *Syntax and semantics: III. Speech acts* (pp. 41–58). New York: Academic Press.

Habermas, T., & Reese, E. (2015). Getting a life takes time: The development of the life story in adolescence, its precursors and consequences. *Human Development, 58*(3), 172–201.

Holmes, J. (1993). *John Bowlby and attachment theory.* London: Routlege.

Langer, E. J. (1992). Matters of mind: Mindfulness/mindlessness in perspective. *Consciousness and Cognition, 1*(3), 289–305.

Main, M. (1991). Metacognitive knowledge, metacognitive monitoring, and singular (coherent) vs. multiple (incoherent) models of attachment: Some findings and some directions for future research. In P. Marris, J. Stevenson-Hinde, & C. Parkes (Eds.), *Attachment across the life cycle* (pp. 127–159). New York: Routledge.

Main, M., Goldwyn, R., & Hesse, E. (2003–2008). *The Adult Attachment Interview classification and scoring system.* Unpublished manuscript, University of California at Berkeley, Berkeley, CA.

Main, M., Kaplan, N., & Cassidy, J. (1985). Security in infancy, childhood, and adulthood: A move to the level of representation. *Monographs of the Society for Research in Child Development, 50,* 66–104.

Markman, A. B. (1999). *Knowledge representation.* Mahwah, NJ: Erlbaum.

McAdams, D. P. (2001). The psychology of life stories. *Review of General Psychology, 5*(2), 100–122.

Neisser, U. (1967). *Cognitive psychology.* East Norwalk, CT: Appleton-Century-Crofts.

Nelson, K. (1986). *Event knowledge: Structures and function in development.* Hillsdale, NJ: Erlbaum.

Nelson, K., & Fivush, R. (2004). The emergence of autobiographical memory: A social cultural developmental theory. *Psychological Review, 111*(2), 486–511.

Petters, D., Waters, E., & Schönbrodt, F. (2010). Strange carers: Robots as attachment figures and aids to parenting. *Interaction Studies: Social Behaviour and Communication in Biological and Artificial Systems, 11*(2), 246–252.

Schank, R., & Abelson, R. (1977). *Scripts, plans, goals, and understanding: An inquiry into human knowledge structures.* Hillsdale, NJ: Erlbaum.

Sroufe, L. A., Egeland, B., Carlson, E., & Collins, W. A. (2009). *The development of the person: The Minnesota Study of Risk and Adaptation from Birth to Adulthood.* New York: Guilford Press.

Sroufe, L. A., & Waters, E. (1977). Attachment as an organizational construct. *Child Development, 48*(4), 1184–1199.

Waters, E., Bretherton, I., & Vaughn, B. E. (2015). Preface. In *Patterns of attachment: A psychological study of the Strange Situation* (pp. x–xxxvi). New York: Psychology Press.

Waters, E., & Cummings, M. (2003). A secure base from which to explore close relationships. *Child Development, 71*(1), 164–172.

Waters, H. S., & Waters, E. (2006). The attachment working models concept: Among other things, we build script-like representations of secure base experiences. *Attachment and Human Development, 8*(3), 185–197.

Waters, T. E. A., Brockmeyer, S. L., & Crowell, J. A. (2013). AAI coherence predicts caregiving and care seeking behavior: Secure base script knowledge helps explain why. *Attachment and Human Development, 15*(3), 316–331.

Waters, T. E. A., Facompré, C. R., Dagan, O., Martin, J., Johnson, W. F., Young, E. S., . . . Roisman, G. I. (2020). Convergent validity and stability of secure base script knowledge from late adolescence to midlife. *Attachment and Human Development, 2020,* 1–21.

Waters, T. E. A., & Fivush, R. (2015). Relations between narrative coherence, identity, and psychological well-being in emerging adulthood. *Journal of Personality, 83*(4), 441–451.

Waters, T. E. A., Raby, K. L., Ruiz, S. K., Martin, J., & Roisman, G. I. (2018). Adult attachment representations and the quality of romantic and parent–child relationships: An examination of the unique contributions of secure base script knowledge and coherence of discourse. *Developmental Psychology, 54*(12), 2371–2381.

Waters, T. E. A., Ruiz, S. K., & Roisman, G. I. (2017). Origins of secure base script knowledge and the developmental construction of attachment representations. *Child Development, 88*(1), 198–209.

APPENDIX 10.1. Alternative (Non-Secure Base) Schemas in the AAI

CAREGIVER AS THE SOURCE OF DISTRESS

The caregiver is described as being causally (either directly or indirectly) linked to the child's distress. In most cases, harsh and threatening caregiving behaviors are consistently described across situations and contexts. As a consequence of recurring and consistent hostile caregiver interactions, an interviewee may develop expectations about the caregiving relationship that become thematically organized in the child, as in the example below.

> INTERVIEWEE: [My mother] wasn't raised emotionally very well, so in turn, she didn't really um, raise me emotionally well in terms of giving me support when I needed it. [. . .] I don't know if I would go to her when I'm upset. Mostly 'cause lots of the time she was the source of it. . . .

AAI_{sbs} coders may naturally wonder whether *all* of the alternative schemas we present, in one way or another, implicate the caregiver as a source of distress. This is largely true; however, we find that cases range in the level of specificity and consistency of the stressful dynamic associated with parent–child interactions. Therefore, if a single or consistent theme emerges from the transcript, coders are able to assign specific alternative schemas. In cases where more than one alternative schema emerges, coders may have difficulty picking a dominant schema and thus assign the more general parent source of distress. The descriptions below are some of the most regularly identified illustrations of alternative schemas that appear in the AAI.

CHILD PUT IN THE MIDDLE

The child notices parental discord on a consistent basis and/or is asked to play an active role in resolving parents' issues (e.g., forced to choose sides, one parent speaks negatively about the other).

> INTERVIEWEE: [What would you do when emotionally upset?] I wasn't in the position to go to one [parent], you know, neither of them spoke very positively about the other one, um, and did not acknowledge that I had a relationship with the other parent.

> INTERVIEWEE: I always thought of [my mother] like she was kind of like my escape 'cause I was like—I hated my dad it was like really—I mean I love my dad but it was just like it was torture and I remember like missing her to death and sometimes he'd let us see her letters that she wrote but sometimes he wouldn't um but he'd always like bad talk her so—and I always felt defensive like that's my mom. . . .

DISMISSING/UNRESPONSIVE

In response to a clear signal for help, the caregiver decides whether the conflict or challenge warrants the provision of secure base support. If the caregiver feels the child's concerns are valid, intervention is provided; if not, the child is dismissed or (as in the example below) explicitly told to resolve the problem on their own.

> INTERVIEWEE: Uh . . . probably I went to my mother first . . . and if she thought that what I was crying about was warranted, then she would help me . . . if she thought that it was because I was being a bit ridiculous . . . she would send me to the bathroom, tell me to wash my face, or ask me to go cry in my room.

Importantly, the Dismissing/Unresponsive alternative schema is not to be confused with the Dismissing attachment classification in traditional AAI coding.

ENMESHED/COMPANIONSHIP

The attachment relationship is defined by explicit mention that the child serves an important role as a source of comfort or companionship to the parent.

> INTERVIEWEE: There was a bond between us. [My mother] could talk to me [about her problems] and I would just sit and listen even if I didn't understand what she was talking about. We were always, always, always, like that.

Although some might argue that the apparent "bond" between the two signifies a healthy attachment relationship, in terms of the secure base concept, this violates the natural order of things. This is because relationships defined by companionship may result in a blurred distinction as to who is the secure base and who should be the recipient of support. Consequently, these kinds of schematic representations make it less likely that the child will seek support from the caregiver due to the absence of a well-established hierarchy (like one might expect in a peer relationship).

Enmeshed characterizations of the relationship can also result in reciprocal or shared inductions of distress owing to the fact that no single figure is effectively resolving the problem (as in the example below).

> INTERVIEWEE: [. . .] it was pretty much always [my mother] and I, so . . . we, we were always together and we, you know, when she was upset, I got upset. When I was upset, she got upset. So we just went through a lotta things together.

ROLE REVERSAL

Unlike the Enmeshed/Companionship alternative schema, the child partly or completely takes on the role of the parent. As illustrated in the example below, we find that trouble usually follows when the parent later tries to act as a secure base.

> INTERVIEWEE: I sort of took over as this role of, like, this parental role. And if I think I'll analyze myself . . . in looking back, I think what had happened was that when [my stepmother] came along, she wanted me to behave like an eleven-year-old. But I had abandoned behaving like an eleven-year-old for two years. So you just can't go . . . I'll never forget um [. . .] after dinner, she handed me a bowl with two cookies in it, like, now we were having snack time. And I thought, "You're not gonna tell me how many cookies I can eat," you know, like things that normal

eleven-year-olds or . . . child . . . children understand . . . you're the parent, I'm the child . . . and this is what yeah . . . I just . . . I just fought her every step of the way. She was not my mother, I told her so on a daily basis . . . and I didn't listen to her, I hated her. . . . I screamed at her [. . .] So, I mean, and that went on for I mean . . . it was very bad . . . very bad.

HARSH AND THREATENING PARENTING

The interviewee expresses a consistent theme of fear of one or both parents, or recounts recurring abuse. Often reflected in these transcripts is the feeling that one constantly needed to "walk on eggshells" or monitor the caregiver's mood in order to avoid conflict.

INTERVIEWEE: [in response to the adjective *distant*] I guess not just a specific time because of all the times [my father] um hit me and my sister. It made me grow distant with him, like it made me not wanna, get close to him, and . . . I don't know, I just always thought he um, didn't wanna get close to us. I don't know if his punishment was his way of um, showing, um love and affection, but . . . Yeah, that's why I don't think I ever tried to um express anything towards him. So that's why I kind of stayed away from him. And, if anything, went towards my mom. And ask for her, like comfort and her love and stuff like that.

INTERVIEWER: And why do you think you weren't as close with your father as you were your mother?

INTERVIEWEE: I think it was because of how he was with my brother, and I was scared like, my brother was kind of like a problem child. Like he would even say that. Um, I was scared that—and him and my dad like, they argued a lot, like yelled at each other and stuff. Um, and I was scared that I would like disappoint my dad and then have the same thing happen to me. Um, so I kind of just avoided that and just tried to like do right by him, where I wasn't as worried about that with my mom. Like I knew that she would take stuff away from me, and—but I wasn't worried that she would ever like, freak. My dad never—I wouldn't say like, ever freaked out at me, but I saw it with my brother, so I didn't want the same things to happen to me.

SELF-INVOLVED

The child comes to learn that the needs of the parent always come first. The implication of this, of course, is that the child is less likely to seek support from the secure base in times of need.

INTERVIEWEE: [in response to the adjective *self-centered*] Well, [my father] put himself before anybody else, you know? It doesn't matter what was going on in the house . . . as long as he got home and had his drink.

INTERVIEWEE: [in response to the adjective *impatient*] My mom played a lot of . . . the father–mother role, but [my father] just had no patience for that, just 'cause he didn't wanna be bothered, he just, he's not, he's not a child person. Never was and never will be.

PARENT DEMANDS EXCELLENCE/STRIVING FOR ACCEPTANCE

The parent–child relationship is defined by a superficial expression of fondness, in which the child is displayed as a trophy or accessory to parents' accomplishments. As a result, the child comes to internalize his or her own successes (i.e., achievement in academics or sport) as being fundamentally linked to their parents' affection. The child with this schema consistently tries to please the parents or live up to their standards, though affirmations that the child has succeeded in this rarely, if ever, appear.

INTERVIEWEE: [in response to the adjective *critical*] My mother was always horning in and trying to give her opinion on things, so that I always felt that I had to be a certain way . . . or meet certain expectations or she would not be satisfied with me.

INTERVIEWEE: Um, [my father] would always, like push me basically to be like the very best possible and like, he would always be the one to sign my test papers, so like in third grade you have those little quizzes. I would have to give it to him to sign and he would always get upset if I got anything less than perfect, so that's one . . . like I don't even remember what my grade was, but I remember my dad like just basically completely like a stone wall, just, you know, signs it and gives it back to me and then asks me what did I do wrong, how can I improve myself, stuff like that.

INTERVIEWEE: I just remember it being really cold one time, and I was like a sophomore in high school or something—or I was a freshman, and I played J.V., and [my father] really wanted me to play varsity the next year, and like the season was over. The season had just ended like, it had been like less than a week, and he already started, like, all right go in the garage and go dribble. And I'm like, our garage isn't heated it—I'm like, and he was like, go put sweats on you'll be fine. And I'm like, it's cold, my season just ended, I have an entire year to get—like, if you don't get started now you're already behind and like all this crap that's like, I just wanna sleep, like I'm still sore, we had like a huge game and like. I like, have some hip problems, so I was sore anyways. He was like, oh you don't have to walk around just stand there and dribble, like if you're good, you won't have to move. . . .

INTERVIEWER: And do you think he realized that you didn't want to do it?

INTERVIEWEE: Yeah, no he totally knew.

SUBJUGATED/SUBORDINATE

The parent–child relationship is defined by a subordinate role, centered around that which is expected of the child (i.e., duties and schedules) rather than what can be expected from the parent as a secure base. Expectations to this effect often describe deep-rooted feelings of worthlessness, helplessness, and inequality.

INTERVIEWEE: [My siblings and I] had certain chores that had to be done. Like every morning there was my mother's coffee in bed. We had to go to the store every day and buy her Pepsi. There's always something. She always has something. She's very, very demanding, very pushy in that way. She wants her things and she wants them now, and that's it.

INTERVIEWEE: The power [my father] had over me was kind of like a king and the peasant relationship, um, where you don't really connect very well, um, I guess you know, a thing like you know, when I was over his house my brother would come and my brother was probably two at the time and so he'd sleep in the room with my father and stepmother and I'd, you know, get a little . . . and they'd shut the door and I'd get the cot that's way in the corner of the living room.

TIT-FOR-TAT

In clear contrast to the "Subjugated/Subordinate" schema, the parent and child both find themselves in equal and competing roles. This can often lead to contentious encounters as might be reflective of sibling relationships.

INTERVIEWEE: Well when I got to 12—I mean my mom's really small, we were like the same size, so like I started wearing her clothes. So, I'd like try to take her clothes and she would yell and scream or fight about it. She would take my clothes. Like, we were like siblings. And since that—we shared so much with each other, including clothes. But then it would have that sib. like, sibling rivalry, whereas she like wants her stuff back and so do I. So, I feel like in that sense we were like siblings.

CHAPTER 11

Laboratory Methods for Assessing Secure Base Use and Support in Adult Relationships

Brooke C. Feeney

All of us, from the cradle to the grave, are happiest when life is organized as a series of excursions, long or short, from the secure base provided by our attachment figure(s).

—BOWLBY (1988, p. 62)

The purpose of this chapter is to discuss laboratory methods for assessing secure base use and support in adult relationships. The chapter is organized into four sections: First, the concept of a secure base, which is central to attachment theory, is defined. Second, laboratory methods that have been used to assess secure base use and support are described. Third, strengths and weaknesses of these methods are identified. Finally, directions for future research are discussed.

THE CONCEPT OF A SECURE BASE

A secure base has been conceptualized broadly as incorporating both the provision of sensitive and responsive support (e.g., comfort) in times of stress and sensitive and responsive support for exploration (e.g., see Crowell, et al., 2002; Crowell & Waters, 2005; E. Waters & Cummings, 2000; H. Waters & Waters, 2006). This chapter focuses solely on the latter aspect (support of exploration). Attachment theory highlights two major caregiving functions that attachment relationships serve: (1) providing a safe haven for the attached person by meeting his or her needs for security and (2) providing a secure base for the attached person by supporting his or her autonomy and exploration in the environment (Bowlby, 1982, 1988). Although these two functions are highly interrelated and may be viewed as part of the same process, in the context of adult relationships, the support of a close relationship partner's exploration in the environment has been vastly understudied relative to the provision of support in times of stress. Thus, laboratory methods for assessing this aspect of secure base use and support are important to highlight, with an eye toward encouraging the development of future research in this area.

Although the emergency/comforting facet of caregiving that involves meeting needs for security will require a great deal more laboratory research as well, this facet of caregiving has been much better represented in the adult literature than has research examining the support of exploration. For example, there have been laboratory studies with adults that involve (1) videotaping couples/dyads as one member deals with a stressful event that was either created in the lab or identified by the couple/dyad member as an ongoing stressor in his or her life (e.g., Collins & Feeney, 2000; Feeney, Cassidy, & Ramos-Marcuse, 2008; Jakubiak & Feeney, 2019; Kane et al., 2007; Monin, Feeney, & Schulz, 2012; Rholes, Simpson, & Orina, 1999; Simpson, Rholes, & Nelligan, 1992; Simpson & Rholes, 2017; Simpson, Rholes, Orina, & Grich, 2002; Simpson, Winterheld, Rholes, & Orina, 2007; Westmaas & Silver, 2001), (2) experimentally manipulating support behavior or expressions of need/distress during a stressful situation to examine its impact on the couple members (e.g., Collins & Feeney, 2004; Feeney & Collins, 2001; Jakubiak & Feeney, 2016a; Jakubiak & Feeney, 2016b; Monin, Schulz, Feeney, & Cook, 2010), (3) identifying attachment differences in physiological responses to stressors (e.g., Feeney & Kirkpatrick, 1996; Carpenter & Kirkpatrick, 1996; Maunder, Lancee, Nolan, Hunter & Tannenbaum, 2006; Pietromonaco, DeBuse, & Powers, 2013), and (4) using virtual reality procedures to assess support provision and use in stressful circumstances (Giglioli, Pravettoni, Martín, Parra, & Raya, 2017; Kane, McCall, Collins, & Blascovich, 2008; Wallach, Safir, & Almog, 2009). In addition, experimental studies have included manipulations of attachment security using priming techniques to show that experimentally induced attachment security increases empathy, the endorsement of prosocial values, and prosocial behavior (Mikulincer et al., 2001, 2003; Mikulincer, Shaver, Gillath, & Nitzberg, 2005; Mikulincer & Shaver, 2005; Mikulincer & Shaver, 2020).

To elaborate on the concept of a secure base, attachment theory stipulates that a secure base functions to support behavior that involves "going out" from the relationship for autonomous exploration in the environment (Bowlby, 1982, 1988; see also Crowell et al., 2002; E. Waters & Cummings, 2000). Good caregivers (support-providers) must know how not only to respond appropriately to attachment behavior and signals of distress but also how to support their partner's exploration behavior (e.g., autonomous goal strivings, personal growth; Bowlby, 1982, 1988). Thus, an important function of caregiving involves the provision of a secure base from which an attached person can make excursions into the outside world (to play, work, learn, discover, create, make new friends) knowing that he or she can return for comfort, reassurance, and/or assistance should he or she encounter difficulties along the way. Bowlby (1988) describes the concept of a secure base as one in which caregivers (support-providers) create the conditions that enable their relationship partners to explore the world in a confident way:

> In essence this role is one of being available, ready to respond when called upon to encourage and perhaps assist, but to intervene actively only when clearly necessary. In these respects it is a role similar to that of the officer commanding a military base from which an expeditionary force sets out and to which it can retreat, should it meet with a setback. Much of the time the role of the base is a waiting one but it is none the less vital for that. For it is only when the officer commanding the expeditionary force is confident his base is secure that he dare press forward and take risks. (p. 11)

Based on Bowlby's early theorizing (Bowlby, 1973, 1980, 1982), attachment researchers have identified important characteristics of a secure base, and they have made important theoretical predictions regarding the consequences of receiving and not receiving secure base support in one's close attachment relationships. For example, key developmental hypotheses associated with secure base use and support include the following: (1) Confidence in caregiver availability and responsiveness (i.e., attachment security) is an advantage in exploring environments and integrating affect, behavior, and cognition during the early years, and (2) the experience of reliable secure base support is an advantage when it comes time to serve as a secure base for one's own children, spouse, and elderly parents (e.g., Dykas, Woodhouse, Cassidy, & Waters, 2006; Vaughn et al., 2007; E. Waters & Cummings, 2000; E. Waters, Crowell, Elliott, Corcoran, & Treboux, 2002; H. Waters & Waters, 2006).

Similarly, recent work in the study of adult attachment has isolated important characteristics of a secure base (extrapolated from Bowlby's description of a secure base) that are presumed to influence exploration behavior and related personal and relationship outcomes (Feeney & Thrush, 2010). These characteristics are described in some depth here as a preface to the types of laboratory studies that have been conducted to examine secure base use and support in adulthood.

First, a secure base supports exploration by being *available* in the event that the base is needed (e.g., to assist in removing obstacles and to respond to needs as they arise). Attachment theory stipulates that throughout the lifespan, the availability of a responsive attachment figure remains the source of a person's feeling secure—and only when a person is feeling secure will he or she be able to explore most effectively, confidently, and autonomously (Bowlby, 1982, 1988). The logic behind this idea is that it is much easier for people to explore and engage in behaviors that enhance their personal growth when they know someone is available for comfort and assistance if things go wrong (see also Feeney, 2007). This is because an individual who feels confident in the availability of his or her "secure base" does not have to cling to that base as much as an individual who lacks such confidence. For example, when Sue is away exploring a potential job opportunity that will help her meet important career goals, her husband Jon may show availability and facilitate her exploration by checking in with her to see how she is doing, and by being responsive to her phone calls and any need for reassurance during this time. Thus, availability may be shown by being attentive to one's partner's needs and responding sensitively to them.

Second, a secure base supports exploration by *not unnecessarily interfering* with it. According to attachment theory, chronically intrusive/interfering behavior is antithetical to sensitive and responsive support provision, and it is a major inhibitor of exploration. We have proposed that intrusive/interfering behavior inhibits exploration, because it communicates a variety of negative messages to the recipient (see also Feeney & Thrush, 2010). It may communicate to the recipient that he or she (1) is not capable of engaging in independent exploration, (2) is not intelligent or competent enough to succeed at exploratory activities, (3) is not deserving or worthy of engaging in independent exploration, and that (4) independent exploration is threatening to close others and one's relationship with close others, (5) close others have negative views of one's abilities, and/or (6) exploration is futile because it is consistently interrupted. Any one of these messages should lead an individual to develop negative perceptions of his or her own abilities regarding exploration, to conclude that exploration is not enjoyable or worth the effort, and to believe that exploration attempts result in negative outcomes and thus should be avoided.

Intrusive/interfering behavior also undermines performance during exploration activities, because it undermines concentration and confidence. For example, when Sue is away exploring a potential job opportunity that will help her meet important career goals, her husband Jon would be unnecessarily interfering if he constantly called her for detailed reports throughout the day, or if he told her (or planned for her) exactly what to do while she is away. Unnecessary interference includes behaviors such as providing support that is not needed or wanted; taking over and controlling a partner's exploration activity; being too directive, forceful, or dominating in support attempts; or impeding the accomplishment of a goal/activity.

Third, a secure base supports exploration by being *encouraging and accepting* of it (Feeney & Thrush, 2010). Encouragement is expected to facilitate exploration and increase the pleasure one is able to take in exploration activities, because it conveys an excitement/enthusiasm regarding exploration, as well as confidence in the explorer's abilities. However, people are unlikely to explore in ways that enhance their learning, personal growth, and self-esteem when the explorations are not encouraged and accepted by their close relationship partners. For example, if Jon would like to take up a new hobby, he will be less likely to pursue this hobby if Sue thinks it is a waste of time or if she resents the time spent apart. However, Jon will be more likely to pursue the hobby if Sue accepts it as being worthwhile and encourages him to try it. Encouraging behavior may involve drawing a partner's attention to an exploratory opportunity (whereas parents may draw their child's attention to a toy, a spouse may draw his or her partner's attention to a career opportunity), expressing confidence in a partner's abilities, complimenting/praising a partner's progress toward a goal, celebrating a partner's successes, encouraging the partner to take initiative, and exhibiting an acceptance of the partner's autonomy.

Thus, the ability to confidently explore the environment stems from having a relationship partner who supports such exploration by encouraging it, not unnecessarily interfering with it, and being readily available and responsive when needed. Insensitive caregivers who do not provide an adequate secure base for their relationship partners are likely to take little notice of their partner's goals and goal-related feelings, to intrude when their partner is trying to solve problem on his or her own, to fail to respect their partner's desire for autonomy by discouraging or impeding exploration, to discourage bids for support and encouragement, or to respond in an ill-timed and unhelpful manner. Nonetheless, the importance of a secure base is evident for individuals of all ages. Just as children can be seen using their parents as a secure base for exploration by keeping track of the parents' whereabouts, exchanging glances, and from time to time returning to the parents to share in mutually enjoyable contact, adults can be seen engaging in similar types of behaviors. For example, an adult is likely to maintain phone contact when exploring away from the spouse for an extended period of time and share details of his or her explorations with the spouse. Bowlby (1988) suggested that individuals who are confident that their base is secure and ready to respond if called upon are likely to take it for granted. Yet should the base suddenly become unavailable or inaccessible, the importance of the base to the "emotional equilibrium" of the individual is immediately apparent. In fact, it is a major postulate of attachment theory that individuals who thrive emotionally and socially, and who make the most of their opportunities, are those who have caregivers, be it a parent in childhood or a spouse in adulthood, who, while encouraging the individual's autonomy, are also available and responsive when called upon.

Attachment theory stipulates that the secure base behavior of attachment figures (i.e., parents, spouses) is likely to be most influential. However, it is important to note that the power of these behaviors may not be limited to attachment figures. For example, authority figures (teachers, employers) and peers, who may or may not be attachment figures, may successfully enact behaviors with the intent of facilitating or undermining exploration attempts. The extent to which attachment figures and nonattachment figures are equally influential may differ among individuals (e.g., secure individuals may be less influenced by attempts to undermine their exploration by nonattachment figures). These are empirical questions that could be addressed in future work. This chapter focuses on laboratory methods for assessing secure base use and support with close others (attachment figures); however, these methods may be extended to nonclose others as well.

LABORATORY METHODS FOR ASSESSING SECURE BASE USE AND SUPPORT

Although adults routinely assign credit for their accomplishments to the support of the significant people in their lives (people who have encouraged them to grow as individuals and strive to reach their full potential), empirical investigations of this important type of support in adult relationships have been sparse. A number of useful laboratory methods recently have been developed for assessing secure base use and support within adult relationships. These include both observational and experimental methods. Examples of studies using each method are described in this section, with the purpose of encouraging researchers to use similar methods to contribute to a relatively sparse literature on the support of exploration in adulthood.

Before considering these methods, however, it is important to note that, historically, the focus of a great deal of adult attachment research has been on measuring attachment orientation and examining correlates of these orientations using self-report methods. This work has often been carried out within the framework of a trait approach; that is, the focus has been more on a person's general attachment orientation (and its predictors) than on the behaviors a person enacts with a particular partner. However, the behavioral research has been growing, and there has been a move toward considering normative attachment processes, as well as individual differences. The methods reviewed below represent some of the research that has been conducted on the topic of secure base use and support.

The observational laboratory methods described below are correlational in nature, and these methods are complemented by the experimental laboratory methods that follow. Each of these methods has characteristic strengths and limitations that offset one another; thus, a multimethod approach to addressing research questions regarding secure base use and support is ideal. For example, behavioral observation and coding has the advantages of allowing researchers to capture process (e.g., characterizing behavior as it unfolds in time), to identify behavioral profiles (e.g., identifying the extent to which particular people behave in particular ways in particular contexts), and to assess behavior as it occurs naturally and spontaneously (enhancing external validity). Limitations of this method are that it is labor intensive, and that much of it tends to be correlational in nature (although observational methods may be used in experiments as well). Although all laboratory methods are subject to concerns related to ecological validity (e.g., effects of being observed), researchers have been very successful in obtaining valid assessments of behavior in the laboratory (e.g., Bakeman, 2000). Experimental methods, on the other hand, have the advantages of permitting causal inferences and increasing internal validity. Although experimental laboratory methods are more limited in terms of external validity, researchers also have been very successful at establishing psychological realism in laboratory experiments (Brewer, 2000). The best solution is a multimethod approach that allows researchers to obtain converging evidence for a particular phenomenon as opposed to embracing one specific procedure as "the diagnostic situation." Following are examples of observational and experimental methods that may be adapted to addressing a variety of research questions regarding secure base use and support in adulthood.

Observational Methods

One of the first observational studies of secure base behavior in adulthood was conducted by Crowell et al. (2002). For this investigation, secure base use and support was conceptualized as incorporating both the provision of sensitive and responsive support (e.g., comfort) in times of stress. and sensitive and responsive support for exploration. Engaged couples participated in a standard problem-solving discussion: The researchers identified a topic with the highest frequency of conflict reported by both partners, then the couple members were asked to discuss the problem for 15 minutes and try to reach a resolution. The couples' interactions were videotaped, and behaviors exhibited during the interactions were coded using the Secure Base Scoring System (SBSS; Crowell et al., 1998), which is a coding system based on Ainsworth's analyses of infant–parent secure base use and support (Ainsworth, Blehar, Waters, & Wall, 1978/2015; E. Waters, Kondo-Ikemura, Posada, & Richters, 1991).

The SBSS targets behaviors that represent secure base use (optimally signaling one's needs clearly and directly) and secure base support (correctly detecting signals and interpreting need, and responding in a timely and sensitive manner). Secure base use is assessed using four theoretically derived subscales, including (1) *initial signal* (the degree of initial clarity of a concern expressed), (2) *maintenance of the signal* (how actively and persistently the individual maintains a clear distress signal), (3) *approach* (degree of direct support seeking toward one's partner and expectation that the partner will be helpful), and (4) *ability to be comforted* (degree to which the individual responds to the partner's support with diminished distress). Secure base support is also assessed using four subscales, and these include (1) Interest in the Partner (degree of willingness and ability to be a good listener and available to one's partner), (2) Recognition of Distress or Concern (degree of awareness of a partner's distress, needs, or concern), (3) Interpretation of Distress (degree of correctness in understanding the partner's concerns and signals), and (4) Responsiveness to Distress (degree of effort and effectiveness in helping one's partner via cooperative means). These scales were theoretically derived and have been shown to have good predictive validity (Crowell et al., 2002).

Also consistent with attachment theory (Bowlby, 1988), our field has viewed the urge to explore the environment as a basic component of human nature (and as a characteristic of most mammals), and has viewed exploration as including a wide range of activities that involve adventure, discovery, learning, novelty, challenge, goal striving, and/or self-enhancement. This conceptualization has formed the basis for our operationalization of exploration in the laboratory. Observational methods provide a particularly useful means for assessing both exploration behavior and support for exploration in the laboratory. These methods allow researchers to observe exactly what caregivers (or support-providers) and support recipients are doing in contexts that elicit secure base use and support. These contexts are those in which one relationship partner is given an opportunity to explore, and the other relationship partner is given an opportunity to provide a secure base. Examples of these observational procedures, used with samples of romantic partners, are described below.

Laboratory Exploration Activity

Laboratory situations have been created to permit the observation of one couple member's exploration behavior as a function of the other couple member's secure base behavior: This is accomplished by giving one member of the couple (the "explorer") a novel exploration activity to try in the presence of his or her partner. To mimic the characteristics of many real-life explorations, laboratory exploration activities should be selected to be novel and challenging (as well as goal-oriented), but performance pressure must be minimized to alleviate any potential concerns about performance or evaluation (and to ensure the elicitation of exploration behavior instead of attachment behavior that is likely to emerge in stressful situations). In one laboratory investigation (Feeney & Thrush, 2010), the following instructions were given to explorers in the presence of their spouses:

> "We'd like for you to try an activity called 'Brick by Brick.' This is an activity that you've probably never tried before—and that you've probably never even heard of before. We'd just like for you to try it out and see what you think. It doesn't matter if you solve the puzzles or not—we just want you to have fun with it and tell us what you think about it afterwards. The object is to arrange these bricks into the patterns illustrated on this stack of cards. [The experimenter demonstrates with the first card.] The solution is on the back of each card in case you get stuck. Again, just check it out and have fun with it."

During this time, the spouse is given a brief questionnaire to complete. The purpose of this questionnaire is to make it clear to both couple members that the exploration activity is not a joint one (that the explorer was the one given the exploration opportunity). However, the spouse remains in the same room, and the spouse's questionnaire is a brief one, to allow the spouse the time and flexibility to exhibit qualities relevant to secure base support provision. After the experimenter leaves the room, the explorer and spouse are unobtrusively videotaped for 10 minutes. The spouse's secure base behavior and the explorer's exploration behavior are later coded by independent observers for content relevant to secure base use and support.

A coding system for assessing secure base use and support in this type of exploration context is as follows: *Support-provider (spouse,* in this example*) behaviors* are coded to reflect each of three theoretically derived qualities of a secure base (availability, noninterference, and encouragement). Two specific spouse behaviors are coded to represent *Availability:*

1. *Attentiveness* is a rating of the extent to which the spouse attended to the explorer (appeared to be focused on him or her) and sensitively responded to his or her requests as he or she engaged in the brick activity.
2. *Avoidance* (reverse-coded) is a rating of the extent to which the spouse ignored the explorer's attempts to engage the spouse, minimized or dismissed the importance or significance to the explorer of solving the puzzles, ignored the explorer's emotional and/or instrumental support seeking, withdrew physically in the room, and/or encouraged the explorer to suppress emotions or concern regarding performance on the activity.

Two additional behaviors are coded to represent spouse *Interference:*

1. *Intrusive Support* is a rating of the extent to which the spouse attempted to provide task assistance that was unsolicited (not requested by the explorer). This includes behaviors such as jumping in and trying to help the explorer with the activity, taking over the task and doing it for the explorer, or giving unsolicited advice/suggestions about what to do.
2. *Controlling Support* is a rating of the extent to which the spouse appeared to be too bossy, too directive, or too dominating in his or her support attempts. Although this code is similar to the intrusive support code, it is important to note that a spouse may provide intrusive support in a manipulative or concerned way (e.g., "Are you sure you want to do that?") without being controlling.

The two behaviors that are coded to represent spouse *Encouragement* are as follows:

1. *Encouragement of Exploration* is a rating of the extent to which the spouse actively encouraged the explorer during the activity. This

includes behaviors such as praising the explorer for solving a puzzle, complimenting the explorer's efforts, providing encouragement (e.g., "You can do it"), and encouraging persistence ("Just keep trying . . . you'll get it").

2. *Confidence in Explorer's Ability* is a rating of the extent to which the spouse conveyed confidence (either directly/explicitly or indirectly) in the explorer's ability to succeed at the brick activity.

The following *exploration behaviors* related to the exploratory task are coded:

1. *Performance* is scored by assigning points related to success at exploration (e.g., amount of puzzles solved). All other exploration behaviors are coded on well-defined rating scales.
2. *Expressed Confidence in Self:* the extent to which the explorer conveyed a sense of confidence and comfort with the activity and with working on the activity without necessarily involving the spouse.
3. *Persistence at Task:* the extent to which the explorer actively worked on the activity and remained focused on it during the activity period.
4. *Expressed Enthusiasm in Process of Task:* the extent to which the explorer seemed to enjoy the activity and to be enthusiastic about it, for example, by smiling while working on the activity, making victory signs upon solving a puzzle, stating that the activity is fun.

The following *explorer behaviors toward the spouse* are coded:

1. *Concern about Spouse Watching:* the extent to which the explorer either verbally or nonverbally expressed a concern about the spouse watching him or her perform the exploration activity (e.g., by telling the spouse not to watch, by blocking the spouse's view of the activity).
2. *Seeking of Task Assistance:* the extent to which the explorer asked for tangible or informational help/assistance in working on the brick activity.
3. *Seeking of Encouragement/Emotional Support:* the extent to which the explorer sought encouragement, compliments, praise, validation, or reassurance from the spouse with regard to the brick activity (e.g., "Look honey, I did it!").
4. *Negativity/Hostility toward Spouse:* the extent to which the explorer exhibited any (verbal or nonverbal) negativity or hostility toward the spouse including criticism, disapproval, annoyance/irritation, contemptuous facial expressions.
5. *Positive Affect toward Spouse:* the extent to which the explorer interacted with the spouse in a warm, friendly, and positive manner.

6. *Receptiveness to Solicited Task Assistance:* the extent to which the explorer was receptive to and accepting of task assistance that was solicited by the explorer.
7. *Receptiveness to Unsolicited Task Assistance:* the extent to which the explorer was receptive to and accepting of task assistance that was unsolicited by the explorer.
8. *Overt Rejection of Solicited Task Assistance:* the extent to which the explorer was overtly rejecting of task assistance that was solicited by the explorer.
9. *Overt Rejection of Unsolicited Task Assistance:* the extent to which the explorer was overtly rejecting of task assistance that was unsolicited by the explorer.

To assess immediate outcomes of secure base use and support in the laboratory, we have assessed changes in the explorer's mood and state self-esteem from before to after the exploration activity. Explorers also report their perceptions of the exploration activity, including the extent to which he or she enjoyed the exploration activity, the extent to which he or she felt knowledgeable or smart during the activity, the extent to which the spouse was helpful or supportive during the activity, and the extent to which the spouse was negative or unsupportive during the activity. The particular outcomes assessed will be tailored to the specific hypotheses under investigation.

Laboratory Goal Discussions

Because exploration also may be conceptualized as goal pursuit, another observational method by which secure base use and support has been assessed in the context of adult relationships involves a Future Goals and Plans Discussion (e.g., Feeney, 2004, 2007). This procedure occurs as follows: Couple members are seated in a laboratory living room, and the person who is implicitly put into the role of an explorer (or support receiver) is given an index card on which his or her personal goals for the future are listed (as identified by the explorer in a prior study session). Couple members are then asked to discuss these goals. The interactions are unobtrusively videotaped and later coded for content relevant to assessing secure base use and support. To assess immediate outcomes of the secure base support dynamics that occur during these discussions, the explorer reports his or her mood and state self-esteem both before and after the discussion. In variations of this procedure, the explorer is asked to identify and discuss the single most important personal goal that he or she wishes to accomplish over a designated time period, such as 6 months or 1 year. This procedure involves following the individual over the designated period of time to determine whether he or she actually accomplishes the goal, and to determine whether goal accomplishment is influenced by the quality of secure base support observed in the earlier laboratory discussion.

Depending on study hypotheses, a variety of *explorer behaviors* reflecting secure base use may be coded from these discussions, including the following:

1. *Confident Exploration of Goals:* the explorer confidently explores avenues for achieving his or her goals and appears comfortable with the autonomous pursuit of goals.
2. *Open Discussion of Goals:* the explorer openly and thoroughly discusses his or her goals (e.g., initiates discussion of various aspects of the goals, elaborates on issues raised by the partner).
3. *Emotional Disclosure:* the explorer openly describes, talks about, and shares emotions and feelings.
4. *Descriptive Disclosure:* the explorer talks openly about the factual details of his or her goals.
5. *Receptiveness to Support Attempts:* the explorer conveys either verbally or nonverbally that the partner's input is welcomed and appreciated.
6. *Avoidance Behaviors:* the explorer exhibits a reluctance to openly discuss his or her goals (e.g., by changing the topic, acting distracted, withdrawing physically).
7. *Warmth/Positive Affect:* the explorer interacts in a warm, pleasant, and positive manner (e.g., by exhibiting positive facial expressions, positive voice tone).
8. *Negative or Hostile Affect:* the explorer exhibits negativity or hostility toward the partner (e.g., by expressing dissatisfaction, criticizing, showing annoyance).
9. *Minimizing Behaviors:* the explorer downplays the significance or importance of his or her goals.
10. *Maximizing Behaviors:* the explorer appears to catastrophize the significance or importance of problems/concerns related to his or her goals.
11. *Modification of Goals:* the explorer changes his or her goals during the discussion.
12. *Blending of Goals:* the explorer appears to merge his or her personal goals with the partner (to include the partner/relationship).
13. *Proximity Seeking:* the explorer initiates and/or seeks physical affection.
14. *Overall Support Seeking:* the explorer openly expresses goal-related concerns and worries, requests understanding or reassurance, and/or asks for assistance in accomplishing goals.
15. *Apparent Security in Relation to Partner:* the explorer engages in an open, easy, and connected interaction with the partner and shows

evidence of being able to explore his or her goals while feeling supported and understood by the partner.

The total number of goals and the nature of the goals discussed are also coded for descriptive purposes.

A variety of *caregiver (support-provider) behaviors* indicative of secure base support also may be coded from these interactions.

1. *Listening/Attentive:* the caregiver displays clear signs of being focused on his or her partner and processing the partner's disclosure of information (e.g., eye contact, nods).
2. *Support of Goals and Autonomous Exploration:* the caregiver supports his or her partner's autonomous pursuit of goals (e.g., by facilitating dialogue about the goals, expressing understanding and respect for the partner and the partner's goals).
3. *Encouragement of Goals and Autonomy:* the caregiver encourages the partner to pursue his or her personal goals.
4. *Communication of Future Availability:* the caregiver conveys that he or she will be available to help as needed in the future attainment of the partner's goals.
5. *Comfort with the Partner's Autonomous Goal Pursuit:* the caregiver behaves in a manner indicating that he or she feels comfortable with the partner's pursuit of autonomous goals.
6. *Avoidance:* the caregiver exhibits a reluctance to openly discuss the partner's goals (e.g., by changing the topic, acting distracted, withdrawing physically).
7. *Intrusiveness/Interference:* the caregiver either overtly or subtly interferes with the partner's goals (e.g., by inserting him- or herself into the goals, trying to change the goals, preventing the partner from pursuing the goals).
8. *Controlling Support:* the caregiver appears to be too bossy, too directive, or too dominating in his or her support attempts (e.g., telling the partner what to do to accomplish a goal instead of offering helpful suggestions).
9. *Warmth/Positive Affect:* the caregiver interacts in a warm, pleasant, and positive manner (e.g., by exhibiting positive facial expressions, positive voice tone).
10. *Negative or Hostile Affect:* the caregiver exhibits negativity or hostility toward the partner (e.g., by expressing dissatisfaction, criticizing, showing annoyance).
11. *Emotional Support:* the caregiver is responsive to the emotional

needs of the partner (e.g., by validating feelings, making empathic remarks, encouraging disclosure of feelings).

12. *Instrumental Support:* the caregiver provides actual, tangible assistance that is focused on fixing a specific goal-related problem or helping to make a plan for how a particular goal may be achieved.
13. *Minimizing Behaviors:* the caregiver minimizes or downplays the significance or importance of the goals.
14. *Maximizing Behaviors:* the caregiver appears to catastrophize the significance or importance of problems/concerns related to the goals.
15. *Proximity Seeking:* the caregiver provides physical affection.
16. *Overall Secure Base Support Effort:* the caregiver demonstrates an active effort to be sensitive and responsive to the partner and his or her goals and goal-related problems throughout the discussion.

Decisions to Embrace Opportunities

Another ideal laboratory method for observing secure base use and support involves creating challenging opportunities that one member of a dyad can choose to embrace or not. The decision made to embrace or forgo a potentially rewarding challenging opportunity can be examined as a function of secure base support behavior provided and received. See Feeney, van Vleet, Jakubiak, and Tomlinson (2017) for a detailed rationale and description of methods and coding procedures. These decision points can also be influenced by experimentally manipulated secure base behavior in the lab. The following section provides examples of some laboratory manipulations of secure base behavior.

Composite variables representing caregiver availability, intrusiveness, and encouragement of exploration may be computed based on these codes.

It is important to note that observational methods are typically labor-intensive, not only because of the time and effort it takes to collect the data, but also because multiple coders must be trained to observe and code behaviors in standardized ways, and issues of reliability must be addressed. However, the benefits of observational laboratory methods far outweigh the costs of relying only on couple members' reports of their typical behaviors (which may be biased and difficult to recall, particularly if couple members do not attend to the specific behaviors that researchers wish to assess).

Experimental Methods

Experimental methods provide an ideal means of assessing the influence on explorers of the presence and absence of secure base support during exploration. Below are examples of procedures that have been used to experimentally manipulate aspects of secure base support to show effects on exploration behavior and immediate outcomes for the recipient.

Manipulating Caregiver (Support-Provider) Intrusiveness

According to attachment theory (Bowlby, 1988), an important function of a secure base is to be available, encouraging, and ready to respond when called on, *but to intervene actively only when clearly necessary.* Attachment theory postulates that noninterference/nonintrusiveness is an important feature of a secure base, and subsequent research examining interactions between parents and children has indicated that intrusiveness is a major inhibitor of exploration and is associated with negative outcomes such as passivity, less competence, and less curiosity on the part of the child (e.g., Ainsworth, Bell, & Stayton, 1974; Cassidy & Berlin, 1994; Egeland & Farber, 1984; Main, 1983; Matas, Arend, & Sroufe, 1978). Although adult attachment researchers have shown that compulsive or intrusive support in stressful situations is associated with attachment insecurity (e.g., Feeney & Collins, 2001; Kunce & Shaver, 1994), the consequences of this type of support in exploratory situations had not been established in adulthood. Therefore, experimental procedures have been developed to manipulate caregiver (support-provider) intrusiveness (which indicates a lack of secure base support) in order to examine some immediate effects of the waiting, noninterfering aspect of secure base support on the recipient.

During this procedure, couple members complete activities in separate rooms. First, they are asked to participate in a communication activity involving instant messaging (1) as a filler activity and (2) to familiarize couple members with the use of the instant messaging system. The username that is established for the person implicitly assigned to the role of an explorer is "romanticpartner1," and the username for the person implicitly assigned to a potential caregiving role is "romanticpartner2." After receiving instructions, couple members are given 5 minutes to interact with one another using the instant messaging system. Second, the explorer is asked to explore a new activity (a computer puzzle game) while the caregiver waits in the other room. A computer puzzle activity provides an ideal exploratory activity for two reasons. First, the goal is to select a novel activity that adults might enjoy exploring in a laboratory situation in a manner comparable to the way in which children are observed exploring toys in laboratory situations in developmental research (e.g., see Grossmann, Grossmann, & Zimmerman, 1999, for a review). The goal is to create an analogue situation in which adults might explore an adult toy. The puzzle activity is selected to be enjoyable and solvable—challenging in a pleasurable, but not in a difficult or stressful, way. Participants are instructed to have fun with it, and there is no pressure for them to perform well. They are instructed to try the activity so that they can report (on a questionnaire) what they think about it afterward. [In prior research (Feeney, 2004), participants have rated the activity as being enjoyable (M = 5.0, on a 7-point scale) and not very difficult (M = 3.2, on a 7-point scale).] The second major consideration in choosing this activity involves the goal of experimentally manipulating partner intrusiveness/interference to examine the effects on the recipient. A computer provides an ideal means of standardizing and delivering support to the explorer during the exploration activity.

The explorer is told that the partner can watch the game on a computer while waiting in the other room if he or she chooses to do so. The experimenter explains that the partner will wait in the other room so that the explorer will not be distracted while playing the game. These instructions are intended to (1) make it unlikely that the explorer will expect any messages given that he or she knows of the experimenter's desire for him or her *not* to be distracted, but at the same time (2) make it possible and believable that the messages sent to explorers in the experimental conditions *could* have come from the partner. Neither member of the couple is told that the explorer might receive messages. The experimenter sets up the game for the explorer by making the puzzle completely visible on the left of the computer screen, and by leaving the instant messenger window (from the previous activity) visible on the right side of the screen. The explorer is given instructions about how to play the game and is then left alone to play for 5 minutes.

Before arriving for the study, explorers are randomly assigned to one of four support conditions (which may vary depending on the particular hypotheses under investigation):

1. *Intrusive/controlling condition:* Explorers receive frequent messages, ostensibly from the partner, that provide the answers to the puzzle (e.g., "1 down—texas") or tell the explorer what to do (e.g., "do 12 down"). The experimenter monitors the explorer's progress from the control room and is careful not to give answers to the puzzle that have already been solved.
2. *Intrusive/supportive condition:* Explorers receive frequent messages, ostensibly from the partner, that are intrusive but emotionally supportive (e.g., "Good luck," "Not bad," "Nice try," "Hard one"). The experimenter monitors the explorer's progress so that delivery of an appropriate message is based on what the recipient actually does.
3. *Nonintrusive/supportive condition:* Explorers receive two messages, ostensibly from the partner, that are nonintrusive and emotionally supportive. One message ("Good luck") is delivered immediately, and another message ("Good job" or "Some of these are hard," depending on how the recipient is doing) is delivered 4 minutes into the game.
4. *Control condition:* Explorers receive no messages. Because no messages are expected, the control condition is intended to provide a baseline, so that outcomes in the experimental conditions can be compared with outcomes that would be present in neutral circumstances (when working alone without any interruption).

The support manipulations are delivered by the experimenter through the instant messaging system. This is accomplished by having the experimenter close the instant messenger in the caregiver's room and take over the "romanticpartner2" username in the control room. After the activity, the explorer is asked to answer a number of questions designed to assess his or her perceptions of the partner's supportiveness during the puzzle activity. Explorers who receive messages also are asked to rate their perceptions of the messages. To provide a supplementary indicator of the way messages are perceived by the explorers, two independent observers later code the explorers' written responses to the messages they receive (for those who respond by sending a message in return). The responses are coded for the degree to which the explorer appears to accept or reject the messages. For explorers in the intrusive/controlling condition (the only condition in which participants receive answers to the puzzle), coders also compute the percentage of answers, out of the total number given, that the explorer fills into the puzzle. Explorers also complete measures of state self-esteem and mood both before and after the exploration activity. Again, the particular outcome measures assessed will depend on the hypotheses under investigation.

Manipulating Task Assistance during Exploration

A similar procedure has been used to test the hypothesis, derived from attachment theory, that individuals whose partners are available to them in times of need (i.e., are accepting of dependency needs) will exhibit more independent functioning as indexed by less receptiveness to experimentally manipulated, unsolicited assistance during a laboratory exploration activity (Feeney, 2007). This procedure occurs as follows: After couple members, who are placed in separate rooms, are given an opportunity to interact through an instant messaging system, the person assigned to the role of explorer is asked to try a new computer puzzle activity. Again, the puzzle activity is selected to be enjoyable and solvable—challenging in a pleasurable but not difficult or stressful way. The explorer is told that the partner can watch the game on his or her computer while waiting in the other room if he or she chooses to do so. Then, the experimenter sets up the game for the explorer by making the puzzle completely visible on the left of the computer screen and by leaving the instant messenger window (from the previous interaction) visible on the right side of the screen. The explorer is given instructions about how to play the game and is left alone to play for 5 minutes. To assess explorers' independent versus dependent exploration, a subset of recipients is randomly assigned to a condition in which they receive unsolicited instrumental support (task assistance) through the instant messaging system during the activity. Again, this assistance is ostensibly provided by the partner but is actually delivered by the experimenter, who takes over the partner's user name. In this condition, explorers receive frequent messages that provide the answers to the puzzle or that tell the explorer what to do to solve the puzzle. The experimenter monitors the explorer's progress from the control room and is careful not to give answers to the puzzle that had already been solved. As a comparison condition, another subset of explorers is randomly assigned to receive unsolicited emotional support during the activity (e.g., "Good luck," "Not bad," "Nice try," "Hard one"). The experimenter monitors the explorer's progress so that an appropriate message is delivered on the basis of what the explorer actually does.

Three indexes of the explorer's independent exploration are obtained: (1) After the activity, explorers report (on a rating scale) the extent to which they paid attention to the messages that were sent by the partner; (2) the experimenter records whether the explorer responded to the support messages that were delivered; and (3) for the subset of explorers who responded to the messages, two independent observers code the written responses for the degree to which the explorer appeared to be rejecting (vs. accepting) the messages. Overt rejection of the messages is coded as the degree to which the explorer was unreceptive to the partner's assistance by conveying that it was not welcomed or appreciated (e.g., by telling the partner to stop sending messages).

Manipulating Encouraging Behavior

Experimental procedures have also been used to experimentally manipulate another aspect of secure base support—caregiver encouragement of exploration (van Vleet & Feeney, 2010). One member of the couple is given an opportunity to engage in a challenging exploration activity, while the other member of the couple waits in another room. Both before and after the activity, explorers are randomly assigned to receive one of three messages from their partners: encouraging messages (e.g., "Have fun . . . you can do it!), discouraging messages (e.g., "Sounds boring . . . hurry, so we can leave"), or neutral messages unrelated to the exploration (e.g., "It's raining outside"). Also, a subset of explorers is assigned to a control condition in which they receive no messages at all. All messages are delivered via handwritten notes from the partner. The partner is asked to copy preprepared notes in his or her own handwriting, similar to methods used in Collins and Feeney (2004) to manipulate support in times of stress. Partners are asked to address their partners the way they normally would and sign the note the way they normally would, but the content of the notes is predetermined according to assigned condition.

The exploration behavior of the explorer is videotaped during the activity and later coded by independent observers. After the activity, measures are obtained of the explorer's perceptions of the notes and of the partner's supportiveness, the explorer's perceptions of the exploration activity, and the explorer's willingness to engage in future exploration activities. A variety of immediate outcomes may be assessed (e.g., changes in the explorer's mood and state self-esteem from before to after the activity), and it will be important for future experimental work to establish the strength and duration of the influence of experimental manipulations on a variety of other theoretically derived outcomes.

STRENGTHS AND WEAKNESSES OF LABORATORY METHODS

There are a number of strengths regarding the use of laboratory methods, such as the ones described earlier, for assessing secure base use and support. First, observational methods allow us to observe actual secure base support behaviors and actual exploration behaviors as they unfold during spontaneous interactions between couple members. Because reports of secure base use and support are likely to be biased by one's personality characteristics, personal motivations, and history of relationship experiences, it is important to obtain independent, observational assessments of these behaviors in order to achieve a complete understanding of these relational dynamics. The importance of obtaining multiple perspectives of the support behavior that occurs within a relationship has been established in prior work (e.g., Collins & Feeney, 2000, 2004). Surprisingly, however, the bulk of research with adults has relied primarily on reports of support that is provided and received.

Second, experimental methods allow us to establish causal relations between aspects of secure base support (or lack thereof) and exploration behavior (as well as other predicted outcomes). Because experimental methods are the only means for establishing causality, it is imperative to include these methods in studies of the effects of secure base use and support. It is unfortunate that the use of experimental methods has been limited in attachment research, because there is a great deal to be gained from experimental analysis. In particular, there has been a limited amount of experimental analysis of normative processes in favor of a heavy focus on individual-difference analysis (comparisons of secure vs. insecure) in the study of adult attachment. This most likely results from the ease of measuring trait constructs (and correlating them with predicted outcome measures), and from the lack of clarity about the normative processes we need to know about (and thus empirically examine). Therefore, important for using the experimental method effectively is a conceptual framework that guides analysis of key secure base skills/components and outcomes. Attachment theory provides such a framework, and many normative predictions (some of which are discussed below) await experimental investigation.

With regard to potential weaknesses of laboratory research, it may be argued that observational and experimental methods lack mundane realism (and therefore lack external validity). This is why it is important to take great care in creating laboratory situations that allow participants to behave both naturally and spontaneously. In the laboratory procedures described earlier, great care is taken to create psychological realism for participants. For example, the lab is set up like a living room (with comfortable sofas, coffee table, bookshelves, and refrigerator), and couple members are given the time to become familiar with, and comfortable interacting in, the lab living room before the procedures of interest occur. Great efforts are taken to ensure that the behaviors assessed are both natural and spontaneous, and experimental manipulations are delivered carefully in ways that do not arouse suspicion.

Careful debriefings are conducted after each study session to (1) educate participants about the scientific purpose of the investigation, (2) inform participants of (and explain) any deception that may be involved in the experimental procedures, and (3) probe participants for suspicion and unnatural responses during the session. Potential weaknesses also may be mitigated by obtaining a convergence of evidence using various procedures and methods, and by undertaking challenging consistency tests to ensure that results can support interpretation of the secure base construct.

DIRECTIONS FOR FUTURE RESEARCH

Many issues regarding secure base use and support await laboratory investigation. As noted earlier, one reason for the limited amount of experimental analysis of secure base use and support thus far is likely to involve a lack of clarity about the specific processes we need to test experimentally. Thus, in this section, we highlight some attachment theoretical predictions regarding secure base use and support that could be tested in experimental and/or observational studies.

Because research examining secure base use and support in adult relationships is still in its beginnings, much theoretical development and empirical research are needed in this area. The laboratory methods described earlier provide a useful foundation for testing some normative predictions derived from attachment theory. It will be important for future research not only to explore the microdynamics of secure base use and support but also to explore the many potential benefits of secure base use and support. For example, individuals whose partners provide them with a secure base from which to explore the world are likely to (1) engage in a variety of exploratory activities; (2) experience increases in self-esteem, self-efficacy, and self-confidence as they gain more knowledge of the world; (3) learn and discover more than they would otherwise; (4) accept challenges and pursue goals; (5) be more healthy emotionally and physically; (6) be more satisfied with their relationships and have better relationship functioning; and (7) hold positive perceptions regarding the benefit of seeking support from others. All of these predictions may be tested in laboratory studies. In addition, observational laboratory methods are likely to provide a beneficial means of uncovering script-like representations of secure base experiences (H. Waters & Waters, 2006). For example, to the extent that some aspects of secure base scripts operate below conscious awareness and are inaccessible for self-report, sequential analysis of behaviors in secure base contexts could assist in identifying if–then sequences of behaviors that reflect secure base scripts. It is my hope the examples of laboratory methods described earlier will provide a springboard for future laboratory research on secure base processes in adult relationships.

It is noteworthy that the discussion of secure base support processes presented here emphasizes explorations of the external world that are likely to have important implications for the relationship and for the inner self in terms of discovery, self-esteem, perceptions of self-competency, and so on. However, effective secure base support in adulthood should include not only the support of a relationship partner's exploration of the physical world but also the exploration of his or her inner, psychological world—for example, the exploration of thoughts, feelings, and emotions related to self-understanding and self-discovery. In fact, Main and her colleagues have described the uninhibited exploration of attachment-related events, thoughts, and emotions as a hallmark of secure attachment (Main, 1995; Main, Kaplan, & Cassidy, 1985). Thus, the support of this type of exploration, in particular, may have important implications for the development of secure attachment orientations in adulthood (e.g., Byng-Hall, 1999). Future research is needed to explore the specific determinants and outcomes of the support of internal versus external forms of exploration.

Also, in future work regarding secure base use and support, it will be important to consider research and theory indicating that individuals must occasionally disengage from an unattainable goal pursuit and reengage in a new one (e.g., Carver & Scheier, 2000; Wrosch, Miller, Scheier, & Brun de Potet, 2007; Wrosch, Scheier, Miller, Schulz, & Carver, 2003); that is, it will be important to consider the attainability of particular exploration pursuits. For example, optimal secure base support processes surrounding a partner's attainable (realistic) goals may be quite different from optimal secure base support processes surrounding a partner's unattainable (unrealistic) goals: Secure base support may involve not only being available, encouraging, and nonintrusive in helping a partner to explore attainable goals, but it also may involve behaviors that assist a relationship partner in disengaging from an unattainable goal and reengaging in another. Specific relational (secure base support) processes involved in helping a partner disengage from a goal must be identified in future work. We suspect that this will be a challenging endeavor given that relationship partners are likely to have different ideas about the attainability of particular goals, and given that support for disengagement may be resisted despite the long-term benefit that disengagement might have for psychological well-being (Wrosch et al., 2003), physical well-being (Wrosch et al., 2007), and quality of life (Wrosch & Scheier, 2003).

Especially important for attachment theoretical predictions, future research is needed to examine the ways in which the attachment, caregiving, and exploration systems function together in the context of everyday interactions with one's relationship partner. We suspect that a delicate balance of encouraging autonomy yet accepting dependence when needed is vital for healthy personal and relationship functioning. We further suspect that some individuals are better at one of these than the other, and that balancing both requires a combination of skills, resources, and motivation (Feeney & Collins, 2001, 2003). Thus, studies that empirically examine this balance (and the underlying mechanisms that influence one's ability to balance both the support of autonomy and the support of dependence) are of paramount importance.

Laboratory methods involving experimental analysis have been especially underrepresented in the literature on secure base use and support, yet this method has much to contribute (see also E. Waters et al., 2002). Much attachment research has focused on individual differences. Although this approach has been crucial to testing and extending attachment theory, limitations include (1) an inability to draw causal inferences, (2) too little attention to the role that context plays in eliciting and organizing attachment behavior, and (3) difficulty in isolating the effects of specific variables that are theorized to produce specific effects. Examples of research questions related to secure base use and support that may be best addressed with experimental methods include the following: Does the receipt of secure base support from a close relationship partner cause one to persist longer and perform better at exploration activities (than those who do not receive such support)? Does a lack of secure base support in an exploration context cause (at least temporary) decreases in feelings of attachment security? Does the receipt of secure base support cause (at least temporary) boosts in feelings of security? Does secure base support from nonclose others have the same effects as secure base support from an attachment figure? Answers to these types of causal questions, and many others derived from attachment theory, can only be tested using experimental methods.

It is also important to emphasize that experimental work should not be limited to examining individual differences in attachment orientation as a function of experimentally manipulated variables. Although quasi-experimental comparisons among attachment classifications are important, it is also important to understand the functioning of the components of secure base use and support in their own right, in normative studies of the effects of context on behavior (e.g., as in the sample questions outlined earlier). Normative attachment research has been especially underrepresented in the adult attachment literature, and experimental methods provide an ideal mechanism for addressing normative questions.

REFERENCES

Ainsworth, M. D. S., Bell, S. M., Stayton, D. F. (1974). Infant–mother attachment and social development: Socialization as a product of reciprocal responsiveness to signals. In M. P. M. Richards (Ed.), *The integration of a child into a social world* (pp. 99–135). New York: Cambridge University Press.

Ainsworth, M. D. S., Blehar, M. C., Waters, E., & Wall, S. (2015). *Patterns of attachment: Psychological study of the Strange Situation*. New York: Taylor & Francis (Psychology Press). (Original work published 1978)

Bakeman, R. (2000). Behavioral observation and coding. In H. T. Reis & C. M. Judd (Eds.), *Handbook of research methods in social and personality psychology* (pp. 138–159). New York: Cambridge University Press.

Bowlby, J. (1973). *Attachment and loss: Separation, anxiety and anger*. New York: Basic Books.

Bowlby, J. (1980). *Attachment and loss: Sadness and depression.* New York: Basic Books.

Bowlby, J. (1982). *Attachment and loss: Attachment.* New York: Basic Books. (Original work published 1969)

Bowlby, J. (1988). *A secure base.* New York: Basic Books.

Brewer, M. B. (2000). Research design and issues of validity. In H. T. Reis & C. M. Judd (Eds.), *Handbook of research methods in social and personality psychology* (pp. 3–16). New York: Cambridge University Press.

Byng-Hall, J. (1999). Family couple therapy: Toward greater security. In J. Cassidy & P. R. Shaver (Eds.), *Handbook of attachment: Theory, research, and clinical applications* (pp. 625–645). New York: Guilford Press.

Carpenter, E. M., & Kirkpatrick, L. A. (1996). Attachment style and presence of a romantic partner as moderators of psychophysiological responses to a stressful laboratory situation. *Personal Relationships, 3,* 351–367.

Carver, C. S., & Scheier, M. F. (2000). Scaling back goals and recalibration of the affect system are processes in normal adaptive self-regulation: Understanding "response shift" phenomena. *Social Science and Medicine, 50,* 1715–1722.

Cassidy, J., & Berlin, L. J. (1994). The insecure/ambivalent pattern of attachment: Theory and research. *Child Development, 65,* 971–981.

Collins, N. L., & Feeney, B. C. (2000). A safe haven: An attachment theory perspective on support-seeking and caregiving in adult romantic relationships. *Journal of Personality and Social Psychology, 78,* 1053–1073.

Collins, N. L., & Feeney, B. C. (2004). Working models of attachment shape perceptions of social support: Evidence from experimental and observational studies. *Journal of Personality and Social Psychology, 87,* 363–383.

Crowell, J. A., Pan, H. S., Gao, Y., Treboux, D., O'Connor, E., & Waters, E. (1998). *The secure base scoring system for adults.* Unpublished manuscript, State University of New York at Stony Brook, Stony Brook, NY.

Crowell, J., Treboux, D., Gao, Y., Fyffe, C., Pan, H., & Waters, E. (2002). Assessing secure base behavior in adulthood: Development of a measure, links to adult attachment representations and relations to couples' communication and reports of relationships. *Developmental Psychology, 38,* 679–693.

Crowell, J., & Waters, E. (2005). Attachment representations, secure-base behavior, and the evolution of adult relationships: The Stony Brook Adult Relationship Project. In K. E. Grossmann, K. Grossmann, & E. Waters (Eds.), *Attachment from infancy to adulthood: The major longitudinal studies* (pp. 223–244). New York: Guilford Press.

Dykas, M. J., Woodhouse, S. S., Cassidy, J., & Waters, H. S. (2006). Narrative assessment of attachment representations: Links between secure base scripts and adolescent attachment. *Attachment and Human Development, 8,* 221–240.

Egeland, B., & Farber, E. A. (1984). Infant–mother attachment: Factors related to its development and changes over time. *Child Development, 55,* 753–771.

Feeney, B. C. (2004). A secure base: Responsive support of goal strivings and exploration in adult intimate relationships. *Journal of Personality and Social Psychology, 87,* 631–648.

Feeney, B. C. (2007). The dependency paradox in close relationships: Accepting dependence promotes independence. *Journal of Personality and Social Psychology, 92,* 268–285.

Feeney, B. C., Cassidy, J., & Ramos-Marcuse, F. (2008). The generalization of attachment representations to new social situations: Predicting behavior during initial interactions with strangers. *Journal of Personality and Social Psychology, 95,* 1481–1498.

Feeney, B. C., & Collins, N. L. (2001). Predictors of caregiving in adult intimate relationships: An attachment theoretical perspective. *Journal of Personality and Social Psychology, 80,* 972–994.

Feeney, B. C., & Collins, N. L. (2003). Motivations for caregiving in adult intimate relationships: Influences on caregiving behavior and relationship functioning. *Personality and Social Psychology Bulletin, 29,* 950–968.

Feeney, B. C., & Kirkpatrick, L. A. (1996). The effects of adult attachment and presence of romantic partners on physiological responses to stress. *Journal of Personality and Social Psychology, 70,* 255–270.

Feeney, B. C., & Thrush, R. L. (2010). Relationship influences on exploration in adulthood: The characteristics and function of a secure base. *Journal of Personality and Social Psychology, 98,* 57–76.

Feeney, B. C., van Vleet, M., Jakubiak, B. K., & Tomlinson, J. M. (2017). Predicting the pursuit and support of challenging life opportunities. *Personality and Social Psychology Bulletin, 43,* 1171–1187.

Giglioli, I. A. C., Pravettoni, G., Martin, D. L. S., Parra, E., & Raya, M. A. (2017). A novel integrating virtual reality approach for the assessment of the attachment behavioral system. *Frontiers in Psychology, 8,* 959.

Grossmann, K. E., Grossmann, K., & Zimmermann, P. (1999). A wider view of attachment and exploration. In J. Cassidy & P. Shaver (Eds.), *Handbook of attachment theory and research: Theory, research, and clinical applications* (pp. 760–786). New York: Guilford Press.

Jakubiak, B. K., & Feeney, B. C. (2016a). A sense of security: Touch promotes state attachment security. *Social and Personality Psychological Science, 7,* 745–753.

Jakubiak, B. K., & Feeney, B. C. (2016b). Keep in touch: The effects of imagined touch support on stress and exploration. *Journal of Experimental Social Psychology, 65,* 59–67.

Jakubiak, B. K., & Feeney, B. C. (2019). Interpersonal touch as a resource to facilitate positive personal and relational outcomes during stress discussions. *Journal of Social and Personal Relationships.*

Kane, H. S., Jaremka, L. M., Guichard, A. C., Ford, M. B., Collins, N. L., & Feeney, B. C. (2007). Feeling supported and feeling satisfied: How one partner's attachment style predicts the other partner's relationship experiences. *Journal of Social and Personal Relationships, 24,* 535–555.

Kane, H. S., McCall, C., Collins, N. L., & Blascovich, J. A. (2008, February). *The effects of social support from a significant other in an immersive virtual environment.* Poster presented at the meeting of the Society for Personality and Social Psychology, Albuquerque, NM.

Kunce, L. J., & Shaver, P. R. (1994). An attachment-theoretical approach to caregiving in romantic relationships. In K. Bartholomew & D. Perlman (Eds.), *Advances in personal relationships* (Vol. 5, pp. 205–237). London: Jessica Kingsley.

Main, M. (1983). Exploration, play, and cognitive functioning related to infant–mother attachment. *Infant Behavior and Development, 6,* 167–174.

Main, M. (1995). Attachment: Overview, with implications for clinical work. In S. Goldberg, R. Muir, & J. Kerr (Eds.), *Attachment theory: Social, developmental, and clinical perspectives* (pp. 407–474). Hillsdale, NJ: Analytic Press.

Main, M., Kaplan, N., & Cassidy, J. (1985). Security in infancy, childhood, and adulthood: A move to the level of representation. In I. Bretherton & E. Waters (Eds.), Growing points in attachment theory and research. *Monographs of the Society for Research in Child Development, 50,* 66–106.

Matas, L., Arend, R. A., & Sroufe, L. A. (1978). Continuity of adaptation in the second year: The relationship between quality of attachment and later competence. *Child Development, 49,* 547–556.

Maunder, L., Nolan, H., & Tannenbaum, D. W. (2006). The relationship of attachment insecurity to subjective stress and autonomic function during standardized acute stress in healthy adults. *Journal of Psychosomatic Research, 60,* 283–290.

Mikulincer, M., Gillath, O., Halevy, V., Avihou, N., Avidan, S., & Eshkoli, N. (2001). Attachment theory and reactions to others' needs: Evidence that activation of the sense of attachment security promotes empathic responses. *Journal of Personality and Social Psychology, 81,* 1205–1224.

Mikulincer, M., Gillath, O., Sapir-Lavid, Y., Yaakobi, E., Arias, K., Tal-Aloni, L., & Bor, G. (2003). Attachment theory and concern for others' welfare: Evidence that activation of the sense of secure base promotes endorsement of self-transcendence values. *Basic and Applied Social Psychology, 25,* 299–312.

Mikulincer, M., & Shaver, P. R. (2005). Attachment security, compassion, and altruism. *Current Directions in Psychological Science, 14,* 34–38.

Mikulincer, M. R., & Shaver, P. (2020). Enhancing the "Broaden and Build" cycle of attachment security in adulthood: From the laboratory to relational contexts and societal systems. *International Journal of Environmental Research and Public Health, 17,* 2054.

Mikulincer, M., Shaver, P. R., Gillath, O., & Nitzberg, R. A. (2005). Attachment, caregiving, and altruim: Boosting attachment security increases compassion and helping. *Journal of Personality and Social Psychology, 89,* 817–839.

Monin, J. K., Feeney, B. C., & Schulz, R. (2012). Attachment orientation and reactions to anxiety expression in close relationships. *Personal Relationships, 19*(3), 535–550.

Monin, J. K., Schulz, R., Feeney, B. C., & Cook, T. (2010). Attachment insecurity and perceived partner suffering as predictors of personal distress. *Journal of Experimental Social Psychology, 46,* 1143–1147.

Pietromonaco, P. R., DeBuse, C. J., & Powers, S. I. (2013). Does attachment get under the skin? Adult romantic attachment and cortisol responses to stress. *Current Directions in Psychological Science, 22*(1), 63–68.

Rholes, W. S., Simpson, J. A., & Orina, M. M. (1999). Attachment and anger in an anxiety-provoking situation. *Journal of Personality and Social Psychology, 76,* 940–957.

Simpson, J. A., & Rholes, W. S. (2017). Adult attachment, stress, and romantic relationships. *Current Opinions in Psychology, 13,* 19–24.

Simpson, J. A., Rholes, W. S., & Nelligan, J. S. (1992). Support seeking and support giving within couples in an anxiety-provoking situation: The role of attachment styles. *Journal of Personality and Social Psychology, 62,* 434–446.

Simpson, J. A., Rholes, W. S., Orina, M. M., & Grich, J. (2002). Working models of attachment, support giving, and support seeking in a stressful situation. *Personality and Social Psychology Bulletin, 28,* 598–608.

Simpson, J. A., Winterheld, H. A., Rholes, W. S., & Orina, M. M. (2007). Working models of attachment and reactions to different forms of caregiving from romantic partners. *Journal of Personality and Social Psychology, 93*, 466–477.

van Vleet, M., & Feeney, B. C. (2010). *Spouse encouragement during a novel challenging activity: Impact on self-perceptions, perceptions of the activity, and performance.* Manuscript in preparation, Carnegie Mellon University, Pittsburgh, PA.

Vaughn, B. E., Coppola, G., Verissimo, M., Monteiro, L., Santos, A. J., Posada, G., . . . Korth, B. (2007). The quality of maternal secure-base scripts predicts children's secure-base behavior at home in three sociocultural groups. *International Journal of Behavioral Development, 31*, 65–76.

Wallach, H. S., Safir, M. P., & Almog, I. (2009). Attachment and sense of presence in a virtual environment. *Virtual Reality, 13*, 205–217.

Waters, E., Crowell, J., Elliott, M., Corcoran, D., & Treboux, D. (2002). Bowlby's secure base theory and the social/personality psychology of attachment styles: Work(s) in progress. *Attachment and Human Development, 4*, 230–242.

Waters, E., & Cummings, E. (2000). A secure base from which to explore close relationships. *Child Development, 71*, 164–172.

Waters, E., Kondo-Ikemura, K., Posada, G., & Richters, J. (1991). Learning to love: Mechanisms and milestones. In M. R. Gunnar & L. A. Sroufe (Eds.), *Self processes and development* (Vol. 23, pp. 217–255). Hillsdale, NJ: Erlbaum.

Waters, H., & Waters, E. (2006). The attachment working concept: Among other things, we build script-like representations of secure base experiences. *Attachment and Human Development, 8*, 185–197.

Westmaas, J. L., & Silver, R. C. (2001). The role of attachment in responses to victims of life crises. *Journal of Personality and Social Psychology, 80*, 425–438.

Wrosch, C., Miller, G. E., Scheier, M. F., & Brun de Pontet, S. (2007). Giving up on unattainable goals: Benefits for health? *Personality and Social Psychology Bulletin, 33*, 251–265.

Wrosch, C., & Scheier, M. F. (2003). Personality and quality of life: The importance of optimism and goal adjustment. *Quality of Life Research, 12*, 59–72.

Wrosch, C., Scheier, M. F., Miller, G. E., Schulz, R., & Carver, C. S. (2003). Adaptive self-regulation of unattainable goals: Goal disengagement, goal reengagement, and subjective well-being. *Personality and Social Psychology Bulletin, 29*, 1494–1508.

CHAPTER 12

The Associative Structure of Adult Attachment Representations

Priming Methods for Assessing Implicit Knowledge and Expectations

Markus Maier, Annie Bernier, and David Corcoran

The working model concept has played an influential role in attachment theory and measurement for over three decades (Bowlby, 1980; Main, Kaplan, & Cassidy, 1985). Nonetheless, attachment theorists are of two minds about the concept (Bretherton, 1985; Bretherton & Munholland, 2008). For some, it is a useful metaphor, a way of highlighting the importance of mental representations—nothing more. For others, it could (should, or does) refer to something more tangible—actual cognitive structures that (in principle) could be measured and mapped, and explain links between attachment history and behavior.

If the internal working model (IWM) concept were merely a metaphor, there would be nothing to measure and little to restrain its taking on excess meaning. The IWM would stand between predictor and criterion, treatment and control, as a "black box" that, as Hinde (1991) pointed out, can explain any result. And at the same time, if it is just a label, not a mechanism, it does not really explain anything at all. An alternative is to treat the IWM concept (and the notion of attachment representations in general) as more than mere metaphors, associating them with specific cognitive structures that were not well known in Bowlby's day but that have since become well understood topics in cognitive psychology. This is the approach we favor—taking the IWM concept seriously as referring to specific kinds of cognitive structures to be measured and mapped, and allowed to explain only what is consistent with demonstrable operating characteristics.

Cognitive psychologists have identified and studied the operating characteristics of several specific modes of representation. These include imagery (e.g., Paivio, 1986), schemes (e.g., Bartlett, 1932; Schank & Abelson, 1977), analogue and logical models (e.g., Johnson-Laird, 1995), associative nets (e.g., Collins & Loftus, 1975), and narratives (e.g., Fivush & Neisser, 1994). All of these likely play roles in representing attachment-related experiences. For example, Main (2000) remarks on the power of family photographs and drawings in clinical and research applications. More formally, H. Waters & Waters (2006) have discussed script-like representations of early secure base experiences. Similarly, Mikulincer and Shaver (2016) reviewed methods from cognitive psychology to probe the meaning structures associated with attachment-related experiences (see also Stupica & Cassidy, 2014, for a review of priming methods with children). Assessing such associative meanings is made somewhat difficult by the fact that they exist (for the most part) outside of awareness. As a consequence, they are not readily or reliably accessed by direct questioning. This chapter focuses on experimental methods for assessing such implicit meanings.

In the following paragraphs we introduce our theoretical framework—the associative network model—and describe how attachment-related representations can be conceptualized as associative structures. We then present selected priming techniques that make it possible to empirically investigate such cognitive structures in order to better understand the meanings people attach to attachment relationships and experiences.

OUR TWO COGNITIVE SYSTEMS

Dual-Process Theories

On a very general level, human information processing reflects activity in two qualitatively different systems. According to dual-processing theories (e.g., Epstein, 1994; Evans, 2003; Schneider & Chein, 2003) a great deal of our cognitive activity is based on an automatic associative system shaped by evolution to react quickly to environmental stimuli and provide simple response tendencies to ensure an individual's survival. This is complemented by a more recently evolved system, specific for human beings, that provides rational thinking and conscious control over behavioral responses.

This distinction between two cognitive systems is not new. It dates back to ancient Greek philosophy. Aristotle in the fourth century B.C.E. postulated the existence of a "sensitive soul," responsible for mobility and sensation, and a "rational soul," capable of thought and reflection (Hamlyn, 1993). Similarly, in the 19th century, when psychology became a scientifically acknowledged discipline, William James (1890) laid the foundations of dual-process theories by describing two different ways of thinking: associative and reasoning. James claimed that associative knowledge was derived from past experiences, describing it as "only reproductive," whereas true reasoning was used for "unprecedented situations" in which past experiences did not provide any solutions.

The Associative and Rational Systems in Memory Networks

Recent approaches to our two cognitive systems have provided a more elaborate theoretical framework. For example, Epstein (1991) postulated the existence of two parallel networks of memory and provided a set of features that distinguish between those. He locates unconscious processing in the experiential system and conscious processing in the rational system. Information processing in the experiential system is based on associationistic connections, whereas the rational system is based on logical connections.

Unconscious processing is mainly affective in nature; that is, it is pleasure–pain oriented and tries to avoid harm and to approach positive outcomes such as safety (see also Elliot, 2008). In contrast, conscious thinking relies on reason-oriented thinking. Unconscious behavioral reactions are mediated by "vibes" from past experiences rather than by conscious appraisals of events. Thus, the experiential system allows for rapid processing and is oriented toward immediate actions as compared to slower more abstract and symbolic processing in the rational system. Associative connections stored in the experiential system are stable and resistant to change, and their operation is context-specific (i.e., they are activated in specific situations only, as opposed to flexible and more general associations based on the rational system). Furthermore, the experiential system operates on the preconscious level outside awareness, whereas the rational system operates consciously and in a more controlled way (see also Bargh, 1994; Posner & Snyder, 1975). Both modes of information processing are based on associative connections but require more or less effort, intentionality, time, and working memory capacity, and are more or less controllable.

Similarly, Evans (2003) described two ways of reasoning that are related to two different systems. System 1 is old in evolutionary terms and shared with other animals: It comprises a set of autonomous subsystems that include both innate input modules and domain-specific knowledge. System 1 processes are formed by associative learning mechanisms of the kind produced by neural networks. They are rapid, parallel, and automatic in nature. System 2 is evolutionarily recent and distinctively human: It permits abstract reasoning and hypothetical thinking but is constrained by working memory capacity. Processing in this system is slow and sequential in nature and makes use of the central working memory system. Despite its limited capacity and slower speed of operation, System 2 permits abstract hypothetical thinking that cannot be achieved by System 1. Some theorists assume that System 2 can cause inhibitory effects on System 1 to resolve conflicts. Schneider and Chein (2003) emphasize the role of a Central Processor in switching between the two systems. This Control System comprises five processors, including a Goal Processor, an Attention Controller, an Activity Monitor, an Episodic

Store, and a Gating and Report Relay. The transition from controlled to automatic processing occurs in this model as environmental or unconscious internal stimulation becomes capable of transmitting output without mediation by the Control System. Thus, any circumstances that shut off the Control System allow for automatic processing based on System 1. Dual-processing theories have also been applied to associative network theories of memory to describe conscious and unconscious associative processing.

With regard to the associative structures underlying internal working models of attachment, representations of a caregiver's availability can be stored in the experiential system in an automatic and unconscious way, and simultaneously represented on a more conscious, controlled level in the rational system. The content of these associations can be the same in both systems or differ depending on how attachment experiences are processed in the mind. An insecure state of mind might comprise unconscious automatic associations of the caregiver as being not available in the experiential system, accompanied by a conscious effortful representation of the caregiver as being accessible in the rational system. On the other side, positive representations of the caregiver's availability might be stored in both systems within a secure state of mind. In other words, secure base and safe-haven representations can be found in both systems and correspond more or less. Bowlby (e.g., 1973, 1979a) has discussed such incompatible representations as a significant source of difficulty in attachment behavior and adjustment.

Cognitive psychologists (e.g., Neely, 1977, 1991) have developed experimental paradigms that allow us to measure the specific content of the representations in the experiential or rational system by manipulating the amount of effort, processing time, controllability, and intentionality available at a specific time. Any experimental conditions under which the available effort, processing time, controllability, and intentionality is low, provide access to the experiential system and therefore measure the content of unconscious associations. Under experimental circumstances in which effort, processing time, controllability, and intentionality is high, the rational system overruns the experiential one, allowing for assessment of the content of the conscious connections stored within this system. Thus, by manipulating these conditions, researchers can deliberately switch between both systems, assessing the connections stored within the two systems independently and comparing them to each other. Some priming paradigms have been developed exactly to serve this goal, and we describe them later in this chapter.

ASSOCIATIVE MEMORY IN COGNITIVE PSYCHOLOGY

The idea that central parts of our memory consist of associative structures has a long tradition in psychology. Associative learning has been widely studied in animal (Pavlov, 1927) and human learning (Watson & Rayner, 1920) through classical conditioning. This research demonstrated that simple associations between neutral and meaningful stimuli can be formed through repeated simultaneous presentations of these stimuli. In line with this, the impact of newly acquired associations on social perception, attitudes, and impression formations has widely been demonstrated in the past (e.g., Gawronski & Bodenhausen, 2006). For example, Carlston and Mae (2007) tested the effects of nonverbal cues on person perception. They paired symbols such as glasses (see also Manz & Lueck, 1968) or graduation caps with pictures of neutral target persons and found significant effects in a later impression-formation task. This effect occurred not only when the person in the picture was described as having intentionally chosen the symbol (Study 1), but also when symbol and person were coincidentally paired together (Study 2), indicating a newly acquired association between a symbol's meaning and a representation of an unknown previously neutral person (see also Callison, Karrh, & Zillmann, 2002). Similar effects have been reported for colors (Elliot & Niesta, 2008; Frank & Gilovich, 1988; Vrij, 1997) or seating positions (Becker, Gield, & Froggatt, 1983). Cognitive psychologists have done a great deal to clarify how these meaningful associations are stored in our memory and how associative information processing works.

Meaning as Associative Networks

The network metaphor was originally developed to describe associative links between different semantic concepts stored in memory (e.g., Anderson, 1983; Collins & Loftus, 1975). Based on these early models, Smith (1998) described from a social-cognitive point of view the fundamental assumptions of associative networks. As illustrated in Figure 12.1, specific concepts, reactions, or evaluations are represented as *nodes* in the network, which, if they are semantically, episodically, or affectively related, are connected via *links*.

Links are formed or strengthened when concepts, reactions, or evaluations are repeatedly experienced or thought about together, or are activated in the context of significant consequences. As Hebb (1949, p. 70) stated: "The general idea is an old one, that any two cells or systems of cells that are repeatedly active at the same time will tend to become 'associated,' so that activity in one facilitates activity in the other."

Activating Associative Links

The strength of an association is represented by the length of the links between the nodes. Each node has a specific activation status that can vary over time. Parts of a network are activated when they are accessed in the course of intentional verbally mediated, rational thinking or problem solving. For example, questioning someone about an attachment figure's availability activates the corresponding representation of the caregiver in mind and also activates a

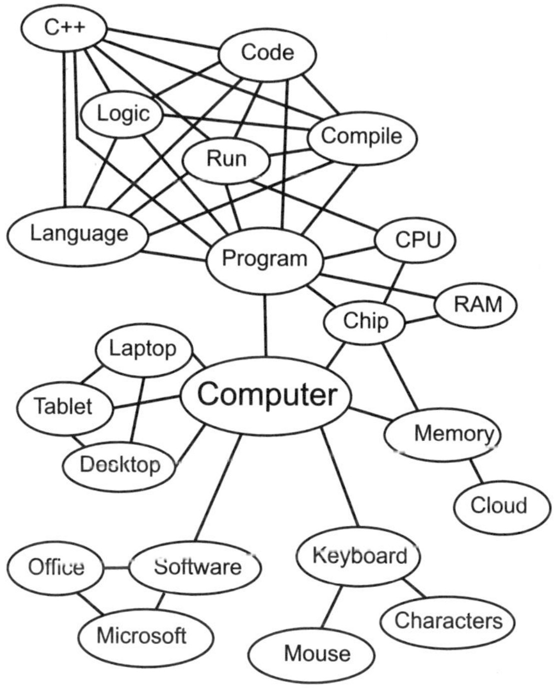

FIGURE 12.1. Example of a semantic network.

related predefined conscious representation of his or her availability. Because this mode of processing is conscious and effortful, it also has high demands on processing capacity in working memory, it needs time, and it can only be processed serially one after another.

Spreading Activation

Another more subtle way that associative links become activated is the spreading activation mechanism (Collins & Loftus, 1975). If an above-threshold activation of one node in the network occurred, activation automatically and effortlessly flows from the activated node to other, related representations. In this way, the related representations become more accessible and thus have a higher probability to influence someone's behavior with only little or no demands on working memory resources. Spreading activation is terminated within a few seconds by decay. Thus, activation does not flow through the whole network but is mostly restricted to nearby nodes. Such spreading activation is the mechanism behind useful implicit measures of associative meaning.

Processing Attachment-Related Information: The Cognitive Unconscious

Bowlby (1969/1982, 1973, 1980) proposed that environmental situations and attachment figures' availability are not appraised anew whenever needed. Rather, starting in infancy, and based on ever-accruing experience, individuals construct models of the world, significant persons within it, and the self. Founded on repeated interactions with the caregiver, these models become "engrained" (Bowlby, 1980, p. 55). In justifying the notion of IWMs, Bowlby (1979b, p. 111) quoted Young (1964): "The idea of a model in the brain is that it constitutes a toy that is yet a tool, an imitation world, which we can manipulate . . . and so find out how to manipulate the real world, which it is supposed to represent."

According to Bowlby (1980) attachment-related IWMs are largely unconscious representations of caregivers' availability and the self in attachment relations and the social environment. As illustrated in Figure 12.2, attachment representations do not stand alone. They cast a net over a wide range of concepts and experiences. They consist of automatic associations that are triggered

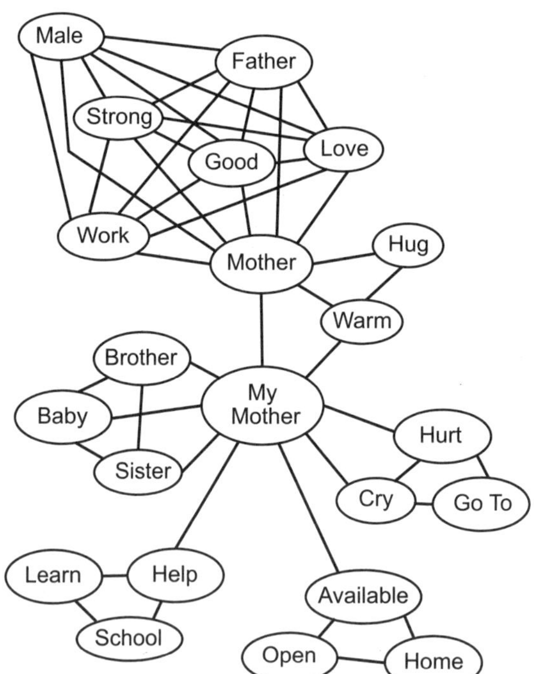

FIGURE 12.2. An associative network with stereotypical attachment-related associations. Association strength is indicated by the length of the connecting lines.

by attachment-relevant situations and automatically guide attachment-related thoughts, behaviors, and affective reactions (see, e.g., Main, 1999; Mikulincer & Shaver, 2003); that is, IWMs are built on preverbally generalized associations about the caregivers and the concept of availability (secure base knowledge; Sroufe & Waters, 1977) and information about a set of situational cues (e.g., specific threats) that associatively trigger the activation of a caregiver representation (safe-haven representation).

Network memory models provide a useful lens through which to view the cognitive structure of these associations, their development, variations in associative strength, and the various ways of becoming active memory. Depending on an individual's attachment state of mind, associations between caregiver representations (e.g., mother or father) and concepts of availability vary in strength and are more or less automatically accessible when activated. It is important to note here that different networks might exist in the experiential system and in the rational system. If the mother concept is activated on the experiential level, activation automatically spreads along the links within this network to nearby nodes, making them more accessible (see Figure 12.3). The structure of associative networks reflects individual experience. Thus, for one person, the concept of *availability* is more accessible after the concept of "my

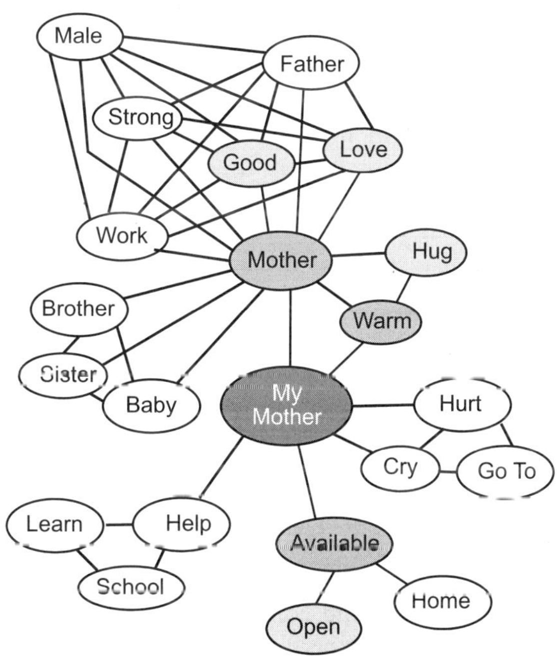

FIGURE 12.3. The spreading activation phenomenon (with My Mother as *context* and *prime*). Denser shading indicates greater activation.

mother" is activated through the presentation of a photograph of the mother or mother-related words/sentences. For another, the same stimuli might activate the concept of *rejection.*

Associations Can Influence Affect, Cognition, and Behavior

It is important to note that associative processing as described in network theories of long-term memory is not restricted to cognitive associations. Automatic associations can also exist between cognitive representations and affect. Bower (1981) assumed that affects such as fear, sadness, or joy can be described as nodes in these networks and be associated with cognitive concepts that activate these affective reactions through spreading activation, as demonstrated in the affective priming research (Fazio, Sanbonmatsu, Powell, & Kardes, 1986). Similarly, basic behavioral tendencies such as approach or avoidance reactions can be described as nodes within these networks having associative relations to all kind of cognitive representations (Chen & Bargh, 1999). Thus, the network metaphor not only explains and predicts the accessibility of cognitive representation when related concepts are activated but it can also be used to describe affective and behavioral processing within these networks. An activation of someone's mother representation might activate not only the concept of availability but also approach (or avoidance) tendencies (e.g., "got to" or "do not go to"; see Figure 12.3) and evoke affective responses such as anticipated joy or fear.

The goals of a cognitive approach to attachment representations include understanding such individual differences in terms of actual experiences and explaining as much as possible of attachment-related psychodynamics in these terms. The claim is not that associative processing accounts for all the phenomena associated with attachment representations, emotions, and behavior—only that because these mechanisms are well understood and empirically accessible, they should be examined in detail before appealing to other types of explanations.

USING PRIMING TO ACTIVATE ASSOCIATIVE MEANINGS

One key method to empirically investigate the associative structures underlying attachment experiences, thoughts, and behaviors is the priming paradigm. This paradigm has the power to experimentally manipulate the circumstances under which associative processing occurs. It allows the experimenter to vary the extent to which conscious and controlled processes contribute to associative processing. Under some experimental conditions such as unconscious activation, limited processing time, and low amount of control, automatic unconscious associations derived from the experiential system dominate an individual's responses in a priming procedure (see Schneider & Chein, 2003).

In the following section we describe some of the most central priming procedures and how they might be used to investigate unconscious attachment experiences.

The term *priming* describes "how recent or current experience passively (without an intervening act of will) creates internal readiness" (Bargh & Chartrand, 2000, p. 255). Generally, in a priming task, two separate phases can be distinguished: The first phase is the *priming phase*. During this, a priming stimulus (typically a word or picture) is presented. This facilitates (or suppresses) a response such as a button press or pronunciation of a target word in the *response phase*. Response speed or strength is taken as an indication of heightened (or diminished) accessibility and thus of associative strength or proximity.

The priming effects obtained in this paradigm result from the spreading activation account in a semantic network (Anderson, 1983; Collins & Loftus, 1975; Collins & Quillian, 1969). Semantically related concepts are connected via links in a memory network. If one node of this network is activated by presentation of a corresponding prime word, activation automatically spreads to all related nodes, making them temporarily more accessible. As a consequence, the target word corresponding to a related node can be more easily recognized as a word and thus more quickly classified or pronounced than a target word belonging to an unrelated node. Thus, the priming effect is caused by a heightened accessibility of the semantic meaning of the target word concept via a common association. Interference with conscious processing from the rational system can be excluded by keeping the interval between the priming stimulus and the response (the stimulus-onset asynchrony [SOA]) short or by using a subliminal prime presentation.

The priming paradigm has proven a very adaptable tool for investigating associative structures in a variety of contexts. Bargh and Chartrand (2000) have summarized strategies used in recent research to investigate associative meanings and their influences on affect, cognition, and behavior.

Conceptual Priming

Conceptual priming refers to experimental techniques in which a prime presentation in one context automatically influences behaviors or mental processes in another context. Typical examples of this kind of priming methods have been applied in trait concept priming. Srull and Wyer (1979) primed the trait concept hostility in one context, then had participants judge an unknown person presented in another context. The unknown person was judged more hostile when participants were primed with hostility compared to a baseline condition (see also Bargh & Pietromonaco, 1982). The conceptual priming method can be used to simulate specific mental states such as hostility to show their transference to other, unrelated situations. This method was not specifically designed to measure associative structures.

Mindset Priming

In this task, people have to actively engage or observe someone's engagement in a goal-directed type of thought (= mindset) in one context. This normally leads to a higher probability that this mindset is also shown in another, unrelated context by the observing person. A specific behavior shown or observed in one situation is more probably shown in another context. Like the conceptual priming techniques, the mindset priming describes a carryover effect of behavioral activation from one situation to another.

Sequential Priming

Another priming method called *sequential priming* and was developed for the assessment of associations between two mental representations. It allows for the measurement of the automatic or controlled nature and strength of an association. A prototype of sequential priming is the semantic priming paradigm (Meyer & Schvaneveldt, 1971; Neely, 1977; for a review, see Neely, 1991). Since the semantic priming is the only technique that allows for the assessment of associative structures, we focus only on this paradigm in the following paragraphs and try to explain its possible usefulness in attachment research.

Semantic Priming

In a semantic priming task, several trials are presented. The number of trials can vary from 40 to 400. Each trial consists of a priming stimulus—that is, a single word that is presented first (e.g., TABLE)—followed by a short delay (the SOA) and then another word, a target stimulus (e.g., CHAIR). Participants have to respond to the target word as quickly and accurately as possible (see Figure 12.4).

Two response tasks can be distinguished: (1) Participants might be asked to classify the target word whether it is a word or a nonword by pressing one of two keys on a response box. Such a design is called the *lexical decision task* (Neely, 1977), or (2) participants have to read aloud the target word, and the response time is measured via voice key. This design is called the *pronunciation task* (Balota & Lorch, 1986). In either task, if the prime word (TABLE) facilitates (i.e., accelerates) the participant's response to the target word (CHAIR) compared to a control trial in which the prime word was unrelated to the target (e.g., DOG), the existence of an association can be assumed. The amount of facilitation measured in millisecond differences between the related and unrelated control condition can hereby serve as an indicator of associative strength (De Groot, Thomassen, & Hudson, 1982; Lorch, 1982; Ratcliff & McKoon, 1981; Fazio et al., 1986; Fazio, Williams, & Powell, 2000; but see Bargh, Chaiken, Govender, & Pratto, 1992).

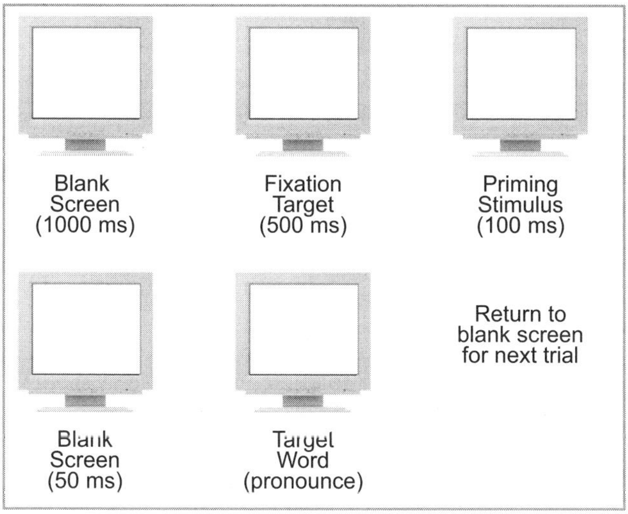

FIGURE 12.4. Semantic priming task.

Contrasting Automatic and Intentional Responses

As mentioned earlier, connections between concepts can be activated consciously and intentionally or automatically. This distinction between the conscious and the unconscious processing in associative memory has been extensively described by several authors and has important implications for our understanding of how information processing works in an associative network (Bargh, 1994; Epstein, 1994; Posner & Snyder, 1975).

To test the automatic nature of the association and therefore to test whether an association is based on the experiential or the rational system, two possible strategies can be undertaken. One possibility is the variation of the SOA. There is evidence from semantic priming research that automatic processes based on the experiential system primarily take place when the SOA is very short, below 500 milliseconds (Neely, 1977; see also Bargh & Chartrand, 2000), because effortful, intentional, and conscious processing needs time. At longer SOAs, strategic, conscious processes based on the rational system can override the automatic priming effect and produce facilitative effects.

Another strategy for comparing unconscious and conscious associations uses subliminal prime presentation. Replicable subliminal semantic priming effects were shown by Greenwald, Draine, and Abrams (1996; Greenwald, Klinger, & Schuh, 1995; but see Klinger, Burton, & Pitts, 2000). To obtain subliminal priming effects, a sandwich masking procedure is recommended. In this procedure, a forward mask consisting of a meaningless letter sequence is presented immediately before the prime word presentation, which is again followed by another meaningless letter string, the backward mask. Under these conditions, unconscious priming effects based on the experiential system are reliably obtained, indicating an automatic association underlying the subliminal priming effect.

The Participant's Response: Lexical Decision versus Pronunciation

The pronunciation task is considered to be a better indicator of spreading activation than lexical decision, since priming effects obtained in the lexical decision can also be explained by an alternative mechanism. This alternative explanation takes into account the fact that for classifying the target word in a lexical decision task there are affirmative (word—yes) and negative (word—no) responses required. According to the compound cue theory, an alternative theory to spreading activation in semantic priming (Ratcliff & McKoon, 1988), individuals use a compound cue that comprises both prime and target to retrieve the target word representation from memory.

This compound cue is checked for familiarity. The information is then used for the lexical decision regarding the target word. Semantically related concepts form a familiar compound cue, as they usually appear together in different contexts. High familiarity facilitates an affirmative response (familiar—yes) and preactivates the yes response to the target. This in turn leads to facilitated classification of the target word as a word. In the case of semantically unrelated items, no match is found, facilitating a no response (familiar—no) that inhibits the yes classification of the target word as a word. According to this model, then, positive priming effects are not based on heightened semantic accessibility of the target word representation in memory caused by spreading activation but by the preactivation of specific response sets. Thus, response facilitation could explain the observation of a positive priming effect in the lexical decision task as well. Such processes are called postlexical matching mechanisms (Neely, 1991). In summary, a priming effect obtained with the lexical decision task can have two alternative explanations; therefore, the exact nature of the association underlying priming effects cannot fully be determined. Such an alternative explanation of the priming effect cannot be applied for the pronunciation task. Thus, this task is considered to be a better and more unambiguous indicator of spreading activation.

Some Precautions

Experimental stimuli have to be carefully selected to guard someone's priming results against alternative interpretations. For example, word length and frequency in spoken language must be controlled and paralleled between the different priming conditions. It is also important to carefully choose between a within-subjects or a between-subjects design. Within-subjects designs have the general advantage of controlling for any a priori differences in response speed or information processing speed unrelated to attachment differences. However, they might put us at risk of any transference effects, as the meaning of an attachment-related prime word through repeated presentation within a sequence of neutral primes can bias the interpretation of the neutral priming stimuli. To avoid such a bias, a between-subjects design might be more useful. Also, each priming study should start with several practice trials to familiarize participants with the task. Instructions should be clear and straightforward to avoid any misunderstandings.

ATTACHMENT EXPERIENCES: NEW PERSPECTIVES ON THEIR UNCONSCIOUS NATURE AND THEIR REPRESENTATION IN MEMORY

Sequential Priming in Attachment Research: An Important Adaptation

Several researchers have used sequential priming to study associative representations of secure base and safe-haven knowledge. In the following paragraphs we present three different priming studies that used either lexical decision or pronunciation tasks to show how associative structures can be assessed in the context of attachment. These studies can, in our view, serve as prototypes for priming techniques in future attachment research.

In one early study, Baldwin, Fehr, Keedian, Seidel, and Thomson (1993) used a supraliminal lexical decision task to determine whether attachment style predicts differences in secure base expectations. Attachment-salient context sentences (e.g., "If I depend on my partner, my partner will . . .") were used to prime positive or negative target outcomes (e.g., support vs. leave). The SOA in this study was 2,000 milliseconds. As predicted by attachment theory, these context sentences primed positive outcome words for secure and negative outcome words for avoidant individuals measured by self-report. Baldwin et al. concluded that interpersonal secure base expectations differ across attachment style in theoretically predictable ways.

Possible problems with these kinds of data could be that people have a "yes—say" tendency to specific compound cues due to idealization. For example, a person might have the conscious view of a partner always being supportive. When the word *support* is presented together with a partner sentence, the key press "word—yes" is facilitated in highly idealizing participants. The priming effect obtained with such a lexical decision design could thus not be produced by unconscious associations but by matching mechanisms predicted by the compound cue theory described earlier (Ratcliff & McKoon, 1988) and the interpretation would be that individuals scoring secure in self-report measures of attachment are idealizing rather than reporting their attachment security.

This could be ruled out by additionally using the pronunciation task as a better indicator of spreading activation. Moreover, the SOA was much higher than 500 milliseconds in this study. The priming effects obtained can thus have been produced by more conscious and controlled processes based on the rational system. However, with some adjustments, for example, by using a short SOA in addition to a long one, this priming procedure could be used to measure secure base knowledge stored in the experiential system (short SOA) and be used to compare those with the connections stored in the rational system (long SOA). Furthermore, by varying the content of the prime sentences, secure base knowledge about several different caregivers can be explored and compared to each other. In addition, different situations varying in threat level and threat content can be used as primes to explore the context-specific nature of the activation of secure base representations across individuals. The priming effect measured in milliseconds would then be an indicator of associative strength, allowing us to assess a hierarchy of caregivers serving as secure bases, and if applied in longitudinal studies, then changes over time could be assessed.

In another series of studies using the lexical decision task, attachment researchers investigated unconscious associations underlying safe-haven representations. According to attachment theory, when individuals are threatened, they seek their attachment figures for comfort and safety (Bowlby, 1969/1982). At the level of unconscious associations, proximity-seeking behavior would be equivalent to faster activation of relevant nodes that indicate closeness to attachment figures after threat priming compared to a neutral prime condition. Attachment theory predicts that threatening stimuli produce heightened mental activity involving contact-seeking with caregivers and partners. In one study, Mikulincer, Birnbaum, Woddis, and Nachmias (2000), using a lexical decision task (LDT) paradigm, primed emergency situations with words such as *death* or *failure* followed by attachment-related target words such as *closeness* or *hug*. The primes were presented either subliminally (20 milliseconds) or supraliminally (500 milliseconds).

The results confirmed that participants were quicker in classifying attachment-related target words in the threat prime condition compared to a neutral condition (e.g., *hat*) both for subliminal as well as supraliminal prime presentations. The data indicate that participants closely associated an emergency situation with proximity seeking. Mikulincer, Gillath, and Shaver (2002) further tested the theory that people associate emergency situations with proximity seeking, specifically focusing on responding to attachment figures (this research also employed LDT methods). In this study, they used a subliminal prime presentation to ensure unconscious processing. Threat words (*separation, failure*) and neutral primes were used and presented for 20 milliseconds, followed by a 20-millisecond mask. Target presentation followed after a 520-millisecond SOA. As target stimuli, names of romantic attachment figures were used. The results showed that participants responded faster to the names of attachment figures (romantic partners' names) when they had been primed with threat words (*separation, failure*) as compared to neutral primes. Furthermore, this interaction was moderated by self-reported attachment avoidance, such that high avoidance scores yielded *slower* reactions to the names of attachment figures following a threatening prime word. Using a subliminal prime presentation ensures that the content of the safe-haven association is based on the experiential system and is therefore an unconscious association.

In a recent study, this finding has been replicated with a different approach to ensure unconscious processing (Selterman, Maier, & Corcoran, 2010). Instead of a subliminal prime presentation, the authors used a supraliminal prime presentation of 200 milliseconds in combination with a short SOA of 250 milliseconds. In addition, instead of romantic partners, mother-related words (*mom, mother*) have been used as target stimuli. Participants responded faster to mother words when being primed with threat primes compared to the neutral prime condition. Again, this main effect was moderated by avoidance scores as in the Mikulincer et al. (2002) study. These data indicate that unconscious safe-haven representations of not only romantic partners but also of mothers are activated under threat activation in adult participants.

The studies reported earlier demonstrated the existence of unconscious safe-haven representations derived from the experiential system with regard to not only romantic but also infant attachment figures. As in the Baldwin et al. (1993) study reported earlier, using the lexical decision task does not provide unambiguous evidence for automatic spreading activation, as the alternative explanation based on compound cue theory cannot be ruled out at this point. However, in future research, a stronger case could be made by using the pronunciation task in replicating those effects. Furthermore, different threat scenarios can be used to determine the situations that evoke unconscious tendencies of seeking an attachment figure, allowing attachment researchers to explore the context-specific nature of safe-haven representations. In addition, using the priming effect measured in milliseconds as an indicator of associative strength could help to describe a hierarchy of attachment figures that serve as safe haven. In longitudinal research these tasks can be used to show transitions from parents to romantic partners serving as a haven of safety from adolescence to early adulthood and beyond.

Context Priming in Attachment Research

In a recent study, Corcoran, Maier, Waters, and Waters (in preparation) used the context priming method to investigate the associative structures of secure base representations and their relation to early attachment experiences by using a pronunciation design. The study addressed several questions:

- Are early representations of caregiver interaction replaced by the more elaborate narrative representations assessed by measures like the Adult Attachment Interview (AAI)?
- Are expectations about sensitive care, cooperation with ongoing behavior, and caregiver availability part of the associative meaning of adult attachment representations?
- Are attachment-related associations based on personal experience or on social norms and observational learning?

In addition to mother primes (MOTHER, MOM) and neutral primes (COOK, ARTIST) a context cue was presented that either activated the individual's own mother representation (MY) or a general mother concept (EVERY). As target words, support- or rejection-related target words were used and had to be pronounced by the participant. The SOA was 250 milliseconds, ensuring the measurement of unconscious associations derived from the experiential system (see Figure 12.5). The design is illustrated in Table 12.1.

Individual differences in secure base representations were measured by the word-prompt method originally developed by H. Waters and Waters (2006). The results indicated that individuals with high script scores had a stronger association between their own mother representation (MY MOTHER) and emotional support than those scoring low in the script method (see Figure 12.6). No differences were found for the EVERY MOTHER condition or neutral prime presentations.

The results demonstrate that associative links to attachment-related expectations are not displaced by the kinds of narrative representations that emerge later and are assessed in the AAI. Instead, they persist, coexisting alongside the narrative representations. The results also indicate that secure base script knowledge is related to the specific components of maternal care that in Ainsworth's Baltimore project were associated with secure infant attachment. Finally, the comparison between MY versus EVERY suggests that these expectations are learned from personal experience (experience with my mother) rather than through observational learning or as cultural norms regarding mothers in general.

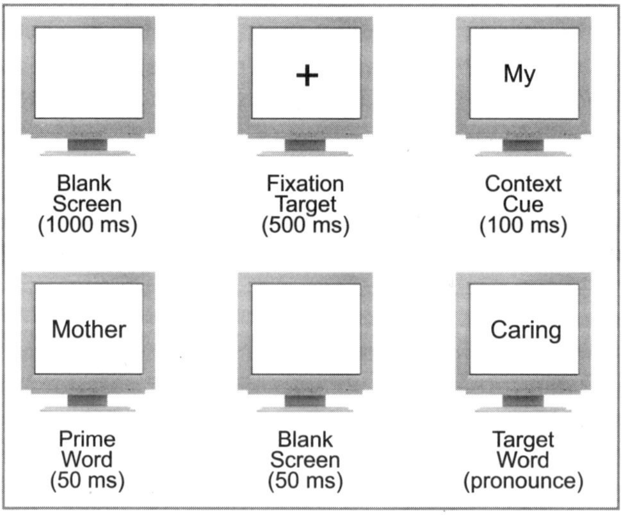

FIGURE 12.5. Context priming task. From Corcoran, Maier, Waters, and Waters (in preparation).

TABLE 12.1. Context Priming Design for Study of Secure-Base Script Knowledge and Attachment-Related Meanings and Expectations

Context word:	My		Every	
Prime word:	Mother	Cook		Artist
	Experiment target words:		*Control study target words:*	
	Available	Rejecting	Wealthy	Bankrupt
	Empathic	Insensitive	Optimistic	Pessimistic
	Helpful	Intrusive	Ambitious	Unattractive
	Caring	Controlling	Patriotic	Disloyal
	Supportive	Selfish	Polite	Vulgar

In future research, this task can be used to test secure base knowledge with different caregivers and their varying strengths. Contrasting long and short SOAs, one could allow for the assessment of conscious secure base knowledge based on the rational system in addition to the ones stored in the experiential system, and the amount of correspondence between the unconscious and conscious associative structures could be compared. Longitudinal studies could explore changes in associative strength over time and the

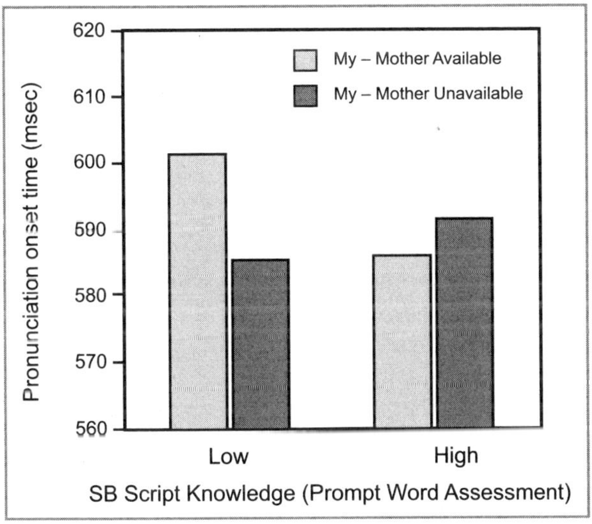

FIGURE 12.6. The effects of secure base script knowledge on pronunciation of caregiving-related words. From Corcoran, Maier, Waters, and Waters (in preparation).

relation of these changes to critical lifetime events. Furthermore, using this paradigm in intervention studies that focus on changing a client's secure base representations might serve as an indicator of the effectiveness of the intervention and its long-term effects. One disadvantage of the pronunciation task, however, is that it produces smaller priming effects than the LDT, making this design less powerful in the statistical analyses.

CONCLUSION

In this chapter we have focused on the associative structures underlying IWMs of attachment and their assessment with the priming paradigm. In our view, much of attachment-related experience, and thus key attachment-related expectations, are stored as associative structures in memory networks. Secure base representations contain associative connections between representations of a caregiver and his or her availability. Safe-haven representations consist of representations of attachment-related threat and a caregiver. Both associative structures can be accessed in automatic and intentional modes. If they are stored in the experiential system, they exist outside of awareness, are stable, resistant to change, fast acting, and need a minimum amount of time and capacity to operate. They are activated, context-specific, and provide basic affective response tendencies to approach positive outcomes and avoid harm. Attachment-related knowledge stored as associations can also exist in the rational system.

The associations based on this system are consciously accessible; they are more flexible and less stable. They need time, intentionality, effort, and capacity to be processed. The contents stored in the two systems can be the same or different depending on an individual's attachment state of mind. Sequential priming techniques allow for the experimental manipulation of the circumstances under which information processing is based in the experiential or the rational system. By using subliminal prime presentations or short SOAs, important information processing parameters such as awareness, processing time, intentionality, and controllability are reduced, making unconscious associative representations derived from the experiential system accessible and measurable. Supraliminal prime presentations or longer SOAs on the other hand foster conscious processing and provide access to the respective associations stored in the rational system. Several examples of priming research used in the past to study attachment representations are described, demonstrating the potential usefulness of these techniques to measure central constructs postulated in attachment theory, such as secure base and safe-haven representations at the unconscious as well as the conscious level. Although demanding considerable effort and care on the part of experimenters and research participants, these methods have the potential to reveal a great deal about attachment representations in theoretical as well as clinical research.

REFERENCES

Anderson, J. R. (1983). A spreading activation theory of memory. *Journal of Verbal Learning and Verbal Behavior, 22,* 261–295.

Baldwin, M. W., Fehr, B., Keedian, E., Seidel, M., & Thomson, D. W. (1993). An exploration of the relational schemata underlying attachment styles: Self-report and lexical decision approaches. *Personality and Social Psychology Bulletin, 19,* 746–754.

Balota, D. A., & Lorch, R. F. (1986). Depth of automatic spreading activation: Mediated priming effects in pronunciation but not in lexical decision. *Journal of Experimental Psychology: Learning, Memory, and Cognition, 12,* 336–345.

Bargh, J. A. (1994). The four horsemen of automaticity: Awareness, intention, efficiency, and control in social cognition. In R. S. Wyer & T. K. Srull (Eds.), *Handbook of social cognition* (Vol. 1, pp. 1–40). Hillsdale, NJ: Erlbaum.

Bargh, J. A., Chaiken, S., Govender, R., & Pratto, F. (1992). The generality of the automatic attitude activation effect. *Journal of Personality and Social Psychology, 62,* 893–912.

Bargh, J. A., & Chartrand, T. L. (2000). The mind in the middle: A practical guide to priming and automaticity research. In H. T. Reis & C. M. Judd (Eds.), *Handbook of research methods in social and personality psychology* (pp. 253–285). New York: Cambridge University Press.

Bargh, J. A., & Pietromonaco, P. (1982). Automatic information processing and social perception: The influence of trait information presented outside of conscious awareness on impression formation. *Journal of Personality and Social Psychology, 22,* 293–311.

Bartlett, F. C. (1932). *Remembering: A study in experimental and social psychology.* Cambridge, UK: Cambridge University Press.

Becker, F. D., Gield, B., & Froggatt, C. C. (1983). Seating position and impression formation in an office setting. *Journal of Environmental Psychology, 3,* 253–261.

Bower, G. H. (1981). Mood and memory. *American Psychologist, 36,* 129–148.

Bowlby, J. (1973). *Attachment and loss: Vol. 2. Separation: Anxiety and anger.* New York: Basic Books.

Bowlby, J. (1979a). On knowing what you are not supposed to know and feeling what you are not supposed to feel. *Canadian Journal of Psychiatry, 24,* 403–408.

Bowlby, J. (1979b). *The making and breaking of affectional bonds.* New York: Methuen.

Bowlby, J. (1980). *Attachment and loss: Vol. 3. Loss: Sadness and depression.* New York: Basic Books.

Bowlby, J. (1982). *Attachment and loss: Vol. 1. Attachment* (2nd ed.). New York: Basic Books. (Original work published 1969)

Bretherton, I. (1985). Attachment theory: Retrospect and prospect. In I. Bretherton & E. Waters (Eds.), Growing points of attachment theory and research. *Monographs of the Society for Research in Child Development, 50*(1–2), 3–39.

Bretherton, I., & Munholland, K. A. (2008). Internal working models in attachment relationships: Elaborating a central construct in attachment theory. In J. Cassidy & P. Shaver (Eds.), *Handbook of attachment: Theory, research and clinical application* (2nd ed., pp. 102–129). New York: Guilford Press.

Callison, C., Karrh, J. A., & Zillmann, D. (2002). The aura of tobacco smoke: Cigars and cigarettes as image makers. *Journal of Applied Social Psychology, 32,* 1329–1343.

Carlston, D. E., & Mae, L. (2007). Posing with the flag: Trait-specific effects of symbols on person perception. *Journal of Experimental Social Psychology, 43,* 241–248.

Chen, M., & Bargh, J. A. (1999). Nonconscious approach and avoidance behavioral consequences of the automatic evaluation effect. *Personality and Social Psychology Bulletin, 25,* 215–224.

Collins, A. M., & Loftus, E. E. (1975). A spreading activation theory of semantic memory. *Psychological Review, 82,* 407–428.

Collins, A. M., & Quillian, M. R., (1969). Retrieval time from semantic memory. *Journal of Verbal Learning and Verbal Behavior, 8,* 240–247.

Corcoran, D., Maier, M. A., Waters, T., & Waters, E. (in preparation). *The secure base script and implicit representations of early attachment related experience.* Unpublished manuscript.

De Groot, A. M. B., Thomassen, A. J. W. M., & Hudson, P. T. W. (1982). Associative facilitation of word recognition as measured from a neutral prime. *Memory and Cognition, 10,* 358–370.

Elliot, A. J. (Ed.). (2008). *Handbook of approach and avoidance motivation.* Mahwah, NJ: Erlbaum.

Elliot, A. J., & Niesta, D. (2008). Romantic red: Red enhances men's attraction to women. *Journal of Personality and Social Psychology, 95,* 1150–1164.

Epstein, S. (1991). Cognitive-experiential self-theory: An integrative theory of personality. In R. Curtis (Ed.), *The relational self: Convergences in psychoanalysis and social psychology* (pp. 111–137). New York: Guilford Press.

Epstein, S. (1994). Integration of the cognitive and the psychodynamic unconscious. *American Psychologist, 49,* 709–724.

Evans, J. S. B. T. (2003). In two minds: Dual-process accounts of reasoning. *Trends in Cognitive Sciences, 7,* 454–459.

Fazio, R. H., Sanbonmatsu, D. M., Powell, M. C., & Kardes, F. R. (1986). On the automatic activation of attitudes. *Journal of Personality and Social Psychology, 50,* 229–238.

Fazio, R. H., Williams, C. J., & Powell, M. C. (2000). Measuring associative strength: Category-item associations and their activation from memory. *Political Psychology, 21,* 7–25.

Fivush, R., & Neisser, U. (1994). *The remembering self: Construction and accuracy in the self-narrative.* New York: Cambridge University Press.

Frank, M. G., & Gilovich, T. (1988). The dark side of self- and social perception: Black uniforms and aggression in professional sports. *Journal of Personality and Social Psychology, 54,* 74–85.

Gawronski, B., & Bodenhausen, G. V. (2006). Associative and propositional processes in evaluation: An integrative review of implicit and explicit attitude change. *Psychological Bulletin, 132,* 692–731.

Greenwald, A. G., Draine, S. C., & Abrams, R. L. (1996). Three cognitive markers of unconscious semantic activation. *Science, 273*(5282), 1699–1702.

Greenwald, A. G., Klinger, M. R., & Schuh, E. S. (1995). Activation by marginally perceptible ("subliminal") stimuli: Dissociation of unconscious from conscious cognition. *Journal of Experimental Psychology: General, 124,* 22–42.

Hamlyn, D. W. (Trans.). (1993). *Aristotle De Anima: Books II and III (with passages from Book 1)*. New York: Oxford University Press.

Hinde, R. A. (1991). Relationships, attachment, and culture: A tribute to John Bowlby. *Infantile Mental Health Journal, 12,* 154–163.

Hebb, D. O. (1949). *The organization of behavior*. New York: Wiley.

James, W. (1890). *The principles of psychology* (Vol. 1). New York: Holt.

Johnson-Laird, P. (1995). Mental models, deductive reasoning, and the brain. In M. Gazzagniga (Ed.), *The cognitive neurosciences* (pp. 999–1008). Cambridge, MA: MIT Press.

Klinger, M. R., Burton, P. C., & Pitts, G. (2000). Mechanisms of unconscious priming: I. Response competition, not spreading activation. *Journal of Experimental Psychology: Learning, Memory, and Cognition, 26,* 441–455.

Lorch, R. F., Jr. (1982). Priming and search processes in semantic memory: A test of three models of spreading activation. *Journal of Verbal Learning and Verbal Behavior, 21,* 468–492.

Main, M. (1999). Epilogue. Attachment Theory: Eighteen points with suggestions for future studies. In J. Cassidy & P. Shaver (Eds.), *Handbook of attachment: Theory, research, and clinical applications* (pp. 845–887). New York: Guilford Press.

Main, M. (2000). The organized categories of infant, child, and adult attachment: Flexible vs. inflexible attention under attachment-related stress. *Journal of the American Psychoanalytic Association, 48*(4), 1055–1096.

Main, M., Kaplan, N., & Cassidy, J. (1985). Security in infancy, childhood, and adulthood: A move to the representational level. In I. Bretherton & E. Waters (Eds.), Growing points of attachment theory and research. *Monographs of the Society for Research in Child Development, 50*(1–2), 66–104.

Manz, W., & Lueck, H. E. (1968). Influence of wearing glasses on personality ratings: Crosscultural validation of an old experiment. *Perceptual and Motor Skills, 27,* 704.

Meyer, D. E., & Schvaneveldt, R. W. (1971). Facilitation in recognizing pairs of words: Evidence of a dependence between retrieval operations. *Journal of Experimental Psychology, 90,* 227–234.

Mikulincer, M., Birnbaum, G., Woddis, D., & Nachmias, O. (2000). Stress and accessibility of proximity-related thoughts: Exploring the normative and intraindividual components of attachment theory. *Journal of Personality and Social Psychology, 78,* 509–523.

Mikulincer, M., Gillath, O., & Shaver, P. R. (2002). Activation of the attachment system in adulthood: Threat-related primes increase the accessibility of mental representations of attachment figures. *Journal of Personality and Social Psychology, 83,* 881–895.

Mikulincer, M., & Shaver, P. R. (2003). The attachment behavioral system in adulthood: Activation, psychodynamics, and interpersonal processes. In M. P. Zanna (Ed.), *Advances in experimental social psychology* (pp. 53–152). New York: Academic Press.

Mikulincer, M., & Shaver, P. R. (2016). *Attachment in adulthood: Structure, dynamics, and change*. New York: Guilford Press.

Neely, J. H. (1977). Semantic priming and retrieval from lexical memory: Roles of inhibitionless spreading activation and limited-capacity attention. *Journal of Experimental Psychology: General, 106,* 226–254.

Neely, J. H. (1991). Semantic priming effects in visual word recognition: A selective review of current findings and theories. In D. Besner & G. W. Humphreys (Eds.), *Basic processes in reading: Visual word recognition* (pp. 264–336). Hillsdale, NJ: Erlbaum.

Paivio, A. (1986). *Mental representations: A dual coding approach.* New York: Oxford University Press.

Pavlov, I. P. (1927). *Conditioned reflexes: An investigation of the physiological activity of the cerebral cortex* (G. V. Anrep, Trans.). London: Oxford University Press.

Posner, M. I., & Snyder, C. R. R. (1975). Facilitation and inhibition in the processing of signals. In P. M. Rabbitt & S. Dornic (Eds.), *Attention and performance* (Vol. 5, pp. 669–682). San Diego, CA: Academic Press.

Ratcliff, R., & McKoon, G. (1981). Automatic and strategic priming in recognition. *Journal of Verbal Learning and Verbal Behavior, 20,* 204–215.

Ratcliff, R., & McKoon, G. (1988). A retrieval theory of priming in memory. *Psychological Review, 95,* 385–408.

Schank, R., & Abelson, R. (1977). *Scripts, plans, goals, and understanding.* New York: Wiley.

Schneider, W., & Chein, J. (2003). Controlled and automatic processing: Behavior, theory, and biological processing. *Cognitive Science, 27,* 525–559.

Selterman, D., Maier, M. A., & Corcoran, D. (2010). *Implicit priming of attachment representations revisited: A replication and clarification.* Unpublished manuscript, Stony Brook University, Stony Brook, NY.

Smith, E. R. (1998). Mental representation and memory. In D. Gilbert, S. Fiske, & G. Lindzey (Eds.), *Handbook of social psychology* (4th ed., Vol. 1, pp. 391–445). New York: McGraw-Hill.

Sroufe, L. A., & Waters, E. (1977). Attachment as an organizational construct. *Child Development, 48,* 1184–1199.

Srull, T. K., & Wyer, R. S. (1979). The role of category accessibility in the interpretation of information about persons: Some determinants and implications. *Journal of Personality and Social Psychology, 37,* 1660–1672.

Stupica, B., & Cassidy, J. (2014). Priming as a way of understanding children's mental representations of the social world. *Developmental Review, 34,* 77–91.

Vrij, A. (1997). Wearing black clothes: The impact of offenders' and suspects' clothing on impression formation. *Applied Cognitive Psychology, 11,* 47–53.

Waters, H. S., & Waters, E. (2006). The attachment working model concept: Among other things, we build script-like representations of secure base experience. *Attachment and Human Development, 8,* 185–197.

Watson, J. B., & Rayner, R. (1920). Conditioned emotional reactions. *Journal of Experimental Psychology, 3*(1), 1–14.

Young, J. Z. (1964). *A model for the brain.* London: Oxford University Press.

CHAPTER 13

The Adult Attachment Projective Picture System

Representational Assessment of Attachment in Adolescents and Adults

Carol George and Malcolm L. West

This chapter describes the development, validation, and use of the Adult Attachment Projective Picture System (AAP; George & West, 2001; George & West, 2012), a free-response picture system measure of adolescent and adult attachment. The AAP fulfills three needs in attachment assessment. First, it provides an efficient means to "observe" attachment representation under conditions that activate the attachment system. Second, the coding system assesses core attachment constructs and processes that are not assessed by other attachment measures (e.g., internalized secure base, goal-corrected partnership, defensive processes). Third, it provides researchers and clinicians with a valid, economical, and efficient classification tool.

We begin the chapter with a discussion of projective methodology and the place of the AAP in this measurement tradition. We then examine the core theoretical constructs that serve as the foundation of the AAP. We next describe how the AAP was developed and the classification coding scheme. Examples of AAP responses from each major classification group are presented. We describe in the final sections of the chapter validity testing and examples of the use of the AAP in basic research, neurobiological, and clinical settings.

PROJECTIVE METHODOLOGY: A WINDOW TO THE MIND

There is a long history of projective methodology in the field of attachment. It is a paradox perhaps that although Bowlby turned away from the dynamic postulates of psychoanalysis (Bowlby, 1969/1982, 1973, 1980), he nonetheless developed a projective technique to examine children's responses to separation and loss (Bowlby, 1973; Klagsbrun & Bowlby, 1976). Kaplan (1984) refined the Klagsbrun–Bowlby method to assess attachment status in middle childhood. Other researchers have developed attachment classification schemes for projective and semiprojective stimulus sets, including pictures (Jacobsen & Hofmann, 1997; McCarthy, 1998; Shouldice & Stevenson-Hinde, 1992; Slough & Greenberg, 1990) and doll play story-stem procedures (Bretherton, Ridgeway, & Cassidy, 1990; Gloger-Tippelt, Gomille, Koenig, & Vetter, 2002; Green, Stanley, Smith, & Goldwyn, 2000; Oppenheim, 1997; Solomon, George, & De Jong, 1995).

The common denominator for free-response projective approaches is how verbal responses to a standardized set of ambiguous visual or play (e.g., family dolls) stimuli provide access to conscious and unconscious thoughts and emotions (Hilsenroth, 2004). Administration is unstructured. Individuals are unencumbered by administrative directives or intrusions and respond freely, guided only by a few basic open-ended questions. They are not contaminated by the self-serving bias of self-report measures, have less risk of the exaggerations and minimizations of experience found in clinical interviews, and are economical and easy to use (Hilsenroth, 2004). The responses provide a rich picture of interpersonal and behavioral dimensions, producing patterns of unconscious and automatic defensive processing for interpretation following standardized guidelines (Leichtman, 2004).

The general accomplishments of this methodology are often dismissed by individuals who prefer what they consider to be more rigorous forms of assessment. Critics argue that projectives do not work well, that they assess poorly defined constructs and are subject to strong interpretive bias, and fail to achieve acceptable validity and reliability standards (Hilsenroth, 2004; Wood, Nezworski, & Stejskal, 1996). However, large scale studies of interrater reliability, test–retest reliability, and predictive validity fail to support these criticisms (Meyer, 2004). Some psychological dimensions have been measured successfully with projective techniques, for example, the achievement motive (McClelland, Atkinson, Clark, & Lowell, 1953).

Projective methods are viable when the concepts measured are tied to a tight theoretical framework and the derived variables have established criteria (Hilsenroth, 2004). The AAP is firmly grounded in theory and research. We drew from two established contributions to attachment assessment when developing the AAP: coherence and defensive processes. Concerning coherence, Main and Goldwyn (1985/1998/2006) established a link between autobiographical discourse coherence in response to the Adult Attachment Interview (AAI; George, Kaplan, & Main, 1984/1985/1996) and a secure state of mind (Main, 1995). This discovery led us to begin the development of the AAP by examining coherence in the story responses to picture stimuli. Regarding defensive processes, Solomon and George (Solomon et al., 1995) operationally defined Bowlby's (1980) model of defensive exclusion and have established validity for this approach in determining attachment status. Defensive exclusion is an AAP critical coding dimension. We discuss this feature of the AAP in detail in the next section.

THE APPLICATION OF ATTACHMENT THEORY TO THE AAP

Coherence and Defense

The representational approach to attachment assessment assumes that we can gain access to the contents and processes of internal working models through individuals' narrative descriptions of attachment experience (Bowlby, 1973, 1980; Bretherton, 2005). Narratives (e.g., stories, biographical accounts) are evaluated concerning the self's description of adequate (responsive, sensitive care) and unsatisfactory (rejection, threatened abandonment, abuse, death) attachment experiences and emotions. Coherence is the sine qua non of attachment status as determined by the AAI. It evaluates the ease with which adults describe their attachment experiences freely and the extent to which autobiographical discourse demonstrates unity or coherence among attachment memories. Narrative discourse is evaluated as maximally integrated or coherent when it is open and natural; restricted, diverted, or uncontrolled discourse is evaluated as incoherent (Main, 1995; Main & Goldwyn, 1985/1998/2006).

The appraisal of coherence and its representational form is measure-specific. The emphasis placed in the field on discourse coherence in assessing attachment representation emerged from the success of the AAI Coherence rating scale in identifying "secure" mothers whose AAI classifications matched their infants' classification as measured by reunion behavior during the Strange Situation (Main, Kaplan, & Cassidy, 1985). However, discourse coherence in response to an interview as an evaluative dimension of attachment state of mind was not derived from attachment theory. Main and Goldwyn (1985/1998/2006) defined AAI Coherence based on Grice's maxims, philosophical rules developed to describe the parameters that regulate human conversation. As such, the AAI is an autobiographical "conversation." The actual experiences described during the interview (e.g., parents as loving, rejecting, or abusive) have relatively little importance when deciding the final classification. Experience is revaluated in relation to coherence. Coherence represents the individual's ability to cooperate in the conversation with the interviewer, stay on task, thoughtfully describe and examine experience, and integrate past and present evaluations of this experience. In short, coherent individuals are secure. Coherent descriptions of attachment failures, disappointments, rejection, and even abuse lead to a secure classification if the individual maintains a thoughtful examination of experience "on the spot" during the interview.

The AAP is a different representational task than the AAI. The AAP is explicitly *not* autobiographical. The individual is instructed to describe the events associated with the hypothetical scenes of children and adults portrayed in a standardized series of theoretically derived attachment situations (hence, the inclusion of the concept of "picture system" in the AAP title). Narrative coherence is not the sine qua non of security in the AAP.[1] Instead, the AAP ultimately evaluates *attachment coherence,* which involves the representation of integrated forms of attachment as defined by theory and developmental research in attachment. Attachment coherence is the yardstick for security in the AAP.

Bowlby (1969/1982) and Ainsworth (Ainsworth, Blehar, Waters, & Wall, 1978/2015) described the parameters of attachment coherence. Attachment-coherent doll-play stories portray children's needs clearly and attachment figure sensitivity as attuned and protective; the coherent self is balanced and capable rather than restricted, confused, or disorganized and dysregulated (Solomon et al., 1995). The hallmark of a coherent caregiver who fosters attachment security combines descriptions of attunement with the desire to flexibly balance the parent's needs with the needs of the child (George & Solomon, 2008; Solomon & George, 1996).

The common integrative elements of these narrative forms in adults and children provide the conceptual foundation for attachment coherence in the AAP. AAP *attachment coherence* is defined as the flexible integration of the attachment and caregiving systems, and the portrayal of an autonomous and integrated self. (These features are delineated more fully in our later description of the coding scheme.) The degree to which individuals achieve attachment coherence in the AAP depends on the shifting balance between adaptive processes and defensive exclusion in their efforts to give meaning to and find meaning in each picture stimulus. The final story product may range from a thoughtful and integrated response to an unreflective, automatic, or even disorganized and dysregulated one.

Defensive processes limit attachment coherence. Bowlby's (1980) thinking regarding defense centered on explaining forms of defensive exclusion that developed in response to extreme threats and ruptures to the attachment relationship. The experiences he described are the core risk factors for attachment disorganization (Lyons-Ruth & Jacobvitz, 2016; Solomon & George, 2011). George and Solomon's (1996, 2008; Solomon et al., 1995) research demonstrated that defensive exclusion is the hallmark of insecure attachment and caregiving (organized–insecure and disorganized). The purpose of defensive exclusion is to suppress the direct expression of attachment thoughts and feeling; attachment assessment attends to defensive substitutions or what

[1]The AAP coding system was originally developed to include a form of the AAI Coherence rating scale. The scale failed to provide information that discriminated among attachment groups and did not add any new or specific information to the AAP coding scheme. As a result, coherence was dropped as an AAP coding dimensions in 2008.

is unleashed when exclusion breaks down. The AAP coding scheme operationally defines story material following Bowlby's three forms of defensive exclusion: deactivation, cognitive disconnection, and the segregated system. Ultimately, the interplay of the forms of defensive exclusion serves as mechanisms that regulate the overall quality of attachment coherence observed in the AAP story responses. Each response is evaluated for defensive processes and combined with other core attachment constructs. These include evaluations of internalization of attachment figures (*internalized secure base*), the goal-corrected partnership (*synchrony*), and the desire for intimate relationships with others (*connectedness*). These evaluations are defined as integrated responses and represent core processes and relationships that are essential to survival in our species. Integrated content defines attachment security, because these representational elements follow the basic tenets of attachment in the Bowlby–Ainsworth model.

Attachment Representation

Activating Attachment

Bowlby's attachment trilogy (1969/1982, 1973, 1980) stressed the importance of observing attachment "in action," that is, when the attachment system is activated. Conditions that activate attachment include those that threaten or compromise physical or psychological safety. Strictly speaking, of course, the internal working model of attachment is not directly observable; therefore, assessment must activate the system to "see" the variations in its representational manifestations. The "contents" and vicissitudes of attachment representation are inferred directly in representational measures (AAI and AAP) or indirectly in self-report questionnaires. Attachment assessments are not equivalent. Self-report forms assess social cognitions that obscure the unconscious processes (i.e., defense, state of mind) (Leak & Parsons, 2001; Maier, Bernier, Pekrun, Zimmerman, & Grossmann, 2004; Riggs et al., 2007).

The AAP stimuli activate attachment by depicting major attachment events, including illness, solitude, separation, death, and threat. The stories represent individuals' attempts to make sense of events and associated affect. In this regard, West and Sheldon-Keller (1994) proposed that the internal working model is an affective category within memory. Affects are the mechanism for reactivating in the present the affective category established in the past. Working models do not evoke affects; rather, affects stimulate a search for applicable working models and meanings in the present based on current reworkings of the past (see also, Bretherton, 2005).

We therefore suggest that the AAP opens and renders amenable to interpretation those personal elements of attachment that individuals may ordinarily keep locked away and excluded from conscious awareness. Individuals make sense of the various depicted attachment scenes by using their perceptual and affective responses to give meaning to the picture stimuli. The external stimulus (the attachment "pull" of the pictures) initiates an internal search for applicable mental concepts.[2]

Representational products provide access only to the presently operating consequences of past attachment experiences, captured succinctly by Main et al.'s (1985) phrase "current state of mind" about attachment. Working models are, in other words, dynamic, associative, affective categories that have the potential to be rediscovered in new situations, such as in response to the instruction to describe what is happening in each AAP picture.

Representation of Family-Based Attachment Experience

In addressing representation, it is important to describe where the AAP picture system falls in relation to other adult attachment measures. The AAP, like the AAI, is firmly grounded in the developmental attachment theory. The AAP picture stimuli have been shown to pull for representation based on experience in the family, that is, the filial attachment–caregiver relationship. AAP attachment classifications were designed and validated to represent the same primary attachment groups identified by the AAI: secure, dismissing, preoccupied, and unresolved. The AAP does not measure a generalized trait and does assess patterns of romantic, dating, or caregiving (i.e., parenting) relationships. Responses do provide information, however, about the intersection of attachment with these other relationships. It also provides indicators of relationship and psychological risk. The AAP has been used increasingly in clinical contexts (e.g., Delvecchio, Di Riso, Lis, & Salcuni, 2016; Bauriedl-Schmidt et al., 2017). We discuss the clinical application of the AAP in more detail at the end of the chapter.

With these theoretical considerations as necessary background, we now describe the AAP and its classification scheme.

THE AAP

The Picture Set and Administration

The AAP is a set of eight black-and-white line drawings. (See West & Sheldon-Keller, 1994, for a complete discussion of the AAP picture selection process.) The drawings contain only enough detail to identify an event; strong facial expressions and other potentially biasing details are absent. Character portrayals are diverse regarding culture, gender, and age. The AAP system includes the following scenes: *Neutral*—two children play with a ball; *Child*

[2]This "unlocking" process was elegantly described by Lis, Mazzeschi, Salcuni, and Di Riso (2008). They described a clinical case in which the AAP unlocked attachment trauma and dysregulation that had been carefully locked away during the AAI by the individual's inability to elaborate on experience (judged dismissing on the AAI and unresolved on the AAP). The analysis of the AAP subsequently led to productive psychotherapy regarding the individual's experience (Lis et al., 2008).

at Window—a child looks out a window; *Departure*—an adult man and woman stand facing each other with suitcases positioned nearby; *Bench*—a youth sits alone on a bench; *Bed*—a child and woman sit opposite each other on the child's bed; *Ambulance*—a woman and a child watch ambulance workers load a stretcher into an ambulance; *Cemetery*—a man stands by a gravesite headstone; and *Child in Corner*—a child stands askance in a corner. Example pictures are provided in Figures 13.1, 13.2, and 13.3.

Two critical features of attachment experience are depicted in the AAP stimulus set. One is the availability of an attachment figure. Only prompt and effective attachment figure responsiveness can successfully "terminate" attachment distress (Ainsworth, 1964; Ainsworth et al., 1978/2015; Bowlby, 1969/1982) and provide "felt security" (Sroufe & Fleeson, 1986). Infants and young children require physical proximity and access to attachment figures. Proximity and access are increasingly balanced by psychological proximity in older children, adolescents, and adults. Individuals in these older age groups can and do appeal to *internalized* attachment figures when attachment needs are activated, and attachment figures are not present (West & Sheldon-Keller, 1994). Some scenes portray an adult or a child alone ("alone" pictures), potentially eliciting representations of internalized attachment figures. Other AAP scenes portray adult–adult or adult–child dyads ("dyadic" pictures) depicting physical proximity and availability of a potential attachment figure. The second critical feature is that the stimuli incorporate a lifespan perspective (Ainsworth, 1989; Bowlby, 1969/1982). The scenes show characters that represent a range of ages, from the young child to the elderly adult.

The AAP should be administered in a private setting, such as a quiet research room or clinician's office. The AAP is preferably administered in person; however, individual or social constraints may be accommodated using the AAP virtual administration procedure. The interviewee should be made comfortable before administration. Welcoming an individual to the administration setting, the process of signing consent forms (if required) or getting settled into a clinical assessment session is typically enough. Use of the AAP with adolescents necessitates a warm-up period (e.g., a nonpressured, nonassessment task or interaction). If possible, the AAP is administered before other assessments. The AAP can be used in conjunction with other attachment measures on the same day, and other assessments (e.g., cognitive, Minnesota Multiphasic Personality Inventory [MMPI]) following the AAP on the same assessment day. We found no administration order effects when assessed the AAP and AAI in the same session. We prefer to administer the AAP first, because the AAI can be exhausting.

The AAP is administered only as a full set of stimuli in the order listed earlier. The stimulus presentation order depicts situations that gradually increase attachment distress. This pattern parallels the design of other developmental attachment assessments, including Strange Situation episodes, children's picture-based assessments, doll-play story stems, and the AAI. Neurobiological evidence has verified the gradual increase in attachment activation associated with the stimulus order (Buchheim et al., 2006).

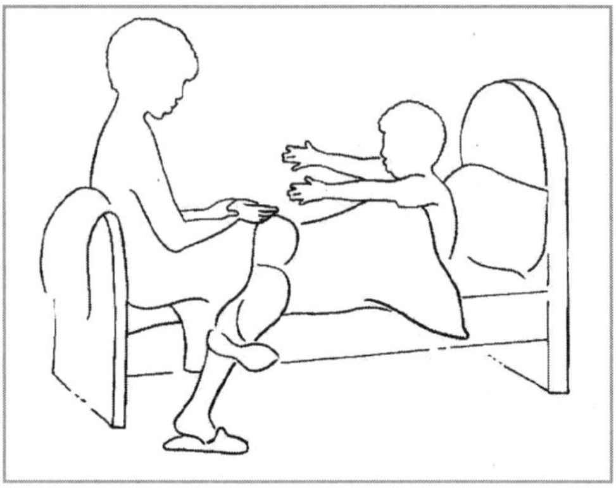

FIGURE 13.1. AAP picture stimulus "Bed."

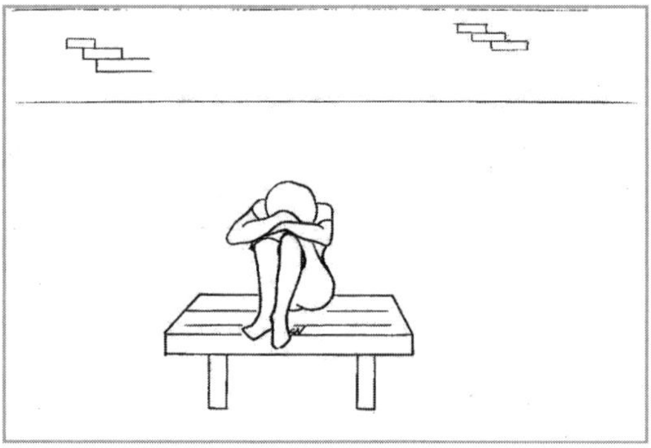

FIGURE 13.2. AAP picture stimulus "Bench."

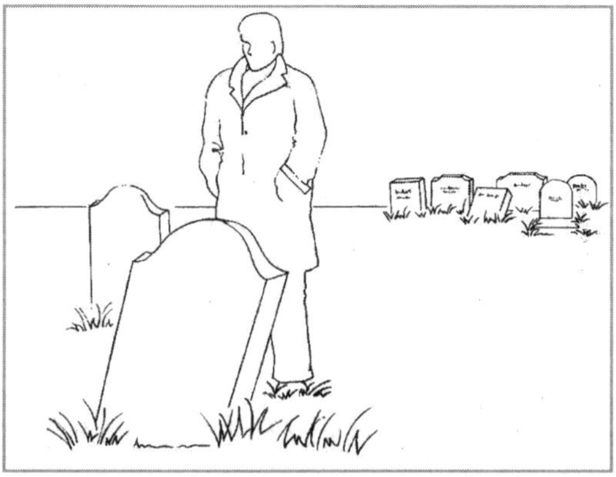

FIGURE 13.3. AAP picture stimulus "Cemetery."

The administration method combines elements of projective and semi-structured interview techniques. The interviewee is seated across from the administrator (or in front of computer or tablet screen if using the Web administration procedure). The administrator begins by stating the instructions: "Describe what is happening in the picture, what led up to the events, what the characters are thinking or feeling, and what will happen next." Performance anxieties are eased by assuring the interviewee that there are no right or wrong answers. The interviewee is handed the first picture as a signal to begin. The administrator waits comfortably for the interviewee to complete the task, asking the previous questions to prompt storytelling when needed.[3] Once completed, the administrator hands the interviewee the next picture stimulus and proceeds similarly through the remainder of the picture set. No debriefing and follow-up is typically required.

Administrators do not need to have a background in attachment theory, assessment techniques, or the AAP coding system. Administrator training requires three to four supervised practice administrations. The AAP has been administered by a range of different individuals, including undergraduate research assistants, experienced researchers, and clinicians. The AAP is tape-recorded and transcribed verbatim for scoring. The standard administration is approximately 25 minutes. AAP transcripts range from two to four pages in length. Coding and classification by a trained, reliable judge usually take between 30 minutes and 2 hours.

Correct administration and ethical use of the AAP is essential for the validity of the instrument and protection of research participants, clients, and patients. The pictures are potent stimuli; however, most individuals respond to assessment with a cooperative, positive attitude. Interviewees typically do not get upset during the "AAP experience" (in contrast to the AAI), although some interviewees tear up or cry. In some situations, the administrator may detect some reluctance in the interviewee's response to the task. On rare occasions, the interviewee asks to stop. We have developed clear guidelines to help interviewers identify defensive resistances compared with cues that would require terminating the administration session. These guidelines have been approved by internal review boards reviewing research using the AAP and meet the standards for professional clinical practice.

Administration guidelines differ for research and clinical application. The rule of thumb for AAP administration that we use in research is not to administer the AAP to individuals who have experienced loss or trauma (witnessing or experiencing a life threatening event) within the past year. Administration within a year of loss or trauma can provide evidence of immediate or short-term responses to these events, which can be useful in clinical and research settings interested in documenting attachment response patterns over time. The AAP has been used successfully with individuals with clinical diagnoses

[3]We use additional neutral pictures to start the AAP with adults with intellectual disabilities to help assuage performance anxieties. See Gallichan and George (2014) for more information.

and abuse, and individuals who are in inpatient settings, institutionalized, or incarcerated.

Training in the coding and classification of the AAP contributes to its ethical use. Evaluation to determine the individual's attachment response and representation cannot be done intuitively, even if one has trained in other attachment assessments. We discuss training at the end of this chapter.

Coding and Classification

Attachment classification using the AAP is based on the analysis of the verbatim transcript of the "story" responses to the seven attachment pictures. Classification is based on coding categories that we have developed to evaluate the patterns and integration of three response dimensions: (1) narrative, (2) story content, and (3) defense. The following discussion provides an overview of these dimensions. The coder evaluates these dimensions separately for each story. Of course, these features of the response are inextricably intertwined; however, the identification of the specific qualities of these features is essential to discriminating among attachment groups.

Narrative

The judge's first task is to evaluate the narrative to identify portions of each response that includes autobiographical personal experience. Personal experience is coded when the individual's response includes information about events that have occurred at any time in that person's life. There are no instructions in the AAP that ask the interviewee to relate the hypothetical events to his or her own life experiences. The AAP instructions direct the individual's attention to the characters in the picture stimuli. The inclusion of personal-experience material in the response indicates a violation of self–other boundaries, which is interpreted as representational blurring or merging of self with other. This state of mind is associated with intense attachment distress, often seen in individuals in the ambivalent–preoccupied or dysregulated/disorganized classification groups (George & Solomon, 2008) or individuals with debilitating self–other boundary problems (e.g., personality and anxiety disorders, Buchheim & George, 2011).

Story Content

The story content dimensions evaluate how the representational narrative conveys meaning to the relationships depicted in the story line. Agency of self and connectedness are coded to evaluate mutuality and integrated attachment in the alone stories; these dimensions are evaluated using the synchrony dimension in the dyadic stories.

Agency of self describes the process by which the character takes productive steps to face the challenges introduced in the story line (i.e., what led up to the scene). Attachment theory holds that these self-capacities are internalized as the product of consistent experiences of sensitive and responsive parental care during infancy and early childhood when the child's attachment system is activated (Sroufe, Egeland, Carlson, & Collins, 2005). Agency of self is required to solve the problem or change the situation when facing distress or threat alone.

The AAP system identifies two integrated forms of agency of self. One is "haven of safety," which applies Ainsworth's concept to the AAP. Haven of safety is coded when the story portrays caregiver sensitivity to the character's attachment need or perceived situation. The other, "internalized secure base," is coded when the story portrays the character as drawing upon internal resources. We developed the internalized secure base concept for the AAP to capture the internal capacity of thoughtful evaluation of self and attachment events, and it is unique in the field of attachment. The character uses solitude to explore feelings and experiences (i.e., the secure base). The secure base concept is central to attachment security (e.g., H. Waters & Waters, 2006); therefore, we pause briefly to clarify how the concept of the internalized secure base in the AAP fits within attachment theory.

The secure base phenomenon in early childhood is dependent on the physical proximity and availability of the attachment figure; the attachment figure is the child's secure base in the real world. In the phase of attachment development that Bowlby (1969/1982) termed the "goal-corrected partnership," the child begins to form enduring internalized models of the relationship with the caregiver. Increasingly, mental representations of the attachment relationship can supplement actual interactions with the caregiver. Separations for secure children are less likely to be threatening, because representations of attachment figures permit "proximity" even in the attachment figure's physical absence. This representational capacity becomes more differentiated over time. The older child's sense of security is increasingly maintained by reference to the internal working model of the attachment figure. Essentially, the secure base effect in adults is a representational process. Internalized representational processes almost exclusively inform and shape mental representations of the self (Bowlby, 1969/1982; Sroufe & Fleeson, 1986). Representation allows the individual to explore the inner world of the self. We thus capture this process in the concept of "internalized secure base," used to refer to that state in which the sense of security and integrity of self is derived from the individual's internal relationship to the attachment figure. The internalized secure base is coded when the story characters have entered and actively explored their internal working models of attachment and self.

The AAP also codes a form of agency of self termed "capacity to act," which represents the character's ability to respond to attachment challenges or distress with constructive action, without assistance from attachment figures. It is helpful to think of capacity to act as functional, problem-focused behavior that maintains attachment regulation.

Connectedness evaluates the representational availability of intimate relationships when a character is alone. Attachment is only one relationship-based behavioral system. Human biology defines additional fundamental behavioral systems that can provide protection, including being a parent (caregiving system), friends (affiliative–sociable system), and sexual relationships (sexual system) (Bowlby, 1969/1982; Hinde, 1982; Marvin, Britner, & Russell, 2016). Connectedness depicts the character's capacity to be in any of these fundamental relationships. Some stories depict successful connections; others depict connections that are blocked (e.g., characters fought) or directed toward strangers or people in social service roles (e.g., teacher, doctor, neighbor); still others depict characters remaining alone. Connectedness is coded only in the two alone pictures in which satisfying interactions with others are plausible: Window and Bench. Connectedness is not coded for stories in which the scene pulls for themes that block connectedness—Cemetery (represents death) and Corner (abuse and threat).

Synchrony evaluates relationship quality in the dyadic pictures. The scenes are drawn to depict a self with a potential attachment figure in a "goal-corrected partnership" following Bowlby (1969/1982). Integrated synchrony is coded when interactions are reciprocal, mutually engaging pleasure or showing sensitivity and care in response to distress and vulnerability. Functional (e.g., give medicine for illness without comfort) or failed interactions (e.g., failure to respond to the child's bid for a hug) do not qualify as integration. The portrayal of functional interactions serves, however, to maintain attachment regulation.

Defensive Processes

As we briefly discussed earlier, defensive processes select, exclude, and transform behavior, thought, and emotional appraisal to terminate the attachment system as much as possible to prevent uncomfortable distress or dysregulation. The AAP provides a framework from which to observe defenses "at work" and to identify the kinds and pervasiveness of defensive operations.

Bowlby (1980) distinguished three forms of defensive exclusion: deactivation, cognitive disconnection, and segregated systems. We followed George and Solomon's (Solomon et al., 1995) defensive processing coding schemes for children's doll play and developed identifying AAP criteria for these three categories. Defense has played a minor role in attachment theory since Bowlby's original writing (Bowlby, 1980; Bretherton, 2005; Bretherton & Munholland, 2016). George and Solomon developed and validated the only coding scheme for identifying defense in assessment (George & Solomon, 2008; Solomon et al., 1995).

Defense is evaluated in all the AAP stories from the words, images, and narrative patterns in the response. It is not possible to describe the complexity of defensive process coding in detail here. Here we describe the general characteristics that define each form of defense.

Deactivation is the process of shifting attention away from events or feelings that activate the attachment system and prevent the individual from becoming distracted by attendant attachment distress. Deactivation serves to exclude the emotional content, especially distress, and contact with attachment figures. Some defensive deactivation maneuvers include emphasis on social rules (i.e., socially correct behavior), materialism, authority, achievement, or romance (diversion of the attachment system to the sexual system). Other forms depict the negative qualities of characters that obscure attending to attachment needs because characters are unworthy, expressed by themes of transgression, punishment, and rejection.

Cognitive disconnection is the process of splitting attachment information and affect from their source (Bowlby, 1980). This form of defense undermines the expression of a unitary, consistent attachment state of mind when the attachment system is activated. The term *cognitive* is a misnomer, because this form of defense excludes intellectual and emotional processes (Bowlby, 1980); thus, we refer to this defense as disconnection to capture its complete defensive quality. Disconnection produces story themes that are vague or confused, or that oscillate between opposite events or feelings (e.g., good–bad, inside–outside, happy–depressed; George & Solomon, 1996, 2008). Individuals are unable to maintain a unitary story line and are confused or ambivalent about events. Characters or the individual telling the story are caught in cycles of waiting, wondering, and wishing for something to happen. Disconnection feeds emotional preoccupation, anger, anxiety, frustration, and attempt to withdraw from or distract attention away from distress.

The *segregated system* is an extreme form of defensive exclusion that develops from a developmental history of severe attachment threats. This defense is the single element in the AAP coding system used to designate representational dysregulation and the unresolved attachment group. The concept of segregated system is complex and has been mostly ignored in attachment theory since Bowlby's (1980) original description. Therefore, we define the concept in more detail here to understand its dynamics and how it is coded in the AAP.

Bowlby (1980) developed the segregated system concept drawing on contemporary cognitive theory to reformulate and update psychoanalytic repression. He applied the concept to explain extreme and psychotic responses to the loss of an attachment figure observed in clinical patients. Experiences and affect associated with the attachment figure and the trauma of the loss (i.e., severed attachment relationship) are "packaged up" and locked away (literally segregated) from consciousness because of the pain of trauma combined with the failure of surviving attachment figures to respond to distress. Two features of this concept are essential to AAP coding: (1) the traumatized self is a repressed, separate self-representation, and (2) activating the attachment system threatens segregating processes. Activation threatens and dysregulates the functioning self. Patients are flooded by pain, anger, and fear, or freeze and constrict in their desperate fight to stave off memories and affect. Research has identified behavioral and representational patterns that are consistent with Bowlby's descriptions. As expected, these patterns differentiate disorganized from organized attachment patterns. Solomon et al. (1995) found that disorganized children described dysregulated, frightening, unmetabolized attachment events in doll play. George and Solomon (1996,

2008) reported that mothers of disorganized children were dysregulated by subjective appraisals of their children and themselves as parents, and as being helpless and out of control. Following doll play (Solomon et al., 1995) and the AAI (Main & Goldwyn, 1985/1998/2006), the AAP evaluates narratives for evidence of segregated systems and evidence of functional containment. Uncontained segregated systems material is the decision criterion used to identify "lack of resolution" and unresolved attachment.

Step 1, then, is to identify the presence of segregated systems material in the response. This material depicts helplessness, fear, failed protection or abandonment, and themes of dangerous events, being out of control, or isolation. Some indices have an eerie quality, a feature that parallels theory and research linking unresolved attachment and dissociation (e.g., Liotti, 2017). Other indices include the sudden intrusion of the individual's own traumatic story (i.e., personal experience), an AAP narrative element that is like the intrusions observed in unresolved AAIs (Main & Goldwyn, 1985/1998/2006).

Step 2 is to evaluate whether segregated system material is contained. Containment or "resolution" means that individuals can regulate attachment distress. Regulation is marked by representational agency, assistance from others, or themes that express confidence that the character has a future. The failure to contain segregated systems indicates that attachment is unresolved, suggesting that the individual remains "haunted" by feelings of abandonment, persecution, fear, helplessness, and vulnerability. On occasion, unresolved individuals freeze and cannot or refuse to respond to a stimulus. This form of constriction is like the behavior of disorganized children in doll play (Solomon et al., 1995).

Classification

The attachment classification group is assigned by evaluating the coding patterns across the entire set of seven attachment stories. The classification procedure uses a hierarchically integrated series of decision points (see Figure 13.4).

The following sections provide examples of prototypical AAP stories and coding elements for each of the attachment groups. We selected stories from different samples to demonstrate the range of AAP use. A detailed description of the classification coding patterns is beyond the scope of this chapter, and interested readers can find a more detailed explanation in the resources listed at the end of this chapter.

There is often interest in how the AAP classification scheme differs from the AAI in determining attachment status. The differences between these two approaches about secure attachment were addressed in the discussion of attachment coherence earlier in this chapter. Differences between the systems are highlighted in the discussion of dismissing, preoccupied, and unresolved groups that follow. The content and defensive processing patterns associated with different attachment classification groups have been shown useful in predicting personality functioning (Gander et al., 2020).

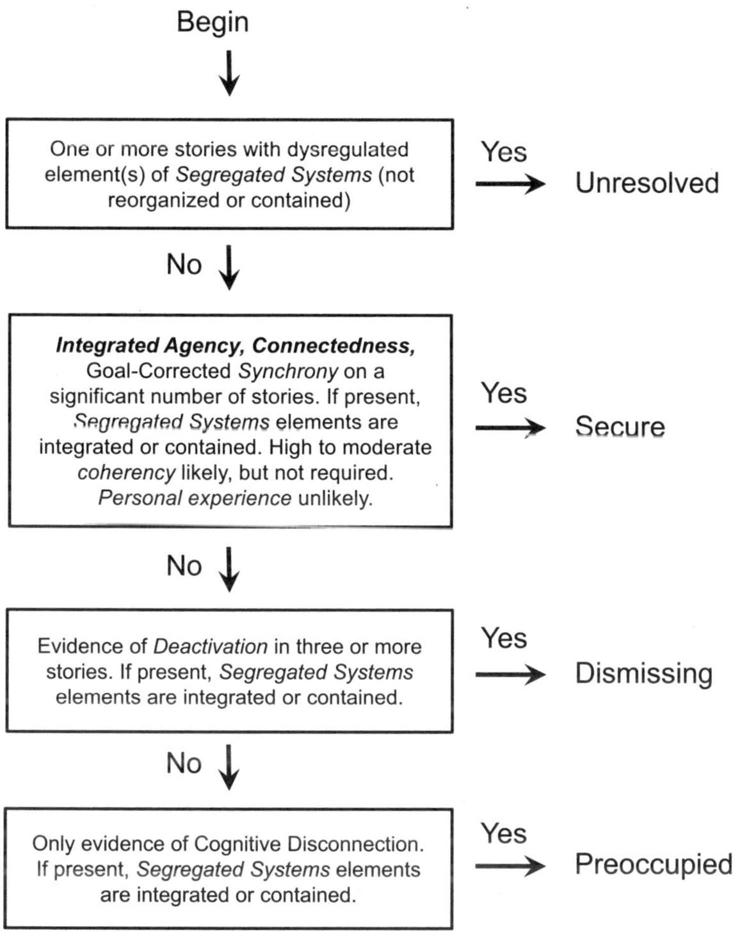

FIGURE 13.4. AAP classification decision hierarchy.

SECURE ATTACHMENT

The hallmark of security in the AAP is the ability to demonstrate the capacity to integrate attachment distress consistent with the concept of attachment coherence we described earlier in this chapter (internalized secure base, haven of safety, goal-corrected synchrony). The relative absence of defense in narratives of secure individuals is striking in direct contrast to the stories of insecure individuals. Secure individuals use defense to navigate and manage tension or distress rather than exclude it.

Many of these qualities are present in the following example of a secure individual's responses to the Bench and Bed stimuli. The narrative response is provided in the left column. AAP coding material is indicated by *italics* and interpreted using the AAP coding system in the right column.

BENCH PICTURE STIMULUS

Hmm, well this looks like a girl who's	
been in a *volleyball tournament*—and	Deactivation
she's just played many games and	Disconnection
she's very *tired*—and the last game	
was a close one and they *lost*. So	Deactivation
she's sitting on a bench to sit and	Agency: internal secure base
regroup, think about the game and, and	
uh, try and reorganize her thoughts and	
get her body and her mind pumped up	Agency: capacity to act
again *to go off and play again*. I think	Agency: capacity to act
then she'll go and uh have a *bite to*	
eat, present herself at the appropriate	
time and, and ahh have the energy she	
needs to *play the next game*, and play	
it well.	

BED PICTURE STIMULUS

Well this looks like bedtime and mum	
has just sat down to say goodnight	
and this young fellow feels *he needs*	
a hug before he goes to sleep * **, *so*	*attachment signal **caregiver
she slides up a little closer to him and	response → Synchrony:
gives him a big hug, and uh strokes his	goal-corrected partnership
head, his back and then tells him to	
roll over onto his tummy and she'll give	
him a bit of a massage and that calms	
him down and gets him ready for *sleep*	
and she kisses him goodnight, and	
leaves the room.	Deactivation

The most striking features of this individual's representation of attachment are stories about available and responsive attachment figures. The girl in Bench demonstrates the internalized secure base, defined earlier as integrated attachment that draws on internalized attachment figures for thoughtful exploration of attachment distress. The AAP codes internalization of attachment figures as integrated connectedness. We note in this story also that the process of integration (internalized secure base) leads to the depiction of the self as having the capacity to act. The girl thinks (internalized secure base), eats, and plays again (capacity to act). In the Bed response, integrated attachment is depicted by a description of maternal sensitivity to the boy's attachment signal (hug). There is no delay. The goal-corrected partnership is evidenced by his mother's prompt and appropriate response.

Defensive exclusion is minimal and is used to move the story along. Individuals demonstrate patterns of preferred defenses in their stories. In Bench, deactivation unveils the distress associated with negative evaluations (losing the game) surrounding achievement (volleyball tournament). Feelings that the self is unworthy lead to agency. In Bed, deactivation plays a different role. We see that sensitive attachment figure care permits "cooling down" and redirecting attachment distress to be able to sleep. Overall, these stories are examples of attachment coherence, in which the coding elements are integrated and combined to represent an autonomous self in a goal-corrected attachment–caregiving relationship.

DISMISSING ATTACHMENT

Dismissing attachment in the AAP is characterized by deactivation levels that interfere with attachment integration. Relationships and interactions are typically described as "getting the job done," that is, functional without assuaging attachment needs. Deactivating portrayals of attachment figures include their roles as authorities, not individuals who provide comfort or care. Stories themes often deflect appealing to attachment figures to other behavioral systems (e.g., friends or lovers) or people in social roles outside the family (e.g., teachers, nurses). The stories of dismissing individuals may demonstrate a failure to deserve care in themes of rejection or punishment. Most dismissing individuals manage the tension of storytelling well, explaining the rationale for events and not slipping personal experiences into the narratives. Many of these qualities are evidenced in the following responses to the Bench and Bed pictures. *Italicized* material represents deactivation.

BENCH PICTURE STIMULUS

This picture the person looks *defeated* and sad um and I would say like maybe has been in um an *athletic competition* or something and they *didn't come in first or didn't come in better their time* or whatever and so they're just sitting on the bench like oh my god you know and next they'll probably I don't know find maybe a little bit of peace or maybe go do something or whatever and so they'll <u>get up</u> from the bench and walk away. Um, I would say they're feeling *defeated,* they're kind of like sad and hopeless not hopeless but sort of disappointed.

<u>Agency: capacity to act</u>

BED PICTURE STIMULUS

Mmm this is a mom waking her son up in the morning but he doesn't want to walk and get out of bed, he wants to get carried out of bed* and he has to go take a shower and brush his teeth and get ready for *school,* and the mom's telling her how good he has to be at *school* today and the daddy's gone for *work* but he's still sleepy and tired and he's crying, well he's whining and the mom is . . . she's being as patient as she can with the kid and *tell him that he has to be a big boy* so . . . he finally gets out of bed but he's asking for a bottle now,* *he's already ten years old and he's in the third grade* and then mom gets ready, he gets ready, *she takes him to school* and he goes to *school* but he doesn't do his *work* and. . . . Umm the little boy's upset because he doesn't like *school,* the mom is frustrated because she doesn't know how to deal with it, and she's trying her best, and the dad's always *working* so the little boy feels annoyed that he has to be there, the mom feeling kind of stuck in the situation where she has no one to help her, and um . . .

*attachment signal

*another attachment signal

The most striking feature of these responses is the sheer quantity of deactivation material, which also blocks integrated attachment. In Bench, there is no evidence of the internalized secure base, and the minimal agency that is described (get up) is undirected action. The self can go forward, but we do not know how. Connectedness was a failure, and the girl remains alone. The Bed story pattern is similar. Deactivation is so interfering that it blocks the attachment figure's response and even when the child signals two times for care. The story elements center on reasons not to provide care, including negative aspects of the boy's development (immaturity) and the mother's emphatic emphasis on her son's achievement (achievement, authority) that deflects attention away from attachment distress. The mother's function is to get her son ready for and take her son to school.

One of the most notable differences between the AAP and the AAI is the absence of material that would be coded in the AAI as *idealization,* which is defined as the discrepancy between the individual's overall view of the parent and the real experience with that parent; it is prototypical for the AAI subgroup labeled "dismissing of attachment" (Main & Goldwyn, 1984/1998/2006). The goal of idealization is to limit the influence of attachment experience and emotion. We find it useful to reframe idealization and the other forms of narrative limiting described in the AAI (e.g., restriction of feeling) in the AAP. Deactivation is the overarching defense mechanism. It shows up in the AAP in a variety of different content forms, including negative evaluation and descriptions of rejection and ignoring that are far from ideal. These latter representational elements closely follow Ainsworth's observations of infant behavior (Ainsworth et al., 1978/2015). We note, too, that there is no evidence of idealization in any of the AAP foundation measures (projective doll play, caregiving interview; George & Solomon, 2008; Solomon et al., 1995).

The prominence of deactivation over idealization per se is likely to be because the AAP is a different kind of measure than the AAI. The task is to interpret the experiences of the hypothetical characters in specified attachment scenes using both conscious and unconscious processes, not to recall one's experience. Speaking hypothetically (i.e., describe what is happening) as compared with instructions to speak about reality is a form of distancing that may relieve individuals from the pressure of creating descriptions of idealized self-deception. The hypothetical story can include elements that clearly identify the rejection, negativity, and problems in attachment that we know are core experiences for dismissing individuals. In the AAI, idealization manifests to exclude and transform autobiographical elements from complete conscious realization, thus, preventing undue distress by "keeping things positive" at the semantic level, while sorting through what to describe in response to interview questions.

PREOCCUPIED ATTACHMENT

The hallmark of the preoccupied group is disconnection. Defensive disconnection interferes with attachment coherence by creating a smokescreen; individuals literally cannot "see" attachment distress if they cannot stay engaged with the affects, events, and people associated with their distress. Preoccupied individuals can portray agency, connectedness, and synchrony on occasion; the problem is that they cannot sustain these forms of integration. Characters in alone stories often appeal to strangers for assistance or remain alone, barely able to demonstrate the agency to go forward. Relationships in the dyadic stories are typically functional, although attachment figures may be portrayed as sensitive in the Bed scene or comforting in the Ambulance scene. These patterns make sense, because preoccupation (analogous to ambivalent–resistant attachment) results from inconsistent attachment figure care (Ainsworth et al., 1978/2015). Overall, the quality of preoccupied responses is confusing and hollow. It is also not uncommon for preoccupied individuals to blur personal experience into the story. Many of these qualities are present in the examples of Bench and Bed responses below. Disconnection is marked in *italics*.

BENCH PICTURE STIMULUS

She's not a happy camper. Sh . . . *I don't know* because I don't know where she is. Ahh *could be a hundred and one reasons why she's sitting like that.* She's not happy. And when a person's tired they usually lie down or you know, maybe lie on the bench but when there's, if you're tired you don't usually sit like this, you know, so it's usually because you're upset. What led up to it *could be anything, depends* on how old she is—is a big factor by the size of her body she could be a teenager which mean—*maybe her boyfriend dumped her or she got in an argument with somebody had a falling out with her parents.* Well she could I guess one would *hope* that if she'd had a problem with some friends it could be *resolved or straightened around uhmm, some kind of reconciliation, I guess* the same w . . . with her parents if it was something that was you know had caused them to not agree on something then one would *hope* that that could you know it could be *reconciled* Well what I is see is that they don't have any shoes on, why don't they have shoes? These people . . . is that a subliminal thing or what? I noticed that with the other one, a silhouette?

Vague reference to relationship by settling a disagreement, does not necessarily involve forgiveness and repair. An oblique attempt at haven of safety.

Oblique attempt at haven of safety.

BED PICTURE STIMULUS

That looks like a mother and a child and the mother doesn't . . . *hard to say whether she going to hug the child or not.* Hmm maybe the child . . . *I don't know,* maybe the child is sad about something and the mother just can't really, you know, can't really enter into the child's sadness. I think maybe the mother, maybe the mother will hug the child but, uhm, *not really understand* necessarily, and the child will go to sleep.

Disconnection in these stories splits off attachment distress from its source by introducing uncertainty and pervasive thematic and narrative fracturing. In the Bench story, the individual repeats statements equivalent to saying "I don't know" throughout the response (a hundred and one reasons; could be anything; depends; two different story lines). There is no productive description of agency because reconciliation does not necessarily include repair or forgiveness and the story line fails to depict constructive action on the character's part. Connectedness to parents or boyfriend is implied as part of the reconciliation but left vague, because there is no image of the self being in contact again with these characters. The only clear conclusion from this story is that the self has a future in these relationships, but we do not know how this happens.

The disconnected quality of the Bed story is similar. The response again includes variations of "I don't know." We note how disconnection has "edited out" of the story a description of the child's attachment signal. The mother is present, struggling with the decision to hug or not, but the child never signals his or her need. Instead, the narrative implies that a sad child needs a hug. The mother waffles and finally hugs the child. Waffling about outcomes interferes with goal-corrected synchrony, creating a pattern of functional interruption that parallels descriptions of the doll-play stories of ambivalent–resistant children (Solomon et al., 1995) and mothers' caregiving experiences (George & Solomon, 2008).

UNRESOLVED ATTACHMENT

The unresolved group is assigned when at least one response fails to integrate or contain segregated systems material. The patterns of other AAP dimensions may resemble any of the three organized attachment groups. The following are examples of unresolved responses to the Bench and Bed picture stimuli. Segregated systems are indicated in *italics*.

BENCH PICTURE STIMULUS

Looks like a *prison.* I had to think of a *prison* because of the bricks here above somehow. A woman, she is in *prison* somehow, she Is sitting somehow on a plank bed and is very *desperate,* that she is *all alone and nobody is visiting her.* She is very *desperate* and. . . . That she is sitting in the prison. Hmm, hmm. She has *stolen* something, she is *kleptomaniac,* that's why she is sitting in *prison.* She has *stolen* something and has, yes. She has not so many relatives or so, there nobody is coming to visiting her, *or so.* And *she has no friends. And she is sitting very desperately alone.* Yes, that is like (laughs). I can't say anything more.	No agency, no connectedness.

BED PICTURE STIMULUS

A mother and a little boy, she's putting him down to go to sleep, doesn't look like he wants her to leave because he's reaching his arms out to her,* and she's just sitting at the foot of the bed, hmm, the little boy probably thinks, maybe he's *scared* of the dark or something, he doesn't want her to leave, he wants her to stay there maybe until he falls asleep so he can feel safer. She's probably thinking, you know he's giving her a hard time about going to bed, um. Maybe, maybe he, or maybe he's going down for a nap from playing um . . . mmm maybe after the situation, maybe the next day he, the little boy might not be so worried about her leaving, the room when he goes to sleep. Yeah. Maybe he had a *nightmare,* or yeah just a bad dream, and maybe he got *scared,* just like doesn't want her to leave, maybe thinks it was more real like think, or maybe thinks he'll have another bad dream and he doesn't want to get *scared* again, that's why he doesn't want her to leave.	*attachment signal
(So what do you think might happen next?) She leaves.	Mother fails to respond to boy's fear.

Segregated systems are signs of attachment dysregulation. Evidence of segregated systems in the Bench story are references to illegal and addictive behavior (kleptomania). The story does not contain character agency; no person comes forward to help the character. Segregated systems in the Bed story are references to the boy's fear. The mother fails to respond; she cannot even take functional steps to help him, such as read him a story or bring him a glass of water. Both stories, and therefore both transcripts, are judged unresolved.

AAP coding for the unresolved classification is not subtle. By contrast, determining the unresolved classification on the AAI requires the rater to pay careful attention to lapses in the monitoring of reasoning and discourse throughout the interview, evaluating the degree to which the individual is confused, disoriented, or frightened by experiences of death or abuse on a 9-point rating scale (Main & Goldwyn, 1985/1998/2996). In the AAP, these "lapses" are evidenced by operationally defined segregated systems indicators. The AAP list of segregated systems coding indices integrates the wealth of theory and research on attachment disorganization available while we were developing the AAP coding system: Main and Solomon's (1990) "fright without solution"; Main and Hesse's (1990) "collapse of behavioral strategies"; Solomon and George's (1999) "failure to terminate hypothesis;" Bowlby's (1973) examination of fear; Bowlby's (1980) description of chronic mourning; and research identifying the correlates and family background related to attachment disorganization (see Lyons-Ruth & Jacobvitz, 2016, for review). The AAP indices for unresolved attachment also include *constriction* (refusing to tell a story). This is a new manifestation of unresolved adult attachment not captured by the AAI. Constriction is observed in the doll play of disorganized children (Solomon et al., 1995) and their mothers' caregiving interviews (George & Solomon, 2008), and is a unique assessment feature for adult attachment only evaluated from the AAP.

Validation

This section provides an overview of the process we used to validate the AAP classification scheme (see George & West, 2012, for a more extensive discussion). Development of the initial AAP classification scheme was based on 13 transcripts of individuals recruited through newspaper advertisements in a community sample of men and women. We created the basic coding categories to match the four standard AAI classification groups: secure, dismissing, preoccupied, and unresolved. AAIs in the development sample were blinded, and we checked our AAP classifications against the AAI classifications, refining our system case by case.

A second step used two samples to test the preliminary coding scheme, again comparing the AAP and AAI classifications. AAPs and AAIs were coded by separate blind judges. The first sample included 25 mothers randomly selected from an ongoing study of infant risk conducted by Dr. Diane Benoit. The second included 24 women drawn from a large-scale study of depression (West & George, 2002). Four-group and secure–insecure classification concordant validity was examined using three independent AAP judges and two independent AAI judges. AAP–AAI concordance rates ranged from 92 to 97%, interjudge reliability ranged from 87 to 97% agreement; kappas ranged from .73 to .82 (all p's $< .001$) (George & West, 2001). Counterbalanced test administration showed no order effect for administration.

A third step was to conduct a large-scale psychometric investigation of AAP concordant and discriminant validity and test–retest reliability (see George & West, 2012, for a complete description of this study). One hundred and forty-four English-speaking adults between ages 19 and 65 (100 women, 44 men) were recruited from community and college settings in Alberta, Canada, and northern California (51% from Canada). The mean age of the women was 36.2 years (SD = 15.2); the mean age of the men was 26.4 years (SD = 8.9), with significantly older women than men in the sample. The mean level of education was 14.7 years. The proportions of women to men and college students to community adults were about equal in the Alberta and California subsamples. The Alberta sample was uniformly White. The California sample was diverse and represented the cultural diversity of northern California (African American, Hispanic, Asian, Filipino, White).

Participants were interviewed individually in a laboratory or office for an initial assessment; 48% of the sample was seen for a follow-up assessment approximately 3 months later. The initial assessment included the AAI, AAP, the Vocabulary and Similarities subscales of the Wechsler Adult Intelligence Scale (WAIS), and a Social Desirability scale (Balanced Inventory of Desirable Responding [BIDR]; Paulhus, 1998). Participants filled out questionnaires following attachment assessments or returned questionnaires mailed in advance before coming to the laboratory. The second assessment included only the AAP retest.

Attachment classifications were made from verbatim transcripts of the AAP and the AAI. Three blind, trained independent coders who did not conduct the interviews classified the AAP. All transcripts were coded and classified by at least two coders. The AAIs were classified blind by two reliable judges. One judge classified all of the AAIs in the sample; a second judge coded 30 transcripts (21%).

Interjudge reliability for the AAP and AAI was compared for four-group and two-group (secure vs. insecure) classification agreement. Four-group agreement kappas were .79–.85, p's < 001). Secure–insecure agreement kappas were .66 and .83, p's < .001). Classification disagreements were resolved through discussion. AAP–AAI convergence for the four major attachment groups was 90% (kappa = .84, $p < .001$); secure–insecure convergent agreement was 97% (kappa = .88, $p < .001$).

Sixty-nine (48%) participants completed the AAP retest (39 females). Fifty-eight (84%) were classified in the same main categories (kappa = .78, $p < .001$). Classification group stability for secure attachment was 82%, 96% for dismissing attachment, 62% for preoccupied attachment, and 80% for unresolved attachment. The most shifts occurred between unresolved and preoccupied classifications. Intelligence and social desirability were not related to AAP classifications.

Other AAP–AAI concordance studies in independent samples have demonstrated strong interjudge and classification concordance with kappas at $p < .001$ levels (e.g., Buchheim & George, 2011; Buchheim, George, & West, 2003; Buchheim et al., 2018). One study did not report satisfactory classification concordance (Jones-Mason, Allen, Hamilton, & Weiss, 2015). Analysis of the AAP transcripts demonstrated incomplete AAP administration. Incomplete administration probing will result in inadequate story material to code agency or other story elements required to contain dysregulation.

APPLICATIONS OF THE AAP: RESEARCH AND CLINICAL SETTINGS

Developed over 20 years ago, the AAP has been used in a wide range of research and clinical settings in North America and Europe. A comprehensive summary of this work is available on the AAP website (*www.attachmentprojective.com*). Here, we illustrate a range of AAP uses.

Studies of basic research and hypothesis testing have included adults and adolescents from a range of samples. These studies establish substantial predictive validity for the AAP. Several studies have examined mothers' adult attachment status concerning caregiving and their children's adjustment and developmental risk. Béliveau and Moss (2005) predicted and found mothers' reported caregiving experiences significantly related to the four standard adult attachment groups judged by the AAP. In their sample of mothers of young school-age children, unresolved mothers reported significantly more parenting stress, stressful life events, parental helplessness, and less child involvement than did secure mothers. Preoccupied mothers reported greater parenting stress than did secure mothers. Adult attachment was were not related to measures of socioeconomic status and psychosocial functioning. Cyr, Béliveau, and Moss (2003) reported a statistically significant match between mothers' AAP classifications and their preschoolers' laboratory reunion classifications.

An area of particular interest has been to examine the correlates of unresolved attachment and complicated grief in basic and clinical research. Joubert, Webster, and Hackett (2012) investigated associations between unresolved attachment, cognitive skills, and dissociation. They found that working memory mediated between unresolved attachment and dissociation. Mazzeschi et al. (2014) reported that unresolved attachment was a major risk factor for child obesity. Pallini, Alfani, Marech, and Laghi (2017) investigated attachment in relation to women who had experienced intimate partner violence as compared with controls. These researchers showed that not only were those in the partner violence group more likely to be unresolved, but they also were unable to demonstrate representations of self with personal agency. The authors concluded that the AAP patterns in addition to the unresolved classification improved the understanding the specific levels of trauma experienced by victims by clarifying their frightening/frightened dynamic typical of the attachment disorganization that undermines mentalization. The Pallini et al. study echoes findings by Fitzke, Buchheim, and Juen (2013) regarding attachment and mentalization. Gander, Sevecke, and Buchheim (2018) demonstrated that variations in the unresolved content of the AAP differentiated among adolescent patient groups. The AAPs of patients with anorexia were characterized by emotional isolation and the inability to maintain self–other boundaries. The AAPs of adolescents with major depression were characterized by fear and attachment figure failed protection. Gander et al. (2020) reported that unresolved attachment mediated between childhood trauma and personality functioning in a study of 199 adolescents between ages 12 and 18. Higher amounts of AAP traumatic material showed greater severity of personality dysfunction, including intimacy, self-direction, empathy, and identity.

The AAP has also been used in neurophysiological research examining how attachment is related to neurophysiological functioning (Fraedrich, Lakatos, & Spangler, 2010). Buchheim and her colleagues (2006) used the

AAP to examine the brain activation patterns associated with resolved versus unresolved attachment status. In this innovative study, the AAP was administered while participants (adult, right-handed women) were in the functional magnetic resonance imaging (fMRI) apparatus. Analyses of the brain activation patterns produced while telling AAP stories showed a significant interaction effect between the sequence of the AAP pictures and unresolved attachment. Unresolved participants, as compared with participants with organized attachments, showed increased activation of the medial temporal brain regions, in particular, areas associated with autobiographical memory and emotion (e.g., amygdala, hippocampus) as attachment activation increased during the AAP task.

Interest in integrating attachment theory in psychotherapy has burgeoned over the past decade. The AAP is user-friendly in psychotherapeutic settings, inexpensive, and can be administered at different points over the course of psychotherapy. It has also been used with clients as the basis for discussion and interpretation. Papers on the AAP in evaluations and psychotherapy address its use in custody evaluations (e.g., Isaacs, George, & Marvin, 2011) and therapy settings, including integrating the AAP in different therapeutic models (e.g., psychodynamic, dialectical behavior therapy, Bernheim et al., 2019; Buchheim, Labek, Walter, & Viviani, 2013; George & Buchheim, 2014). Other discussions address using the AAP in multimodal assessment (e.g., Rorschach, Thematic Apperception Test [TAT], MMPI-II), family-based interventions (e.g., Finn, 2011; Gallichan & George, 2014; Joubert, 2007) and early intervention programs, such as the Circle of Security (Pazzagli, Laghezza, Manaresi, Mazzeschi, & Powell, 2014).

CONCLUSION

The AAP provides the field with a valid, economic, user-friendly measure of adult attachment that can be used in basic and clinical research and psychotherapy settings. The representational assessment of attachment is a complex process requiring the description and understanding of the patterns among several variables. The unique AAP dimensions define major theoretically derived concepts not measured in any other adult attachment assessment. These elements have been shown in studies such as those summarized earlier to augment the understanding of attachment processes beyond the classification group designation. We look forward to future work in basic, clinical, neurobiological research, and therapeutic application opened by the AAP.

REFERENCES

Ainsworth, M. D. S. (1964). Patterns of attachment behavior shown by the infant in interaction with his mother. *Merrill–Palmer Quarterly, 10,* 51–58.

Ainsworth, M. D. S. (1989). Attachment beyond infancy. *American Psychologist, 44,* 709–716.

Ainsworth, M. D. S., Blehar, M., Waters, E., & Wall, S. (2015). *Patterns of attachment: A psychological study of the Strange Situation.* New York: Taylor & Francis (Psychology Press). (Original work published 1978)

Bauriedl-Schmidt, C., Jobst, A., Gander, M., Seidl, E., Sabaß, L., Sarubin, N., . . . Buchheim, A. (2017). Attachment representations, patterns of emotion regulation, and social exclusion in patients with chronic and episodic depression and healthy controls. *Journal of Affective Disorders, 210*(1), 130–138.

Béliveau, M. J., & Moss, E. (2005). Contribution aux validités convergente et divergente du Projectif de l'Attachement Adulte [Convergent and divergent validity of the Adult Attachment Projective]. *La Revue internationale de l'éducation familiale, 9,* 29–50.

Bernheim, D., Gander, M., Keller, F., Becker, M., Lischke, A., Mentel, R., . . . Buchheim, A. (2019). The role of attachment characteristics in dialectical behavior therapy for patients with borderline personality disorder. *Clinical Psychology and Psychotherapy, 26*(3), 339–349.

Bowlby, J. (1973). *Attachment and loss: Vol. 2. Separation.* New York: Basic Books.

Bowlby, J. (1980). *Attachment and loss: Vol. 3. Loss.* New York: Basic Books.

Bowlby, J. (1982). *Attachment and loss: Vol 1. Attachment.* New York: Basic Books. (Original work published 1969)

Bretherton, I. (2005). In pursuit of the internal working model construct and its relevance to attachment relationships. In K. E. Grossmann, K. Grossmann, & E. Waters (Eds.), *Attachment from infancy to adulthood: The major longitudinal studies* (pp. 13–47). New York: Guilford Press.

Bretherton, I., & Munholland, K. A. (2016). Internal working model construct in light of contemporary neuroimaging research. In J. Cassidy & P. R. Shaver (Eds.), *Handbook of attachment: Theory, research, and clinical applications* (3rd ed., pp. 63–88). New York: Guilford Press.

Bretherton, I., Ridgeway, D., & Cassidy, J. (1990). Assessing internal working models of the attachment relationship: An attachment story completion task for 3-year-olds. In M. T. Greenberg, D. Cicchetti, & E. M. Cummings (Eds.), *Attachment in the preschool years* (pp. 273–308). Chicago: University of Chicago Press.

Buchheim, A., Erk, S., George, C., Kaechele, H., Ruchsow, M., Spitzer, M., . . . Walter, H. (2006). Measuring attachment representation in an fMRI environment: A pilot study. *Psychopathology, 39*(3), 144–152.

Buchheim, A., & George, C. (2011). The representational, neurobiological and emotional foundation of attachment disorganization in borderline personality disorder and anxiety disorder. In J. Solomon & C. George (Eds.), *Disorganized attachment and caregiving* (pp. 343–382). New York: Guilford Press.

Buchheim, A., George, C., & West, M. (2003). The Adult Attachment Projective (AAP)—Psychometric properties and new research. *Psychosomatics Psychotherapy Medical Psychology, 53*(9–10), 419–427.

Buchheim, A., Labek, K., Taubner, S., Kessler, H., Pokornoy, D., Kächele, H., . . . Karch, S. (2018). Modulation of gamma band activity and late positive potential in patients with chronic depression after psychodynamic psychotherapy. *Psychotherapy and Psychosomatics, 87*(4), 252–254.

Buchheim, A., Labek, K., Walter, S., & Viviani, R. (2013). A clinical case study of a psychoanalytic psychotherapy monitored with functional neuroimaging. *Frontiers in Human Neuroscience, 7,* 677.

Cyr, C., Béliveau, M.-J., & Moss, E. (2003, March). *Maternal attachment representations: Links with child attachment and externalizing behavior problems.* Paper presented at the Society for Personality Assessment, San Francisco, CA.

Delvecchio, E., Di Riso, D., Lis, A., & Salcuni, S. (2016). Adult attachment, psychological adjustment, and well-being in drug-addicted inpatients. *Psychological Reports, 118*(2), 587–607.

Finn, S. (2011). Use of the Adult Attachment Projective System (AAP) in the middle of long-term psychotherapy. *Journal of Personality Assessment, 93*(5), 427–433.

Fitzke, E., Buchheim, A., & Juen, F. (2013). Activation of the attachment system and mentalization in depressive and healthy individuals—An experimental control study. *Psihologija, 46*(2), 161–176.

Fraedrich, E. M., Lakotos, K., & Spangler, G. (2010). Brain activity during emotion perception: The role of attachment representation. *Attachment and Human Development, 12*(3), 231–248.

Gallichan, D. J., & George, C. (2014). Assessing attachment status in adults with intellectual disabilities: The potential of the Adult Attachment Projective Picture System. *Advances in Mental Health and Intellectual Disabilities, 8*(2), 103–119.

Gander, M., Buchheim, A., Bock, A., Steppan, M., Sevecke, K., & Goth, K. (2020). Unresolved attachment mediates the relationship between childhood trauma and impaired personality functioning in adolescence. *Journal of Personality Disorders, 34,* 468–488.

Gander, M., Sevecke, K., & Buchheim, A. (2018). Disorder-specific attachment characteristics and experiences of childhood abuse and neglect in adolescents with anorexia nervosa and a major depressive episode. *Clinical Psychology and Psychotherapy, 25*(6), 894–906.

George, C., & Buchheim, A. (2014). Use of the Adult Attachment Projective Picture System with a severely traumatized patient: A psychodynamic perspective. *Frontiers in Psychology, 5,* 865.

George, C., Kaplan, N., & Main, M. (1984/1985/1996). *The Adult Attachment Interview.* Unpublished manuscript, University of California, Berkeley, Berkeley, CA.

George, C., & Solomon, J. (1996). Representational models of relationships: Links between caregiving and attachment. *Infant Mental Health Journal, 17*(3), 18–36.

George, C., & Solomon, J. (2008). Attachment and caregiving: The caregiving behavioral system. In J. Cassidy & P. R. Shaver (Eds.), *Handbook of attachment: Theory, research, and clinical applications* (2nd ed., pp. 833–856). New York: Guilford Press.

George, C., & West, M. (2001). The development and preliminary validation of a new measure of adult attachment: The Adult Attachment Projective. *Attachment and Human Development, 3*(1), 30–61.

George, C., & West, M. (2012). *The Adult Attachment Projective: A new assessment of adult attachment.* New York: Guilford Press.

Gloger-Tippelt, G., Gomille, B., Koenig, L., & Vetter, J. (2002). Attachment representations in 6-year-olds: Related longitudinally to the quality of attachment in infancy and mothers' attachment representations. *Attachment and Human Development, 4*(3), 318–339.

Green, J., Stanley, C., Smith, V., & Goldwyn, R. (2000). A new method of evaluating attachment representations in young school-age children: The Manchester Child Attachment Story Task. *Attachment and Human Development, 2*(1), 42–64.

Hilsenroth, M. J. (2004). Projective assessment of personality and psychopathology: An overview. In M. J. Hilsenroth & D. L. Segal (Eds.), *Comprehensive handbook of psychological assessment: Vol. 2. Personality assessment* (pp. 283–296). Hoboken, NJ: Wiley.

Hinde, R. A. (1982). *Ethology*. New York: Oxford University Press.

Isaacs, M., George, C., & Marvin, R. S. (2011). Utilizing attachment measures in custody evaluations: Incremental validity. *Journal of Child Custody, 6*(1–2), 139–162.

Jacobsen, T., & Hofmann, V. (1997). Children's attachment representations: Longitudinal relations to school behavior and academic competency in middle childhood and adolescence. *Developmental Psychology, 33*(4), 703–710.

Jones-Mason, K., Allen, I. E., Hamilton, S., & Weiss, S. J. (2015). Comparative validity of the Adult Attachment Interview and the Adult Attachment Projective. *Attachment and Human Development, 17*(5), 429–447.

Joubert, D. (2007). The Adult Attachment Projective. In S. R. Jenkins (Ed.), *Handbook of clinical scoring systems for thematic apperceptive techniques.* Hillsdale, NJ: Erlbaum.

Joubert, D., Webster, L., & Hackett, R. K. (2012). Unresolved attachment status and trauma-related symptomatology in maltreated adolescents: An examination of cognitive mediators. *Child Psychiatry and Human Development, 43*(3), 471–483.

Kaplan, N. (1984). *Internal representation of the separation experiences in six year olds: Related to actual experiences of separation.* Unpublished master's thesis, University of California, Berkeley, Berkeley, CA.

Klagsbrun, M., & Bowlby, J. (1976). Responses to separation from parents: A clinical test for young children. *British Journal of Projective Psychology, 21*(2), 7–21.

Leak, J. K., & Parson, C. G. (2001). The susceptibility of three attachment style measures to socially desirable responding. *Social Behavior and Personality: An International Journal, 29*(1), 21–30.

Leichtman, M. (2004). Projective tests: The nature of the task. In M. J. Hilsenroth & D. L. Segal (Eds.), *Comprehensive handbook of psychological assessment: Vol. 2. Personality assessment* (pp. 291–314). Hoboken, NJ: Wiley.

Liotti, G. (2017). Conflicts between motivational systems related to attachment trauma: Key to understanding the intra-family relationship between abused children and their abusers. *Journal of Trauma and Dissociation, 18*(3), 304–318.

Lis, A., Mazzeschi, C., Salcuni, S., & Di Riso, D. (2008, January). *The use of the Adult Attachment Projective (AAP) in collaborative assessment.* Paper presented at the international congress Attaccamento: Metodi a Confronto. Padova, Italy.

Lyons Ruth, K., & Jacobvitz, D. (2016). Attachment disorganization from infancy to adulthood: Neurobiological correlates, parenting context, and pathways to disorder. In J. Cassidy & P. R. Shaver (Eds.), *Handbook of attachment: Theory, research, and clinical applications* (3rd ed., pp. 667–695). New York: Guilford Press.

Maier, M. A., Bernier, A., Pekrun, R., Zimmerman, P., & Grossmann, K. E. (2004). Attachment working models as unconscious structure: An experimental test. *International Journal of Behavioral Development, 28*(2), 180–189.

Main, M. (1995). Recent studies in attachment: Overview, with selected implications for clinical work. In S. Goldberg, R. Muir, & J. Kerr (Eds.), *Attachment theory: Social, developmental, and clinical perspectives* (pp. 407–474). Hillsdale, NJ: Analytic Press.

Main, M., & Goldwyn, R. (1985/1998/2006). *Adult Attachment Interview scoring and classification system.* Unpublished manuscript, University of California at Berkeley, Berkeley, CA.

Main, M., & Hesse, E. (1990). Parents' unresolved traumatic experiences are related to infant disorganized attachment status: Is frightened and/or frightening parental behavior the linking mechanism? In M. T. Greenberg, D. Cicchetti, & E. M. Cummings (Eds.), *Attachment in the preschool years* (pp. 161–182). Chicago: University of Chicago Press.

Main, M., Kaplan, N., & Cassidy, J. (1985). Security in infancy, childhood, and adulthood: A move to the level of representation. In I. Bretherton & E. Waters (Eds.), Growing points in attachment theory and research. *Monographs of the Society for Research in Child Development 50*(1–2, Serial No. 209), 66–104.

Main, M., & Solomon, J. (1990). Procedures for identifying infants as disorganized/disoriented during the Ainsworth Strange Situation. In M. T. Greenberg, D. Cicchetti, & E. M. Cummings (Eds.), *Attachment in the preschool years* (pp. 121–160). Chicago: University of Chicago Press.

Marvin, R., Britner, P. A., & Russell, B. S. (2016). Normative development: The ontogeny of attachment. In J. Cassidy & P. R. Shaver (Eds.), *Handbook of attachment: Theory, research, and clinical applications* (3rd ed., pp. 273–209). New York: Guilford Press.

Mazzeschi, C., Pazzalgi, C., Laghezza, L., Radi, G., Battistina, D., & De Feo, P. (2014). The role of both parents' attachment pattern in understanding childhood obesity. *Frontiers in Psychology, 5,* 791.

McCarthy, G. (1998). Attachment representations and representations of the self in relation to others: A study of preschool children in inner-city London. *British Journal of Medical Psychology, 71*(1), 57–72.

McClelland, D. C., Atkinson, J. W., Clark, R. A., & Lowell, E. L. (1953). *The achievement motive.* East Norwalk, CT: Appleton-Century-Crofts.

Meyer, G. (2004). The reliability and validity of the Rorschach and Thematic Apperception Test (TAT) compared to other psychological and medical procedures: An analysis of systematically gathered evidence. In M. J. Hilsenroth & D. L. Segal (Eds.), *Comprehensive handbook of psychological assessment: Vol. 2. Personality assessment* (pp. 315–342). Hoboken, NJ: Wiley.

Oppenheim, D. (1997). The Attachment Doll-play Interview for Preschoolers. *International Journal of Behavioral Development, 20*(4), 681–697.

Pallini, S., Alfani, A., Marech, L., & Laghi, F. (2017). Unresolved attachment and agency in victims of intimate partner violence. *Psychology and Psychotherapy: Theory, Research and Practice, 90*(2), 177–192.

Paulhus, D. L. (1998). *The Balanced Inventory of Desirable Responding.* Toronto: Multi-Health Systems.

Pazzagli, C., Laghezza, L., Manaresi, F., Mazzeschi, C., & Powell, B. (2014). The Circle of Security parenting and parent conflict: A single case study. *Frontiers in Psychology, 5,* 887.

Riggs, S. A., Paulson, A., Tunnell, E., Stahl, G., Atkison, H., & Ross, C. A. (2007).

Attachment, personality, and psychopathology among adult inpatients: Self-reported romantic attachment style vs. Adult Attachment Interview states of mind. *Development and Psychopathology, 19*(1), 263–291.

Shouldice, A., & Stevenson-Hinde, J. (1992). Coping with security distress: The Separation Anxiety Test and attachment classification at 4.5 years. *Journal of Child Psychology and Psychiatry, 33*(2), 331–348.

Slough, N. M., & Greenberg, M. T. (1990). Five-year-olds' representations of separation from parents: Responses from the perspective of self and other. In I. Bretherton & M. W. Watson (Eds.), *New directions in child development: Vol. 48. Children's perspectives of the family* (pp. 67–84). San Francisco: Jossey-Bass.

Solomon, J., & George, C. (1996). Defining the caregiving system: Toward a theory of caregiving. *Infant Mental Health Journal, 1*(3), 183–197.

Solomon, J., & George, C. (1999). The place of disorganization in attachment theory: Linking classic observations with contemporary findings. In J. Solomon & C. George (Eds.), *Attachment disorganization* (pp. 3–31). New York: Guilford Press.

Solomon, J., & George, C. (2011). Dysregulation of maternal caregiving across two generations. In J. Solomon & C. George (Eds.), *Disorganization of attachment and caregiving* (pp. 25–51). New York: Guilford Press.

Solomon, J., George, C., & De Jong, A. (1995). Children classified as controlling at age six: Evidence of disorganized representational strategies and aggression at home and at school. *Development and Psychopathology, 7*(3), 447–463.

Sroufe, L. A., Egeland, B., Carlson, E. A., & Collins, A. W. (2005). *The development of the person.* New York: Guilford Press.

Sroufe, L. A., & Fleeson, J. (1986). Attachment and the construction of relationships. In W. Hartup & Z. Rubin (Eds.), *The nature and development of relationships* (pp. 51–71). Hillsdale, NJ: Erlbaum.

Waters, H. S., & Waters, E. (2006). The attachment working models concept: Among other things, we build script-like representations of secure base experiences. *Attachment and Human Development, 8*(3), 185–197.

West, M., & George, C. (2002). Attachment and dysthymia: The contributions of preoccupied attachment and agency of self to depression in women. *Attachment and Human Development, 4*(3), 278–293.

West, M., & Sheldon-Keller, A. E. (1994). *Patterns of relating.* New York: Guilford Press.

Wood, J. M., Nezworski, M. T., & Stejskal, W. J. (1996). The comprehensive system for the Rorschach: A critical examination. *Psychological Science, 7*(1), 3–10.

CHAPTER 14

Measuring Attachment

Legacy and Prospects

Everett Waters, Brian E. Vaughn,
and Harriet Salatas Waters

A first-year graduate student related this story to us. It was her freshman year at a distinguished West Coast university, and she was excited to be taking Introductory Psychology from a renowned developmental psychologist. After an excellent lecture on social development, discussion turned to career prospects in developmental psychology. Asked about possibilities for an academic career in attachment study, the professor granted that there had been some very innovative work in the area. Nonetheless, in his view, attachment study had more or less run its course; something new might be a better bet. This was the mid-1980s. Fortunately, our student was not dissuaded. For most of the work covered in this volume was initiated and bore fruit after that lecture. Clearly, attachment study was nowhere near having run its course. With increasingly sophisticated theoretical and measurement tools, we continue to have great expectations for the future of attachment study.

LEGACY

Attachment study was born in the twilight of behaviorism and operationalism. Both were influential in developmental psychology into the mid-1970s. Many of our own graduate instructors were confident that psychology must keep to observable phenomena and that theoretical concepts must be defined in terms of the operations by which one measures them. Today's students, though, find it impossible to imagine that the study of emotion was, so recently, an anathema in influential circles. Or that these waning paradigms could have mounted such a determined defense against emerging cognitive, biological, and evolutionary perspectives. Yet this was the context in which John Bowlby was trying to formulate a new perspective on emotional bonds, and Mary Ainsworth was offering up naturalistic observations of infant care in Uganda. What we know as attachment theory was yet to be formulated. Moreover, the only data were clinic and field observations. There were no measures or measurements, only Mary Ainsworth's observations. Yet here we are, four decades on, with much to report and much to do.

We are not sure how interested John Bowlby was in measurement per se. But he clearly appreciated the value of empirical evidence. Mary Ainsworth was quite familiar with classical measurement theory. Indeed, her PhD thesis was a scale construction project on the measurement of Blatz's security construct in adults. Moreover, she worked for years as a psychodiagnostician and psychometrician at the Sheppard and Enoch Pratt Hospital, and in private practice in Baltimore. She clearly viewed ethological observation as a complement to psychometric methods. Interestingly, Ainsworth rarely discussed psychoanalysis or used psychoanalytic terminology around her laboratory. Yet it seems likely that her familiarity with the complexities of psychoanalytic theory contributed to her skills as an observer. Not that she looked at attachment behavior through a psychoanalytic lens; she did not. But the way in which psychoanalytic theory incorporates context, complex connections, requires convergent evidence, and so forth, and most of all, its focus on meaning, is mirrored in Ainsworth's ethological perspective on behavior—both reflect a systems perspective.

Theory and Measurement

The success of the attachment paradigm is attributable in large part to John Bowlby's recognition that biology, rather than physics, is the better model for developmental science in general and for attachment in particular. Cambridge afforded Bowlby a solid scientific education, and he saw no way forward for attachment theory other than a solid scientific framework grounded in empirically accessible concepts. At the same time, he recognized that attachment is a biological phenomenon, a product of evolution, the solution to a puzzle. We are not free to define or measure it to fit some idealized view of science or methodology. The theory had to meet the phenomenon on its own terms. This meant a back-and-forth between theory and measurement. This is central to the construct orientation described by Cronbach and Meehl (1955). One section of this classic article, "Specific Criteria Used Temporarily: The Bootstraps Effect," describes a dynamic in which preliminary construct definitions suggest initial measurement strategies and criteria. These serve well enough to test predictions from the preliminary theory and support revisions. The revised theory points to more adequate measurement and more refined tests of increasingly refined predictions. And on we go, pulling ourselves up by our own bootstraps—from only a sketch of a theory and uncertain measurements to better measurement and better-defined constructs. Toward a more comprehensive, parsimonious, internally consistent, testable, empirically supported theory. Importantly, there is nothing random about this process. Strategy is critical at every step; this is what makes it interesting. Nor is the goal a perfect or permanent theory. We hope only to build a solid enough foundation for useful understanding and perhaps a usefully coherent defense in the face of a new paradigm (see Kuhn, 1962/2012) or as Imre Lakatos (1970) would have it, to maintain a progressive research program.

The contributors to this volume all understand and play this game quite well. Their own work and their contributions here reflect sophisticated perspectives on behavior, key constructs such as security, and measurement. Each of the chapters illustrates the value of focusing on meaning, as well as methodology, in research design and interpretation of results. The effort is not to publish the most articles but to move the theoretical ball down the field. There is little room here for instrument-driven research or a mere search for significant correlations. Theory and measurement, theory and measurement. Tests of hypotheses that would require significant theoretical change if they failed—what Meehl called "dangerous tests." These, as much as anything, account for the good health and good prospects of attachment study (see Waters, Bretherton, & Vaughn, 2015).

Conveying Implicit Knowledge

Much of the shared knowledge that defines a paradigm is implicit—recognizable, but not necessarily verbalizable, by every seasoned practitioner. For the first decade or two, attachment theory seemed a somewhat closed affair. One heard reference to an "attachment mafia," which we accepted as a play on "Minnesota mafia," a reference to the leadership roles of Institute of Child Development faculty in the Society for Research in Child Development. In fact, it was more likely an allusion to the fact that Mary Ainsworth and her students dominated the field of play. Even seasoned researchers were finding it difficult to succeed in an entirely new paradigm.

In retrospect, the problem was not that attachment theory and research were poorly presented. Both Bowlby and Ainsworth wrote with exceptional clarity. The problem was communicating across paradigms. Indeed, Sroufe and Waters (1977) were truly surprised when more than a few readers received their essay "Attachment as an Organizational Construct" as a virtual *Rosetta Stone*. Perhaps, situated as they were at Minnesota's Institute of Child Development, squarely on the solid middle ground of developmental psychology, their language was more accessible. More likely, the paper worked because it conveyed quite a bit of information that was in the air, implicit, common currency, readily available in the hallways of Mary Ainsworth's lab and at the Institute—but had not found a place in scholarly writing.

It is easy to underestimate how much such implicit knowledge contributes to a paradigm's coherence. Now, researchers who had the advantage of being, so to speak, present at the creation are retiring. It is important to make sure that this information is not retired with them. Next generations would simply have to spend time rediscovering it. Thus, a primary goal of these chapters has been to make explicit the relation to theory, the premises, strategies, and expectations underlying the development and use of key attachment measures.

Posada, Waters, Vaughn, Pederson, and Moran (Chapter 1), Vaughn, Waters, and Teti (Chapter 2), and Waters, Vaughn, and Bernard (Chapter 3) have provided valuable information about the thinking and insights underpinning maternal sensitivity scales, the Strange Situation, and the Attachment Q-set. In doing so, they have gone well beyond the information in training manuals and research reports. Yet their most valuable contribution may be their characterizations of attachment behavior as it looked through Mary Ainsworth's eyes and in her best descriptive writing. Similarly, Carlson (Chapter 4) and Solomon, Duschinsky, Bakkum, and Schuengel (Chapter 5) convey a great deal of information about disorganized attachment and their struggle to view such unexpected behavior in own right, while also trying to find its place in current attachment theory. Much of this work depends on intuition and tentative hypotheses that may only serve as bridges to empirical tests—information that may never find its way into scholarly reports but is critical to appreciating, conceptualizing, and measuring attachment disorganization, whether within the ABC (avoidant, secure, ambivalent or resistant) attachment framework or otherwise.

Early on, critics often dismissed attachment study as "Strange Situation research." Bowlby had always recognized the relevance of attachment across the lifespan and was keen to preserve psychoanalytic insights about the relevance of early experience to later relationships. However, without age-appropriate measures, Ainsworth and her students gave little thought to following infants into adulthood. The emergence of the Adult Attachment Interview (AAI; Main & Goldwyn, 1985–1995) opened the door to testing hypotheses about attachment across the lifespan and focused attention on Bowlby's ideas about attachment representation and defensive processes. It also opened the door to criticisms that attachment theory was a theory of close relationships in infancy and in adulthood, with a great deal in between left to the imagination (see Waters, Kondo-Ikemura, Posada, & Richters, 1991). Kerns and Siebert's (Chapter 6) and Allen's (Chapter 7) discussions of measurement for middle childhood and adolescence demonstrate how much has been done to develop measures after infancy, and how much more there is to do. They also convey valuable information about the importance of keeping the secure base center stage in attachment theory, and the ways in which doing so has facilitated the design of innovative, age-appropriate measures beyond the separation–reunion paradigm.

H. Waters and T. Waters (Chapter 8) have addressed address an issue that arises with cognitive development in middle childhood and reaches forward to the AAI. What do attachment representations represent? Although work on script-like attachment representations is rooted in cognitive psychology rather than attachment theory, H. Waters and T. Waters provide another example of how keeping the secure base concept center stage, even when it is not initially clear how to implement this, is a powerful strategy.

First encounters with the AAI often leave an impression of overwhelming complexity. This fades in the course of formal workshops on AAI scoring. However, many researchers and practitioners want first to understand the goals of such extensive training. In addition, even greater numbers of developmentalists and researchers from other disciplines need only to understand the AAI well enough to follow the research literature or to evaluate it for inclusion as a secondary measure in projects that are not primarily focused on attachment. Crowell (Chapter 9) specifically addresses these audiences. Details give way to meaning in this clear portrayal of the measurement strategy, its goals, and key insights that are both measurement-related and contributions to attachment theory.

Also focusing on adult attachment narratives, T. Waters and Facompré (Chapter 10) have highlighted the question, "What happened to the secure base concept when attachment moved to the level of representation?" They note that the use of different core constructs (secure base in early years and narrative coherence in the AAI) poses a significant problem for the coherence of attachment as a lifespan theory. Looking at attachment narratives much the way Mary Ainsworth looked at behavior, they find that they are replete with secure base-related expectations and vignettes. Moreover, the script-like structure of this material facilitates an individual's conformity with Grice's maxims of conversational cooperation, which is the favored explanation for AAI coherence. Thus, script-like representations of early secure base experience are not displaced by narrative coherence; they play a significant role in creating it. This elegant solution to a difficult problem again illustrates a view to complexity and organization that was characteristic of Mary Ainsworth's ethological observations and rating scales. It demonstrates again the value of keeping the secure base concept center stage and of focusing on ordinary (as opposed to attachment-specific) cognitive processes. The problem solving illustrated here is a useful template for new research on different modes of attachment representation. But, again, research journals have little room for the implicit knowledge underpinning such work.

Feeney (Chapter 11) and Maier, Bernier, and Corcoran (Chapter 12) have illustrated the use of methods from social and experimental psychology to study the secure base concept. Behaviorists and learning theorists criticized early generations of Bowlby–Ainsworth attachment researchers as muddle-headed for their dependence on naturalistic observation and correlational/individual-differences analyses. As a result, the first generations of attachment researchers acquired something of an aversion to experimental methods and the roles of learning in attachment development. Paradigm shifts take time. Fortunately, recent generations of attachment researchers are entirely comfortable exploiting the full range of methods and tools from both individual-differences and experimental paradigms, and are becoming more sophisticated about the roles of associative and social learning. They also feel comfortable exploring the different facets of attachment representation. Good experimental design is as much a skill as good behavioral observation. It can be hard to convey to attachment researchers who have focused primarily on individual differences. Much as earlier chapters help us see attachment behavior through Mary Ainsworth's eyes, Feeney and Maier et al. illustrate how experimentalists can peer into attachment behavior under controlled conditions, without doing violence to its organization or meaning.

Finally, George and West (Chapter 13) have illustrated the value of exploring different facets of attachment representation and the importance of remaining open to multiple methodologies. Although the projective method is associated with the psychodynamic perspective, in the hands of George and West, it is primarily a method for exploring associative meaning, more open-ended but ultimately not unlike the priming methods discussed by Maier et al. Most importantly, Chapter 13 conveys a great deal about the intuitive sense for the secure base phenomenon and attachment representations that underpins the AAI and other narrative methods. This is valuable information for both experimentalists and clinicians. It also opens new doors for convergent and discriminant validation of attachment measures from middle childhood to adulthood.

Each of our authors has worked hard to explicate implicit information that we too often take for granted and that is not easily accessible outside their research groups. They have also highlighted and clarified the roles of theory and strategy in attachment measurement. In doing so, they have illustrated the advantage of some background in psychometrics and philosophy of science. (See Nunnally & Bernstein, 1994; Ghiselli, Campbell, & Zedeck, 1981; Godfrey-Smith, 2003; Okasha, 2016.) We find that we depend on such material every day. Yet neither is standard fare in current developmental psychology graduate programs.

PROSPECTS

Research on attachment measurement has far outpaced anything John Bowlby or Mary Ainsworth could have expected. This success ensures the continued good health of attachment study in general. Although the chapters in this volume represent only a subset of the most widely used measures and measurement strategies, the commonalities speak to core aspects of the attachment paradigm—a perspective on behavior, the secure base phenomenon, naturalistic observations as a validity criterion, and a focus on meaning rather than on mere procedures. The contributors have done a great service by explicating premises, strategies, and intuitions that are important to new generations of attachment researchers but find little room in formal reports.

Multiple Facets of Relationships

Looking forward, several tasks seem to deserve high priority in attachment measurement research. These include expanding theory and measurement to address facets of attachment relationships beyond maternal sensitivity and confidence in caregiver/partner's availability and responsiveness. Robert Hinde (1976) addressed the multifaceted architecture of close relationships in his paper "On Describing Relationships." Although he is addressing relationships in general, his discussion of relationship patterns including diversity in interaction content, reciprocity versus complementarity, qualities of interactions, exclusivity, intimacy, and so forth. These are easily adapted to attachment relationships across age. For example, we might find, at any age, reliable differences among relationships in (1) the extent to which they focus on emergency support versus support for exploration and enrichment, (2) the limits of trust, (3) the contexts in which friction and ruptures arise, their function in the relationship, and how they are resolved, or (4) schemas and script-like representations that reflect individual or relationship history (see T. Waters & Facompré, Chapter 10, this volume; Young, Klosko, & Weishaar, 2003). If we could instantiate multiple relationship facets as measures, we could determine whether they point to a single latent security construct or to distinct facets. We could also see whether the hypothesis that early experience establishes a prototype for later relationships is better supported in some facets than in others. The possibilities here should be a significant impetus to renew interest in observing relationships in naturalistic settings.

Additional tasks highlighted in this volume include the need for (1) more comprehensive information on the correlations among attachment measures; (2) additional observations of secure base behavior in various contexts and at the full range of ages now covered by laboratory assessments; (3) attention to the consistency, coherence, and motivation of secure base support across age; (4) attention to attachment's role as a moderator in studies of other processes and mechanisms (logically, the opportunities here far outnumber cases in which attachment is a primary causal mechanism); and (5) expanded integration with cognitive science and computational modeling.

Attachment measures are often a student's first encounter with the practical meaning of key attachment concepts and issues. As they become skilled using a particular measure to address research questions, they also learn to recognize the contexts in which attachment theory is relevant. Eventually, with much experience across many trials, often augmented by teaching and training their own students, they acquire the expectations and fluency characteristic of experts. In addition to compiling a great deal of technical information, the contributors to this volume would have gone to great lengths to articulate insights and intuitions essential to attachment study. In sharing the crown jewels of attachment study, they have done much to ensure its continuing good health. We are pleased to have afforded them the opportunity and the space to do so.

REFERENCES

Cronbach, L. J., & Meehl, P. E. (1955). Construct validity in psychological tests. *Psychological Bulletin, 52*(4), 281–302.

Ghiselli, E., Campbell, J. P., & Zedeck, S. (1981). *Measurement theory for the behavioral sciences.* New York: Freeman.

Godfrey-Smith, P. (2003). *Theory and reality—An introduction to the philosophy of science.* Chicago: University of Chicago Press.

Hinde, R. A. (1976). On describing relationships. *Journal of Child Psychology and Psychiatry, 17,* 1–19.

Kuhn, T. S. (2012). *The structure of scientific revolutions* (50th anniversary ed.). Chicago: University of Chicago Press. (Original work published 1962)

Lakatos, I. (1970). Falsification and the methodology of scientific research programmes. In I. Lakatos & A. Musgrave (Eds.), *Criticism and the growth of knowledge: Proceedings of the International Colloquium in the Philosophy of Science* (Vol. 4, pp. 91–195). New York: Cambridge University Press.

Main, M., & Goldwyn, R. (1985–1995). *The Adult Attachment Interview Classification and Scoring System.* Unpublished manuscript, University of California at Berkeley, Berkeley, CA.

Nunnally, J. C., & Bernstein, I. (1994). *Psychometric theory* (3rd ed.). New York: McGraw-Hill.

Okasha, S. (2016). *Philosophy of science: A very short introduction* (2nd ed.). New York: Oxford University Press.

Sroufe, L., & Waters, E. (1977). Attachment as an organizational construct. *Child Development, 48,* 1184–1189.

Waters, E., Bretherton, I., & Vaughn, B. E. (2015). Preface. In M. D. S. Ainsworth, M. Blehar, E. Waters, & S. Wall (Eds.), *Patterns of attachment: A psychological study of the Strange Situation* (pp. x–xxxvi). New York: Taylor & Francis/Psychology Press.

Waters, E., Kondo-Ikemura, K., Posada, G., & Richters, J. (1991). Learning to love: Mechanisms and milestones. In M. Gunner & L. A. Sroufe (Eds.), *Minnesota Symposium on Child Psychology: Vol. 23. Self processes and development* (pp. 217–255). Minneapolis: University of Minnesota Press.

Young, J. E., Klosko, J. S., & Weishaar, M. E. (2003). *Schema therapy: A practitioner's guide.* New York: Guilford Press.

Index

Note. f or *t* following a page number indicates a figure or a table.